COMPLETE BOOK OF MEDICAL SCHOOLS

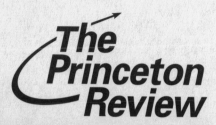

The Princeton Review

COMPLETE BOOK OF MEDICAL SCHOOLS

2001 EDITION

Random House, Inc.
New York
www.randomhouse.com/princetonreview

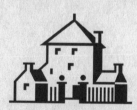

Malaika Stoll

Princeton Review Publishing, L.L.C.
2315 Broadway
New York, NY 10024
E-mail: comments@review.com

ISBN: 0-375-76153-5
ISSN: 1067-2176

Manufactured in the United States of America on partially recycled paper.

Editor: Julie Mandelbaum
Account Manager: Kevin McDonough
Designers: Chris Thomas and Meher Khambata

9 8 7 6 5 4 3 2 1

2001 Edition

Acknowledgments

Malaika Stoll would like to thank Pam and John for their hospitality. Also, thanks to Jeff and Cele for their flexibility, Andy for his assistance, Gretchen for her support, David from the Berkeley Princeton Review office for his idea, and Dr. Goober for being an inspiration.

Special thanks must go to the hundreds of med students and scores of admissions officers who have supplied information for this book over the years. This year's edition owes a great debt to the efforts of many: to Amy Kinney and Kevin McDonough for their data collection panache; to Robert Franek, Director of Guidebook Publications, for his enthusiasm; to Julieanna Lambert, Greta Englert, Rachelle Nashner, and Jason Kantor for their patience and understanding; to Julie Mandelbaum for her last-minute contribution; and to Chris Wujciak for putting up with the rest of us. And finally, to all of our deweys for their hard work: Yojaira Cordero, Melissa Fernandez, Michael Palumbo, Chris Blazier, Alex Simon, Charlie Looker, Jessica Allen, Melissa Kay, and Megan Ritchie.

Contents

Preface

For the past nineteen years, The Princeton Review has offered preparatory courses and tutoring for standardized tests such as the SAT, MCAT, LSAT, GRE, GMAT, USMLE, and MBE. More than 70,000 students took our courses last year, and hundreds of thousands have bought our "Cracking" series test-prep books. At the center of our approach is the desire to help students tear away the anxiety and sense of helplessness that have surrounded these entrance exams for so many years. The Princeton Review has long been an advocate of students' right to be informed consumers.

Besides being consumers of entrance exams, students are also consumers of education. Before investing in a graduate degree, they have the right and the need to gather as much information as possible. We hope that this publication will provide students with a viable means of achieving this goal. The *Complete Book of Medical Schools* contains the essentials students will need to answer both basic and advanced questions regarding their list of prospective medical schools. The 2001 edition is our most complete medical school handbook to date; it contains all of the 124 accredited allopathic schools in the United States, 16 in Canada, 3 in Puerto Rico, as well as 19 accredited osteopathic schools.

When viewing individual schools listed in this year's guide, you will find the union of painstakingly researched school profiles coupled with school-specific statistical data. Each profile has been sent to the medical school itself for review prior to publication so that we may provide our readers with the most accurate and current information about the programs. We hope this book will serve as an important guide as you research, gather, and consider information before embarking on your medical career.

We wish you good luck as you pursue your career in medicine. If you have questions, comments or suggestions, we welcome them. Please give us you insights:

The Princeton Review
Complete Book of Medical Schools
2315 Broadway
New York, NY 10024
RobertF@review.com

We appreciate your input and want to make our books as useful to you as they can be.

Sincerely,

Robert Franek
Director, Guidebook Publications

1 How to Use This Book

Although some people describe medical school education as somewhat canned—and downplay the differences between schools—real, concrete differences do exist. Some differences, like the fact that a family medicine clerkship is two weeks at one school and eight at another, might not seem like a big deal, but such details may help convey a school's priorities. The school profile section of this guide will help you to discern such differences, and in doing so match your interests with the school that can best fulfill them. But don't just use this book to decide where to apply, also use it as a preparation for interviews. Learn the detailed information about course offerings and facilities to demonstrate knowledge about a school and formulate relevant questions. Look at the descriptions of such pertinent information as each program's fundamental academic approach and resources, the student body, and the school's emphasis as evident in the path its graduates take—all good points to bring up in an interview and to aid in your decision of where to attend.

As you review the school profiles, keep the following in mind:

- *Just as admissions offices rely too heavily on quantitative measures to evaluate candidates (MCAT and GPAs), applicants probably rely too much on school ranking in deciding where to apply and where to go to school. Often, the criteria for ranking have little to do with how well a school will train you or how enjoyable your experience will be (NIH research dollars for example). Thus, you will find no quantitative rankings in this book.*

- *Our goal is to present accurate and complete descriptions of medical schools. Note that the Admissions Offices of each medical school had the opportunity to read and edit our write-ups. In deciding where to apply or where to go, you should use this book as part of your research. Take every opportunity to meet with medical students at the schools in which you are interested. Speak with more than just one student at each school, and with students in different years at each school.*

- *In response to managed care and other trends, many medical schools that traditionally focused on research or specialty medicine claim now to focus on primary care. Whether a school really has changed its focus may be partially gleaned from the percentage of graduates who enter primary care fields. Schools' definitions of primary care vary (some include Ob/Gyn for example). Thus, national statistics vary in determining the percentage of medical school graduates entering primary care residency programs, anywhere from 25–55 percent. So, keep this variance in mind when researching medical schools and deciding how your education will affect your medical career course.*

- *In the Graduates section, under Student Life, we purposely left out a statistic that often comes up in the literature. This stat tells what percent of students match within their top one, two, or three choices in residency programs. It is interesting that the less prestigious schools often have impressive rates. This is in part because students only rank schools that they have a good chance of getting into (and at which they were successful in obtaining an invite to interview). In addition, students at less prestigious schools are less likely to enter highly specialized residency positions that are typically the most competitive. We left this stat out because we believe it is misleading.*

- *For most schools, we list their website addresses—they are often helpful and some include candid student opinions, so try to visit them before you make a commitment to apply, interview, or attend.*

HOW THIS BOOK IS ORGANIZED

The 2001 edition of *Complete Book of Medical Schools* includes all U.S., Canadian, and Puerto Rican accredited medical schools. The profile of each school is broken down into five text sections—Overview, Academics, Student Life, Admissions, and Cost. The general data in the allopathic profiles is supplemented by three categories of hard stats—Student Body, Admissions, and Cost and Aid—listed in the shaded sidebar column. We also created a supplementary chapter of a complete list—including a general overview and admissions requirements—of the 19 accredited osteopathic schools.

Here's what you will find in the various text and statistic sections for each allopathic school profile:

PROFILE

The opening paragraph is reserved for general information about the school and the medical program. You will find the school's objective stated here, as well as information about its faculty and unique features of the program. Does your top choice have a special program for Native Americans who live in Minnesota? You'll find that information here.

ACADEMICS

First we give you a basic look at the academic program—quarter system or semester, pass/fail or honor, and USMLE requirements. Then we break it down in accordance with how your own studies will be broken down—Basic Sciences and Clinical Training—outlining the academic requirements and path of each. Here you will find out how much time you have to spend hunched over a book vs. the fun part—hunched over, say, a cadaver. We will often use the term "selective" to describe certain clinical requirements. It means that students have some choice within a specified area. Selective courses are less "free" than an "elective" (which might also have some restrictions).

STUDENTS

Discover where your potential classmates call home and who they are—percentage-wise. In the Student Life section we describe what kind of recreation facilities are available, where you might live, where you might go out. We also include information about the graduates. Who are the grads of this school—primary care physicians, surgeons, public health administrators—and in what type of community do they choose to practice?

ADMISSIONS

Pretty straightforward: The Requirements section details what the school is looking for in its prospective students. Pay special attention to Suggestions for some hints about how to impress the school. Then whip out your date book—the Process section will tell you the dates you need to know and key stats about who gets interviews and then who the lucky recipients of the fat envelopes are.

Cost

This is the stuff you really need to know—can you even possibly afford this school? What is the cost of living? Do you need a car or not? Does your budget allow for off-campus housing, or will you forever be stuck in dorm-like conditions? We also outline financial aid: Who gets it? How much? And what resources are available?

SIDEBAR

The shaded column next to each school listing contains the following information:

STUDENT BODY

Type: Is the school private or public?

Enrollment: Total number of students enrolled in the medical school.

% male/female: Gender breakdown based on total enrollment.

% underrepresented minorities: Percentage of African Americans, Native Americans, Mexican Americans, and mainland Puerto Ricans in the total enrollment.

 # applied: The number of people who applied to the school in the most recently reported year, presented as the total number and the number of out-of-state/province residents who applied.

% interviewed: The percentage of applicants who interviewed at the school in the most recently reported year. Also broken down in terms of total interviewed versus out-of-state/province applicants interviewed.

% accepted: The percentage of applicants who were accepted at the school in the most recently reported year. Also broken down in terms of total and out-of-state/province.

% enrolled: The percentage of people who were accepted who actually entered the school as first-year medical students in the most recently reported entering class, in terms of total and out-of-state/province.

Average age: The average age of entering class.

ADMISSIONS

Average GPA

Overall undergraduate grade point average of the students who matriculated in the most recently reported entering class. Wherever possible, this figure is broken down to reflect the grade point average of these students in science courses.

Average MCAT

Average MCAT scores of the students who matriculated in the most recently reported entering class, broken down into the following areas: Biology, Verbal, Physics, and Essay.

MCAT Score Release Policy

The school's admissions policy regarding withheld MCAT scores. (The MCAT score release system is explained in more detail on page 13.) Note: Not all schools responded to our inquiries about this policy, and those who didn't are thus noted.

Application Information

Outlines all the dates and facts you need to know:

Regular application: The latest date by which the school must receive all application materials for regular admission.

Regular notification: The latest date by which the school will notify prospective students its decisions concerning regular admission.

Early application: The latest date by which the school must receive all application materials for the early decision plan.

Early notification: The latest date by which the school will notify prospective students of its decisions concerning admission to the early decision plan.

Transfers accepted?: Yes or No.

Admissions may be deferred?: Yes or No.

AMCAS application accepted?: Yes or No—Does the school participate in the American Medical College Application Service?

Interview required?: Yes or No.

Application fee: How much to apply?

COSTS AND AID

Tuition & Fees

Most recent yearly tuition figures available for both state residents and nonresidents. The amount of money students can expect to spend on books and fees is listed here as well.

Financial Aid

% students receiving aid: Percentage of medical students at the school receiving some sort of financial aid.

Average grant: The amount of money in grants students receive on average.

Average loan: The amount of money lent to students on average.

Average debt: How much do students owe when they get out?

2 So You Want to Be a Doctor . . .

Congratulations! You are attempting to enter one of the most competitive career fields on the planet, in the toughest applicant pool in decades, in a country with the best and most sought-after medical education in the world. You're going to need all the help you can get, which is probably why you're reading this book. The bad news is that even armed with all the information we can give you, and the help of a pre-med advisor, the application process is still going to be brutal. The painful reality is that there are about 42,000 applicants for approximately 16,000 spots. The good news, however, is that if you are persistent and have worked hard for the past several years to make yourself a competitive candidate, you have a good chance at a certified letter and a career that will keep you challenged and fulfilled for the rest of your life.

WHAT MAKES A COMPETITIVE APPLICANT?

Well, that's the $200,000 question (about what it will probably cost you to go to medical school after all the interest adds up). In 1998 the average matriculated (accepted) medical student had an undergraduate science GPA of 3.52, a nonscience GPA of 3.64, and an overall GPA of 3.57; their average MCAT scores were 9.5 verbal, 9.9 physical sciences, 10.2 biological sciences, and a P on the writing sample. So, roughly, to be a competitive student in 1998 you needed about a 3.6 GPA and around a 30 combined score on the MCAT. You also probably needed to have some volunteer time, possibly some experience in scientific academic research, demonstrated leadership roles, interesting extracurricular activities, a well-written personal statement, excellent communication skills, and maybe a recommendation letter from the Surgeon General. This year, it will probably be worse.

But what you have to keep in mind is that, despite the odds, there are always large numbers of normal, sane people who actually didn't get straight A's and haven't designed the health care system of a developing country who still manage to get into medical school. You can be one of them. First, however, you have to decide whether you will only consider applying to allopathic schools or if you would consider applying to osteopathic medical schools or to foreign med schools if none of your U.S. attempts pan out. Many of the Canadian schools listed in this book only accept Canadian applicants, so look into this as you are researching schools.

ALLOPATHIC MEDICINE

Allopathic schools confer the M.D. on their graduates, and allopathic training is by far the most widely available and recognized type of medical training. Both the Canadian and Puerto Rican Medical schools in this book are fully accredited allopathic institutions and are part of the AAMC. Allopathic programs usually concentrate in the first two years on the basic sciences needed to practice medicine. In recent years, medical schools have begun experimenting with different ways of going through the material; this has resulted in programs that may teach systems- or case-based science in small, independently directed study groups instead of separate disciplines delivered in a lecture hall setting. Most schools have made a concerted effort to get students together with patients at a much earlier stage in their education—it used to be that medical students might not come in contact with any actual sick people until they'd already been through two years of school. The last two years of medical school are mainly spent doing clinical rotations. Even if you're sure that your calling in life is plastic surgery, you're going to have to do a pediatrics rotation. Most medical students really enjoy having a chance to delve into the various specialties, although you are usually rotated out of an area a few minutes after you actually learn enough to be useful.

Allopathic training will give you the option to practice in any of the medical specialties, and unlike the D.O. (Doctorate of Osteopathic Medicine), the M.D. is universally recognized worldwide as a medical degree. For an abundance of information on all aspects of allopathic training and practice, visit the AAMC website (www.aamc.org). If you are interested in practicing overseas, the M.D. is a far easier degree to negotiate with than the D.O. Otherwise, the best way to decide which path is right for you is to spend time with both M.D.s and D.O.s, and talk to them at length about their practices.

OSTEOPATHIC MEDICINE

Osteopathic medicine in the United States got its start in the late 1800s. Its founding father was Dr. Andrew Taylor Still, who established the American School of Osteopathy in Kirksville, Missouri, in 1892. The various regulatory bodies (osteopathic versions of AAMC and the AMA) were well under way by the early 1900s, and are now the American Osteopathic Association (AOA) and the American Association of Colleges of Osteopathic Medicine (AACOM). There are currently nineteen colleges of osteopathic medicine throughout the United States; the D.O. is only issued in the United States. Visit the AOA's website at www.am-osteo-assn.org and the AACOM's website at www.aacom.org to find out more information about these organizations.

Osteopathic medicine has an interesting history; until fairly recently, its insistence on preventive care, communication with the patient, and a holistic approach to health was considered to be somewhat radical. Now, of course, much of what osteopathic medicine has always espoused is rapidly becoming part of all medical training. The major difference today between osteopathic and allopathic training is that osteopaths are taught an additional modality of treatment called manipulation (not to be confused with chiropractic manipulation, which has an entirely different system of education and is not recognized as a fully licensed medical degree). The osteopathic philosophy posits that there is a unity between a living organism's anatomy and physiology. Osteopathic medicine includes "the behavioral, chemical, physical, spiritual, and biological knowledge related to the establishment and maintenance of health as well as the prevention and alleviation of disease. Osteopathic concepts emphasize the following principles: 1. The human being is a dynamic unit of function; 2. The body possesses self-regulatory mechanisms which are self-healing in nature; 3. Structure and function are interrelated at all levels; 4. Rational treatment is based on these principles." (AOA *Yearbook of Osteopathic Physicians* 1996, Chicago: AOA, pg. 732.) These principles translate into more work for students of osteopathic medicine: They have to learn all of the same science as their allopathic counterparts, plus osteopathic diagnosis and treatment, in the same amount of time. To practicing osteopathic doctors, their training gives them a way of helping their patients that allopaths do not have. The last state to grant osteopathic doctors full practice rights was Mississippi in 1973, although some states certified D.O.s to practice in all public hospitals as complete physicians and surgeons much earlier.

As you might guess from their philosophy, many osteopathic doctors choose to become primary care physicians. Most work in Family Practice, Internal Medicine, Pediatrics, Ob/Gyn, and General Surgery. In the words of one osteopathic dean, they tend to be generalists first and specialists second. However, there are D.O.s in just about every area of modern medical practice, from Neurological Surgery to Psychiatry, Oncology, and Emergency Medicine. Traditionally, D.O.s are not accepted in droves into some surgical subspecialties, and if you have your heart set on esoteric medical research, the D.O. degree is probably not for you. Although osteopathic research used to be something of an oxymoron, the AOA is becoming much more active in encouraging research activities, particularly in primary care.

Although applicants for D.O. school used to be less competitive numerically than most allopathic applicants, this is no longer really the case. At most osteopathic schools, matriculates have undergrad GPAs of about a 3.4 and combined MCAT scores of just under 25. Last year, there were 55,000 applications from 9,500 applicants for 2,500 seats. However, osteopathic schools do have a reputation for "looking past the numbers" and put a very strong emphasis on looking at the whole picture of the candidate. This often makes osteopathic school an attractive choice for nontraditional, older students whose GPAs from their first trek through undergraduate school prove prohibitive in most allopathic programs. If you have a few blemishes on your academic record but a life that suggests you'll make a dedicated physician, you should strongly consider applying to osteopathic schools.

Most pre-meds trying to decide whether or not to apply to osteopathic schools worry about what will happen to them after they graduate and apply for a residency. Osteopathic graduates participate along with allopaths and foreign medical graduates (both American and nonresident) in the National Resident Matching Program (NRMP)—the Match. D.O.s can apply for either osteopathic or allopathic residencies, and for that reason many take both the USMLE (United State Medical Licensing Examination) and the COMLEX (Comprehensive Osteopathic Medical Licensing Examination, which is a series of exams administered by the National Board of Osteopathic Medical Examiners). Louisiana is the only state that does not recognize the COMLEX and requires D.O.s to pass the USMLE to be licenced. Osteopathic doctors have a much harder time obtaining residency spots than allopaths, so consider this when deciding whether or not to apply to osteopathic schools. The NRMP also points out that the lower residency match rate for osteopathic doctors is partly due to the fact that they can be appointed outside of the Match. If you want a high-profile residency or career, you should think carefully before applying to an osteopathic medical school, because there is still some prejudice about the prestige of the D.O. degree. On the other hand, if you want to practice primary care (as most D.O.s do), a D.O. degree could be a good choice.

FOREIGN MEDICAL SCHOOLS

The third option, if you aren't accepted to either kind of U.S. medical training, is to go overseas. Traditionally, most American students attend schools in Mexico and the Caribbean. If you are seriously considering attending a foreign school but want to practice in the U.S., make sure you take a hard look at the prospective school's USMLE pass rate. Although foreign schools are much easier to get into, they will put you in just as much debt—if not more—as U.S. schools, without the same assurance of a career that will render you capable of paying it off. Another consideration is that the U.S. now legislatively restricts the number of residencies available to graduates of foreign medical schools, and has stopped reimbursing hospitals for services rendered by foreign-trained residents. Even if you successfully pass the USMLE Steps 1 and 2, you may not be able to find a residency to complete your licensure with Step 3.

THE NUMBERS GAME

Because of the sheer volume of applications they have to wade through, admissions officers have to make some initial decisions based on GPA and MCAT scores—deceptively simple acronyms for the arcane processes they represent.

Your GPA, for the purposes of applying to medical school, consists of your science GPA (biology, chemistry, physics, and math), your nonscience GPA (every other class you ever suffered through), and your cumulative GPA. These are calculated for your undergraduate career, any nondegree-seeking post-secondary work, and any degree-seeking post-secondary programs. In other words, you could conceivably have nine GPAs. Each medical school has its own policies for deciding which GPA means the most to them when they're choosing which applicants to interview and/or matriculate. The average GPA of all applicants (not necessarily accepted) in 1998 was a 3.31 science, a 3.52 non-science, and a 3.4 overall.

Although community college classes count as part of your GPA, they may not always be acceptable as prerequisite, pre-medical course work. If you are planning to take some of your core pre-med courses (biology, chemistry, physics, etc.) at a community college, it's an extremely good idea to do some advance planning and call some of the schools that you're interested in to make sure that they have no qualms about community college credit. Similarly, if you took an AP class in high school and then tested out of a core class, such as physics, you may run into trouble when you apply unless you've taken upper-division course work in that subject. Again, it is very much to your advantage to check with a few medical schools and your pre-health advisor to make sure that your academic record doesn't have any holes in it.

Your MCAT score is made up of four separate marks: verbal reasoning, physical sciences, biological sciences, and the writing sample. Verbal reasoning and the science sections are scored from 1 to 15, although in recent years the top verbal score has been designated as 13 to 15. The writing portion of the MCAT requires that you write two essays, which generate a single score. This score is reported as a letter J–T, where J is low and T is high, presumably to emphasize its almost total lack of usefulness of the writing sample. The average score for all applicants on each section in 1998 was 8.6 verbal, 8.9 physical sciences, 9.2 biological sciences, and an O on the writing sample. As noted above, a competitive score is probably much closer to a 30 than a 24.

The writing sample, added to the MCAT a few years ago in an attempt to ensure the applicant's ability to communicate, is largely ignored by admissions committees. They don't get to ask the questions, so they're not particularly interested in the answers. Virtually the only time the writing sample is looked at very carefully is in the case of a disconnected application—a beautifully written personal statement with low verbal scores and/or a low writing sample score. Some schools will also consider the writing score if they are evaluating the English ability of English as a Second Language applicants. This does not mean that you can take a nap during the writing sample. You should make every effort to answer the questions in a coherent and focused way on the off-chance that the committee decides to look at your score, or that you happen to be applying to one of the very few schools in the country that does take note of the writing sample grade.

THE SUM OF YOUR EXPERIENCE

Although your GPA and MCAT score play a large role in your application, admissions committees are also looking for several other attributes. They are quite interested in who you are, why you want to be a physician, and whether or not you have a clue about what being a doctor is really like.

EXPOSURE TO THE HEALTH CARE FIELD

Although students with no discernible exposure to health care still matriculate, the vast majority of successful pre-meds have some experience, usually volunteer work, in a hospital, clinic, hospice, or other health care setting. Some pre-meds are lucky enough to find paying positions as EMTs, nurse's aids, or organ and blood bank workers. You should try to find a volunteer or paid position to stick with for at least six months. Many pre-medical programs have specific classes you can take that include organized volunteer time as part of their course work—even if you are a returning adult student and not officially registered as pre-med. You can often get college credit for community service work in the medical field. Although it may seem difficult to find the time to volunteer, it will make a huge difference as you work on your personal statement and get through your interviews.

You will have stories to tell, and will be able to speak far more effectively about the reasons that you want to become a physician.

LEADERSHIP EXPERIENCE AND COMMUNITY SERVICE

Leadership is often in the eye of the beholder, but one of the simpler ways to prove your abilities is to join a club or campus organization and get elected to office. You can also lead youth- or religious-affiliated organizations, or participate in a variety of community service organizations such as food banks, literacy programs, and mentoring. The key is to have some longevity with whatever cause you decide to embrace, so that you can achieve a measure of responsibility. If you are serious about practicing primary care medicine, for example, this is your chance to build your resume and to start proving yourself. Find a clinic that needs a dedicated volunteer, and get your feet wet.

RESEARCH

Academic research is quite a bit easier to get involved with than you might think. Research labs are always looking for drones—read "undergrads"—to help with the unlovely business of test-tube cleaning and organism counting. With any luck, however, you should be able to find a program in which you will actually be able to conduct experiments and write about the results. If you are considering a career in academic medicine, you should try to get involved in research projects as early in your undergraduate career as you can convince someone to take you. One of the best ways to find out about cool research projects and psychotic professors is to bribe a teaching and research assistant with a cup of coffee and ask about the various projects in their departments. They will inevitably know who is a kind and supportive teacher of nascent research genius, and who will work you into the ground without ever bothering to learn your name.

HUMANITY

Medical schools are interested in training bright, empathic, communicative people who have a strong interest in science and a wide-ranging intellect. They are not interested in students with perfect grades who have clearly never done anything else with their lives than try to break the curve in chemistry class. The schools want to graduate physicians who will listen to their patients and be able to effectively use the myriad tools available to heal them. What this means is that there is no magic system that will create an unbroken path into medical school. You can major in Art History, Modern Dance, or Biochemistry—it doesn't matter, as long as you take the classes you need to fulfill medical school requirements. You can take a few years off and join the Peace Corps or go straight through school. Admissions committees will be trying to discern what you have learned from your experiences, and how the things you have seen and done have led you to become a physician.

THE APPLICATION PROCESS

There are many factors to consider when applying to medical schools. Besides the obvious clinical and scholastic goals, it is important to look for a school in a location that you like. Although you may think that you won't see the light of day for four years, you should apply to schools that are in geographic areas that appeal to you and will provide outlets for your hobbies and interests.

APPLYING TO ALLOPATHIC MEDICAL SCHOOLS

Most allopathic medical schools use AMCAS®, the American Medical Colleges Application Service, which is a centralized and standardized application that is handled by the AAMC, the Association of American Medical Colleges. (Schools that do not use AMCAS are noted in the sidebar of each school profile in the next section of this book. You need to contact these schools individually for their application procedures.) You can use either an electronic (called the AMCAS-E®) or paper copy of

AMCAS. In general, it is much easier to use the electronic application, because very few people own typewriters anymore (much less remember how to line up all the little blank spaces), and the forms themselves are quite lengthy. You can get a copy of the application directly from the AAMC or from your pre-health advisor. The AMCAS application costs $55 for the first school; the more schools you apply to, the less you pay for each application. If you have significant financial hardship, you can apply directly to AMCAS for a fee waiver on their services. You will also need to prepare transcript requests, so that your undergraduate school or schools will only have to forward one copy of your transcripts directly to AMCAS. You will need to get transcripts from every post-secondary school you ever attended, even if you only took one class there or the credits transferred elsewhere. AMCAS begins accepting transcripts on March 15 each year and completed applications on June 1. It will take a couple of weeks for AAMC to process everything, at which point you'll receive a "transmittal notification." You can call and use AAMC's voicemail to check your status. You can reach AAMC on the Web at www.aamc.org or by phone at 202-828-0600. At most universities and colleges, your pre-health advisor will help you navigate the AMCAS application, which can be fairly baffling. One of the toughest parts of the application is the "Personal Comments" page, where you have exactly one typewritten, single-spaced page to explain your life and convince them that you should be one of the chosen few. Needless to say, this part of the application takes time and patience—be sure to read through the suggestions and advice for working on it that are included later in this chapter.

When you are choosing which schools to apply to, make sure that you check their in-state residency requirements. Although many allopathic schools are private, there are quite a few public schools that receive free money every year from out-of-state applicants they are prohibited from accepting into their programs; it doesn't matter how qualified you are, if you aren't a state resident, you can't get in.

APPLYING TO OSTEOPATHIC SCHOOLS

Osteopathic schools use their own internal system, called AACOMAS, which in many respects works exactly the same way as AMCAS. They have both paper and electronic applications. You can request an application from their website at www.aacom.org, or call 301-968-4100. Like the AMCAS application, AACOMAS takes some time to fill out, so make sure you get started early. It also includes a personal statement, but it's even shorter than AMCAS's—you only have half a page to explain why you want to be an osteopathic physician. You will also need to get a recommendation from a D.O., a fact that takes some applicants by surprise. If you are serious about osteopathic school, search for a mentor D.O. as early as possible. One of the nice things about AACOMAS is that all osteopathic schools use it—you don't have to worry about tracking down additional applications. Because osteopathic schools are private institutions, they don't have residency requirements (although some may have tuition breaks for residents of particular states). If you are interested in going to osteopathic school, investigate all of the colleges and choose based on your interest in the program and living conditions in the area.

WHEN TO APPLY TO MEDICAL SCHOOL

Whether you're applying to osteopathic or allopathic medical schools, you need to apply as early as you can in the process. In general, pre-medical students begin the application process in the spring semester of their junior year, or approximately a year and a half before they want to enter medical school. The vast majority of medical schools engage in some type of rolling admissions, which means that they read and evaluate applications as the folders arrive. Admissions officers are only human. Even though they make every effort to give the same consideration to applicant number 1 and applicant number 6,005, the sheer volume of applications takes its toll on their patience and enthusiasm. In practical terms, this means that if you take the April MCAT (Medical College Admission Test) and get your applications in by late June, you will have a distinct advantage over someone taking the August test. Even if you turn in your AMCAS or AACOMAS application early, the vast majority of medical schools will not look closely at your application until they have a copy of your MCAT scores. Each year, many students are accepted with August test scores and applications that arrived late in the process. Unfortunately, there are also large numbers of students who are not accepted but would have had a decent chance had they applied earlier. Basically, you should try to get every advantage you can. Turning in your application early can certainly help to give you an edge in what has become an incredibly competitive applicant pool. Also, procrastinators take note: AMCAS is serious about its deadlines. If an application is late, you'll get it back.

WHEN TO TAKE THE MCAT

As far as we know, all U.S. osteopathic and allopathic medical schools require the MCAT, which is given in April and August of each year (University of Rochester now requires the MCAT, although it didn't in the past). Many of the Canadian schools do not require the MCAT. According to the "AMCAS Survival Guide" (an official publication of the AAMC) you should "if possible, take the Medical College Admissions Test (MCAT) on the April test date." As evidence, they cite the admissions cycle—earlier is better. Of course, not all applicants' academic schedules realistically allow them to take the April test. There are three ways to get the forms you need to register for the MCAT. You can request them at the AAMC website, pick them up from a pre-med advisor, or contact the MCAT program office at the following address:

MCAT Program Office
P.O. Box 4056
Iowa City, IA 52243

If you have not finished most of the prerequisites for the test—two semesters each of biology, physics, general chemistry, and organic chemistry—you probably should not sit for the exam. If you are determined to try the test without being fully prepared, take advantage of the fact that you can take a practice test at any Princeton Review office. It is much, much better to find out precisely what your current scoring levels are on a practice exam than to have to explain a woefully low score on a later medical school application.

There are varying levels of readiness you can be at when you decide to sit for the MCAT. For many would-be medical students, trying to juggle core classes, jobs, and other obligations means that they might not be finished with the last semester of one of the subjects before the April test rolls around. This is not too much of a disaster, even though in many cases the gap in their education is the last semester of organic chemistry—and since recent Biological Sciences sections have been made up of between 40 and 60 percent organic chemistry, it's not a gap that's easy to ignore. It is possible, although it's certainly not the best idea, to take the last semester of one of the necessary courses concurrently with studying for the MCAT. If you find yourself in this situation, it is vitally important to lighten your course load so that you will be able to adequately study for the exam while keeping good grades in your courses. Thoroughly studying for the MCAT should take about as much time as taking organic chemistry with a lab.

HOW TO STUDY FOR THE MCAT

You are correct in assuming that since you're reading a book published by The Princeton Review, we're a little biased as to how we think you should study for the MCAT. The short answer here is that for most people, taking a course to prepare for the MCAT is worth the investment in both time and money. This is simply because studying for the MCAT is a tedious and wretched business, and having a class full of fellow sufferers at least makes you feel less alone in your pain. A class also forces you to study in a reasonable way, cover the material effectively, get plenty of practice, and gives you the resources to shore up any gaps in your academic preparation.

There are some people who do not need much preparation for the MCAT, and you'll meet them in medical school. They'll be getting honors designations in all of their classes while maintaining their world rankings as premier ice climbers/Sanskrit poets/master chefs. You'll like them, because they're inevitably nice people as well as hopelessly talented, but unless you're pretty sure you're one of them (you might qualify if you're reading this while skydiving) you'll need some help with the test.

First, assume that you will be spending about twenty hours a week for several months studying for the MCAT. Although it doesn't test everything you've learned in school, it will feel that way. And, if you're rusty or haven't studied one of the subjects in awhile—physics, general chemistry, organic chemistry, and biology—you're going to have to do some in-depth review. At the same time, you have to keep in mind that this is a standardized test, and even though it's one of the better ones available, it still suffers from the same flaws as all other standardized tests—a fact that you can use to your advantage. And given the level of competition for seats in medical school, you need every edge you can get.

The key to doing well on the exam is to know the material, and then to know the test. The MCAT consists of four timed sections administered over a period of more than seven hours.

As you can see from the grid below, the MCAT tests basic sciences—but don't assume that the exam is a science test similar to the kind you have learned to take as an undergraduate. Fundamentally, the MCAT is a verbal test, which is why on average, humanities majors tend to get slightly better scores in all of the sections than any other major. They are seeing a test format that they are used to: passages and questions. Science majors, on the other hand, are generally used to manipulating formulas and answering questions that may have a setup, but are not embedded in a long series of paragraphs.

In practice, it is much easier to raise your score if you start with low science numbers but a high verbal score. Unfortunately, most examinees are in exactly the opposite position. This is of real concern because more and more medical schools have come to regard scores that are out of balance as undesirable. They will often look more favorably on a candidate with three tens than someone with an eight verbal and two twelves. In order to change your verbal score you will have to practice the type of causal, linear logic that it tests. AAMC has released three previous MCATs and a couple of books of practice items (any formal test preparation course should give you reams of additional practice material). AAMC Test Three comes closest to approximating the MCAT as it has recently appeared, so you should save that test until the end of your preparation. If you live somewhere where you don't have access to test preparation courses, you will probably find yourself rapidly running out of verbal practice material, although most college bookstores are reasonably well stocked with practice materials relating to the science portions of the MCAT. You can use reading comprehension sections from other graduate-level standardized tests such as the GRE or LSAT to supplement your verbal study, but keep in mind that the passages in these tests were not written to be read under the same time constraints as were the MCAT passages.

The MCAT			
Section	**Questions**	**Time**	**Score**
Verbal Reasoning	65	85 minutes	1–15
Physical Sciences	77	100 minutes	1–15
Writing Sample	2	60 minutes	J– T
Biological Sciences	77	100 minutes	1–15

THE MCAT SCORE RELEASE OPTION

The MCAT Score Release Option is available to students on the day of the test. Your answer sheet will contain a space to indicate whether you choose to have your scores sent only to yourself or to all AAMC schools as well as your selected non-AAMC medical schools. If you choose to have your scores sent only to yourself, you will receive a score report after approximately fifty days. You can then decide when, if ever, you want medical schools to receive these scores. This means that if you are not pleased with your scores, you do not have to release them. You can then take the test again. If you are pleased with your scores, you can choose to have them released to your medical schools of choice. There is no charge for releasing scores to AAMC schools. If a student needs scores released to non-AAMC schools, the charge is six dollars per test per school. Students are given six free reports to non-AAMC schools if requested on the day of the test.

Students who choose not to release their scores should know that their AMCAS file will contain their test history. This means that AAMC schools will know when a student decided not to release her scores. This is a basic flaw in the AMCAS score release system.

Although the score release system seems to provide a nice option for testers, admissions officers may look at withheld scores with suspicion. Indeed, there has been an ongoing debate in the pre-med advising community about score release. Since every advisor has different contacts, each one comes up with a different opinion as to the advisability of withholding scores. The school-by-school information on score release that you will find in the sidebars of this book comes from our direct inquiries to medical school admissions offices. As you will see, many schools chose not to respond to our repeated requests for information on their policy toward withheld MCAT scores. We urge you to use caution in choosing to withhold your scores from schools that have not explicitly stated a policy on the matter.

Schools know when you withhold your scores, and as you might imagine, this can be interpreted in many different ways. Withholding your scores could work to your disadvantage in presenting yourself as a candidate for admission to a particular medical school. Although some schools told us that they do not hold it against you if you withhold your scores, others said they were inclined to look negatively on withheld scores and would rather see your entire test history. It's important that you make an informed decision. Where information is not available, your safest option is to release your scores.

YOUR BUDDING CAREER AS A NOVELIST

If you've ever harbored any fantasies of becoming a writer, now is your chance. If you've ever harbored fantasies of wiping the art of composition from human memory in retaliation for the suffering you endured in your Freshman English class, you're going to have to find a way to cope. The personal comments section of the ACOMAS and AMCAS application is your chance to convince the committee that you are more than the sum of your numbers and that you deserve a chance at an interview.

Idea Generators

It is extremely difficult to write about anything important in a page or less, so assume that you will be spending some quality time with your computer. To get started, you can try a couple of different approaches to get your fingers moving:

Clustering

You may remember this from Freshman Comp. You probably thought it was silly back then, but it just might save you now. Get a large blank piece of paper and write down a few words to describe some of the experiences that have led you to pursue medical school. You don't have to write them down in any particular order, and you should scatter them across the page. After you have several topics to work with, see if you can spot any patterns. Some of them will probably be interrelated.

Next, generate longer descriptions of the words you wrote. For example, try to explain what you mean by "intellectual challenge." Was there a particular class you took? A paper you wrote? After you have some ideas on paper, try pulling them together based on the patterns of relationships you see between the topics. For example, telling a story about helping to clean a wound while volunteering in the ER might be a good way of letting them know that compassion is one of your qualities.

Free Writing

This is particularly helpful if you find that you are having trouble figuring out where to start. All you have to do is sit down and force yourself to write about anything that comes into your mind. Don't worry about punctuation or grammar—just write for several pages. Take a break and look back at what you wrote. Most of the time, you'll be surprised to discover the beginnings of an idea.

Talk, Talk, Talk

One way to avoid writer's block and get started is to talk into a tape recorder, or bribe a friend to write as you speak. Sometimes, an empty screen or page can be intimidating in and of itself. You can get started on your essay by telling your story to a tape recorder, or by having a friend write down what he or she thinks is interesting or important as you explain why you want to go to medical school. Don't expect to have suddenly generated your essay in this way. However, you can generate some material with which to start writing.

Three Basic Approaches

There are many different ways to structure the personal essay, but there are three basic approaches that can be used alone or in combination.

"My History in School"

This essay focuses on college experiences. It works well for people whose grades are fairly high and who feel the need to demonstrate their maturity. The essay should be about your development, specialties, and strengths. The best essays usually have specific examples. It helps to have a specific class, professor, paper, or experience that crystallizes your experiences and ties into your goals. One of the benefits of this essay is a built-in chronology and organizational structure.

"My Life History"

In this essay, focus on a few events or main ideas that illustrate the qualities you can bring to medicine. If your whole life clearly leads up to being a physician (even if it might not have seemed that way at the time) this can be a good choice. One of the pitfalls of this structure is that it can let you ramble and lose coherency. Although you need to give a brief overview of your life, you also need to concentrate your paragraphs around individual ideas.

"The Story"

This is often the most effective essay if it's done correctly. Focus on one or two stories that illustrate some of the points listed above. The story essay is the most fun for admissions officers to read, and is the most likely to be coherent and cohesive. You don't have to go overboard with adjectives and turns of phrase to write effective narrative. Just pick a few moments that most clearly define why you want to be a physician.

Key Bragging Points

No matter the subject you plan to focus on, the following are points that you should consider incorporating into the finished essay:

Academic Strength

You can discuss this generally, or with a specific example of a moment in which you enjoyed an intellectual challenge.

Commitment to Ideals

No one expects you to be Albert Schweitzer, but most good physicians have a streak of empathy and altruism.

Careful, Complex Thinking

It is very difficult to explain something as complicated as your motivation to be a physician. Most people, when writing about a defining moment in their lives, assume that the audience is right there with them. This is not the case. You have to explain what you think and feel after you describe the event. Don't assume that the admissions committee is going to fill in the blanks for you.

Why You Want to Be a Doctor

The question you should ask yourself is why—when many other people who've had similar life/career/academic experiences take one look at the horrendous hours involved in medical training and decide that teaching or counseling are perfectly good alternatives—you want to be a doctor. For instance, although many physicians decide to be doctors because of an early experience with the illness of a family member, there are far greater numbers of people with the same background who never consider medicine—but would still describe themselves as compassionate and moved to help people. You have to force yourself to ascertain what odd mixture of qualities—intellectual and emotional—have convinced you that going into more than $100,000 in debt in the era of HMOs is a good idea.

Reasons, Not Excuses, for Weakness

Do not attempt to cover up or gloss over any deficiency, academic or otherwise. You will earn yourself points by honestly and openly dealing with your less than sterling qualities. If you have a couple of low grades or if you had a bad semester, briefly explain what happened, discuss what the experience taught you, and move on.

Good, Clever, Interesting Writing

Translation: Lots and lots and lots of drafts. Everybody has a distinct voice, and you're not going to survive medical school without a sense of humor. Find a way to get both qualities across without resorting to clichés. Prohibited phrases include: Lifelong learning, challenge of a lifetime, healing the mind as well as the body, childlike wonder, frail hands, quiet desperation, and any variations on these themes. Lots of essays turn melodramatic in desperate moments and end up containing such hackneyed characters as grief-stricken relatives, precious children, and heroic doctors. Just say what needs to be said—most of the time, less is more.

Overall Conservative Tone

Shock value doesn't work, despite the tales you might have heard about cartoons and poems. Admissions committees expect you to take the exercise seriously, and to treat the process with respect. Humor is fine, but it needs to be subtle.

Show, Don't Tell

One of the traps of the personal statement is to rewrite your resume in prose. Instead of listing your accomplishments, explain what they mean to you and show how they have affected your life. For example, if you really want to practice primary care, it is far more effective for you to explain in detail what motivates you than to simply state your goal.

The Evolution of the Essay

Good essays tend to evolve, and often bear very little resemblance to rough drafts. Don't be afraid to start over, or to let the essay build on itself. If you write something that doesn't use any of the forms described above but that you feel gets across the points you want to make, than that is the essay you should stick with. Don't force yourself into a mold.

No matter what your eventual essay looks like, however, there are a few general issues that you should think about.

Focus

Generalizing is always really bad. (See what I mean?) Your essay must communicate specific points clearly and effectively. This means that every time you write a sentence that could be used in any other essay, you need to cross it out and start over. For example, "I truly enjoy working with people" could be the opening line in an application for Fry Guy at McDonald's just as easily as it could be a statement about the profound impact you want to have on your patients' health.

Editing

No mistakes. If you are not one of those people who go around making a pest of themselves by correcting everyone else's grammatical errors, you need to find one. Most colleges and universities have writing centers with free editorial assistance, or you can check the local college paper for teaching assistants who are willing to edit for food. No matter what, make sure someone else reads your essay.

Interest

Everyone has an interesting style, and you need to write until you find it. You are who you are for a reason; you have to write until that reason becomes apparent to anyone reading the essay.

Relevance

At some point, the reader will have to have a very clear sense of just why they should let you into their medical school. Don't get so caught up in explaining your inner child that you forget to mention your desire to become a doctor.

Coherence

Make sure your essay fits together. You shouldn't be able to move a paragraph or a sentence when you're finished.

Remember that your entire personality is not going to be reflected in this essay, nor can you entirely offset an otherwise weak application. But this is your big chance to talk to the committee, so make the most of it. Spend the necessary time to draft and rework your essay until it is the best measure of your writing ability and candidacy for medical school.

SECONDARIES AND LETTERS OF RECOMMENDATION

After medical schools receive your application, they will send you what's called a "secondary." Some schools send all of their applicants a secondary, and some go through an initial cut (usually based totally on GPA and MCAT score). One of the reasons that schools like to send secondaries is that they usually charge you about fifty dollars for the privilege of filling them out. Secondaries usually include a variety of essays that are slightly more directed than the "personal comments" in either the ACOMAS or AMCAS. Some typical secondary questions are:

- *What is your favorite novel?*

- *What are your hobbies?*

- *Where do you see yourself in ten years?*

- *Name a leadership role that you've taken and what it taught you about yourself.*

- *What has been your greatest academic achievement? What has been your greatest academic failure?*

- *What type of medicine do you think you might want to practice?*

As you can see, most of these essays seem fairly simple, but that doesn't mean you shouldn't spend time thoughtfully filling them out. Many secondaries are quite lengthy, so it's a good idea to fill them out as you get them, unless you've decided for some reason not to continue with your application to the school. If you find that the cost of sending back secondaries rapidly becomes prohibitive, you can call the individual schools and request a fee waiver. If you were eligible for a waiver from AMCAS, for example, you will probably be able to have most of your secondary fees waived.

You should also take care of your letters of recommendation at the secondary stage. If you are a student who is still in school and you have access to pre-health advising, your letters will probably be handled by that office, and at least one of your letters will probably be from the pre-health advisor. Usually, your recommenders will write one letter that the advising office will copy and send to your list of schools. If you are a returning adult, you may have to take care of all the requests and letters yourself.

Letters of recommendation for medical school work in much the same way as any other such letters; you will have much better luck if you approach your potential recommender with a copy of your resume, transcript, and personal statement. Try to make an appointment to speak to the person to explain to them about the various schools to which you are applying, and to make your case. Even if you have been out of school for awhile, you should try to get at least one letter from a former professor. Medical schools are interested in your character, your desire to be a physician, your academic preparedness, and your intellectual ability. Although most employers could attest to some of those qualities, you will probably need a letter from a professor that discusses your academic abilities. As an undergrad or in your post-bacc program, try to build relationships with faculty members so they can write something meaningful about you. Don't ask for a letter from someone famous unless they know you pretty well. Name dropping is not considered to be particularly attractive in a prospective medical student.

Although many returning adults feel awkward approaching professors they might not have spoken with in several years, most are pleasantly surprised to discover that for the most part, professors do tend to remember their students, and most are happy to write them letters of recommendation. Both current and former students should also consider asking for letters from doctors with whom they have worked or volunteered—and remember that if you're applying to osteopathic school, you have to have a letter from a D.O.

Once you discover how painless it really is to get a letter of recommendation, you may be tempted to go into overdrive on the theory that inundating the committee with reams of stationary will force them to recognize your worthiness. Resist this! Do not send more letters than the school asks for. The committee will not read them, and you will not have done yourself any favors. The only time you might consider sending extra letters is if you are placed on hold after an interview, and have in the meantime been working with someone who you feel would be able to contribute some additional information about your abilities.

MINORITY RECRUITMENT

Minority recruitment has been a thorny issue for years, and, given the current state of race relations in the U.S., the whole question of who gets in and why has become increasingly complicated and contentious. Each year, because competition is so fierce, qualified candidates are turned down at both private and public medical schools. Many of them mistakenly blame their rejections on race. It is very much the case that lots of people are rejected for a far less concrete reason than ethnicity: bad luck. When medical schools routinely receive 4,000 applications or more for 100 seats in the fall class, at least several hundred of those people are going to be roughly equivalent in terms of their academic preparation, communication skills, aptitude for the profession, etc. The admissions committee then has to sit down and make some fairly arbitrary decisions.

It is at this point that minority status can tip the scales. Minority status in this case refers to *underrepresented* minorities, such as Native Americans, African Americans, Latinos, and some other specific groups. If you are not sure whether or not you are a minority in this narrow sense, you should contact AMCAS. Most public and private medical schools are under pressure to produce primary care physicians for underserved areas and communities. If they have a candidate with a background that suggests he or she will fill this need, that person will have an advantage over someone coming from an adequately served area. In many cases, this amounts to a preference for candidates with specific ethnic backgrounds—but it is a preference that occurs after a field of equally qualified applicants is generated from the initial pool. Medical schools are simply too competitive—not to mentioned ethically bound to turn out competent physicians—to accept candidates who are not up to the intellectual challenge of medicine. This selectivity advantage, however, extends to people of any ethnicity who come from rural areas and seem inclined to return to practice. Even that perennial bugbear of affirmative action—the white male—has an advantage if he comes from a small town and can convincingly show that he wants to be a primary care physician.

There is also a type of minority status that AMCAS recognizes that deals only with economic factors, and does not take into account ethnicity or country of origin. To be considered a "financially disadvantaged" minority, you need to have been under financial strain for a long period of time, and to have been the recipient of federal aid in the form of AFDC, welfare, food stamps, or other such programs. Your financial situation needs to have had an ongoing and persistent negative effect on your ability to procure education, housing, food, etc. In other words, the average two-job-struggling-to-make-ends-meet college student does not qualify. This minority status is reserved for those who have struggled uphill their entire lives, and have somehow managed to make it through undergraduate school. The basic rule of thumb here is: If you are a financially disadvantaged minority, you probably know it. If you're in doubt, you probably aren't.

Medical schools are faced with a problem that is actually a boon for the quality of health care in the U.S.—they literally have more good applicants than they can take. What this means for the hopeful pre-med is that if he comes from a community—ethnic or regional—that needs physicians, the odds of acceptance are somewhat less daunting than they are for everybody else. What it absolutely does not mean, however, is that underqualified minority candidates are getting into medical school, while their better-qualified counterparts from middle-class suburbia are being kept out. Medical schools are still predominantly white and largely populated with students whose socioeconomic backgrounds gave them access to first-class undergraduate education, and they continue to get into school in much higher numbers than any other group. Currently, about 43 percent of enrolled medical students are women, 57 percent are men, and about 30 percent are minorities. Of that minority population, however, some groups (such as Asian Americans) have achieved statistical parity with their representation in the population. Other groups, such as African Americans, Latinos, and Native Americans, are still underrepresented. The AAMC has sought to increase enrollment of underrepresented minorities in recent years. AOA has recently instituted a minority scholarship, the Sherry R. Arnstein Minority Student Award, to boost minority recruitment at osteopathic schools. Although all U.S. medical schools are trying harder to find physicians who will fit the needs of the diverse population, they have the luxury of choosing from among the most highly competitive and well-prepared applicant pool they've ever seen.

In other words, if you don't get into medical school the first time around, it probably will have had less to do with the color of your skin than whether or not you had a good day during your interview, how early or late you turned your application in, the quality of your recommendations, or a whole host of other factors. Work hard on continuing to make yourself the best possible candidate, and apply again the next year.

WHAT HAPPENS AFTER YOU'VE BEEN ACCEPTED

So you've achieved the impossible, the best-case scenario . . . multiple acceptances. First, congratulations. Second, it's probably not a good idea to share your good fortune with too many of your pre-med friends, unless you don't particularly want to keep them and you've first removed all the sharp objects from the room.

BACK TO REALITY

After the giddiness wears off, you will have to deal with the best problem you will ever have: choosing which school to attend. Remember that you have lots of time to choose the medical school that best fits your goals and lifestyle. You can hang on to your acceptances until May 15, at which point schools will begin dropping your name off of their acceptance lists if you have not committed. Remember, however, that most of your fellow pre-meds do not share your enviable position. If you are accepted by a school that you know you will not attend, notify them before the deadline so that they can offer the seat to someone else.

Factors to Consider

So, while you are basking in your acceptance, think seriously about the following factors, but don't selfishly hold onto too many acceptances while you are deliberating.

How much does the school emphasize and reward teaching?

This is a huge concern and often overlooked. Look into how much the school values teaching vs. how much they emphasize research. This can be the difference between being taught and being forced to teach yourself.

What are community, social life, and support systems like?

Talk to current students to determine the overall community of the school. You'll be there for four years, and you certainly won't be studying all—OK, most, but not all—of the time. Do the students seem to be accepting the rigors of med school with a positive view or do they waste all extra energy complaining? What is the quality of life in general like at this school?

What's the quality of the residents?

The residents are the ones who will be teaching you when you're a med student, so of course you want them to be good. You should presumably be able to approximate the quality of residents based on the quality of post-graduate training programs (residency programs) at the hospitals affiliated with the school.

How family-friendly is the school?

If you're a returning adult student with a family, check into the spouse/partner support available at the schools you're considering. Getting through medical school will be hard on you and your family, and many places have begun programs that allow spouses/partners to attend special seminars and support groups that acclimate you to the pressures of your chosen educational and career path.

Where will you be living?

Believe it or not, you will occasionally escape to the outside world. Make sure that the activities and hobbies you enjoy are available somewhere in the general vicinity. If you come from one climate and are moving to another, consider how that will affect you. Quite literally, a sudden lack of sun can really change how you feel and how well you will be able to study. Also, find out how close the clinical facilities are to the school and housing. The closer the better.

What kind of research opportunities are available?

Some schools are much better equipped than others, and it's not always the "name" schools that are doing the most cutting-edge research. Different schools have different specialties, and it is not uncommon to find a public school with an excellent program in a given field.

Traditional or systems-based?

Actually, there are now a variety of approaches to the first two years of medical training. Two of the most prevalent approaches, however, are the traditional two years of hard science in lecture format (similar to the way you were taught as an undergraduate), and systems-based study, which looks at "the hard sciences" in the context of a particular biological system.

What kind of financial aid offer are they making?

If you are one of the chosen few, you may actually be able to negotiate a bit on your financial aid offer. Most medical students get through school on federal loans, but if you have several acceptances you may be able to contact the schools you are most interested in and bargain for the best deal.

How much will you owe?

No matter what kind of financial package you get, you will most likely owe a staggering sum when you graduate, and it all eventually has to be paid back. As an intern and resident, you won't be making much in the way of a salary. Although most physicians eventually achieve a comfortable living standard, the practice of medicine is in such a state of flux that it is impossible to predict what kinds of jobs and compensation will be available ten years from now. A public university education, while perhaps not carrying quite the cachet as a private school, may save you tens of thousands of dollars.

BEHIND DOOR NUMBER 1 . . . MORE STANDARDIZED TESTS!

Most medical students take the USMLE Step 1 (and/or the first COMLEX—the COMLEX exams go in the same order as the USMLEs) in June at the end of the second year of medical school. Osteopathic students must pass the USMLE to obtain allopathic residency spots. You can also take it in October. Step 1 is often used to determine whether or not a student has "passed" their course work and can continue into their third and fourth years of training. Step 2 is usually taken during the third or fourth year of school during clerkships. It is offered in August and March. At this point, the vast majority of senior U.S. medical students go through the Match. Very few contract privately for their first year of graduate medical training. Most programs in the Match now use ERAS (Electronic Residency Application Service), which is administered by AAMC, rather than a traditional paper application. Step 3 is usually taken after at least one year of residency (most physicians do at least three years of residency, but still take the test after the first year), and is offered in June and December. The USMLE is written and scored by the National Board of Medical Examiners, which administers Steps 1 and 2. Step 3 is administered by the state. The state confers the license; the USMLE is a prerequisite.

INTERNATIONAL MEDICAL GRADUATES

International medical graduates (IMG) go through a special process to be granted licensure in the U.S. Before you can start a residency program, you need to be certified by the Education Commission for Foreign Medical Graduates (ECFMG). To be certified, an IMG must complete the following five steps:

- *Take USMLE Steps 1 and 2.*

- *Send medical credentials and fill out the paperwork necessary to show proof of medical education.*

- *Take the English test administered by the ECFMG.*

- *If you don't pass the English test, you can take the Test of English as a Foreign Language instead.*

- *Take the Clinical Skills Assessment, which is a live "standardized patient" exam.*

After this, you go to the board of the state you want to practice in and find out what the requirements are for taking the Step 3 (each state determines its own passing score). You can get a residency either through the NRMP Match or through a private contract. After you pass Step 3 and follow any other state guidelines, you are granted a temporary license to practice in that state.

If you are currently in a medical program abroad and thinking about transferring, you need to contact the schools that you're interested in applying to and ask about their transfer policies. In general, it is extremely difficult to transfer into U.S. medical schools.

HIGH SCHOOL STUDENTS

If you've picked up this book and you're still in high school, you're very much ahead of the game. You can get started on the road to medical school by participating in volunteer activities and researching potential college choices to find out what kind of pre-medical training they offer. Remember, you can major in any subject that interests you as long as you take your pre-medical courses. In fact, you are likely to have a higher GPA if you choose a subject you enjoy than if you force yourself to study something like electrical engineering. A few schools have special programs that funnel students through their undergraduate education directly into medical school. If you are interested in these programs, you should contact the following schools directly for more information:

Boston University

Brown University

Case Western University

East Tennessee State University

George Washington University

Howard University

Louisiana State University—New Orleans

Louisiana State University—Shreveport

Michigan State University

New York University

Northwestern University

University of Alabama

University of Miami

University of Michigan

University of Missouri, Kansas City

University of Rochester

University of South Alabama

University of Southern California

University of Wisconsin

IMPORTANT CONTACT ORGANIZATIONS

AMERICAN OSTEOPATHIC ASSOCIATION (AOA)
142 E. Ontario Street
Chicago, IL 60611-2864
800-621-1773
www.am-osteo-assn.org

AMERICAN ASSOCIATION OF COLLEGES OF OSTEOPATHIC MEDICINE (AACOM)
5550 Friendship Boulevard
Suite 310
Chevy Chase, MD 20815-7231
301-968-4100
301-968-4101 (fax)
www.aacom.org

AMERICAN ASSOCIATION OF MEDICAL COLLEGES (AAMC)
2450 N. Street, NW
Washington, D.C. 20037-1126
202-828-0400
202-828-1125 (fax)
www.aamc.org

EDUCATION COMMISSION FOR FOREIGN MEDICAL GRADUATES
3624 Market Street
Fourth Floor
Philadelphia, PA 19104-2685
215-386-5900
www.ecfmg.org

FEDERATION OF STATE MEDICAL BOARDS
400 Fuller Wiser Road
Suite 300
Euless, TX 76039-3855
817-868-4000
817-868-4099 (fax)
www.fsmb.org

NATIONAL BOARD OF MEDICAL EXAMINERS
3750 Market Street
Philadelphia, PA 19104
215-590-9500
215-590-9555 (fax)
www.nbme.org

THE UNIVERSITY OF TEXAS SYSTEM FOR MEDICAL AND DENTAL APPLICATIONS CENTER
702 Colorado, Suite 6,400
Austin, TX 78701
512-499-4785
www.utsystem.edu/mdac
(Texas public schools do not use AMCAS)

3 Advice for the "Nontraditional" Applicant

Forty years ago, most medical school applicants shared certain traits. The "traditional" medical school applicant was white, male, and just older than twenty. Most likely, he majored in biology or chemistry while in college. Although he knew that medical school would be difficult and that his career would be challenging, he looked forward to choosing from a wide range of medical specialties and being financially secure. As a trained professional, he would possess real skills and expertise and, as a result, could expect to enjoy authority and autonomy.

The past few decades have seen substantial changes both in the composition of the medical school applicant pool, and in the professional opportunities available to medical school graduates. Based on the previous idea of the "traditional" medical student, women and minority applicants could be considered "nontraditional," but the term is currently used to describe applicants who are older than most med students. Of the applicants to the 1996 entering medical school class, about 50 percent were between twenty-one and twenty-three years old, with this age group representing the statistical mode. However, the mean age of applicants nationwide was almost twenty-five. About 30 percent of applicants were between twenty-four and twenty-seven years of age, and 16 percent were older than twenty-seven. Thus, although most people apply to medical school during or directly after college, a significant and increasing proportion of applicants are several years older.

Some of these older applicants, always intending to apply to medical school, completed pre-medical requirements during their years as undergraduates, and simply postponed medical school to work, travel, or start a family. Others were unsuccessful at gaining admission directly out of college and are attempting a second or third time. Another group considered medical school in college, but did not complete requirements or the application process. Some older applicants never seriously considered medicine until after they graduated college and were involved in another occupation. Whatever the reason for postponing, older applicants now represent a significant proportion of the medical school candidate pool.

Aspiring doctors who did not take the prerequisite science courses in college or did not excel in them face a formidable challenge. These individuals have a minimum of seven years of medical school and residency on the horizon and, in addition, must complete (and do well in) one to two years of basic science courses before even applying to medical school. Nonetheless, thousands of adults, despite the arduous path ahead of them, decide to tackle this challenge. This chapter is intended as a source of information and support for nontraditional applicants in all stages of the application process. It is written by a nontraditional applicant with the input of others who are or were in the same category. Follow eight nontraditional applicants through the entire process—from decision-making, to post-bacc training, to MCAT preparation, and acceptance. The group is comprised of real individuals[1] coming from a wide range of backgrounds, some elements of which will

[1] Names have been changed.

hopefully resemble aspects of your own situation. When these people decided that medical school was their goal, this is who they were and what they were doing:

- *Becky, a 28-year-old who completed two years of college and had worked as a medical assistant for ten years.*

- *Pete, a 28-year-old with a law degree who was unhappy in his field.*

- *Tina, a 27-year-old art history major who was working in a gallery and dating a medical student.*

- *Bob, a 35-year-old chemistry professor at a small college.*

- *Mitch, a 30-year-old former Peace Corps volunteer, who was working in international development.*

- *Jacob, a 24-year-old volunteer firefighter. A car accident and subsequent hospitalization kept him from completing organic chemistry while in college. Discouraged, he dropped out of the pre-medical track.*

- *Eve, a 42-year-old wife and mother of three who graduated college twenty years ago, and had little experience working outside of the home.*

- *Donald, an engineering graduate student who decided that he needed more human contact in his work.*

DECIDING THAT MEDICINE—AND MEDICAL SCHOOL—IS WHAT YOU WANT

Some of these people were absolutely sure about going to medical school. Jacob, for example, had always known. Tina, who was fascinated by what her boyfriend studied in medical school, had a strong hunch. Donald imagined that being a physician would give him what he felt was missing from his career, but he had limited contact with the medical field and had not fully considered other options that would give him more personal interaction.

Being reasonably sure about medicine is important because you will invest time, money, and energy into the medical school preparation and application process. It is also important because admissions officers will look for indications of your commitment. If you are sure of it, your commitment is more likely to come through in your personal statement and your interview.

If you have never worked or volunteered in a medical setting, you should explore your opportunities. You might arrange to informally shadow a physician or to volunteer in a hospital that has a formal program. Some volunteers find that they are given more responsibility at a small clinic than they are in a large hospital, so look into clinic programs as well. Explore opportunities to volunteer in overseas medical projects. Of our eight subjects, those who had more than one medically related experience felt that it was beneficial because they were exposed to the variation that exists within the field. Not only are volunteer activities helpful in your decision-making process, but they will become significant resume builders should you decide to apply to medical school. In addition, they are likely to be valuable and, hopefully, enjoyable experiences.

One way to help determine if medicine is the right career for you is to talk to others who have made the choice. Interview as many people as you can. Talk to practicing physicians, residents, medical students, and those involved in academic medicine such as researchers. Find out what they love and hate about their work. Ask questions that will help you put their comments about medicine in perspective. For example, if you come across someone who positively hated medical school and dislikes being a physician, ask him what part of medical school he hated the least. If his favorite part of the experience was the relaxing cruise-ship vacation he took after his first year, he probably could have made a better career choice for himself. His views of medical school may not be an indication of what the experience will be like for you.

If possible, talk to medical students, physicians, and residents who are or were nontraditional. Find out whether they feel that they made the right decision. What were the biggest sacrifices they had to make? Visit the pre-medical and medical student discussion pages on the Internet where many nontraditional applicants and students share their thoughts.[2] Although we are unaware of books documenting the experiences of nontraditional medical students, at least one book does give accounts of nontraditional applicants.[3] A commonly held view is that nontraditional medical students have more difficulty with the pre-clinical medical curriculum, but excel during the clinical years.[4] Based on our own discussions, however, nontraditional medical students express fewer doubts about their decision to go to medical school than those who went directly from college. Perhaps this is because they appreciate having a second "chance" at a career, or perhaps it is because they gave the decision more thought.

Bob's decision to apply to medical school was influenced by his sister-in-law. She works in medical equipment sales and is five years older than Bob. She encouraged him to follow his dream, saying that she, too, had entertained the idea of becoming a physician when she was thirty. She decided against it and at forty still dreams about doing it today. But with two young children, she feels that it would be too difficult. Bob decided that it would be more painful to spend his life wondering if he should have gone to medical school than to go and—in the worst-case scenario—drop out and return to teaching.

Mitch also found it helpful to talk to people working in totally unrelated fields. He had worked for two years in a clinic in rural Africa, and thought that he wanted to become a pediatrician. However, he became discouraged while talking to his friends who were medical students, residents, or newly graduated practicing physicians because it seemed that few people loved everything about what they were doing. Many of his friends warned him of the burden of debt and the prospect of having little free time. One friend told him that in comparison to Mitch's current job, which involved traveling around the world, he would be *bored* in medicine. Mitch then took an informal poll of all his friends who included teachers, writers, business owners, software designers, lawyers, and full-time parents. He found that people in all occupations both love *and* hate certain things about their work.

Although medical students and physicians complain about debt, teachers complain about low salaries, and business owners complain about financial insecurity. All of Mitch's friends in their early thirties complain about working too hard, and about the difficulty of balancing their personal and family lives with their careers. Mitch concluded that, despite the initial discouragement he got from friends in the medical profession, people in medicine are among the *most* professionally fulfilled. Although medical students and physicians had complaints, they were engaged in their work and most couldn't imagine a better career. He also noticed that a significant number of nonphysicians he spoke to, although unhappy with their own jobs, still discouraged him from going into medicine. He realized that some of these people had, at one point in their lives, entertained the idea of becoming a doctor. They had successfully talked themselves out of medical school and were sold on all the reasons why *not* to go into medicine. As far as his friend's comment about being bored,

---

[2] Try: Medworld at www.med.stanford.edu/MedSchool/MedWorld/welcome_g1.html and The Interactive Medical Student Lounge whose address is falcon.cc.ukans.edu/nwseen.

[3] Goss, Bryan. *Applying to Medical School for the Nontraditional Student.* 1997: Lakeshore-Pearson Publications. Contact Mountain Books, Albuquerque, NM.

[4] Some studies indicate that nontraditional students do less well in basic science courses. See Blacklow HM et al. *Postbaccalaureate Preparation and Performance in Medical School.* Academic Medicine 1990 June; 65 (6). Other studies refute the claim. See Hall ML, Stocks MD. *Relationship Between Quantity of Undergraduate Science Preparation and Preclinical Performance in Medical School.* Academic Medicine 1995 March; 70:3.

Mitch realized that others tended to glamorize his current work because it involved travel. He knew that being a pediatrician would, on a day-to-day basis, be more interesting than the paperwork he dealt with in his current job. Furthermore, he could probably work overseas as a physician if he found himself yearning for travel.

After you follow Mitch's example and grill everyone you know, ask yourself some serious questions. What jobs and experiences have you loved most in your life? Do you foresee medicine providing similar satisfaction? Have you enjoyed some aspects of your medically related work? Do you have the skills it takes to become a physician? To be fulfilled as one? Whether or not to pursue a career in medicine is an important decision that will affect many years of your life. Give yourself time, both for information gathering and personal reflection. Write down your thoughts on what is influencing your decision. Whether or not you decide to go for it, if you carefully weigh the decision now, you will be less likely to doubt it later on.

Resist feeling that, because you are "older," you should make your decision to enter medical school as quickly as possible. Medical school, internship, and residency require at least seven years to complete. Moreover, medicine is a career of lifelong learning. Start finding things to enjoy about the process of becoming a doctor now. Deciding to go to medical school is part of the process. Try not to stress too much about the decision, and find some satisfaction in your information gathering and self-reflection.

GETTING INTO MEDICAL SCHOOL AS A NONTRADITIONAL APPLICANT

If you are reading this, you have probably decided to move forward with your plan to become an M.D. or a D.O. Hopefully, your level of maturity and your life experience have allowed you to make a well-informed decision that a student just out of college may not be in a position to make. Between 20 percent and 30 percent of applicants in the 24- to 37-year-old age range are admitted to medical school, while approximately 45 percent of 21 to 23 year olds are admitted. Although these statistics suggest that the odds are against older applicants, age itself is not regarded as a disadvantage, and may in some cases be a plus. The smaller percentage of older applicants admitted may be partially due to lower GPAs[5] and test scores. Even the most exciting and unique older applicant must have a competitive GPA and MCAT score.

The timing of the admissions process is often an issue for nontraditional applicants. Donald started thinking about medical school mid-way through his first year of graduate school. It was January 1995. He realized that he had prerequisites to fulfill and that he wouldn't be eligible to enter medical school the following fall, but thought he would be able to matriculate in the fall of 1996. Donald quit his graduate program and entered an intensive pre-medical curriculum, completing his requirements by January 1996. He took the MCAT in April 1996. If Donald had taken pre-medical courses part-time rather than full-time, he could not have adhered to this schedule. Had he done poorly on the MCAT the first time, he could have been delayed an entire year and postponed entrance until 1998. As a result of the timing of the admissions process, it takes two to four years to matriculate after deciding to pursue medical school. The following are the important dates to remember as you think about timeframe and requirements:

- *April: MCAT is given. You should have completed all prerequisite science courses by this date.*

- *June: AMCAS (preliminary) applications are accepted. Filling out the AMCAS application requires all undergraduate, graduate, and post-bacc transcripts (they accept transcripts beginning on*

[5] Smith, SR. *A Two-Year Experience with Premedical Postbaccalaureate Students Admitted to Medical School.* Academic Medicine; 1991: 66:1.

March 15, but the completed application isn't accepted until June 1). You will need your own copies, and you will need to have copies sent directly to AMCAS. It is important to submit AMCAS applications as soon as possible because most schools offer rolling admissions.

- *August: MCAT is given. Use this test date only if you need to improve your scores from the April test. You will indicate on your AMCAS application whether you intend to take (or retake) the test on this date. If so, many schools will not look at your application until August scores are available (some time in October). The penalty for this delay may very well outweigh your score improvement. Thus, unless you anticipate significant score improvement, the August MCAT is not advised.*

- *August: Medical schools to which AMCAS applications have been submitted begin sending secondary applications. Some schools will review AMCAS applications closely, and send secondary ones to a limited number of applicants. Others send them to everyone who applies through AMCAS. There is almost always an additional fee. In some cases, secondary applications require essays or short-answer questions that focus on motivation, personal characteristics, values, and experiences. In other cases, the application is very simple and similar to the AMCAS application. Thus, receiving a secondary application may be an indication that a school is interested in you. When you return the application and fee, you demonstrate your interest in the school. Schools often want these back within two to four weeks. You will also need to submit recommendations at this time. Some schools ask for a photo.*

- *August–May: Based on AMCAS and secondary applications and recommendations, applicants are invited to interview during this period. Some schools conduct all their interviews during one or two months, while others spread them out. Most schools accept 25–50+ percent of interviewed candidates. Thus, getting an interview is an excellent sign. Most admissions decisions are also made during this period, with the exception of applicants who fall into a "hold" or "wait list" category.*

- *June–August: Wait-listed candidates may be accepted.*

ACADEMIC REQUIREMENTS

Most medical schools require or strongly prefer that applicants have a B.A. or B.S. degree from a four-year accredited college or university. All medical schools require a minimum level of science preparation that includes approximately one year each of biology, chemistry, organic chemistry, and physics. Some nontraditional candidates meet these requirements by taking night courses while simultaneously working part- or full-time. Others enroll full-time at private or public undergraduate institutions. Some choose to enroll in special "post-baccalaureate pre-medical" programs (we call them post-bacc programs) offered by a surprisingly large number of colleges and universities (see chapter 8 for a comprehensive listing of post-bacc programs). Post-bacc programs vary widely in terms of cost, rigor of course work, grading system, percentage of graduates admitted to medical school, structure and flexibility of curriculum, duration, size, and class composition. Unlike medical schools, post-bacc programs are neither accredited as such, nor ranked.

Becky needed to complete her B.A. in addition to fulfilling science prerequisites. When she decided it was time take a shot at fulfilling her long-time dream of becoming a physician, she lived and worked in California, which has some of the most selective state-affiliated medical schools in the country. Becky decided to move to another state and complete her B.A. there so that she would be qualified for admission to the state's medical school. Becky enrolled full-time for three years to complete her B.A.—not all of her previous college credits transferred—and fulfill all her science requirements.

Becky's strategy is interesting and may be advisable for others in similar situations who are prepared to relocate. Before moving across the country, be sure that you understand your new state's criteria for determining residency. In some states, being a full-time student does not ensure resident status. Becky might have saved herself a year of schooling had she looked at more colleges and possibly uncovered schools willing to award her credit for all her previous college work.

Tina graduated from a prestigious college, but had taken neither science nor math classes while in school. She was also concerned about her undergraduate GPA, which was 2.9. To make herself a more competitive applicant, she wanted to demonstrate both competence in the sciences and overall improved study skills. Some post-baccalaureate pre-medical programs are quite structured and involve only the minimum science prerequisites; Tina felt that she needed more than this to make up for her undergrad GPA. One of Tina's options was to apply to a post-bacc program that allows participants to take additional courses beyond those in the required scientific disciplines. This type of program tends to be somewhat flexible, allowing students to spend as much time as needed to fulfill requirements and take any additional courses. Students get the opportunity to learn foreign languages, improve writing or math skills, or take courses often recommended—but not required— by medical schools such as biochemistry or statistics. Other post-bacc programs apply students' course work toward a master's degree.

Tina decided not to enter an organized post-bacc program. Instead, she enrolled full-time as a non-degree candidate at a local, private university. This gave her access to larger course offerings. One of the advantages of post-bacc programs is that they are compact, scheduling courses and labs so students may complete all requirements within a year. Tina was less worried about speed, and more interested in earning excellent grades. Another important consideration for Tina was letters of recommendation. Medical schools usually prefer that applicants submit a composite letter from their pre-medical advisor who is typically an administrator or dean, a department head, a specified faculty member, or some type of counselor. The letter discusses the student's qualifications and incorporates comments from his or her pre-medical professors. Because Tina chose a small school, she had the opportunity to get to know her professors and, presumably, to secure meaningful comments from them. At some colleges, only degree-earning students have full access to pre-medical and other advisors, but Tina was able to secure one who agreed to write a letter for her. One advantage to true post-bacc programs is that the pre-medical advisors are able to write appropriate letters of recommendation for nontraditional applicants.

Some pre-medical candidates are highly concerned with getting through the application process quickly and have no interest in prolonging pre-medical course work. Pete had a 3.7 GPA in college and an excellent record in law school. He had no need to prove himself scholastically, but just wanted to "get the sciences out of the way." He was a good candidate for a highly selective post-bacc program. To be admitted to one of these programs, applicants must submit detailed information including personal statements, prior standardized test scores, and several recommendations. Interviews are often required. These programs seek to admit students who will not only complete the course work, but who are likely to be accepted to medical school. Often, the brochures for these programs boast the percentage of graduates who have been admitted into medical school. Although a high acceptance rate is partially a reflection of the quality and resources of the program itself, it also indicates that they accept well-qualified students. In one year, Pete was able to complete all his sciences and study for and take the MCAT.

Pete took advantage of an arrangement between his post-bacc program and a medical school, allowing him to enter medical school in the fall following completion of pre-medical course work. Thus, he avoided an "in between" year generally devoted to the medical school application process. Several selective post-bacc programs offer this type of arrangement, affiliation, or linkage with a number of medical schools. In some cases, the medical school and the post-bacc program are part of the same university. Many nontraditional candidates are disappointed to discover that top medical schools such as Harvard, University of Pennsylvania, and Columbia do not offer these arrangements with their own university's post-bacc program.

Pete took the shortest path possible to medical school. In the fall of 1996 he left the law firm where he was working, and in the fall of 1997, he was beginning medical school. He was happy to skip the long and stressful medical school application process, having been through a similar experience with law school. While ideal for some, Pete's path is neither available nor advisable for everyone. The short, intensive post-bacc programs are grueling and may be too fast-paced for some people. Graduates of these programs often claim their post-bacc work was more demanding than medical school itself. Although these programs can serve as excellent preparation for medical school, they may discourage people who could have succeeded had they enrolled in a more relaxed program.

Earning acceptance to a post-bacc program with affiliated medical schools does not assure your acceptance to medical schools. Post-bacc students in these programs usually apply to the affiliated schools, but acceptances are only provisional, and based on securing a minimum GPA and MCAT score. Only a handful of medical schools participate in these linkages, and each school limits the number of positions available through the direct admissions route. Pete chose his post-bacc program in part because one of the linked medical schools interested him. If none of the medical schools that allow admission through this route appeal to you, saving one year now is probably not worth spending four years someplace you don't want to be. Generally, medical schools agree to these arrangements as a means of enrolling students who they would otherwise not attract. Thus, if you are accepted as a post-bacc student to one of these schools, you are not likely to be accepted to other schools if you apply through the regular admissions process. Another disadvantage to these arrangements is that they are usually binding: if you get in, you must go. If you earn a perfect score on the MCAT, you cannot withdraw and apply to your dream school for the following year. Additionally, you have no opportunity to compare financial aid packages.

While Donald, Tina, Pete, and Becky quit their jobs to enter pre-medical studies full time, Mitch, Jacob, and Eve opted for part-time schooling. Eve wanted to ease into school, and decided to take one course at a time. She enrolled in a general chemistry class through the extension office of a local public university. Her children spent summers at camp and with relatives, allowing her to take a compact organic chemistry course during the summer. The following school year, she enrolled in a two-semester biology course, and she took an intensive physics course the next summer. Eve was concerned that her age would hurt her chances of being accepted to medical school. Some pre-medical advisors believe that being older than forty may be a slight disadvantage.[6] However, had she crammed all of the required science courses into just one year, she would have only been one year younger when she applied to med school, but a whole lot more frustrated and perhaps not as appealing a candidate because her grades could have suffered. In retrospect, Eve's only regret about taking courses "on her own" is that she missed the camaraderie and support that she might have had in a post-bacc program. An advantage to post-bacc programs is that you will meet people facing challenges similar to your own.

Most medical schools advise nontraditional applicants to demonstrate success in *recent* course work. Bob had fulfilled all the prerequisites in college about fifteen years earlier. Since Bob had a graduate degree in science, and remained active in an academic environment, the fact that he completed his prerequisite courses years earlier did not hurt him. His hurdle was the MCAT, for which he reviewed intensely.

The grading systems vary tremendously among undergraduate institutions and post-bacc programs. Some material that you learn as a pre-med, such as the basic biochemical processes, will serve you in medical school. Other topics, like whether your rowboat sinks or rises if you fall into the

[6] See the article, "Is It Too Late For Me To Go To Medical School?" by Leon C. Dorosz, Professor and Chair, Department of Biological Sciences, San Jose State University.

water, might not. As a pre-medical student, your goals should be to figure out whether you enjoy studying science, to learn the material for the MCAT, and to get good grades.

Some colleges and universities with post-bacc programs assign nontraditional students to regular, undergraduate science courses. You attend lectures, labs, and exams alongside undergraduates, and may or may not be graded on the same curve as your younger classmates. Most likely, the mean score of post-bacc students is somewhat higher than that of the rest of the class. Undergraduates shouldn't be penalized by your presence since, after all, you already have your B.A. Thus, schools with significant numbers of post-bacc students are likely to separate them from the undergraduates for grading purposes. Unfortunately, this practice could hurt you because you may be competing with your undergraduate classmates for positions in medical schools. Your cumulative test score of 90 percent put you in the middle of the post-bacc curve and earned you a C, while your classmate's 90 percent put him at the front end of the undergraduate curve and earned him an A. Although a letter of recommendation could explain that you did in fact maintain a 90 percent average, a C is still a C.

Some post-bacc programs address this issue by setting the post-bacc curve higher. The mean score will represent a B grade rather than a C grade. Highly selective post-bacc programs usually recognize that all their students were strong in college, and will set the mean somewhere in the A– or B+ range. If a college that does not have a formal post-bacc program allows you to enroll in science courses, your GPA might be slightly higher because you will be graded with your classmates, many of whom are probably less focused and less serious than you about maintaining excellent grades. Note, however, that many medical schools consider the caliber of undergraduate institutions when evaluating GPAs. This applies to traditional and nontraditional applicants alike.

THE MCAT

The MCAT is a day-long exam that is offered twice yearly at locations throughout the country. It is composed of four sections. An individual's raw score (number wrong out of number possible) on each section is compared with those of test-takers nationwide and is converted to a scaled score. Because most MCAT takers have never sat through an all-day exam, many find the experience a test of endurance and concentration as much as a test of knowledge (see page 11 for more information on the MCAT).

All medical schools, with the exception of one or two, require the MCAT. Schools evaluate MCAT scores in different ways. Some have devised formulas that incorporate MCAT results and GPAs and produce numerical scores. In some cases, if an applicant's score falls above a cutoff, he will receive a secondary application or perhaps be invited to interview. Although certain sections of the MCAT may be weighted more heavily than others by some admissions offices, most schools regard all sections except the essay as equally important. In some formulas, the MCAT and GPA carry roughly equal weight, while in others one is weighted more heavily. A number of schools claim that GPA is more important than MCAT. Although this may be true, consider such statements in light of the recent outcry against standardized tests. A school that admits to using test scores as its primary means of weeding out applicants could be regarded as lazy and discriminatory.

Most schools claim not to use specified formulas or cut-off points and indicate that they might consider an applicant with a very low MCAT score if other aspects of his application are extraordinary. But generally, admissions committees rely heavily on MCAT scores because they are considered a strong indicator of success in the first two years of medical school, and because they are the easiest part of an application to judge. Examining the average MCAT scores of accepted students at a school gives you a rough idea of what you will need to gain admission there.

The MCAT is important for all applicants, but may be especially so for nontraditional applicants. Eve's college grades were twenty years old. Over the years, colleges and universities have made changes and adjustments to grading scales and curricular requirements. Thus, her GPA might not be comparable to that of someone who graduated from the same school in 1998. Furthermore, how she performed in college twenty years ago is probably not a great indicator of how she will fare in medical school today. Grades in post-bacc courses are important, but as mentioned earlier, there is wide variation in grading policies among post-bacc programs and between regular undergraduate courses and the same courses within post-bacc programs. The benefit of the MCAT is that it is standardized, supposedly allowing admissions committees to compare the aptitude of people with different backgrounds.

When preparing for the MCAT, consider that the results of that one day of work are nearly as important as all your other academic achievements. Beyond striving for a sound academic background, most medical school applicants—both traditional and nontraditional—take some sort of MCAT preparation course like the ones offered by The Princeton Review. For some, a test-prep course teaches material never learned, or never absorbed, in class. For others, it relieves some anxiety associated with standardized tests, and thereby allows for an improved performance. For those lacking self-motivation, taking a course is a good way to encourage studying.

Some post-bacc programs offer an MCAT review along with pre-medical courses. Usually, such a review will be much less intensive than a course offered by an outside organization. In Pete's post-bacc program, most students enrolled in a private course that met twice weekly for three months prior to the April MCAT. Since the post-bacc program itself was so intensive and required many hours per day of studying, the students needed to be pushed to devote time to MCAT preparation. Pete did not take the course because he felt confident that he would enter medical school the following fall through the arrangement he had made with an affiliated medical school. The medical school required Pete to take the MCAT and to score at least a nine in all subjects. By January of his post-bacc year, Pete was scoring eights or higher in all sections, and reasoned that, by finishing his pre-medical courses and studying for the MCAT on his own, he could score nines.

Formal MCAT courses typically include three or four practice, full-length MCATs. The exams are scored, giving students an idea of their strengths, weaknesses, and overall progress throughout the course. Pete obtained practice MCATs through the Association of American Medical Colleges (AAMC), and set aside three Saturdays prior to the April exam to take them. For those who do not take a course, it is important to order these practice exams and to be disciplined about taking them.[7] The exams come with tables that allow you to convert your raw score to the scaled score that gives you an accurate idea of how you'll score on an actual MCAT. There are a number of books available that review important MCAT topics and offer tips for taking the exam.

Review books and courses are a good idea for both nontraditional and traditional students, although nontraditional students who have been out of the standardized test scene for many years may particularly need the help. For example, when Becky took her first practice exam, she was discouraged because she was barely able to complete half of the questions in the science sections. MCAT questions are not arranged in order of difficulty, and Becky was spending too much time on really tough passages that appeared early in the sections. She improved her score significantly on the science sections just by training herself to skip and go back to difficult passages.

Some nontraditional applicants have an advantage on the verbal section. Just being older, you may have had more time than a college student to read a wide variety of books. Eve loves reading, and found the verbal section to be a confidence builder. Becky, who did not read extensively for work or pleasure, found the verbal section very difficult. Donald, who learned English as his second language, studied more for the verbal section than for both science sections combined. Becky improved her verbal score by focusing on concentration skills. One way to do this is to read slightly complicated or technical magazine and journal articles every day for several months before the MCAT. Force yourself to concentrate for an extended period of time each day.

[7] Practice exams are real MCATs from years past. Order from: AAMC, Membership and Publication Orders, 2450 N. St. NW, Washington, D.C. 20037-1129. Phone: 202-828-9416.

THE PERSONAL STATEMENT AND INTERVIEW

Health care has changed dramatically in the United States, and some argue that physicians in the twenty-first century will have to possess a wider range of skills than was previously considered adequate. Not only must physicians be experts in their respective fields, but it is advantageous to understand the financial, legal, ethical, and political issues surrounding health care provision. Medical schools recognize the need for well-rounded physicians. The schools now offer revised curriculums that include nonscience courses, and they admit more and more nonscience majors.

As a nontraditional applicant, you have unique experiences and skills. These will differentiate you from other applicants and can be an important strength. The AMCAS personal statement, essays for secondary applications, and the interview are opportunities for you to shine. Although you are probably tired of being asked why you want to become a doctor, you will have to figure out how to answer the question with sincerity and enthusiasm. As a nontraditional applicant, your motivation is an extremely important consideration for admissions committees.

Despite recognizing the value of nontraditional students, admissions committees may be skeptical of applicants who are embarking on their second or third career. Essays and interviews also allow you to address their concerns and doubts about your motivation. In interviews, Donald was often asked what made him so sure he wouldn't drop out of medical school as he had engineering school. The concern is partially that poor judgment with respect to your first career choice suggests the possibility of poor judgment in your decision to apply to medical school. Or, perhaps the worry is that some people are eternally unfulfilled, and will therefore be unfulfilled by a career in medicine. Many people believe that if you are good at something, you enjoy it. Thus, not liking your previous job suggests to some that you were bad at it and that you may possess some hidden faults.

All medical school applicants—both traditional and nontraditional—must figure out how to package themselves. Like wrapping a present that is oddly sized, some nontraditional applicants have to be creative in their packaging. Donald's strategy was to maintain a positive attitude. He told interviewers that some of what attracted him to engineering, such as the analytic thinking required, also applies to medicine. He asked interviewers whether some of the principles in engineering would translate to physiological issues. He emphasized his excellent academic record, his success in science courses, and his demonstrated willingness to work hard in school. He also stressed how much he enjoyed volunteering at a clinic. He did his best to be personable and talkative, thereby showing off his "people skills" rather than restating what was written in his essay—that he was switching fields because he wanted to work directly with people.

Tina's story—that she was bored working in an art gallery and envious of her boyfriend's career—would not get her into medical school without clarification. Tina enjoyed certain aspects of her job, such as interacting with artists and clients. She loved much of the art with which she worked, particularly the pieces that were highly expressive and revealed human emotion. On the other hand, she missed a sense of social purpose in her gallery work, and she felt that she wasn't being intellectually challenged. Tina packaged herself as passionate, people-oriented, and interested in helping others. She was good at her job, but knew that it would not engage her for life. Through her work, she came to know what she liked and disliked, what fulfilled her and what did not. Unlike children of physicians who are likely to consider medicine as a potential career from an early age, Tina never thought about it as a realistic pursuit until her twenties when her boyfriend entered medical school. Now that she had an idea of what medical school and medicine were like, and now that she knew herself better, she was ready to commit to the career. Because she enjoyed working with people, she envisioned a career in primary care. She believed that as a result of her studies and work in the art world, she had good insight into the mental capacity and emotions of people. She wondered if psychiatry was the field for her.

Packaging Jacob was relatively straightforward. He had a reasonably consistent interest in medicine, demonstrated by earlier pre-medical courses and more recent firefighting work that involved some emergency medical skills. In Jacob's personal statement, he needed to address the reasons he dropped out of the pre-medical track in college. Jacob had been hospitalized, and this experience was emotionally difficult for him. Being in a hospital and being around sick and dying people was enough to make him question whether he really could be a physician. When he returned to school, he was less committed to going to medical school and decided to focus on completing his major and general requirements with good grades. After graduation, he fully recovered and had regained his interest in medicine. He took several first aid courses, volunteered in an emergency room, trained to become a fireman, and looked around for post-bacc programs. In his essay, Jacob brought up the doubts that he had about becoming a physician, and discussed how he overcame them. Had he glossed over his hospital experience and the fact that he only took one semester of organic chemistry in college, admissions committees may have concluded that he "just couldn't cut it" as a pre-med. By addressing the situation, he presented himself as someone who matured and grew from a difficult experience.

Some medical schools read the essays and personal statements of all applicants and use them, along with grades and scores, for initial screening. Others only read essays after some applications have been weeded out. If you are filling out applications, you are at the point where you can't do much about your grades or scores. However, you can write an excellent personal statement. Enlist a friend, relative, advisor, or coworker who is well read and writes well to review your statement and make suggestions. Have someone who really knows you read it to be sure that you have conveyed your strengths. On the AMCAS application, exactly one page is provided for an applicant's personal statement. The resume of a nontraditional applicant is probably longer than that of a college senior, and limiting your statement to one page may seem difficult. However, you need not mention all of your accomplishments, experiences, or reasons for pursuing medicine. Choose your most impressive accomplishments, your most meaningful experiences, and your most compelling reasons for pursuing medicine (see page 13 for more advice on how to compose a good essay).

There are countless approaches to writing a personal statement. Becky wrote about learning. By focusing on a concept, she subtly brought up her relevant accomplishments and experiences, and explained her motivation for wanting to go to medical school. During her career as a nurse, she learned a tremendous amount from doctors, other nurses, patients, and families. She loved applying her knowledge to her daily work, and seeing her work pay off in the people she helped. However, she felt that her formal education did not enable her to really understand disease, treatments, and the healing process. Having worked closely with physicians, she understood that they didn't always know everything. She felt, however, that they had the tools to ask the right questions. Asking and answering questions, addressing problems and solving them, observing others, and analyzing their techniques are among the activities Becky looked forward to in medical school.

Eve concentrated on the doctor-patient relationship, discussing vivid memories of her own pediatrician and comparing the relationship she had with him to that of her children and their current pediatrician. She was able to elaborate on her accomplishment of raising three well-adjusted children, a feat that involved serving as caretaker, healer, friend, manager, teacher, advisor, and so on. Mitch described a few of his work experiences in Africa and Latin America, focusing on the ones that were most directly related to health care issues. He wrote that although he enjoyed working overseas, he felt that he would be able to contribute more as a physician than as a project manager. Jacob's prose included personal accounts of saving peoples' lives as a firefighter, and how fulfilling he found that aspect of his work.

The secondary application may have general questions that allow you to elaborate on topics mentioned in the AMCAS essay. Some secondaries contain questions about particular experiences that you may have had, such as research, community service, or employment. Some questions focus on your values and personal experiences. Chapter 6 of this book includes a profile of each medical school. In the "Application Process" section of each description, we give the percentage of AMCAS applicants who generally receive secondaries. Some schools send secondary applications to a very limited number of applicants, and receiving a secondary from these schools means that you made it through a significant screening.

All schools limit the number of applicants that they interview. If you have been invited to interview, it is a sign that you are a "competitive" applicant and you should be pleased. If you receive several interview invitations, the odds are that you will get into medical school. Nontraditional applicants who have interesting life experiences have an advantage in interviews because there is more to talk about than college courses or summer jobs. In addition, you may have had more experience interviewing for jobs and other educational programs than a college student. Hopefully, this will allow you to be more relaxed during the interview process.

In writing a personal statement, you are able to edit, rewrite, rethink, and start over. In an interview, you don't have this luxury. Being relaxed is important, but so is being prepared. Interviewers may ask about courses you have taken. Before going into an interview, review your academic transcripts. Which courses were your favorites? Your least favorite? Why? How do your preferences relate to your desire to go to medical school? If there are any particularly low or high grades, be prepared to discuss what went on in those classes. Review your AMCAS and secondary applications. Be sure that you can discuss every experience you have listed or discussed. Think of some sort of interesting, impressive, (tastefully) funny, or meaningful comment for each experience. Be prepared to answer questions about your childhood. What aspect of yourself do you really hate talking about? Be ready to talk about it, or figure out a good way to divert the conversation from it. What (of relevance) do you know about and enjoy talking about? Think about ways to introduce this subject into an interview.

Although most interviews are one-on-one, some schools use panels of more than one interviewer. Some schools offer group interviews where you interview alongside other applicants. Interviewers may be faculty members, administrators, medical students, or members of the community. Older applicants may find that interviewing with current students, who could be somewhat younger, challenging. An important part of being a physician is the ability to communicate and to get along with all types of people in all types of positions. The interview is an opportunity to demonstrate your skills in this area.

There are predictable interview questions, such as, "Why do you want to go to medical school?" Others are much less predictable, and may even be surprising or shocking. You may be asked about your strategy for balancing personal/family life and medical school, or whether you intend to have children. These questions might seem to be inappropriate, particularly to women. However you choose to answer such questions, it is probably best *not* to get defensive. It is reasonable to have concerns about these issues. Tina found that she got a good response when she turned the questions around and asked the interviewer whether *he* felt being a medical student/resident/physician was stressful on a marriage and what *he* felt about having children while in medical school. For more advice on interviewing techniques, turn to chapter 5.

CHOOSING YOUR MEDICAL SCHOOL

In the early and mid-1990s, the volume of applications to U.S. medical schools reached an all-time high. Although this increase in the number of applications has ceased and the number appears to have leveled off, the process remains highly competitive. As a result, most pre-medical advisors recommend that applicants apply to at least ten schools. Some applicants, particularly those from states with competitive state-affiliated medical schools and whose grades and test scores are below average, should apply to thirty or more schools. In deciding which and how many schools to apply to, it is valuable to talk to a pre-medical advisor. They will help you determine how strong your application is.

The average MCAT scores of students at a particular school are an indicator of how difficult it is to get in. Be sure to apply to a few "safety" schools to which you have a better chance of being admitted. Medical school admission and rejection decisions don't always make sense. Donald was accepted to some of the most prestigious schools in the country, but not to his own state school. This element of chance is a reason to apply to a number of schools, and not to set your hopes on a single school.

For legal reasons, most schools claim that "age is not a factor in admissions." One way to evaluate a school's attitude toward nontraditional students is to look at its student body. Are there a significant number of nontraditional students? What is the average age of incoming students, and what is the age range? Typically, a school's student body reflects its applicant pool, and some schools with fewer nontraditional students simply have fewer nontraditional applicants. If a school that interests you has few nontraditional students, you may want to ask why. It is possible that the school is looking to diversify its students, and will be particularly interested in your application. Medical schools that have arrangements with post-bacc programs are clearly interested in nontraditional students. You should explore them carefully.

Some people argue that all the medical schools in the United States are very good and that there is no particular reason to aspire towards a "top" school. An important difference between medical school and many other graduate or professional degree programs is that medical training does not end at graduation. Rather, a physician's formal education continues during internship, residency, and possibly into fellowship experiences. In terms of job opportunities, where you do your residency could be more important than where you go to school. While attending a well-reputed school will help in residency placement, doing very well at a lesser-known school will also allow you to secure a desirable residency. On the other hand, an advantage to attending a well-reputed school is the comfort of knowing that you don't necessarily have to graduate at the top of the class.

For those who want to practice strictly clinical medicine, there are factors to consider that may be equally, if not more, important than a school's general reputation, which is often based largely on the research associated with the institution. In evaluating the training you will receive, some of the issues to consider are the school's location, the patient population to which students are exposed, the extent to which first and second year students learn clinical medicine, the format of the basic science curriculum,[8] interdisciplinary aspects of the curriculum,[9] the learning resources available to students, the school's role in the community and as a health care provider, the emphasis on primary care, the grading system, and the accessibility of faculty. Even if you are uninterested in a career in medical research, there are educational benefits to becoming involved in research efforts while in medical school, and you may be interested in schools that facilitate faculty/student collaboration and encourage student participation in research.

Rather than focusing on prestige or a published ranking,[10] concentrate on what you want from a school. Among other features, Mitch wanted access to a school of public health so that he could continue working in public and international health issues. Eve looked for schools that devoted significant resources to primary care. Donald looked for more structured programs, while Becky was interested in programs that allowed flexibility. Jacob applied primarily to schools with strong repu-

[8] Some schools use lectures and labs while others have an entirely case-based approach. A number of schools fall somewhere in the middle, incorporating some of each educational methodology. There is no evidence that a particular curriculum is "best." You need to consider your own learning style.
[9] Presumably, nontraditional students bring an interdisciplinary perspective and benefit from this approach.
[10] There is no definitive ranking. *U.S. News & World Report* publishes a yearly report ranking graduate schools. Be sure to understand the methodology used when reading their findings.

tations for emergency medicine. Bob hoped to continue teaching part-time or during summers while in school. He looked for schools that would allow this.

Beyond academic features, there are lifestyle issues to consider that may be quite different from those faced by recent college graduates. In college, Mitch enjoyed being part of a cohesive student body at a small, remote, private school. As a thirty-year-old who had spent significant time overseas, he wanted to live in a more multicultural environment. He hoped to have a social life that, to some degree, involved people other than his medical school classmates. Most of the schools he applied to were either in urban areas or were closely associated with a larger university. Tina wanted to remain near her boyfriend, and decided to limit her applications to schools in the region of the country where he was studying. Because of her family, Eve had location issues as well. As a nontraditional student, you are likely to have more responsibilities and complexities in your life than a recent college graduate. As a result, you may find that lifestyle issues play a more important role in determining where you apply and where you go to school.

Interview day is a rare opportunity to hear first-hand what it is like to be a student at a particular medical school. During the course of the day, you will probably speak with current students, either formally or informally. Ask the students you meet for the names of nontraditional students within the class. If you have a spouse and/or children, ask for the names of students in similar situations. While interviewing, you will be focused on making a good impression and getting in. Later, however, you might have some choices to make and you may be desperately trying to differentiate one school from the next. Input from current students, particularly those with backgrounds similar to your own, will be invaluable (for more advice on how to choose a school, turn to page 18).

FINANCIAL ISSUES

The cost of a medical education is daunting for traditional and nontraditional students alike. With the exception of those who have accrued savings in former careers, financing medical school as a nontraditional student involves challenges. Nontraditional students often have higher living expenses associated with off-campus living, dependents, debt, and other financial responsibilities. With few exceptions, financial aid offices will look at your parents' income and assets in determining assistance packages. This applies to all students, regardless of their age and whether they themselves are parents. If you are married, medical schools will expect your spouse to contribute to the extent that he or she can. If your parents and/or spouse are less than thrilled about supporting you in this endeavor, financial questions can translate to personal/emotional issues. Older medical students will have less time in the workforce to pay off educational debt, and it is unclear whether financial aid offices consider this in making awards (for more information on financial issues, turn to page 37).

Consider the financial implications of going to medical school, and try to come up with a strategy for dealing with them. If your heart is set on going, financial issues alone should probably not stop you. When deciding where to apply, add to your list of considerations the average debt of graduating students. Even if this figure is not published, financial aid offices will probably provide it. Look very closely at your state-affiliated medical school because in-state tuition is typically much less than private school costs. Ask financial aid offices about loan repayment programs. Think about ways to trim your budget, such as living with relatives or giving up your car. The material possessions you forego now, and as a result of future loan payments, will be irrelevant if you truly love and are fulfilled by your future career.

4 Financing Medical School

HOW MUCH IS ALL OF THIS GOING TO COST?

There's no doubt that med school is expensive. For the 1998–1999 school year, the average first-year tuition for an out-of-state student attending a U.S. private medical school was $26,476; in-state was $24,917. The average at public schools was $9,263 for in-state students and $22,391 for out-of-state students. When planning for the cost of attending medical school, however, tuition is only part of the picture. You must also pay for books, equipment, housing, utilities, food, insurance, transportation, and miscellaneous costs. All of these expenses add up quickly; depending on where you attend school, they may equal or exceed the price of tuition.

The cost of a medical education is daunting, but once in practice, physicians are among the most highly paid professionals. Currently, the average physician earns just less than $200,000 annually. Although it will be years before today's first-year students make that kind of money, they can assume the financial burden of their education with the confidence that they will one day make enough money to justify the investment.

AND HOW CAN I PAY FOR IT?

Since the medical student of today will be the well-paid physician of tomorrow, medical schools expect the students and their families to be responsible for the cost of their education. Except in cases in which a student has exceptional financial resources, it is essential to rely on outside sources of financial assistance to pay the bill.

FINANCIAL AID PROGRAMS

There are two general types of financial assistance: loans and scholarships/grants. Loans must be repaid, and have varying interest rates, deferment options, and repayment periods. Many loans will be available to you only if you have documented need, but some funds are available regardless of your financial situation. Most medical students borrow heavily, relying on the potential of a generous salary once they begin practice. For 1997 med school graduates, the average debt was $80,462, and by all indications, that amount will continue to increase. Scholarships, or grants, are gifts that you don't need to repay. They can be awarded on the basis of any of three factors—financial need, outstanding academic merit, or a promise of future service—or a combination of those factors.

Loans

Anyone with good credit, regardless of financial need, can borrow enough money to finance a medical education. If you have financial need, you will most probably be eligible for some types of financial aid if you meet the following basic qualifications:

- *You are an American citizen or a permanent U.S. resident.*

- *If you are a male 18 years of age or older, you are registered for Selective Service or you have documentation proving that you are not required to register.*

- *You are not in default on student loans obtained prior to applying to medical school.*

- *You have a good credit history.*

If you have financial resources that disqualify you for some types of aid, but you meet the above requirements, you are still eligible for assistance. The loans for which you are qualified, however, usually have higher interest rates, offer less favorable repayment schedules, and often require that interest payments be made during school.

Following is a description of each of the four basic types of loans: federal, state, private, and institutional.

Federal

Federal loan programs are funded by the federal government. The amount available each year is based on the national budget and is affected by the priorities of the executive and legislative branches of the government. Federal loan resources have been declining for the last several years, and the downward trend will probably continue. Even so, federal loans, particularly the Stafford Loan, are usually the "first resort" for borrowers. Most federal loans are need-based, but some higher-interest loans are available to a student or his family regardless of financial circumstance.

State

Students who are residents of the state in which they attend medical school may be eligible for state loan programs. Like federal loan funding, state funding has been decreasing. Eligibility is usually based on need and may be further tied to specific segments of the population (e.g., minority or disadvantaged students, or students who are interested in practicing family medicine in underserved areas of the state). Individual schools can provide you with information about state loan programs.

Private

Private loans are funded by contributions from foundations, corporations, and associations. A number of private loans are targeted to aid particular segments of the population (e.g., minority or disadvantaged students, women, or students who are interested in practicing family medicine in underserved areas of the state). You may have to do a good deal of investigation to identify all of the private loans for which you might qualify. The best place to begin your search is in public, undergraduate, and med school libraries. There are also a number of commercial financial aid search services available, but beware—financial aid officers warn that search services sometimes charge hefty fees for information that, in the majority of cases, students can obtain themselves. Private financial aid resources are also available on the World Wide Web. FastWEB is the largest free scholarship database on the Web; you can find it at web.studentservices.com/fastweb.

Institutional

The amount of loan money available, and the method by which it is disbursed, varies greatly from one school to another. As part of the shift toward emphasizing primary care, some schools offer assistance to students who are committed to providing primary care after graduation. Private schools, especially those that are older and more established, tend to have larger endowments and, therefore, can offer more assistance. To find out about the resources available at a particular school, refer to its catalogue or contact its financial aid office.

We have compiled a table of the most commonly used loan programs. Included in this table is information about the characteristics of each loan. The following defines each category.

Name: The full name of the loan and the acronym, if applicable, by which it is most commonly known.

Source: Information about who funds and who administers each loan.

Eligibility: Some loans are need-based. Others are open to people regardless of their financial situation. A few federal and private schools require that a student fit a specific demographic profile.

Maximum Allocation: There is a maximum amount of money you can borrow from any one program, so many medical students find it necessary to borrow from more than one source. Most loans have both maximum yearly and aggregate loan amounts. Amounts you borrowed from the same loan program for your college education are deducted from the aggregate amount you can borrow in medical school.

Repayment and Deferral Options: Important considerations in structuring your educational debt are how long you have to pay back loans and whether principal and/or interest may be deferred until you have completed your education. This column provides information about the repayment period and deferral options for each loan. It is important to remember that, no matter what the source of a loan, the responsibility for keeping track of loan activity is yours.

Interest Rate: This column provides information about the current interest rate of the loan. Fixed-rate loans use the same interest rate throughout the life of the loan. Variable-rate loans base their interest rate on established financial values, usually ninety-one-day Treasury Bills (T-Bills) or the prime lending rate. Since these rates fluctuate greatly, you should check with a bank to find out the exact interest rate.

Pros: Listed in this category are factors that make this an attractive loan source. Attractive features include long repayment terms, deferral policies that waive both interest and principal throughout medical school and all or part of residency training, and low, fixed-rate interest.

Cons: Listed in this category are factors that make a particular loan unattractive. Such features include short repayment times, limited deferral options, or variable, high-interest rates.

Scholarships/Grants

Some grant, or gift money, comes with no strings attached; these are nonobligatory scholarships. Although such scholarships may be available on the basis of outstanding academic merit alone, others are based on a combination of merit and need. In fact, all federal, nonobligatory scholarships are based on need and may also require that you fit a particular demographic profile. Scholarship amounts vary, and they are administered by the same groups as loans: federal and state governments, private foundations, and institutions. For more information about state and institutional scholarships, contact the financial aid offices at some of the schools to which you are going to apply. The private scholarship opportunities available to you depend on such diverse factors as your ethnic identity, your socioeconomic background, and your field of interest. You can find out about private scholarship or grant opportunities at your public or university library.

Obligatory Scholarships

Some federal scholarships are available to students who agree to serve at the Public Health Service, at the Veterans Administration, or in the Armed Forces. These scholarships provide full tuition, some or all expenses, and a monthly stipend. Service-based scholarships, which are not based on need, all carry an obligation to serve at least one year for every year of support. The advantage—a "free" medical education—is obvious, but this is not an option to take lightly. Time spent in residency—which is often restricted to only military residencies—does not count toward your service debt, so you may be out of medical school for seven to twelve years before you're free of your obligation. Some states and counties also have some service-based scholarship programs ortuition remission programs available. Despite their lengthy obligations, service-based scholarships are in high demand. To increase your chances of obtaining one, apply as early as possible. Ask the financial aid offices of schools in which you are interested who to contact locally for more information.

TABLE OF LOANS

NAME OF LOAN	SOURCE	ELIGIBILITY	MAXIMUM ALLOCATION
Federal Stafford Student Loan (SSL, formerly GSL) Call 888-888-3469 for more information	Federal, administered by participating lender.	Demonstrated financial need.	$18,500/year (at least $10,000 of this amount must be in unsubsidized Stafford loans). The maximum aggregate total is $138,500, no more than $65,500 of which may be in Subsidized Stafford Loans. The maximum aggregate total includes any Stafford loans received for undergraduate study.
Unsubsidized Stafford Student Loan Call 888-888-3469 for more information	Federal, administered by participating lender.	Not need based.	$18,500/year (at least $10,000 of this amount must be in unsubsidized Stafford loans). The maximum aggregate total is $138,500, no mor than $65,500 of which may be in Subsidized Stafford Loans. The maximum aggregate total includes any Stafford loans received for undergraduate study.
Health Professions Student Loan/Primary Care Loan (HPSL) Contact school for more information	Federal, administered by school.	Exceptional financial need; commitment to primary care.	Tuition plus $2,500 stipend.
Perkins Loan (formerly NDSL) Contact school for more information	Federal, administered by school.	Demonstrated financial need.	$5,000/year, with aggregate of $30,000. Aggregate amount includes undergraduate loans.
Alternative Loan Program (ALP) Call 800-858-5050 for more information	AAMC, administered under MEDLOANS division of AAMC.	Not need based.	Cost of attendance minus other aid received. Aggregate: original principal of debt may not exceed $189,125.

PAYMENT AND DEFERRAL OPTIONS	INTEREST RATE	PROS	CONS
10 years to repay. Begin repayment 6 months after graduation. Forbearance possible for up to three years of residency training.	Variable, 91-day T-Bill plus 2.5%. Capped at *8.25%.	Most common medical school loan. Interest is paid by the government during school. Once you get a loan, later loans are at the same rate.	None.
10 years to repay. Interest begins to accrue from day loan is disbursed; you can pay the interest or have it capitalized (added to principal). Begin repayment 6 months after graduation. Forbearance possible for up to 3 years of residency training.	Variable, 91-day T-Bill plus 2.5%. Capped at *8.25%.	Not need based. Same interest rates as Federal Stafford. Once you get a loan, any later loans are at the same rate.	Interest is not paid by the government while you're in school.
10 years to repay, beginning one year after graduation. Deferrable during residency and under special circumstances.	Fixed, 5%.	Low interest rate.	Very limited funding.
10 years to repay. Begin repayment 9 months after graduation. Can be deferred for 2 years during residency.	Fixed, 5%.	Low interest rate.	Low maximum allocation; primarily restricted to first- and second-year students.
Standard: 20 years of interest and principal payments. Altenative: 3 years of interest only and 17 years of interest and principal. Repayment generally begins 3–4 years after graduation, depending on length of residency.	Variable, based on 91-day T-Bill plus 2.5% adjusted quarterly. After graduation, rate is 91-day T-Bill plus 2.85% adjusted quarterly.	High maximum allocation; not need based.	Also a "loan of last resort." High interest rate. Interest accrues upon disbursement and is compounded during residency.

*Call to confirm most recent interest rate. They are variable.

THE FINANCIAL AID PROCESS

PREPARING TO APPLY

Many students miss out on assistance they are eligible for by making some basic, avoidable mistakes. Top financial aid officers supplied the following common errors and their suggestions to avoid them.

Missing Deadlines and Keeping Poor Records

Like your applications for admission, your financial aid applications should be submitted as early as possible. To make sure that you have the data required by the financial aid office, file your income tax forms early and encourage your parents (even if you are an independent student) to do the same. Photocopy all forms that you submit and note the date you send them. Make a financial aid file of these forms and any material related to the decisions of the financial aid committees of the schools to which you apply. Keep careful track of deadlines—if you miss them, you miss out on the opportunity for most aid.

Submitting Information to the Wrong Needs Analysis Service

There are three different needs analysis services: ACT (American College Testing), CSS (College Scholarship Service), and GAPSFAS (Graduate and Professional School Financial Aid Service). Each medical school uses one of these services to determine how much financial assistance their prospective students require. Many applicants assume that because they have submitted information to one of the services for one school, they have done everything they need to do for all the schools they are considering. Making this assumption can have serious repercussions. Until the proper service completes the needs analysis, the financial aid office cannot package your financial aid. To avoid making this mistake, check with the financial aid offices of all the schools you are applying to, to see which service they use. Submit the proper materials to the appropriate service. More detailed information on the needs analysis services and their function can be found under "Calculating Your Contribution."

Having a Poor Credit History

People are often unpleasantly surprised when they see their credit histories. Even relatively minor financial problems, like making a couple of late payments on loans or credit cards, can lower your credit rating. Also, credit bureaus sometimes make mistakes, causing negative, but false, information to show up on your record. Since a bad credit history will make you ineligible for many, if not all, loan programs, it is a good idea to check your credit history before you apply for financial aid. Because it usually takes several weeks to obtain a copy of your history, you should order one well in advance of the time you will begin to submit your applications. There is usually a fee for this, but it's worth the few dollars to check to make sure it is accurate.

Defaulting on Undergraduate Student Loans

If you haven't been keeping up with your student loan payments, you will have a very hard time qualifying for loans, especially those funded by the federal government. Clear up any problems with prior student loans well before applying for additional assistance. If you are still in school and have not yet begun repaying your loans, talk to your undergraduate financial aid officer to clarify repayment and deferral options on your loans. Remember that the burden of keeping track of your loan activity is on you, and that once you start medical school, you must keep the lenders apprised of your whereabouts.

APPLYING FOR AID

Students who seek financial aid must go through additional steps in the admissions process to find out whether or not they qualify for assistance. Schools' policies may vary somewhat, but they all follow the same general lines. To determine whether or not you qualify for aid, and if you do, how

TABLE OF GRANTS

NAME OF GRANT	SOURCE	ELIGIBILITY	SERVICE OF OBLIGATION	AMOUNT OF GRANT
National Health Service Corps (NHSC)	Federal.	Need-based; former EFN recipients and students with interest in primary care are preferred.	Two to four year contract. Years spent in residency do not count toward fulfilling obligation.	Maximum amount is full tuition and fees plus stipend.
Financial Assistance for Disadvantaged Health Professions Students (FADHPS)	Federal, administered through school.	Exceptional financial need and disadvantaged background; family contribution not to exceed the lesser of $5,000 or one-half the cost of education.	None.	Varies; up to $10,000/year.
National Medical Fellowship Scholarship (NMF)	Private.	First- or second-year underrepresented minority, female, rural, or disadvantaged background with documented financial need.	None.	Varies.
Scholarship Program for Students of Exceptional Financial Need (EFN)	Federal, administered through school.	Exceptional financial need and disadvantaged background; family contribution not to exceed the lesser of $5,000 or one-half the cost of education.	None.	Varies; tuition and other educational expenses.
Armed Forces Health Professions Scholarship	U.S. Army, U.S. Navy, and U.S. Air Force.	Able to serve in military; age restrictions; U.S. citizens only.	One year for every year of support. Years spent in residency do not count toward fulfilling obligation.	Full tuition, "reasonable" fees, and stipend. Student becomes officer in service branch upon matriculation and receives all benefits of rank.

much aid you need, schools must first determine how much it will cost for you to attend, and then how much of that cost you and your family can bear.

How Schools Determine Their Cost

Each medical school prepares a student budget that includes the expenses associated with being a first-year medical student. Included in this budget are items such as tuition and fees, books, equipment, housing, utilities, food, insurance, transportation, and personal expenses. To figure out how much assistance you will need to pay this cost, schools must determine the amount that you and your family can reasonably contribute.

Calculating Your Contribution

To determine how much you and your family can contribute, medical schools use one of the three federally approved needs analysis services (GAPSFAS, CSS, or ACT). All of these services require you to submit a FAF (Financial Aid Form) or FFS (Family Financial Survey), tax information, and other relevant financial data. You should submit the needs analysis information as soon after January 1 as possible. To make sure you have all the required information, you should file your previous year's income tax returns early. Because some federal loan programs and some institutions require parental information even from independent or married students, your parents should also file their income tax forms as early as possible.

In 1993 an additional step was introduced to the process. All students who wish to be considered for federally funded loans must submit the Free Application for Federal Student Financial Aid (FAFSA). You can get a FAFSA from the financial aid office of the schools to which you apply. Again, you should submit this form as soon after January 1 as possible to maximize your chances of getting the financial aid for which you are eligible.

On the basis of the information you give them, GAPSFAS, CSS, or ACT calculates your financial need by subtracting your expected personal and family contribution from the total student budget furnished by the school. If expenses are higher than the estimated contribution, you show financial need.

Your Tentative Financial Aid Package

Once the existence and amount of need has been determined, the financial aid office of each school to which you apply puts together a tentative financial aid package to meet that need. The package can include loans, scholarships, grants, or a combination of these elements.

Accepting Your Financial Aid Package

Once you matriculate at a school, the financial aid office will put together your actual financial aid package. At this point, you should take a close look at what you are offered. In most cases, loans will make up a portion of the package. Remember, loans must be repaid—with interest—and the amount of this debt will affect your lifestyle far beyond medical school and residency. For instance, if you borrow a large sum of money for medical school, you may have trouble later obtaining a loan for a large purchase like a car or a house. You are not required to accept all the aid you are offered, so it is in your best interest to borrow only what you need to meet your expenses.

CUTTING COSTS

Medical schools formulate their student budgets by using average expenses for everything except tuition. By making some adjustments to your lifestyle, it is usually possible to undercut this budget, and therefore decrease the amount of money you borrow. Following are some strategies recommended by financial aid professionals to reduce debt.

BOOKS AND EQUIPMENT

Buy good-quality used textbooks and equipment whenever possible. Selling books and equipment you no longer need is a good way to earn extra cash.

TRANSPORTATION

Automobile loan payments, insurance premiums, licensing fees, fuel, and maintenance really add up. Evaluate your need for a car before taking one to medical school. If you attend school in a place where public transportation is available or where you can bike or walk to school, leave the car behind. If you must have a car, you can save by raising insurance deductibles and carpooling with fellow students.

INSURANCE

Most medical schools require you to carry medical and, in some cases, disability insurance. Before you buy into the school's plan, check your existing coverage. If your parents still claim you as a dependent, or if you have a spouse whose medical benefits extend to you, you may already have adequate coverage.

OTHER EXPENSES

Millions of Americans find themselves in financial straits each year because of revolving credit. Medical students are no exception. If you find that you have trouble avoiding the temptation of pulling out the plastic for purchases you can't afford, cut up your cards. Remember, if you can't afford to pay for something with cash or a check, you probably can't afford to charge it, either. To keep discretionary expenses from getting out of hand, set up a detailed budget and stick to it. If you've never used a budget before and need help, there are many computer software programs that help you set up a budget, track expenses, and give you reports on how you're doing.

A FINAL WORD

YOUR FINANCIAL AID RIGHTS

- *You have the right to expect that the financial aid office will assist you in obtaining financial aid and information about financial aid opportunities.*

- *Financial aid officers who you give information to about your/your family's financial profile can not publicize this information.*

- *You have the right to accept or decline all or part of the aid offered.*

- *You have the right to appeal your financial aid package if your financial aid picture changes for the worse. (This does not necessarily mean, however, that the amount of aid will increase.)*

- *You have the right to examine your financial aid file at any time.*

- *You are entitled to treatment that does not discriminate on the basis of race, creed, age, handicap, gender, or national origin.*

YOUR FINANCIAL AID RESPONSIBILITIES

- *You are responsible for meeting the expenses related to attending medical school.*

- *You are responsible for reading and understanding the conditions and terms of all of the elements in your financial aid package.*

- You are responsible for submitting financial aid applications on time.

- You are responsible for obtaining and filling out financial aid forms and supplying accurate and complete information on these forms.

- You are responsible for reporting to your financial aid office any outside scholarships or loans that may affect your amount of need.

- You are responsible for using loan funds to pay tuition.

- You are responsible for repaying all loans.

- You are responsible for notifying all lenders of all changes of address during and after medical school.

- You are responsible for keeping accurate and complete records of all financial aid applications and transactions.

5 The Interview:

Separating the Merely Qualified from the Truly Worthy

Be proud if you're invited to an interview. You've made it through two initial screenings, one before and one after the supplemental application. Usually, this means that the Admissions Committee thinks you're qualified to attend their school. Unfortunately, they also invite a lot of other qualified people, and they don't have space to admit all of you. The object is to convince everyone who interviews you that the school would be a better place with you in it. Easy to say, a little harder to do.

Because almost everyone has heard horror stories about someone else's interview, most people start to worry about the interview before they even submit their applications. Try to relax. A good interview begins with good preparation. You can start by becoming familiar with the interview process.

WHO CONDUCTS INTERVIEWS?

Different schools have different policies about who conducts the actual interview. In general, schools have a Medical Selection Committee made up of professional admissions or student affairs people and faculty members. Often, especially in more progressive schools, upper-level med students also participate. At some schools, you'll have a couple of separate, one-on-one interviews; at others, you'll be interviewed by a panel. You may be the only applicant in front of a panel (this really seems like an inquisition), or you may be joined by other candidates.

At many schools, the person or people you speak with become your advocates in the final selection process. When all the interviews in a certain time period are finished and the Selection Committee meets, these people share their observations about you and sometimes recommend a particular action. The final decision, of course, is up to the entire committee.

WHAT CAN I EXPECT?

Since med schools are trying to revise their curricula to make medical education more people-focused, you can assume that the interview process will also reflect this change. Eventually. For the time being, though, a number of schools still design the process to see how well you function under stress.

Stress interviews can take a lot of different forms, but their main characteristic is that the interviewer puts you in a position where he or she can observe how you act—and how you speak—under pressure. Proponents of stress interviews argue that they get you to drop your carefully studied "med school interview facade" and reveal what you're really like. Typical tactics include asking questions about sensitive or controversial topics, delving into extremely personal matters, rattling off a series of game show-like trivia questions, or showing disapproval—through challenging remarks or negative body language—at almost everything you say.

The way to handle this type of interview is to try to relax and try not to get defensive or confused. Generally, a stress interview is not intended to elicit a particular response, but to judge how you handle all of your responses. If an interviewer asks you a question that you think moves beyond the limits of acceptability, you should say so. You are perfectly within your rights to say in a polite tone of voice, "I'm sorry, but I don't feel comfortable answering that type of question. Is there something else you'd like to talk about?" In some cases, the interviewer might be testing how you handle personal boundaries.

Before you get too worked up over the stress interview, you should be aware of two things. First, students we surveyed who reported being flabbergasted by an aggressive interviewer were often accepted at that school anyway. So don't place too much importance on a bad experience. They expect you to be stressed, and you probably didn't do nearly as badly as you think. Second, and more important, most interviews aren't like this. People don't often talk about their good experiences, but there are plenty of them.

In the vast majority of cases, the interviewers are trying to build up an honest picture of you beyond the numbers, and most do not use stress interviews. They are used to seeing "mediclones": a species of pre-med who bores everyone who will listen about their research accomplishments, volunteer experiences, and commitment to practicing family medicine in a rural area. As long as you don't spend the entire interview second guessing what it is you think they want you to say, you should do perfectly well.

HOW SHOULD I ACT?

The golden rule for interviews is "Be Yourself." Interviewers have been through all of this before, and they're pretty good at spotting people who are putting on an act or reading from a mental script. What they're trying to find out from this interview is what kind of person you are and how you relate to others. Up until now, you've been only a few sheets of paper, a bunch of numbers, and (probably horrible) photograph. Now's the time to show them your stuff. But, remember no lying and no b.s.

BE PREPARED

Although there is no way to prepare yourself for every question you may be asked (and, as you'll see, some of the questions may be bizarre), you should be ready to answer questions about your motivation to become a physician, your academic background, your extracurricular and leisure activities, your job or research experience, and your views on medical problems and ethical issues. Later in this chapter is a sample of questions that current medical students were asked in their interviews. Some of them are typical; others are truly strange. As you get ready to interview, try to answer some of these questions to yourself, and then to a friend, parent, or professor. In addition, you may want to audiotape or videotape mock interviews to see how you sound and look. When you choose a guinea pig to be your surrogate interviewer, select someone who will be honest with you about the strengths and weaknesses of your responses. Don't try to memorize answers word for word; canned responses, no matter how valid, are stiff and unconvincing (just look at a tape of a presidential debate). Come up with general responses and, where appropriate, cite facts to support your opinions and conclusions.

APPROACH WITH CONFIDENCE

Like dogs, interviewers seem to smell fear. The tone of your interview is often set in the first few seconds, so approach with confidence. Greet your interviewer with a firm handshake and look him in the eye. During the interview, be positive. Think of it as a pleasant conversation with someone you'd like to get to know better. A good interview is a dialogue, where there is considerable "give and take." Unless your interviewer brings them up, avoid controversial or emotionally charged subjects like abortion. If you're asked your views, state them and move on.

TAKE YOUR TIME

In the course of your interviews, you will be asked scores of questions, some on issues to which you haven't given a great deal of thought. Your interviewers don't expect you have a ready answer for every one of these questions, but they do expect you to come up with a coherent, well-thought-out response. Many applicants are afraid that if they hesitate, it will seem that they are unprepared. Not so. Good physicians don't rush to a conclusion without considering the facts; rather, they think through a problem before they decide how to act. If a question catches you off guard, take a second to think it through. If it seems ambiguous, don't be afraid to ask for clarification. If you don't know, admit it and ask the interviewer to share the answer. By taking the time to make sure that your response is well conceived and well spoken, you will impress the interviewers as thoughtful and articulate—two characteristics essential in a good doctor.

ASK QUESTIONS

Although the interview is the time for medical schools to find out about you, it is also an excellent opportunity for you to find out more about the school. Before you go to an interview, make sure you've studied the school's information packet and are ready to ask intelligent questions about the program. Do a search at your undergraduate or public library to see if the school has been in the news and, if so, for what. Unless you are a great actor, ask questions only about those things you are truly interested in; you don't want to look like you're sucking up.

BE ON TIME

Make sure that you get detailed directions before you make the trip, and arrive with enough time to park and find the office. If you are invited to interview at several schools in the same geographic region, you might save on travel costs and time by making an interview "circuit," visiting several schools on the same trip. This can mean that you have several interviews in the same week or even the same day. Give yourself as much time as possible at each, so that you have time to make the transition, both physically and mentally, from one school to the next. If you can, try to get to each campus early enough to walk around, talk to students, and formulate questions that are specific to the school.

DRESS FOR SUCCESS

Like it or not, looks count. No matter what your usual mode of dress, you should dress conservatively and professionally for your interviews. For men, this means a suit, or a blazer and nice slacks (and, of course, a tie); for women, a suit, blazer and skirt or dress slacks, or a business-style dress is appropriate. Regardless of your gender, keep an eye to detail; even the most beautiful suit looks shabby if your shoes are scuffed and worn, and the effect of a great-looking blazer is ruined by a ragged backpack. Polish your shoes, invest in a nice portfolio or case for your papers, and by all means, iron your clothes. If you are generally somewhat less than conservative in your dress, you may want to tone it down: men, replace the big hoop earring with a stud; women, take off the gold glitter polish and paint on clear. After all, you don't want to be asked, as one of the respondents to our survey was, "Why are you dressed the way you are? Why did you come here looking the way you do?"

CONDUCT YOURSELF PROFESSIONALLY

Admissions committees can see from your application that you are smart, accomplished, and highly regarded by your professors. The interview is an opportunity for them to gauge things that are not so easily conveyed on paper. Medical schools are looking for students with maturity, empathy, and superior interpersonal skills. All of these things come through in the interview. In a group setting, where the committee talks with more than one candidate at a time, you will be observed not only when you answer a question, but also when your fellow applicants are speaking. Keep alert, and show interest. After all, you never know what you may learn that you can use in your next interview.

HOW AND WHEN TO FOLLOW UP ON YOUR INTERVIEWS

First, don't forget to send a thank you note after each set of interviews. You can write several different notes to each of your interviewers, or send just one addressed generally to the interview committee. Don't write a novella in your thank you note. It's fine to mention a particular question or topic you found interesting during your interview, but you should confine yourself to only a few lines. As you might have guessed, it's a good idea to take a few brief notes, such as the interviewer's names and some of the topics they covered, right after you leave the interview. For the thank you notes themselves, you can use any nice stationary paper.

If the school is not entirely certain of the strength of your application relative to other candidates after your interviews, you may be placed on a "hold" list. Don't despair. You made it as far as the interview process, which (except in the case of some public schools who interview every candidate) means that you have survived some of the initial cuts. Being placed on hold after your interview means that your candidacy is strong, but not so compelling that the school is ready to accept you without seeing what the rest of the applicant pool looks like. You can, however, send supplementary information to further support your application. For example, if you have been doing research, volunteer work, or taking classes that didn't appear on your initial application, and if you didn't get a chance to talk about your new activities during the interview, you can write a short—less than one page—letter outlining your recent accomplishments and send it to the school. This shows that you are still working hard to better your chances of acceptance into medical school.

WHAT ARE THEY GOING TO ASK?

Over the past several years, The Princeton Review has surveyed current medical students about their schools and the medical school application process. The sample interview questions in this section come from those surveys. Although the following list of questions is by no means exhaustive, it is a good sampling of questions that were asked in real interviews in the recent past. When we first decided to ask current med students what they were asked in their interviews, we had no idea how strange—and it some cases disturbing—some of their responses were going to be. Get ready, because, while some of the questions are pretty standard, others are truly bizarre.

So You Want to Be a Doctor?

Some of the students we surveyed were unprepared for questions like those that follow, thinking them so mundane that they wouldn't be asked. From our research, however, we can say with confidence that if you're granted even one interview, you're almost sure to be asked several questions about your motivation and suitability for medical school.

- *Why do you want to be a doctor?*
- *The future of medicine looks bleak. Why do you want to go into it?*

- *What articles have you read recently that relate to the reasons you want to become a doctor?*

- *What do you see yourself doing with a medical degree?*

- *Were you influenced by relatives to pursue a career in medicine?*

- *How do you know you want to be a doctor if your parents aren't doctors?*

- *How will you be a better doctor than your [family member]?*

- *Why do you want to attend [name of school]?*

- *Why should we accept you?*

- *How are your accomplishments better than those of the other candidates in this interview?*

- *Evaluate yourself based on the required evaluation of the interviewer.*

- *Why on earth did they give you an interview?*

- *Do you think you are motivated enough for medical school?*

- *Would you give up a body part to gain entrance to medical school?*

- *When you don't get into medical school, what will you do?*

- *What would you do if Saddam Hussein took over our country and wouldn't allow women in medical school?*

- *What career path would you follow if all the medical schools closed today?*

- *You've taken an odd, nontraditional path to get here. Why are you interested in medicine?*

- *What disadvantages do you see in being an older student?*

- *Can you afford to come here?*

- *How will you finance your medical education?*

- *Describe what you believe to be the financial rewards of medicine.*

- *If doctors were paid as much as teachers, would you still want to be a doctor?*

- *Come on, don't you see yourself driving a Mercedes convertible in ten years?*

- *Doctors have the power to give or take life. How do you feel about "playing God"?*

- *Why didn't you become a veterinarian?*

TELL ME A LITTLE BIT ABOUT YOURSELF . . .

Selection committees use the interview as an opportunity to find out what makes you tick. Prepare yourself for personal questions about your character traits, your coping mechanisms, and your life experiences. You may also be asked to comment on your interpersonal relationships. Always be honest.

- *What is your worst quality?*

- *If you could change anything about yourself, what would it be?*

- *Are you aggressive?*

- *What makes you a fun person?*

- *Do you have a good sense of humor? Tell me the funniest joke you ever heard.*

- *What makes you angry?*

- *What makes you sad?*

- *What scares you?*

- *Do you like sick people?*

- *Are you afraid of death?*

- *What are you ashamed of?*

- *What are you the most proud of?*

- *One of the people who wrote a letter of recommendation for you described you as [adjective]. Do you agree with that description?*

- *Was there a time in your life when you had tremendous responsibility?*

- *What is the wackiest thing you've ever done?*

- *What was the biggest mistake you ever made?*

- *What is the worst thing that has happened to you in the past four years?*

- *Tell me something you wanted to achieve but did not, or something you've failed at. How did you cope with failure?*

- *What role has stress played in your life?*

- *How could you prove to me that you can perform well under stress?*

- *What do you do to alleviate stress?*

- *What support structure do you have in [town in which school is located]?*

- *Tell me about your family.*

- *Tell me about your mom.*

- *What does your father do for a living?*

- *What does your brother do for a living?*

- *What role do you play in your family dynamic?*

- *How is your relationship with your parents?*

- *What is the physical health of your parents, and how would you handle an illness of theirs while attending school?*

- *Who is the person in the world to whom you are closest?*

- *Describe your best friend.*

- *What does your closest friend think about your relationship with him or her?*

- *Give one word that a friend would use to describe you.*

IT'S ALL ACADEMIC

Grades, MCAT scores, and courses are fair game for the inquisitive interviewer. You may be asked to explain your performance in a course or to tell what you learned. A hint: To be better prepared for questions of this type, get a copy of your transcript and take a look at it. Look for things that might cause an interviewer to ask a question. Lower than normal grades stick out, as do courses with funny names (like Rocks for Jocks). Then, again, only be honest.

- *What do you think of the GPA as a valid method of categorizing students?*
- *Why were your first-year grades so bad?*
- *Why do you have so many C grades on your transcript?*
- *Explain your low math grade.*
- *Why are your grades high compared to your MCAT scores?*
- *Do you realize that your MCAT scores aren't anything special?*
- *Tell me about your research.*
- *Have you taken any humanities classes, and what papers did you write in them?*
- *What did you learn in [name of course]? (It's worth noting that some people were asked about normal courses like "Philosophy 101" and others were asked about bizarre courses like "The Art of Murder," "Fairy Tales," and "Play, Games, Toys, and Sports.")*
- *Who was the author of your biochemistry textbook?*

EXTRA, EXTRA, READ ALL ABOUT IT!

Whatever your extracurricular activities and work experiences, you will most likely be asked how they relate to your commitment to and preparedness for studying medicine. Think about your extra-curricular experiences and what you learned about yourself, the medical field, and/or working with people as a result of participating in these activities. If you've been out of school for a while and have worked extensively in another field, be ready for questions about why you decided to change fields. Scientific or medical research experience is a plus, but can be a real liability if you're not able to discuss it in detail.

- *What are your hobbies?*
- *How does your hobby relate to being a doctor?*
- *Have you taught yourself to do anything, and if so, what?*
- *How has working as a [name of job] made you a better candidate for medical school?*
- *What volunteer work contributed to your commitment to become a doctor?*
- *What did you do with your job earnings?*

MEDICAL ISSUES AND ETHICS: WHERE DO YOU STAND?

Interviewers love to ask students about a medical issue or about an ethical dilemma related to medicine. In general, there is no wrong answer to these questions. You should know the terminology (for example, what is the difference between euthanasia and euthenics?), and be aware of some pros and cons for each of these issues. Since the health care crisis and attendant problems in reforming the health care delivery system have been grabbing headlines, you should be prepared to discuss the issues intelligently. No one expects you to be an expert on this or any other issue, but you should do some research before your interviews. Don't be surprised if an interviewer challenges your view on an issue; usually, he is trying to see how well you support your argument.

- *What is the greatest problem facing medicine today?*
- *What do you consider the most important thing medicine has done for mankind?*
- *What do you think will be the most significant scientific breakthrough in the next ten years?*
- *If you could find a cure for AIDS or for cancer, which would you choose and why?*
- *If you were Surgeon General, what is the first thing you would do?*
- *If you were the Health Commissioner of [a large city], what would you do?*
- *What is preventive medicine?*
- *What is the biggest problem family practitioners face?*
- *What are your views on euthanasia?*
- *What do you think about euthenics (not euthanasia)?*
- *What would you do about the alcoholism problem in this country?*
- *What do you think about condoms being distributed in high schools?*
- *What are your views on mandatory HIV testing for doctors and patients?*
- *Current AIDS education programs aren't working; what should we do?*
- *Why will organ rationing be the problem of the future in medicine?*
- *If brain transplants were possible, what would be your opinion of them?*
- *Should people have the right to sell their own organs?*
- *Do you think it's ethical to take the life of a fetus for a cell line to save the life of a sibling with cancer?*
- *Should we spend so much time and effort trying to keep premature infants alive?*
- *Should retarded people be sterilized without their consent?*
- *If a cure were invented for aging, what repercussions would it have on society in general and the medical profession in particular?*
- *How do you feel about animal research?*
- *What is the proper treatment of laboratory rats?*
- *What role should politics play in medicine?*
- *Is health care a right or a privilege?*
- *What is your opinion of socialized medicine?*
- *How would you organize health care in an ideal world?*
- *Discuss the health care system of Australia.*
- *What do you think should be done about patients who can't pay for treatment?*
- *What is the difference between Medicare and Medicaid?*
- *What is your opinion of HMOs and PPOs?*
- *How will you react to the death of your first patient?*

- *Who would you go to if your mom needed surgery: a surgeon with good hands and a bland personality or a surgeon with not as good hands with a great personality?*

- *If your father was dying of cancer and you were an attending resident, how would you break the news?*

- *How would you tell your best friend's wife (who is your patient) that she has cancer? What would you do if she then refused to tell her family?*

- *Pretend to tell me a loved one of mine has died.*

- *You have to amputate one of the legs of an eight-year-old child. How would you tell him?*

- *Would you give a transfusion to a child whose parents were Jehovah's Witnesses?*

- *If a Hindu, for example, comes in and refuses surgery on the basis of religion, and the surgery is his only hope, what would you do? Also, what if the patient is this man's child?*

- *Would you refer a terminal patient to a "suicide doctor"?*

- *If you diagnosed a patient with a terminal illness as having only two months to live and the family and the patient wanted to end the turmoil ("pull the plug"), would you allow it or strongly disagree?*

- *What would you do if you saw a bleeding child on the side of the road?*

- *What would you do if you had a female patient who was trying to conceive, and your colleague had that patient's husband, and the husband was HIV positive?*

- *If one of your colleagues refused to treat a patient with AIDS, how would you address that colleague?*

- *How would you react if a fellow medical student had AIDS and entered surgery with you?*

- *Would you perform a hair transplant on an AIDS patient?*

- *Would you let a surgeon with AIDS operate on you?*

- *Would you treat a white supremacist, and should physicians be forced to treat such a patient?*

- *If you made a mistake as a physician, how would you handle it?*

TO CHOOSE, OR NOT TO CHOOSE

Abortion is not only a hot political topic, it also seems to be a hot topic for interviews. Some schools are affiliated with hospitals where abortions are performed; some are not. Don't try to guess if the interviewer is hoping you will espouse a particular position; honesty seems the best policy on this issue. If you are asked about your willingness to perform an abortion (as a large number of those we surveyed were), you may want to mention that it is not only your conscience but also the rules of the hospital or laws of the land that you must consider.

- *What should a physician's role be in the politics of abortion?*

- *What are your views on abortion?*

- *What would you do as a physician if you were asked to do something contrary to your stand on abortion?*

- *Would you perform an abortion for a teenager, and would you tell her parents?*

- *How do you justify being a Catholic and going to an institution that allows abortion?*

- *If you wouldn't perform an abortion because of your religious beliefs, but you would refer a patient to another physician who would perform an abortion, are you not just as guilty in God's eyes?*

HAVE YOU HEARD THE NEWS?

Good doctors are aware of, and involved in, the world around them. You may be asked about current events, even things completely unrelated to medicine. The questions that follow are only examples; in most cases, these events are no longer current. To prepare for questions like these, keep up with what's happening. If you get most of your news from the TV or radio, start reading newspapers and news magazines for more in-depth coverage.

- *Who is the U.S. Secretary of State?*

- *What do you think about the current situation in Bosnia?*

- *What do you think about the current social climate in Mozambique?*

- *What do you think about the political situation in Iraq and surrounding countries?*

- *What is your opinion on the confirmation hearings of Clarence Thomas?*

- *Why did Margaret Thatcher resign?*

- *Do you think the Israelis beat up on the Palestinians?*

PHILOSOPHY 101

From the serious to the silly, questions interviewers ask can make you stop and think. (And, for some of these questions, one of the things you might think is, "What does this have to do with med school?")

- *What are the top five priorities of society?*

- *What is your purpose for living?*

- *How do you resolve the apparent dichotomy between the cruelty and suffering in the world and your belief in a loving God?*

- *Do you see any parallels between medicine and the priesthood?*

- *Do you feel Catholics are morally superior?*

- *What is Zen Buddhism?*

- *Explain Hinduism.*

- *Are you a racist?*

- *Do you have trouble working with black people?*

- *Do you believe that racism still exists?*

- *How do you feel about affirmative action?*

- *Would you move to Canada to avoid serving active duty during a military conflict abroad?*

- *What is your view on censorship in the arts?*

- *What would you do if you saw a classmate cheating on a test?*

- *Do you believe in drug legalization?*

- *Do you believe that volunteerism could help eliminate greed from society's social structure?*

- *Is altruism ever pure, without some kind of motive?*
- *Do you believe in life after death?*
- *What is your opinion about natural law ethics?*
- *Explain the mind-body problem.*
- *Are you a vertical or horizontal thinker?*
- *If you could be any cell in the human body, what would you be?*
- *If you were to build a human being, what would you include and exclude?*
- *Define hope.*

TRIED AND TRUE

Some questions sound more like pickup lines than med school interview questions. Although none of those surveyed was asked, "What's your sign?" there were plenty of old favorites that you may as well be prepared for.

- *Are you a person who thinks a glass is half empty or half full?*
- *If you could go back in history and meet anyone, who would it be and why?*
- *If you could talk to someone from the future, what would you ask him?*
- *If a genie were able to grant you three wishes, what would they be?*
- *If you were stranded on a desert island, what five books would you want?*
- *If your house was burning down, and you could save only one thing, what would it be?*
- *If you could be any vegetable, what would you be?*
- *If you could be any kind of fruit, what would you be?*
- *If you could be any kind of animal, what would you be?*
- *If you could be any inanimate object, what would you be?*
- *If you could be any cartoon character, who would it be?*
- *What is your favorite color?*
- *What was the last book you read, and how did it influence your life?*
- *What was the last good movie you saw?*
- *Tell me what you see when you look in the mirror.*
- *What was the most embarrassing moment in your life?*
- *Who is your hero?*
- *If you could invite three role models to dinner, who would they be and why, and what would you serve them?*
- *When you die, what would you like your tombstone to read?*

I'LL TAKE POTPOURRI FOR $500, ALEX

The students we surveyed were asked some trivia worthy of "Final Jeopardy." The bad news is that, because of the very nature of these questions, you can't prepare for them. The good news is that a simple "I don't know" seemed to satisfy the interviewers. For bonus points, ask for the answer, or, as one student did, tell them you'll check and get back to them. He did and, subsequently, he got in.

- *What is the largest lobbyist group in the U.S.?*
- *Which state first had women's suffrage?*
- *What language did Abraham (of the Bible) speak?*
- *When did Iraq become an independent nation?*
- *How many numbers that contain 9 are there between 1 and 100?*
- *What is the capital of Vietnam?*
- *When and how was Pakistan formed?*
- *Who won the 1969 World Series?*
- *Name a seven-letter word with three u's in it.*
- *What is the difference between European and American eighteenth-century poetry?*
- *Why was the Civil War fought?*
- *What is the origin of the name "Cincinnati"?*
- *What do the e's in e.e. cummings' name stand for?*
- *When and why was the March of Dimes founded?*
- *When did Istanbul become Istanbul?*
- *Name the four non-Arabic-speaking countries in the Middle East.*
- *What was Thomas Aquinas famous for?*
- *Who was the architect who built the Great Wall of China?*
- *Where was Millard Filmore born?*
- *Give a brief history of the Jesuit order.*
- *Define the Apollonian and the Dionysian as they figure in the philosophy of Nietzsche.*
- *Who was the head of NATO during World War II?*
- *What size tippets do you use on your fly lines with a 14X fly?*

A Corollary: I'll Take Science & Medicine for $1,000, Alex

A few interviewees were asked trivia questions that actually related to science and medicine. For the most part, they knew the answers. When they didn't, and the question was obscure, it didn't seem to hurt their chances of getting in. Your undergraduate coursework and MCAT review should be preparation enough for a lot of these questions.

- *What was the first industrialized country to practice socialized medicine? The second?*
- *How much does the U.S. spend each year on medical care?*
- *How does a lightbulb work?*
- *What would be the physiological effects of performing the high jump in Mexico City?*
- *Why don't fish die in winter?*

- *Why does ice float on the top of water?*
- *How do you make a protein?*
- *So, what is Alzheimer's disease anyway?*
- *Where is your hamstring region?*
- *Tell me what you know about DNA.*
- *What is the Grignard Reaction?*
- *What is Poisson's equation?*
- *Describe protein structure.*
- *What is PKU?*

ANITA WHO?

Despite the media attention focused on the issues of gender discrimination and sexual harassment, medical school interviewers are still asking questions that, if they were asked in a job interview, would be deemed inappropriate or illegal. These kinds of questions are more common than you would expect. The students who told us they'd been asked these questions (and there were lots of them, mostly female) expressed emotions from confusion to outrage. Still, most admitted to being intimidated that they would be rejected if they did anything but reply calmly, and therefore they answered honestly and without additional comment. How you handle a question like this is up to you. At this point, you too might feel that there is too much at stake to make waves, but, on the other hand, it is certainly within your rights to ask how the question is relevant or even to politely decline to answer.

- *How did you get such a high score in math? I've never seen such a high score from a woman!*
- *Do you know that you have extraordinarily good looks?*
- *Why is a pretty young girl like you wasting her time and money applying to med school?*
- *Why do you want to be a doctor rather than a nurse?*
- *Will you faint if I take you into surgery?*
- *Would you feel uncomfortable being alone with a male patient?*
- *How did taking a nude art class make you feel?*
- *What would your ideal date be?*
- *Do you find it hard to find educated black men to date?*
- *What was the strangest sexual position you have ever employed?*
- *Who do you think is the best model in this year's* Sports Illustrated *swimsuit issue?*
- *How frequently do you masturbate?*
- *Are you gay?*
- *Why don't you like men?*
- *Do you have a boyfriend?*
- *How does your boyfriend feel about your going to medical school?*
- *Would having a boyfriend affect your decision in choosing a medical school and career?*

- *Are you prepared to handle possibly losing your boyfriend over the stress and distance?*

- *Are you married?*

- *What kind of person would you like to marry?*

- *Do you plan to marry while in medical school?*

- *Why aren't you married?*

- *How will you deal with being married while in medical school?*

- *What does your husband do?*

- *Why did you get divorced?*

- *Do you plan to remarry?*

- *Do you expect to have a family? If so, why are you applying to medical school?*

- *If you become pregnant, what will you do?*

- *Have you ever gotten a girl pregnant?*

- *How do you plan to manage a family and a career? After all, you are a woman.*

- *How would you raise your children if you were a doctor?*

- *What would you do if you were sexually harassed at any time during school, residency, or your career?*

- *Are you prepared for the sexual discrimination you are most likely to face as a student, resident, intern, and so on?*

EXPECT THE UNEXPECTED

Although most of the questions fall into one of the previous categories, some of the questions are just plain off the wall. Some of the following questions were logical from the perspective of the candidates' background, so be prepared to answer questions about the leisure activities you listed on your application or the experiences you related in your essays. Other questions came straight out of left field. These are unlikely to be repeated, but they give you an idea of the kind of things interviewers ask to catch you off balance. If you're asked a question like this, take your time and think it through. If all else fails, remember, it's better to say "I don't know" than to try to "baffle 'em with bull." As one of those surveyed said after an unsuccessful attempt at bluffing, "It doesn't work—they've heard it all before."

- *Why didn't you bring me a doughnut?*

- *What would you do if I dropped unconscious right now?*

- *What would you do if you ran me [the interviewer] over as you left the campus?*

- *What would you say if you smashed your finger with a hammer?*

- *How tall are you?*

- *How did you get your hair to do that?*

- *Is that your natural hair color?*

- *What bar or dance club did you get that hand stamp from?*

- *Where did you buy your suit?*
- *Why are you dressed the way you are? Why did you come here looking the way you do?*
- *What's that stain on your sleeve?*
- *Can you sing the blues?*
- *Do you think that anyone can become a singer?*
- *Do you know how to play an instrument?*
- *How do you play your guitar and harmonica at the same time?*
- *Who is your favorite classical music composer?*
- *What's your favorite Beatles album?*
- *Do you like Axl Rose?*
- *What is your favorite college football team?*
- *What do you think the chances are that the [team name] will make the playoffs?*
- *Why are the majority of NBA players black?*
- *How much can you bench press?*
- *If you're accepted, will you play on our softball team?*
- *What was your opinion of the rich, yuppie Greek students on your undergraduate campus?*
- *How much do you drink?*
- *Have you ever cheated?*
- *Have you ever tried an illegal substance?*
- *Have you ever stolen a car?*
- *What kind of car do you drive?*
- *What is your opinion of Charlie Brown?*
- *Do you prefer the old Star Trek or the new one?*
- *Why didn't you take Latin?*
- *Do you dream in Chinese or English?*
- *Do you know how to surf?*
- *Are you most like Madonna, Margaret Thatcher, or Mother Theresa, and why?*
- *What is your favorite card game?*
- *Do you play bingo?*
- *Does your mother know where you are?*

6 Allopathic Profiles

United States Medical School Profiles

UNIVERSITY OF ALABAMA

SCHOOL OF MEDICINE

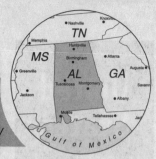

Office of Medical Student Services, VH100, Birmingham, AL 35294

Admission: 205-934-2433 • Fax: 205-934-8724

Email: admissions@uasom.meis.uab.edu • Internet: www.uab.edu/uasom/

The University of Alabama School of Medicine is a state-sponsored institution, structured to serve the needs of the entire state. It uses three campuses—one in Birmingham, one in Tuscaloosa, and one in Huntsville. Students study basic sciences at the Birmingham campus, where they benefit from affiliated schools of Dentistry, Medicine, Nursing, Optometry, Health-Related Professions, and Public Health. The proximity of these schools to the School of Medicine facilitates a comprehensive approach to medical training. The University of Alabama emphasizes patient care and trains medical students in the physical, behavioral, and social aspects of health care. Clinical rotations take place at all three campuses, allowing students to work with a diverse patient population. The Medical School promotes primary care, community involvement, and overseas experience.

Academics

Basic sciences are taught during the first two years, primarily through lectures and small group case studies. Clinical techniques are introduced early and are often taught in small groups. The curriculum is particularly rich in relevant Humanities and Social Science courses such as Ethics and Behavioral Sciences. Joint M.S./M.D. degrees are offered in many fields, notably the Masters in Public Health/M.D. combination. About 8 students a year are accepted into joint M.D./Ph.D. programs, usually as M.S.T.P. candidates. A combined undergraduate/medical school program is offered at the University of Alabama at Birmingham to which high school seniors who are Alabama residents may apply.

BASIC SCIENCES: The academic year is organized into quarters. During the fall quarter of the first year, students take the following: Biochemistry, Biostatistics, Gross Anatomy, Medical Ethics, and Behavioral Sciences. Winter quarter includes the following: Cell and Tissue Biology and Medical Physiology. Spring curriculum is Pharmacology, Neuroscience, and Nutrition. Throughout the first year, students participate in a course called Introduction to Clinical Medicine, which covers the patient interview and addresses doctor/patient interaction. During the fall of year two, Pharmacology continues and Microbiology is introduced. Pathology is a year-long course, taken throughout year two. Clinical Medicine continues in year two, focusing on physical diagnosis. The Lister Hill Library at the Birmingham campus houses 240,000 volumes and uses computer online search services. Pre-clinical performance is evaluated on an A–F scale. The USMLE Step 1 is required following completion of pre-clinical studies.

CLINICAL TRAINING: Clinical training begins well before the required clerkships of the third year. In addition to the introductory clinical course work of the first two years, some students are involved in community programs, which provide patient exposure to public health programs, such as the AIDS Care Team and other projects aimed at young or homeless populations. The final two years are essentially combined, with required clerkships filling all of the third year and part of the fourth year. Students choose a primary campus for clerkships a few students will ultimately rotate to all three campuses. Each campus has unique strengths. Required clerkships are Medicine; Surgery; Pediatrics; Ob/Gyn; Family Medicine; Rural Medicine; Neurology; and Psychiatry. Each campus is affiliated with several teaching hospitals, and rotations take students to a variety of learning environments ranging from large Veterans Affairs Hospitals to small, rural clinics. For required rotations, grading is A–F and for electives, Pass/Fail. The School of Medicine established a Medical Student Enrichment Program in 1995, which encourages and facilitates overseas clinical experience. In addition to providing elective opportunities to medical school seniors, medical students may apply to the program for placements during the summer between their first and second years. In 1996, 14 out of 22 applicants were accepted into the program, which took them to Russia, Guatemala, Jamaica, and South and West Africa. The USMLE Step 2 is required for graduation.

Students

One-seventh of the members of a typical class are considered out-of-state residents, but a much greater percentage of the student body went to college out of state. About 75 percent of matriculates majored in a scientific field during their undergraduate studies. Generally, 10–15 percent of the students are underrepresented minorities, mostly African and Native Americans. There is a wide age range among students. Class size is 160.

STUDENT LIFE: Outside of class, students are often involved in recreational and volunteer activities. Some are active in student organizations, such as national medical groups. The Student Government Association consists of elected members of each class. The Birmingham campus with its many departments provides a community beyond that of medical students alone. Most students choose to live off campus, where housing is ample and relatively affordable. Most students have cars.

GRADUATES: Family practice and internal medicine are particularly popular fields among graduates. Although graduates are competitive for residencies nationwide, a significant number enter residency programs in Alabama, at University-affiliated hospitals or other locations in the state.

Admissions

REQUIREMENTS: Undergraduate requirements are Biology or Zoology (8 semester hours); Chemistry with lab (8 semester hours); Organic Chemistry with lab (8 semester hours); Physics with lab (8 semester hours); Math (6 semester hours); and English (6 semester hours). Academic work accomplished overseas may be acceptable, depending on the institution and the course. The MCAT is required, and it must not be more than two years old at the time of application. If taken more than once, the school uses the most recent MCAT scores. The AMCAS application is required.

SUGGESTIONS: The Admissions Committee values experience with patient care and exposure to health care environments. The University of Alabama School of Medicine welcomes nontraditional applicants and has admitted several students who are older than 40. Due to the state-mandated preference for Alabama residents, out-of-state applicants are required to have an overall GPA of 3.5 or higher and MCAT scores of 30 or higher.

PROCESS: All Alabama residents receive a secondary application. Generally, about 70 percent of this group are interviewed. About 12–14 percent of out-of-state applicants are interviewed. Of those out-of-state applicants interviewed, about 42 percent are accepted and 5 percent are wait-listed. Notification begins in October, and the class is generally filled by April. Interviews consist of three, 30-minute sessions with faculty members.

Costs

The University estimates that a student's yearly expenditures will be about $15,000. This includes more than $2,000 for transportation, suggesting that students will need to own a car. Tuition is not included in this figure, but is relatively low, at around $10,409 per year in-state including all fees.

FINANCIAL AID: The financial aid policies of the Medical School at The University of Alabama differ from those of most medical schools in that factors beyond financial need are considered in determining awards. Most scholarships are based primarily on merit (60%), although financial need is also considered (40%). After scholarships are granted, students are expected to borrow up to $18,500 per year in a combination of subsidized and unsubsidized loans.

UNIVERSITY OF ALABAMA

STUDENT BODY

Type	Public
*Enrollment	691
*% male/female	61/39
*% underrepresented minorities	11
# applied (total/out)	1,530/1,083
% interviewed (total/out)	70/14
% accepted (total/out)	NR/NR
% enrolled (total/out)	31/12

ADMISSIONS

Average GPA and MCAT Scores

Overall GPA	3.59	Science GPA	3.62
MCAT Bio	10.2	MCAT Phys	9.8
MCAT Verbal	9.8	MCAT Essay	NR

Score Release Policy

The school has not responded to our inquiry regarding withheld MCAT scores. Therefore, we advise caution. Contact the Admissions Office before witholding any scores.

Application Information

Regular application	11/1
Regular notification	10/15 until filled
Early application	6/1–8/1
Early notification	10/1
Admissions may be deferred?	Yes
AMCAS application accepted?	Yes
Interview required?	Yes
Application fee	$65

COSTS AND AID

Tuition & Fees

Tuition (in/out)	$7,069/$21,207
Cost of books	NR
Fees	$3,340

Financial Aid

% students receiving aid	76
Average grant	NR
Average loan	NR
Average debt	$67,268

*Figures based on total enrollment

ALBANY MEDICAL COLLEGE

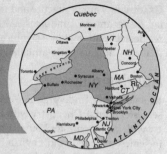

Office of Admissions, 47 New Scotland Avenue, Mail Code 3
Albany, NY 12208
Admission: 518-262-5525 • Fax: 518-262-5887
Internet: www.amc.edu

Albany Medical College has responded to the nationwide increase in managed care, and resulting demand for primary care providers, with an educational program that trains outstanding generalist and well-rounded specialist physicians. The curriculum teaches students to practice in a complex, cost-cutting environment while maintaining patient needs as the foremost concern. Albany is a private school, credited with training nearly 40 percent of the region's physicians. It is located in the capital of New York State, an active, comfortable, and student-friendly city. The nearby Catskill and Adirondack Mountains provide year-round recreational activities and New York City, Boston, and Montreal are just a few hours away by car or train.

Academics

Albany Medical College responded to the changing health care needs in the United States by restructuring its curriculum in 1993 to better address contemporary issues in health care, while simultaneously providing a solid clinical and scientific education. The curriculum focuses specifically on the principles and practices of comprehensive care—health care that addresses the full spectrum of patient needs from medical and preventive to palliative and psychosocial. Grades of honors, excellent, good, marginal, and unsatisfactory are used to evaluate student performance. In the clinical years narrative assessments of performance are also used as an important evaluation tool. Graduation requirements include recording a score on the USMLE Step 1 and Step 2 and passing a clinical skills exam.

BASIC SCIENCE: Basic science education is coordinated and integrated in a manner that spans all four years of medical school, systematically increasing basic science knowledge within the context of clinical medicine. By teaching within a clinical context, the college offers a learning environment that focuses on developing problem-solving skills. Basic science concepts are divided into themes or modules that are most often organ based. Taught in conjunction with clinical case experience, these modules come together to form the foundation for the clinical education. In the first year students combine basic science instruction with clinical cases to focus on normal function. In the second year students further expand their knowledge and focus primarily on abnormal function and the disease state. Students learn clinical skills beginning in their first year by working within small groups and interacting with patients. Standardized patients who are trained to simulate evaluation purposes. Students explore legal, ethical, and humanistic concerns in a four-year module called Health Care and Society. Systems of health care, epidemiology, biostatistics, and evidence-based medicine are concurrently studied in a four-year module called comprehensive Care Case Study. Fundamental knowledge of nutrition also begins in year one and is integrated in all

four years of the curriculum. Managing information is a key component throughout all thematic modules. The Schaffer Library of Health Sciences houses more than 127,000 volumes and 1,000 journals, contains 3,000 multimedia programs and has 25 new computer stations in the independent learning center. Throughout their medical education, students rely on these resources as well as the support of the library faculty.

CLINICAL TRAINING: An innovative experience, Orientation Clerkship, transitions students from the first two years of the curriculum to the clinical and rotation requirements of the final two years. This two-week clerkship occurs during the summer prior to year three. These learning opportunities on standardized patients enable medical students to develop, practice, and enhance their clinical skills and abilities. Students participate in mock preceptor rounds, assess their own clinical skills and perform basic medical procedures. The third year required clinical clerkships are in the process of changing from hospital-based experiences to hospital- and ambulatory-based experiences. The third-year required clerkships are Medicine (includes Radiology, 12 weeks); Surgery (8 weeks); Ob/Gyn (6 weeks); Pediatrics (8 weeks); Family Practice (6 weeks); and Psychiatry (6 weeks).

Fourth-year rotation requirements are Surgery (4 weeks); Emergency Medicine (4 weeks); Neuro/Opthomology (4 weeks); Critical Care (4 weeks); and an elective in either Family Practice, Medicine, or Pediatrics (4 weeks). Required rotations take place primarily at Albany Medical Center Hospital as well as regional and local community hospitals, community health centers, psychiatric inpatient units, nursing homes, adult homes, and in patients' homes. The remainder of fourth year includes electives chosen by the students.

Students

Of students in the 1998 entering class, 9 percent were underrepresented minorities. Geographic representation was as follows: Northeast (65%); South (6%); Midwest (3%); West (24%); foreign countries (1%). There is usually a wide range of ages within the student body. Class size is 124.

Student Life: The student community is very active both on and off campus. There are about thirty campus clubs and organizations, including a student newspaper, outdoor and athletic clubs, support groups for students with similar backgrounds or situations, and groups focused on community activities. For example, one student organization arranges activities for the Medical Center's pediatric cancer patients, while another brings AIDS education programs to local schools. Residence halls in the vicinity of the School are available for single students. Off-campus housing is generally comfortable and affordable.

Graduates: Typically, more than half of a graduating class enters training programs in primary care. Eighty-nine percent of the 1999 graduating class secured one of their top three choices in the National Residency Match Program.

Admissions

Requirements: Requirements are six semester hours each of Biology, Chemistry, Organic Chemistry, and Physics. All courses should include associated labs. When assessing GPAs, the Admissions Committee considers the intensity of each student's course load as well as his or her undergraduate institution. The MCAT is required of all applicants. For those who have retaken the exam, the best set of scores is used, though all scores should be submitted.

Suggestions: Community service and medical-related activities are valued. College courses should be varied, and demonstrate breadth and depth. There is no preference for New York State residents.

Process: All AMCAS applicants are sent secondary applications. About 15 percent of those completing secondaries are interviewed, although some applicants are put in a hold category and interviewed later in the year. Interviews take place from September through April, and consist of two sessions with faculty, students, administrators, or local physicians. The interview day also features a group orientation and the opportunity to meet with deans, faculty, and students. Candidates are notified on a rolling basis, and are either accepted, rejected, or wait-listed. About 35 percent of interviewees are accepted. Albany Medical College offers combined degree programs with Sienna College, Union College, and Rensselaer Polytechnic Institute. Interested students should apply during their senior year in high school. The MCAT is waived for students admitted through these joint programs. Students admitted to the programs earn both degrees in seven or eight years depending on the undergraduate institution.

Costs

The expected yearly budget for a single student is about $10,642. This allows for either on- or off-campus housing and car ownership for a first-year student.

Financial Aid: The FAFSA and institutional forms are used to determine financial need. Most financial aid is need-based and consists of grants and loans. Some merit scholarships are also available.

ALBANY MEDICAL COLLEGE

STUDENT BODY

Type	Private
*Enrollment	517
*% male/female	49/51
*% underrepresented minorities	5
# applied (total/out)	7,859/6,004
% interviewed (total/out)	8/7
% accepted (total/out)	3/67
% enrolled (total/out)	33/68
Average age	24

ADMISSIONS

Average GPA and MCAT Scores

Overall GPA	3.40	Science GPA	3.30
MCAT Bio	10.48	MCAT Phys	10.00
MCAT Verbal	10.09	MCAT Essay	P

Application Information

Regular application	11/15
Regular notification	10/15 until filled
Transfers accepted?	No
Admissions may be deferred?	Yes
AMCAS application accepted?	Yes
Interview required?	Yes
Application fee	$75

COSTS AND AID

Tuition & Fees

Tuition	$30,797
Cost of books	$1,168
Fees	$0

Financial Aid

% students receiving aid	84
Average grant	$1,000
Average loan	$40,224
Average debt	$100,175

*Figures based on total enrollment

ALBERT EINSTEIN COLLEGE OF MEDICINE
OF YESHIVA UNIVERSITY

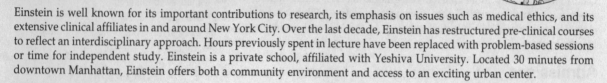

1300 Morris Park Avenue, Bronx, NY 10461
Admission: 718-430-2106 • Fax: 718-430-8825
Email: admissions@aecom.yu.edu • Internet: www.aecom.yu.edu

Einstein is well known for its important contributions to research, its emphasis on issues such as medical ethics, and its extensive clinical affiliates in and around New York City. Over the last decade, Einstein has restructured pre-clinical courses to reflect an interdisciplinary approach. Hours previously spent in lecture have been replaced with problem-based sessions or time for independent study. Einstein is a private school, affiliated with Yeshiva University. Located 30 minutes from downtown Manhattan, Einstein offers both a community environment and access to an exciting urban center.

Academics

In addition to the requirements described below, all students conduct research projects through the Independent Scholars Program. Such research often leads to publication or to distinction at the time of graduation. Projects involve a faculty mentor, and can be in traditional or nontraditional medical science fields. Students may apply for joint Ph.D./M.D. programs at the time of initial application or while enrolled in the M.D. program. Those accepted into this program receive stipends, either through the M.S.T.P. program or from institutional sources. The Ph.D. may be earned in the following fields: Anatomy, Biochemistry, Biophysics, Cell Biology, Genetics, Immunology, Microbiology, Molecular Biology, Neuroscience, Pathology, Pharmacology, and Physiology. Evaluation of student performance uses Honors, Pass, and Fail. Passing the USMLE Steps 1 and 2 are requirements for graduation.

BASIC SCIENCES: Throughout the first and second years, Introduction to Clinical Medicine complements the basic science curriculum by addressing practical and personal issues related to the patient interview and examination. About forty entering students participate in a Generalist Mentorship program, which involves shadowing a primary care physician. First-year courses, taught primarily with lectures and labs, are: Histology, Anatomy, Cardiovascular Physiology, Principles of Pharmacology, and Disease Mechanisms. The course Molecular and Cellular Foundations of Medicine uses both lectures and small group sessions. During the second part of year one, and throughout all of year two, instruction is organ-based, is carried out in small groups, and uses a case-based approach. Courses are Renal Physiology and PathoBiology; Nervous System and Behavior; Endocrine System; Reproductive System and Human Sexuality; Cardiovascular System; Respiratory System; Gastrointestinal System and Liver; Hematology; and Rheumatologic and Orthopedic Disease. Other second-year courses are Microbiology and Infectious Disease and Parasitology. On average, students spend about twenty hours per week in class. A Cognitive Skills Program offers reviews for the USMLE and tutoring for students who will benefit from it. Basic science instruction takes place in the Arthur B. and Diane Belfer

Educational Center for Sciences, which is open 24 hours a day and contains classrooms, laboratories, study areas, a student bookstore, and computer rooms. The D. Samuel Gottesman Library has 250,000 volumes, 2,400 journal subscriptions, computer databases, and other informational technology. Electronic search mechanisms allow easy access to several large collections in the New York area.

CLINICAL TRAINING: Third-year required clerkships are Medicine (11 weeks); Pediatrics (7 weeks); Psychiatry (6 weeks); Ob/Gyn (6 weeks); Surgery (8 weeks); Family Medicine (6 weeks); Geriatrics (2 weeks); and Neurology (2 weeks). During the fourth year, two months of a subinternship in either Medicine or Pediatrics is required, as are two months in an ambulatory care program. For clinical training, Einstein students have access to six prominent hospitals in New York, comprising a total of 6,988 beds. These are Jacobi Medical Center (537 beds); Montefiore Medical Center (745 beds); Long Island Jewish Medical Center (829 beds); Beth Israel Medical Center (212 beds); and the Bronx-Lebanon Medical Center (two centers, 540 beds). Training also takes place at mental health facilities and long-term care centers primarily for older populations. Several nationally recognized research institutes are part of Einstein's resources and provide further opportunities for students. Fellowships are available for up to 20 fourth-year students, enabling them to fulfill elective requirements overseas. Numerous organized exchange programs also exist, with countries such as Germany, Sweden, Israel, France, Japan, and Cuba.

Students

Students come from around the country. Undergraduate institutions that are particularly well represented are Yeshiva, State Universities of New York, private northeastern colleges and universities, and public universities in California. In a typical entering class, about 9 percent of students are minorities, most of whom are African American. Students who have taken time off after college account for about one-third of entering classes, and those over 30 years old account for about 5–10 percent. Class size is 180.

Student Life: Central meeting areas, such as the Lubin Student Lounge and the Max and Sadie Friedman Lounge, feature music, food, television, and an opportunity for interaction outside of the academic environment. There are full athletic facilities for student use. School-sponsored activities include class parties, clubs focused on films or the outdoors, and organizations based on cultural, religious, or ethnic affiliations. Einstein has its own symphony orchestra. The beaches of Long Island and the culture, entertainment, and excitement of Manhattan are easily accessible by car or public transportation. Most students live on campus, in the Eastchester Road or Rhinelander Residences, where studios and one- and two-bedroom apartments are available.

Graduates: Among the 1999 graduates, the predominant residency choices were Internal Medicine (45%); Pediatrics (12%); Surgery or General Surgery (10%); Ob/Gyn (6%); Emergency Medicine (6%); Psychiatry (5%); Family Practice (4%); and Ophthalmology (3%). Einstein has the largest post-graduate training program in the country, and is the destination of about 40 percent of Einstein School of Medicine graduates. Programs at other New York institutions, in the Philadelphia area, and in California are also popular choices.

Admissions

Requirements: Requirements are Biology (8 semester hours); Chemistry (8 hours); Organic Chemistry (8 hours); Physics (8 hours); College Math (6 hours); and English (8 hours). The MCAT is required and should be no more than 3 years old. For those who have retaken the MCAT, the best score is counted. Thus, there is no advantage to withholding scores.

Suggestions: College students should pursue studies in their area of interest, as no particular major is considered more appropriate than the next. Course work in the Humanities and Social Sciences is important. Statistics is useful, and computer literacy is necessary. Einstein looks closely at the personal interaction skills of its applicants and at their ability to work with people from diverse backgrounds.

Process: All AMCAS applicants are sent secondary applications. Of those returning secondaries, about 20 percent are invited to interview. Interviews are with faculty members, last for about an hour, and take place between August and May. On interview day, there is a tour of the campus, and a lunch period with current Einstein students. Notification begins in January, at which point applicants are accepted, wait-listed, or rejected. Wait-listed candidates may submit additional material.

Costs

Beyond tuition, yearly expenses are about $14,000. This assumes campus housing and does not necessarily cover the cost of owning a car.

Financial Aid: Most but not all financial aid is need-based, as determined by the FAFSA and institutional forms. Students may apply for scholarships, awarded to students based on a range of factors, through the financial aid office.

ALBERT EINSTEIN COLLEGE OF MEDICINE OF YESHIVA UNIVERSITY

STUDENT BODY

Type	Private
*Enrollment	723
*% male/female	52/48
*% underrepresented minorities	6
# applied (total/out)	7,954/6,085
% interviewed (total/out)	20/13
% accepted (total/out)	NR/NR
% enrolled (total/out)	11/9
Average age	22

ADMISSIONS

Average GPA and MCAT Scores

Overall GPA	3.61	Science GPA	3.58
MCAT Bio	10.8	MCAT Phys	10.8
MCAT Verbal	9.7	MCAT Essay	NR

Score Release Policy

The school has not responded to our inquiry regarding withheld MCAT scores. Therefore, we advise caution. Contact the Admissions Office before withholding any scores.

Application Information

Regular application	11/1
Regular notification	1/15 until filled
Early application	6/1–8/1
Early notification	10/1
Transfers accepted?	No
Admissions may be deferred?	Yes
AMCAS application accepted?	Yes
Interview required?	Yes
Application fee	$85

COSTS AND AID

Tuition & Fees

Tuition	$29,950
Cost of books	$1,000
Fees	$1,775

Financial Aid

% students receiving aid	75
Average grant	$8,500
Average loan	$20,000
Average debt	$65,000

*Figures based on total enrollment

UNIVERSITY OF ARIZONA

COLLEGE OF MEDICINE

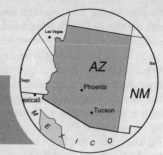

PO Box 245075, Tucson, AZ 85724

Admission: 520-626-6214 • Fax: 520-626-4884

Internet: www.ahsc.arizona.edu/pre-med

The University of Arizona is a public institution whose Board of Regents works closely with the state's leadership to ensure that the University serves the needs of the Arizona population. In support of this objective, the College of Medicine directs resources towards training primary care physicians who are likely to remain in Arizona and who, ideally, are interested in working with underserved groups. In Arizona, these groups are often Hispanic and Native American. The College of Medicine benefits from its association with the numerous professional health schools, including Colleges of Pharmacy and Nursing, and a range of departments within the University. It offers modern facilities and a modern approach to learning. Tucson is a growing, culturally rich city that provides a diverse patient population for clinical training. Students also gain clinical experience in hospitals and smaller health care provider units located in other parts of the state.

Academics

Students may apply to joint Ph.D./M.D. programs in the following: Anatomy, Biochemistry, Cell Biology, Genetics, Immunology, Microbiology, Molecular Biology, Neuroscience, Pharmacology, and Physiology. Combined studies in other fields are possible as well, including a collaborative program of Arizona State University, Northern Arizona University, and the College of Medicine at the University of Arizona. This program focuses on the health needs of underserved communities and leads to a Master's in Public Health along with the M.D. Through this and other venues, medical students at the University of Arizona take advantage of the resources of the academic and medical institutions throughout the state.

BASIC SCIENCES: The basic sciences are taught in the Basic Science Building of the Tucson campus. Traditional lectures with labs are the primary mode of instruction, occupying about 24 hours per week. Alternative teaching methods, including small-group and case-based learning, account for the remaining six hours per week of structured classroom time. First-year courses are Anatomy; Histology and Cell Biology; Physiology; Neuroscience; Biochemistry; Medical and Molecular Genetics; Preparation for Clinical Medicine; and Social and Behavioral Science. During year two, students take Microbiology; Pathology; Pharmacology; Preparation for Clinical Medicine; and Social and Behavioral Science. In the course Preparation for Clinical Medicine, students focus on clinical problem-solving and learn patient evaluation skills. This course links basic science principles with clinical applications. Computers, located in the Learning Resource Center, supplement lectures and are an important component of the basic science education. The Arizona Health Science Library houses nearly 200,000 volumes, operates extensive online database and informational services, and is connected electronically to the library system of the greater university. To accommodate the study schedules of all students, the library is open 24 hours a day. Students are evaluated with an Honors/Pass/Fail scale.

The USMLE Step 1 is required upon completion of basic science course work.

CLINICAL TRAINING: Patient contact begins during year one in Preparation for Clinical Medicine. Throughout the four years, there are opportunities for clinical exposure through volunteer and outreach programs. In addition, clinical research is often community based and gives medical students a chance to help others while they learn. The Commitment to Underserved People (CUP) is a program through which many medical students volunteer. In CUP, students are involved in health education for, and supervised treatment of, people in underserved communities. The formal clinical curriculum begins in year three, when students rotate through the following clerkships: Medicine (12 weeks); Pediatrics (6 weeks); Family Medicine (6 weeks); Ob/Gyn (6 weeks); Psychiatry (6 weeks); Surgery (6 weeks); Specialty Surgery (3 weeks); and Neurology (3 weeks). Year four is composed of electives, many of which can be taken at alternate locations throughout the state. Clinical facilities in Tucson are the University Medical Center, the University Outpatient Clinic, the Children's Research Center, and the Arizona Cancer Center. The hospitals serve managed care participants, and the medical school seeks to respond to the ongoing changes in the economics of health care, as seen in the public health/health policy components of medical school training. Evaluation of clinical performance is Honors/Pass/Fail. Passing the USMLE Step 2 is a requirement for graduation.

Students

Students are either Arizona residents, or are from western states that do not have their own medical schools. Generally, about 15 percent of the student body are underrepresented minorities, most of whom are of Mexican American descent. Older students comprise about one-third of each class. A wide range of undergraduate institutions and majors are represented in a typical class. Class size is 100.

Student Life: With access to both the campus community of over 36,000 students, and a medium-sized urban community, students have active social lives. Recreational facilities are extensive at the University. The Medical School's emphasis on community involvement promotes extra-curricular activities that are medically related. Student clubs also provide mechanisms for support and social interaction. The Chicano/Latino Club is linked to similar organizations at California universities, providing a larger network for those involved. On-campus housing options include apartments and dorms. Most students, however, opt to live off campus.

Graduates: At least 60 percent of graduates enter primary care fields, which include Family Medicine, Ob/Gyn, Internal Medicine, and Pediatrics. About 50 percent of graduates enter residency programs within the state.

Admissions

Requirements: Applicants should have completed one year of each of the following subjects: Biology, Physics, Chemistry, Organic Chemistry, and English. In addition, at least 30 hours of upper-division course work as part of the undergraduate record is required. For older applicants, recent science course work is necessary. The MCAT is required, and only the best scores are considered, suggesting that applicants should not withhold scores. Together, the MCAT and college record are used for initial screening.

Suggestions: Hands-on clinical experience is important, as are other activities that demonstrate an applicant's commitment to community service. The Admissions Committee is interested in applicants whose undergraduate records include significant course work in the Humanities and Social Sciences. Applicants are advised to take the April rather than August MCAT.

Process: All AMCAS applicants receive secondary applications, and virtually all who meet residency requirements are interviewed. Interviews are conducted from September through March and consist of three short meetings with faculty members and one longer session with a practicing clinician from the area. About one quarter of those who interview are accepted, with notifications occurring on a rolling basis. A ranked wait list is established, but those who find themselves on this list are not encouraged to send additional information.

Costs

The estimated yearly budget for a single student is $8,000–$9,000, which includes room, board, and expenses associated with school. This is in addition to tuition. Most students own cars.

Financial Aid: The University of Arizona offers institutional, state, and federal loan and scholarship programs. Most financial aid is based on need and requires parental income disclosure, but some scholarships are awarded solely on merit. In particular, five merit scholarships are awarded each year to graduates of Arizona high schools.

UNIVERSITY OF ARIZONA

STUDENT BODY

Type	Public
*Enrollment	406
*% male/female	52/48
*% underrepresented minorities	15
# applied (total/out)	608/71
% interviewed (total/out)	82/1
% accepted (total/out)	NR/NR
% enrolled (total/out)	20/25

ADMISSIONS

Average GPA and MCAT Scores

Overall GPA	3.62	Science GPA	NR
MCAT Bio	NR	MCAT Phys	NR
MCAT Verbal	NR	MCAT Essay	NR

Score Release Policy

The Admissions Committee will take into consideration unusual circumstances that led to the student choosing to withhold scores.

Application Information

Regular application	11/1
Regular notification	1/31
Admissions may be deferred?	Yes
AMCAS application accepted?	Yes
Interview required?	No
Application fee	$0

COSTS AND AID

Tuition & Fees

Tuition (in/out)	$8,360/NR
Cost of books	NR
Fees	$76

Financial Aid

% students receiving aid	87
Average grant	NR
Average loan	NR
Average debt	NR

*Figures based on total enrollment

University of Arkansas

COLLEGE OF MEDICINE

4301 West Markham Street, Slot 551, Little Rock, AR 72205
Admission: 501-686-5354 • Fax: 501-686-5873
Email: SouthTomG@exchange.uams.edu • Internet: www.uams.edu

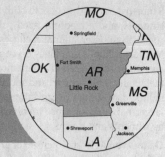

Over the past 10 years, the University of Arkansas College of Medicine has expanded its focus and, as a result, has greatly increased its federal research dollars. The College of Medicine's primary mandate to train health professionals who will serve the state has remained intact. Quality instruction in primary care and exposure to rural patient populations are two of the school's strengths.

Academics

The College of Medicine, along with the schools of Nursing, Pharmacy, Health Related Professions, and Graduate Studies, comprise the University of Arkansas for Medical Sciences, one of five campuses of the University of Arkansas system. Most students complete the M.D. curriculum in four years, but a few students each year take part in joint M.D./Ph.D. or M.D./M.S. programs with the Graduate School. Joint degrees can be pursued in the following fields: Anatomy, Biochemistry, Immunology, Microbiology, Neuroscience, Pharmacology, and Physiology. Students may apply for a program, organized in conjunction with the School of Public Health and Tropical Medicine at Tulane University in New Orleans, which leads to an M.H.P. along with an M.D.

Basic Sciences: Throughout year one, students learn skills related to patient care in Introduction to Clinical Medicine. Fall semester courses are Genetics, Gross Anatomy, and Microscopic Anatomy. Spring semester courses are Biochemistry, Neuroscience, and Physiology. In the fall semester of year two, students take Behavioral Sciences, Medical Ethics, Microbiology, and Pathophysiology I. In the spring, classes are Introduction to Clinical Medicine II, Pathophysiology II, and Pharmacology. Scheduled class time accounts for about 20 hours per week, most of which is devoted to lecture and lab. Alternately, for perhaps two hours per week, small groups are used as the instructional format. Grading uses an A–F scale. Passing the USMLE Step 1 is a requirement for promotion to year three, and USMLE 2 for graduation. Basic-science teaching facilities, including libraries and labs, are part of the medical complex, which includes the main hospitals as well as residence halls

Clinical Training: Patient contact begins in year one, in Introduction to Clinical Medicine. The third year consists of required clerkships in the following: Internal Medicine (12 weeks); Surgery (8 weeks); Ob/Gyn (6 weeks); Psychiatry (6 weeks); Pediatrics (8 weeks); Specialties (4 weeks); Geriatrics (unspecified); and Family Medicine (4 weeks). During year four, students choose among Primary Care Selectives (8 weeks) and Specialties Clerkships (4 weeks). The remainder of the year is designated as elective study, some of which may be taken off

campus, out of state, or overseas. Training takes place primarily at the University Hospital (400 beds), located in the Medical Center complex. Other training sites are the Arkansas Children's Hospital (the 6th largest children's hospital in the country) and two VA hospitals (500 and 2000 beds). In addition, outreach-training sites in small communities around the state provide exposure to rural medicine. The primary care clerkships involve rotations to these sites, located in El Dorado, Fayetteville, Fort Smith, Jonesboro, Pine Bluff, and Texarkana. Specialized research institutes in Little Rock include The Child Study Center, The Ambulatory Care Center, The Arkansas Cancer Research Center, and the Jones Eye Institute. Evaluation of clinical progress in required clerkships uses an A–F scale, and electives are graded as Pass/Fail. Students must take the USMLE Step 2, though passing is not a requirement for graduation.

Students

Virtually all students are Arkansas residents. About 65 percent of students earned undergraduate degrees in Arkansas. Approximately 78 percent of incoming students in a recent class had undergraduate majors in science disciplines. Classes include a significant number of older students, including some who were older than 40 years old at the time of admission. Class size is 150.

Student Life: Little Rock is a small but lively city, with indoor and outdoor recreational activities. Students take part in volunteer and community activities, such as the Fighting AIDS Through Education Program, which introduces health education programs into junior and senior high schools, or the Alliance for Recovery, which meets the needs of tornado victims. Most single first- and second-year students live on campus in residence halls. Upperclass students and married students live either off campus or in university-owned apartments.

Graduates: Many graduates enter post-graduate programs in Arkansas. Programs in about 20 specialty areas are offered at university-affiliated hospitals in Little Rock. In addition, a number of family practice residencies are available at rural locations around the state. At least half of the graduates of the School of Medicine enter primary care fields.

Admissions

REQUIREMENTS: Within each class, 70 percent of students must be equally divided from among the four congressional districts in the state. The College of Medicine is allowed to admit a few out-of-state applicants each year, but only if they do not displace Arkansas residents with equal qualifications. Out-of-state applicants should be highly qualified and have close ties to Arkansas. Students must have successfully completed the following courses prior to matriculation: Biology (one year); Chemistry (one year); Organic Chemistry (one year); Physics (one year); English (1.5 years); and Math (one year). The MCAT is required, and scores must be no more than 4 years old. Scores from all sections of the MCAT, including the writing sample, are considered.

SUGGESTIONS: Other courses deemed helpful are Biochemistry, Zoology, Botany, Embryology, Genetics, Histology, Calculus, Physical Chemistry, Statistics, Sociology, Speech, Anthropology, Psychology, Human Ecology, Composition, Literature, History, and Logic. For students who graduated from college several years ago, some recent course work is useful. All medically related extracurricular activities are valued.

PROCESS: Virtually all AMCAS applicants are asked to submit secondary applications. All Arkansas residents, and highly qualified out-of-state residents are interviewed, with interviews taking place between August and January. Team interviews consist of a one-hour session with faculty. All applicants are notified by February, and approximately one-quarter of interviewees are accepted. A ranked wait list is established, and about 30 students from the list are usually admitted. Wait-listed candidates who commit to practicing in underserved areas of Arkansas may improve their chances of admissions.

Costs

In addition to tuition, anticipated costs for a single student are about $12,000 yearly. This includes all academic and living expenses and assumes on-campus housing.

FINANCIAL AID: Most aid is need based. Need is determined by the FAFSA form and additional information requested by the College of Medicine. Average indebtedness is relatively low ($62,000) due to the low cost of tuition and the scholarships available.

UNIVERSITY OF ARKANSAS

STUDENT BODY

Type	Public
*Enrollment	568
*% male/female	60/40
*% underrepresented minorities	10
# applied (total/out)	541/280
% interviewed (total/out)	NR/NR
% accepted (total/out)	NR/NR
% enrolled (total/out)	NR/NR

ADMISSIONS

Average GPA and MCAT Scores

Overall GPA	3.60	Science GPA	3.57
MCAT Bio	9.40	MCAT Phys	8.90
MCAT Verbal	9.50	MCAT Essay	O

Score Release Policy

The school has not responded to our inquiry regarding withheld MCAT scores. Therefore, we advise caution. Contact the Admissions Office before withholding any scores.

Application Information

Regular application	11/1
Regular notification	12/15 until filled
Transfers accepted?	Yes
Admissions may be deferred?	Yes
AMCAS application accepted?	Yes
Interview required?	Yes
Application fee	$50

COSTS AND AID

Tuition & Fees

Tuition (in/out)	$9,596/$19,192
Cost of books	$800
Fees	$203

Financial Aid

% students receiving aid	84
Average grant	NR
Average loan	NR
Average debt	$62,000

*Figures based on total enrollment

BAYLOR COLLEGE OF MEDICINE

One Baylor Plaza, Room N104, Houston, TX 77030
Admission: 713-798-4842 • Fax: 713-798-5563
Email: melodym@bcm.tmc.edu • Internet: www.bcm.tmc.edu

Baylor recently implemented a revised curriculum that coordinates and integrates basic and clinical sciences throughout the four years. Patient contact begins in the first year; clinical rotations start mid-way through year two, and interdisciplinary perspectives are incorporated into the fourth year. Baylor is located in Houston's Texas Medical Center, a 675-acre medical complex consisting of 42 nonprofit member institutions. Baylor's clinical facilities are expansive, and the diverse patient population reflects the urban surroundings of Houston, the largest city in Texas.

Academics

Students enjoy a flexible curriculum with various opportunities for individualized experiences. For all students, grading in basic science courses is Honors, Pass, Marginal Pass, and Fail. During clinical training, students are evaluated with Honors, High Pass, Pass, Marginal Pass, and Fail. The USMLE is not a specified academic requirement.

About 12 students each year enter a combined M.D./ Ph.D. program, earning the doctorate degree in Biochemistry and Molecular Biology, Cardiovascular Sciences, Molecular and Cellular Biology, Developmental Biology, Immunology, Molecular and Human Genetics, Molecular Physiology and Biophysics, Molecular Virology and Microbiology, Neuroscience, or Pharmacology. Interdisciplinary programs at Baylor and the University of Houston, and an engineering program with Rice University are also options. Nineteen M.D./Ph.D. students are funded annually by the NIH M.S.T.P. training grant. Other students are supported by private or institutional sources.

BASIC SCIENCES: Complementing basic science courses are clinical experiences, behavioral sciences, and social/ethical perspectives. Throughout the first year and a half, students take Integrated Problem Solving (IPS) and Patient, Physician, and Society (PPS). The IPS course develops lifelong learning skills by focusing on problem-solving and the use of modern informational systems. The PPS course introduces, basic clinical skills such as the physical diagnosis and examination along with principles of patient care. Other first-year subjects are organized into blocks. Courses are: Gross Anatomy and Embryology; Cell Biology and Histology; Biochemistry; Physiology; Immunology; General Pharmacology; Bioethics; Nervous System; Behavioral Sciences; Infectious Disease; and General Pathology. The first semester of the second year is organized around body/organ systems: Immunology/Rheumatology; Cardiology; Genetics; Respiratory; Gastroenterology; Dermatology; Renal; Genitourinary/Gynecology; Endocrinology; Age-related Topics; and Hematology/Oncology. Both faculty and student tutors are available for additional instruction outside of the classroom. Basic sciences are taught primarily at the DeBakey Biomedical Research Building. The Learning Resources Center provides study areas and edu-

cational aids such as computers with medical software and Internet access, videotapes, and interactive learning programs. The Houston Academy of Medicine—Texas Medical Center Library contains more than 260,000 volumes, making it one of the largest medical libraries in the country.

CLINICAL TRAINING: Clinical rotations begin in January of year two. Required clerkships are: Pediatrics (8 weeks); Ob/Gyn (8 weeks); Psychiatry (8 weeks); Family and Community Medicine (4 weeks); Medicine (12 weeks); Surgery (12 weeks); Surgical Subspecialties (4 weeks) and Neurology (4 weeks). Throughout year three, students participate in Longitudinal Ambulatory Care Experience (LACE) that requires one half-day each week. Other requirements include four weeks of Selectives and 20 weeks of Electives in addition to a year-long course on the Mechanisms and Management of Disease (MM.D.). The MM.D. course is comprised of modules that correlate basic science principles with clinical concepts. At the end of the fourth year, students may elect a two-week course in Integrated Clinical Experiences (ICE), which serves as a transition to post-graduate training. Students train in the Baylor Affiliated Teaching Hospitals in the Texas Medical Center complex and at other sites around the city. In total, Baylor's teaching facilities hold approximately 5,000 beds. Elective credits may be earned at institutions throughout the United States as well as overseas.

Students

Approximately 70–75 percent of students are Texas residents. Students in the class that entered in 1999 came from 64 undergraduate institutions. About 16–20 percent of students are underrepresented minorities, and a wide age range is seen within the student body. Entering class size is 168.

STUDENT LIFE: A two-day orientation introduces entering students to the school's academic and nonacademic resources and promotes a supportive atmosphere from the beginning. First-year students also benefit from peer counseling groups and professional advising. Numerous organizations promote extracurricular, professional, community service, and religious interests, or offer support for minority or other groups of medical students. Some examples include the Family Practice Club, the Texas Medical Association Medical Student Section, and the Baylor Association of Minority Medical Students. An athletic center with exercise equipment and weights, basketball, racquetball, aerobics, and volleyball is available to medical students. Houston is home to almost two million people and is a center for commerce, industry, arts, and recreation. A dormitory operated by the Texas Medical Center is located near Baylor, although most medical students opt to live off campus in nearby residential areas.

GRADUATES: Graduates are successful in securing residencies in all generalist and specialty areas. Baylor also administers post-graduate programs.

Admissions

REQUIREMENTS: Prerequisites are one year each of Biology, Chemistry, Organic Chemistry, and English. Science courses must include associated labs. The MCAT is required and must be from within the past five years. For applicants who have taken the exam on more than one occasion, the most recent set of scores is weighted most heavily.

SUGGESTIONS: Approximately 70–75 percent of the positions in each class are reserved for Texas residents, making non-resident positions highly competitive. The April, rather than August, MCAT is recommended. Beyond intellectual ability, Baylor is interested in personal integrity and demonstrated interest in medicine.

PROCESS: Baylor does not participate in AMCAS. Institutional applications are available in June preceding the year of anticipated entrance. Approximately 15 percent of applicants are interviewed between September and February. Interviews usually consist of three 30-minute sessions each with a faculty member or medical student. The interview weekend features a group orientation session, a campus tour, and the opportunity to meet informally with students and faculty members. Of interviewed candidates, about 40 percent are accepted on a rolling basis.

Costs

In addition to tuition and fees, the estimated yearly cost of living for a single student is about $15,000. This budget allows for off-campus room and board.

FINANCIAL AID: Most financial aid is need-based, with need determined by the FAFSA form. Students who do not qualify for resident tuition rates are often eligible for scholarships, which serve to reduce the price of tuition. Merit-based scholarships are available.

BAYLOR COLLEGE OF MEDICINE

STUDENT BODY

Type	Private
*Enrollment	666
*% male/female	56/44
*% underrepresented minorities	18
# applied (total/out)	2,357/1,067
% interviewed (total/out)	26/9
% accepted (total/out)	12/4
% enrolled (total/out)	59/38
Average age	23

ADMISSIONS

Average GPA and MCAT Scores

Overall GPA	3.80	Science GPA	NR
MCAT Bio	11.30	MCAT Phys	11.20
MCAT Verbal	10.20	MCAT Essay	Q

Score Release Policy

Applicants must have scores sent from all MCAT exams taken. However, only the most recent score is considered.

Application Information

Regular application	11/1
Regular notification	Rolling
Early application	8/1
Early notification	10/1
Transfers accepted?	Yes
Admissions may be deferred?	Yes
AMCAS application accepted?	No
Interview required?	Yes
Application fee	$50

COSTS AND AID

Tuition & Fees

Tuition (in/out)	$6,550/$19,650
Cost of books and supplies	$2,331
Fees	$968

Financial Aid

% students receiving aid	81
Average grant	$11,725
Average loan	$16,955
Average debt	$65,263

*Figures based on total enrollment

BOSTON UNIVERSITY
SCHOOL OF MEDICINE

715 Albany Street, Boston, MA 02118
Admission: 617-638-4630
Internet: med-amsa.bu.edu

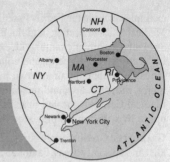

Boston University (BU) is a large, urban institution that encompasses fifteen Schools and Colleges, including schools of Medicine, Dentistry, and Public Health. Although the University is independent and attracts a national student body, it is integrated into the city of Boston and responds to the needs of the local community. The School of Medicine, located in the South End of Boston along with the B.U. Medical Center, originated from what was the first medical school in the world for women. B.U. medical students benefit from the clinical exposure provided by the urban area and also enjoy its cultural, historical, and recreational offerings. The curriculum includes some problem-based learning.

Academics

Several combined degree programs are offered, including the M.D./M.P.H., to which all students accepted into the medical school may apply. Qualified students may pursue a joint M.D./Ph.D. program, earning the doctorate degree in Anatomy, Biochemistry, Biomedical Engineering, Biophysics, Behavioral Neuroscience, Cell Biology, Genetics; Immunology, Microbiology, Molecular Biology, Pathology, Pharmacology, or Physiology. Most students take part in a four-year curriculum of basic and clinical science, leading to the M.D. However, up to ten students each year enter an Alternative Curriculum which spreads out the first year of study into two years, thereby freeing up time for academic or personal interests. Evaluation uses Honors, Pass, and Fail in addition to narrative reports when possible. Passing the USMLE Step 1 is a requirement for promotion to year three.

BASIC SCIENCES: An Integrated Problems course supplements the traditional lecture/lab format of first- and second-year courses. Integrated Problems meets in small groups, and uses an interdisciplinary approach to tackle case studies that relate to subjects discussed in other courses. First-year courses are: Gross Anatomy; Histology; Biochemistry; Physiology; Endocrinology; Neuroscience; Principles of Psychiatry in Medicine; Essentials of Public Health; Immunology; Genetics; and Introduction to Clinical Medicine I (ICM I). ICM I develops an understanding of the doctor-patient relationship and discusses sociocultural issues related to it. Second-year courses are: Pathology; Pharmacology; Microbiology and Infectious Diseases; Biology of Disease I; Biology of Disease II; ICM II; Psychiatry; and Integrated Problems. In ICM II, students learn to conduct patient interviews and physical examinations. A benefit of the ICM continuum is that instruction involves mentorships with practicing physicians, often in primary care settings. Most basic science instruction takes place in the Instructional Building, which has classrooms, administrative offices, and a library with 117,000 volumes and 1,300 periodicals. This building connects to the Housman Research Building, which offers a learning center and a computer room.

CLINICAL TRAINING: Required third-year clerkships are: Family Medicine (6 weeks); Medicine (11 weeks); Surgery (11 weeks); Ob/Gyn (6 weeks); Pediatrics (6 weeks); and Psychiatry (6 weeks). More than half of the fourth year is reserved for electives. Required fourth-year clerkships are: Home Medicine/Geriatrics (4 weeks); Neurology (4 weeks); Radiology (4 weeks); Primary Care (4 weeks); and a Subinternship (4 weeks). Clinical training takes place at the Boston Medical Center (633 beds), the Veterans Affairs Administration Medical Center (535 beds, in Jamaica Plain), and at least eighteen other affiliated hospitals and health care facilities. Several research centers are part of the Medical Center, and also serve as educational facilities for medical students.

Students

Underrepresented minorities account for about 10 percent of the student body. At least one-quarter of students took time off after college, and the average age of entering students is 24. Although a large number of states and colleges are represented, a significant proportion of students graduated from the undergraduate institutions of Boston University, Harvard, and other schools in the area.

STUDENT LIFE: Students are involved in many medical student organizations ranging from the Creative Arts Society to volunteer efforts like the Domestic Violence Awareness Project or The Outreach Van that provides medical care to the poor and homeless. Medical student housing is convenient to instructional facilities and promotes cohesion among students. Medical students have access to the facilities of the greater university, including the student union and several athletic facilities that offer swimming pools, an ice skating rink, dance and other classes, and sailing or rowing on the Charles River. As part of the ICM courses and clinical rotations, medical students travel in and around Boston and more than 50 miles outside of the city. This gives students an opportunity to explore Boston and other parts of New England.

GRADUATES: In the 2000 graduating class, the most prevalent specialty areas were Medicine (21%); Pediatrics (10%); Emergency (9%); Surgery (9%); Obstetrics/Gynecology

(7%); Diagnostic Radiology (5%); Internal Medicine-Primary Care (5%); and Anesthesiology (4%).

Admissions

REQUIREMENTS: Prerequisites are one year each of English, Humanities, General Chemistry, Organic Chemistry, Physics, and Biology. In evaluating GPA, factors such as the intensity of the undergraduate workload are considered. The MCAT is required and should be from within three years of the date of matriculation. For applicants who have taken the exam more than once, the committee looks at the best set of scores.

SUGGESTIONS: In addition to requirements, Calculus is recommended, as is a broad background in the Humanities and Social Sciences. The April MCAT is strongly urged. For applicants who have been out of college for a period of time, some recent course work is advised.

PROCESS: BU does not have a secondary application. About 10 percent of the approximately 10,000 AMCAS applicants are invited to interview, with interviews held between October and March. Interviews consist of one one-hour session with a faculty member. With only eighty positions available for applicants to the four-year program, admission is very competitive. There are several alternate paths to gaining admission. A seven-year program, leading to the B.A. and M.D. degrees is offered in conjunction with BU's undergraduate college. Engineering undergraduates at BU are also eligible to apply for a joint B.S./M.D. program with the School of Medicine. Sophomores at accredited colleges may apply to the BU College of Medicine for entrance upon completion of their B.A. requirements, as long as specified minimum GPA and MCAT scores are achieved. This relieves some of the pressure of the medical school application process. Selected colleges enrolling predominantly underrepresented minorities participate in a similar eight-year program with BU.

Costs

In addition to tuition, the yearly cost of living for a single student is about $17,000. This allows for on-campus or shared off-campus housing and includes car ownership.

FINANCIAL AID: Students applying for financial aid are expected to use personal and family resources, in addition to federal, state, and outside assistance. The Office of Financial Aid offers loans, with only limited grant money available. Most assistance is based on financial need, as determined by the FAFSA form and the College Scholarship Service needs analysis. Some assistance is offered on the basis of special criteria, such as commitment to primary care, ethnic background, or outstanding achievement.

BOSTON UNIVERSITY

STUDENT BODY

Type	Private
*Enrollment	619
*% male/female	62/38
*% underrepresented minorities	10
# applied (total/out)	10,674/9,225
% interviewed (total/out)	NR/NR
% accepted (total/out)	NR/NR
% enrolled (total/out)	NR/NR
Average age	24

ADMISSIONS

Average GPA and MCAT Scores

Overall GPA	3.52	Science GPA	3.53
MCAT Bio	10.31	MCAT Phys	10.17
MCAT Verbal	9.25	MCAT Essay	NR

Score Release Policy

The school has not responded to our inquiry regarding withheld MCAT scores. Therefore, we advise caution. Contact the Admissions Office before withholding any scores.

Application Information

Regular application	11/15
Regular notification	Rolling
Early application	8/1
Early notification	10/1
Transfers accepted?	Yes
Admissions may be deferred?	No
AMCAS application accepted?	Yes
Interview required?	Yes
Application fee	$95

COSTS AND AID

Tuition & Fees

Tuition	$36,530
Cost of books	$2,032
Fees	$450

Financial Aid

% students receiving aid	80
Average grant	$1,900
Average loan	$17,000
Average debt	$115,000

*Figures based on total enrollment

BROWN UNIVERSITY
SCHOOL OF MEDICINE

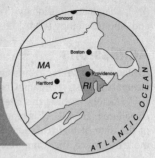

97 Waterman Street, Box G-A212, Providence, RI 02912
Admission: 401-863-2149 • Fax: 401-863-2660
Email: MedSchool_Admissions@brown.edu • Internet: www.brown.edu

Brown uses a decidedly interdisciplinary approach to the study of medicine. The School of Medicine ensures that students have had an excellent liberal arts background by primarily enrolling students who were Brown undergraduates. The diversity of the student body is enhanced through inclusion of several other selected applicant groups, including nontraditional applicants from post-baccalaureate programs, medical students enrolled in the Brown/Dartmouth program who complete basic science course work at Dartmouth, joint M.D./Ph.D. candidates, and selected students identified by premedical advisors at Providence College, Rhode Island College, the University of Rhode Island, and Tougaloo College through the Early Identification Program.

Academics

Most students enter the School of Medicine after the fourth year in an eight-year B.A./M.D. curriculum to which they were admitted out of high school. Although curricula of this type are offered at other schools, Brown is unique in that it admits the majority of its medical students through this program, called the Program in Liberal Medical Education (PLME). Brown/Dartmouth participants study basic sciences at Dartmouth, and join Brown students for clinical training. They receive their M.D.s from Brown. Applicants may be considered for M.D./Ph.D. programs in conjunction with Brown graduate departments in the following fields: Artificial Organs, Biomaterials, Cellular Technology, Ecology, Epidemiology, Gerontology, Molecular Biology, Biochemistry, Molecular Pharmacology, Physiology, Neuroscience, and Pathobiology.

BASIC SCIENCES: Principles of patient care, and of the social and behavioral aspects of medicine, are integrated into the basic science curriculum. Throughout years one and two, students are exposed to clinical environments through Affinity Groups, which bring students with shared interests together for research, community projects, and close contact with mentor physicians. Examples of Affinity Groups are Marine Medicine, Alternative Medical Therapies, and Women's Reproductive Health. The first two years are organized into semesters. During the fall semester of year one, students take Physiology, Anatomy, Histology, and Medical Interviewing. During the spring semester of year one, Biochemistry, Microbiology, Pathology, and Neurobiology are taken, as is Human Development in Health and Illness, which uses small-group instruction. The basic science courses are taught primarily through lectures and labs. Pathophysiology provides a structure for year two, which is organized around organ systems or concepts such as: Cardiovascular, Renal, Hematology, Pulmonary, Nutritional, Gastroenterology, Infectious Diseases, Supporting Structures, and Endocrine. Pharmacology, Pathology, Introduction to Clinical Medicine, and Clinical Psychiatry are also part of the second-year curriculum. Pre-clinical instruction takes place in the Biomedical Building, which is central to the Brown campus. The Science Library is fully computerized, with online database systems. Medical students have access to all of Brown's academic facilities, including the main library, which houses two million volumes. Grading is Honors/Pass/Fail. Passing Step 1 of the USMLE is not a requirement for promotion.

CLINICAL TRAINING: Patient contact begins in the first year, fall semester, with Medical Interviewing. Formal clinical training, consisting of required core rotations and electives, occupies years three and four. In total, 48 weeks are devoted to core clerkships and 32 weeks to electives. Requirements are: Medicine (12 weeks); Surgery (12 weeks); Pediatrics (6 weeks); Ob/Gyn (6 weeks); Family Medicine (6 weeks); Psychiatry (6 weeks); Medicine or Pediatrics Subinternship (4 weeks); and Longitudinal Ambulatory (one half-day per week for 26 weeks). Community Health is integrated into Medicine and Family Practice Clerkships. Clinical training takes place at seven affiliated teaching hospitals in the Providence area: Bradley Hospital; Butler Hospital; The Miriam Hospital; Memorial Hospital of Rhode Island; Rhode Island Hospital; Hasbro Childrens; V.A. Medical Center; and Women and Infants Hospital. The hospitals attract an ethnically and socio-economically diverse, urban population. Noteworthy areas of clinical care and research include Child/Adolescent Medicine, Psychiatric Care, International Health, Cancer, AIDS, Artificial Organs, and Diabetes. Evaluation of clinical performance uses an Honors/Pass/Fail scale supplemented by narratives. The USMLE Step 2 is a requirement for graduation.

Students

Fifty-five percent of the students majored in a scientific field as undergraduates. About 14 percent of students are underrepresented minorities, mostly African Americans and Puerto Ricans. About 14 percent of entering students are over 25 years old upon matriculation.

STUDENT LIFE: PLME students make up about 71 percent of the student body. Students who studied basic sciences at Dartmouth account for 11 percent. Rhode Island residents who entered through the EIP make up 7 percent of students, and those who attended post-bacc programs make up about 7 percent of each class. The remaining 4 percent of students are either M.D./Ph.D. candidates or former Brown students. Medical students have full access to the school's recreational activities and facilities. Brown has over 200 student clubs and organizations that unite students. Although most students choose to live off campus, residence halls and housing co-ops are available.

GRADUATES: In recent years, 16 percent of graduates entered residency programs at hospitals affiliated with Brown. About half of each class enters primary care residencies.

Admissions

REQUIREMENTS: Eligibility requires either: Participation in the PLME program; completion of a post-baccalaureate, pre-medical program at Columbia, Brown, or Bryn Mawr; selection through the EIP from Providence College, Tougaloo College, Rhode Island College, or the University of Rhode Island; enrollment as an undergraduate or graduate student at Brown; or acceptance to the Brown/Dartmouth program. It is recommended that entering students should have completed: Biology (four one-semester courses, including both a two-semester introductory sequence and advanced-level courses in genetics and introductory Biochemistry; a laboratory experience in at least two courses); Chemistry (one semester of general chemistry and organic chemistry); Physics (usually a one-year, two-course sequence); Calculus (one semester); Probability and Statistics (one semester); Social and Behavioral Sciences (at least two courses). The MCAT is required only for students applying to the Brown/Dartmouth program.

SUGGESTIONS: For a typical medical school applicant, the only way to gain admission to Brown is through the Brown/Dartmouth program or as an M.D./Ph.D. candidate. About 15 students each year enter the Brown/Dartmouth program.

PROCESS: The PLME application is part of the undergraduate application package. The deadline is January 1, and notification is April 1. Those attending schools that are part of the EIP program should contact their pre-medical advisors for application procedures. The EIP deadline is March 1, and notification is early April. Those who must complete science requirements before applying to medical school should consider postbacc programs at Columbia, Brown, and Bryn Mawr. Interviews are required of Brown/Dartmouth and M.D./Ph.D. applicants. The deadline for the M.D./Ph.D. program for applicants interested in applying for the 2000 school year is November 15. M.D./Ph.D. applicants are notified of the admissions decision in early January. The Advanced Standing and Fifth Pathway application deadline is February 1 and notification is in the beginning of March. The Brown Avenue application deadline is March 1 and notification is in early April.

Costs

Tuition and student fees for a first-year student for the 1998–1999 school year is approximately $28,900. The anticipated yearly budget for books, apartment rent, utilities, and other living expenses for a single student living on campus is $11,000, assuming the use of public transportation.

FINANCIAL AID: The basis for awards is financial need. Financial aid is available from both internal (institutional) and external sources. Actual awards depend on federal funding levels as well as institutional resources. Once federal loans are secured, Brown may offer grants and loans to students who are eligible to apply for institutional aid. Parental information is required for students applying for institutional aid.

BROWN UNIVERSITY

STUDENT BODY

Type	Private
*Enrollment	315
*% male/female	47/53
*% underrepresented minorities	14
# applied (total/out)	2,099/2,042
% interviewed (total/out)	1/1
% accepted (total/out)	8/7
% enrolled (total/out)	56/55
Average age	23

ADMISSIONS

Average GPA and MCAT Scores

Overall GPA	3.52	Science GPA	3.71
MCAT Bio	10.21	MCAT Phys	9.84
MCAT Verbal	9.89	MCAT Essay	P

Score Release Policy

School does not require MCAT for all programs.

Application Information

Regular application	11/1–3/1
Regular notification	12/1 until early April
Transfers accepted?	Yes
Admissions may be deferred?	Yes
AMCAS application accepted?	No
Interview required?	Yes
Application fee	$65

COSTS AND AID

Tuition & Fees

Tuition	$26,896
Cost of books	NR
Fees	NR

Financial Aid

% students receiving aid	71
Average grant	$13,475
Average loan	$21,724
Average debt	$76,406

*Figures based on total enrollment

UNIVERSITY AT BUFFALO
SCHOOL OF MEDICINE AND BIOMEDICAL SCIENCES

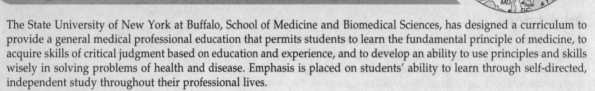

45 Biomedical Education Building, Buffalo, NY 14214-3013
Admission: 716-829-3466 • Fax: 716-829-3849
Email: jjrosso@acsu.buffalo.edu • Internet: www.smbs.buffalo.edu/ome

The State University of New York at Buffalo, School of Medicine and Biomedical Sciences, has designed a curriculum to provide a general medical professional education that permits students to learn the fundamental principle of medicine, to acquire skills of critical judgment based on education and experience, and to develop an ability to use principles and skills wisely in solving problems of health and disease. Emphasis is placed on students' ability to learn through self-directed, independent study throughout their professional lives.

Academics

In addition to the M.D., the School of Medicine and Biomedical Sciences awards the Ph.D., M.A., M.S., and the combined M.D./Ph.D. There are four M.S.T.P.-sponsored M.D./Ph.D. positions available each year. Departments awarding graduate degrees include: Anatomy, Biochemistry, Biophysics, Cell Biology, Genetics, Immunology, Microbiology, Molecular Biology, Neuroscience, Pathology, Pharmacology, and Physiology. A new joint-degree program, leading to the M.D./M.B.A. began in 1997. Evaluation of medical students uses Honors/Pass/Fail. Passing the USMLE Step 1 is required before matriculants can enter third year.

BASIC SCIENCES: Basic sciences are taught through a combination of lectures, labs, small group sessions, problem-based learning and clinical experiences. On average, students are in class or scheduled sessions for about 27 hours per week. First-year courses are: Gross Anatomy; Biochemistry; Human Behavior; Histology; Embryology; Physiology; Neuroscience, Medical Genetics; Scientific Basis of Medicine; Social and Preventive Medicine; and Clinical Practice of Medicine, which provides early patient-contact experiences. Second-year courses are: Hematology; Pathology; Microbiology; Pharmacology; Scientific Basis of Medicine; Social and Preventive Medicine; Genetics; Human Behavior; and the continuation of Clinical Practice of Medicine. Summer externships, which allow up to 60 first- and second-year medical students to shadow primary care physicians are available with stipends. Stipends are also available on a limited basis for summer research projects. The Health Sciences Library features a Media Resources Center with approximately 2,000 multimedia items, a History of Medicine Collection with 12,000 volumes, and a comprehensive general medicine/scientific book and journal collection.

CLINICAL TRAINING: Third-year required rotations are: Internal Medicine (8 weeks); Surgery (8 weeks); Ob/Gyn (7 weeks); Pediatrics (7 weeks); Psychiatry (7 weeks); and Family Medicine (7 weeks). The Family Medicine Clerkship includes six sessions in a community-based family physician's office, two sessions in a problem-based learning format, one session focusing on a community project, and one session devoted to independent learning. During the third year, students also choose a week-long seminar from diverse selective offerings. Fourth-year requirements are four weeks each of Neurology, Medicine, and Surgery, and four weeks of an ambulatory experience. Four-year electives are also available. Training takes place at: The Buffalo General Hospital; Children's Hospital of Buffalo; Erie County Medical Center; Mercy Hospital; Millard Fillmore Health System; Sisters of Charity Hospital; Roswell Park Cancer Institute; and the Buffalo VA Medical Center. The Community Academic Practice Program identifies community-based sites for clinical training. With faculty approval, up to 16 weeks of electives may be taken at other academic institutions.

Students

All but one or two students in each class are New York residents. About 20 percent of entering students are over 25 years old. Approximately 5 percent of students are underrepresented minorities. Class size is 135.

STUDENT LIFE: The first year begins with a relaxed orientation week that allows students to get acquainted with each other and their new surroundings. Several student centers serve as focal points for student life on campus. The Student Union houses more than 75 clubs and organizations in addition to recreational facilities, dining areas, and a theater. The Oasis Recreation Center features pool tables, music, and a TV room. The Harriman Student Activities Center is an alternate student union, and the Creative Craft Center provides ongoing craft programs and courses. The Living Well Center (LWC) is dedicated to improving students' overall health and wellness. It offers a range of services to students, including counseling, health education, fitness assessments, seminars on personal health issues, relaxation services such as massage, and special events with outside speakers. For medical students, the LWC also provides opportunities for volunteer work in areas related to preventive medicine. Buffalo is an affordable and student-friendly community. Residence Halls and graduate student apartments are available close to campus.

GRADUATES: Among graduates in a recent class, the most prevalent specialty fields were: Internal Medicine (28%); Pediatrics (25%); Family Practice (15%); Ob/Gyn (10%); Surgery (11%); and Emergency Medicine (5%). Approximately half of graduates entered residency programs in New York State.

Admissions

REQUIREMENTS: Prerequisites are Biology (two semesters); Chemistry (four semesters, including two of Organic Chemistry); Physics (two semesters); and English (two semesters). The MCAT is required, and must be from after 1996. For applicants who have taken the exam on multiple occasions, the best set of scores is generally considered. Thus, there is no advantage in withholding scores.

SUGGESTIONS: In addition to science requirements, two years of course work in Social Sciences and one year in the Humanities are advised. For applicants who have taken time off after college, some recent course work is recommended. Medically related experience is important.

PROCESS: All applicants are sent secondary applications. Between 400 and 500 applicants are interviewed from September through February. These candidates are selected from a pool of about 2,500, meaning that about 20 percent of applicants make it to the interview stage. Interviews consist of two sessions each with a faculty member or medical student. On interview day, there are also group informational sessions, a campus tour, and the opportunity to have lunch with current medical students. The first acceptance letters are mailed in October, with subsequent batches of letters sent at 4–6-week intervals throughout the year. Approximately 30 percent of interviewees are accepted initially. Others are rejected or placed on a wait list. Supplementary material from wait-listed candidates is not encouraged. Usually 60–70 percent of interviewees are eventually offered an acceptance before orientation begins.

Costs

The estimated yearly cost of living for a single New York State Resident is $27,000. This budget allows for housing, car ownership, and tuition.

FINANCIAL AID: Assistance is based on financial need as determined by the FAFSA form. In addition to federal programs, state financial aid is available. Regents Scholarships for economically disadvantaged and underrepresented minority students provide up to $10,000 per year in the form of grants. A Regents Physician Loan Forgiveness Program will pay off $10,000 per year in student loans in return for practicing in underserved areas within New York. Need-based, partial tuition scholarships are also offered to 35–40 matriculants annually.

UNIVERSITY AT BUFFALO

STUDENT BODY

Type	Public
*Enrollment	575
*% male/female	49/51
*% underrepresented minorities	9
# applied (total/out)	1,687/376
% interviewed (total/out)	15/3
% accepted (total/out)	11/1
% enrolled (total/out)	47/29
Average age	23

ADMISSIONS

Average GPA and MCAT Scores

Overall GPA	3.60	Science GPA	3.53
MCAT Bio	9.80	MCAT Phys	9.60
MCAT Verbal	9.10	MCAT Essay	P

Score Release Policy
We use the highest score obtained. No advantage to withholding any score.

Application Information

Regular application	10/15
Regular notification	10/15 until filled
Early application	6/1–8/1
Early notification	10/1
Transfers accepted?	Yes
Admissions may be deferred?	Yes
AMCAS application accepted?	Yes
Interview required?	Yes
Application fee	$65

COSTS AND AID

Tuition & Fees

Tuition (in/out)	$10,840/$21,940
Cost of books	$3,048
Fees	$950

Financial Aid

% students receiving aid	85
Average grant	$3,000
Average loan	NR
Average debt	$60,000

*Figures based on total enrollment

University of California, Davis

SCHOOL OF MEDICINE

One Shields Avenue, Davis, CA 95616

Admission: 530-752-2717

Internet: www-med.ucdavis.edu

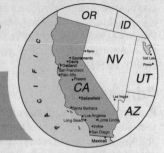

The University of California Davis (UC Davis) School of Medicine has a record for training outstanding physicians and for its contributions to research. The School of Medicine is on the UC Davis campus, which also features Schools of Agriculture, Veterinary Medicine, and Management, in addition to comprehensive undergraduate and graduate school programs. The school's primary clinical facility, the UC Davis Medical Center, is located in Sacramento, the state capital, and serves an expansive region of thirty-two counties and 5 million residents. Davis is a two-hour drive from some of the best hiking and skiing in the country and an even shorter distance to San Francisco, the Napa Valley wine country, and the Pacific Ocean.

Academics

The School of Medicine is well-integrated into the UC Davis Campus and benefits from the academic programs of the University. About 20 percent of each class extend their first two years into three, extend their fourth year, or take time off from the standard curriculum at some point. This "Enrichment Option" allows students to pursue research or attend to other academic and personal goals. Joint-degree programs organized in conjunction with graduate departments at UC Davis lead to an M.B.A., M.A., or Ph.D. along with the M.D. degree. In addition, the M.P.H. degree may be earned at UC Berkeley School of Public Health. Those interested in careers as physician-scientists may apply for programs leading to doctorates in the following fields: Biochemistry, Biomedical Engineering, Cell Biology, Genetics, Immunology, Molecular Biology, Neuroscience, Pathology, Pharmacology, Physiology.

BASIC SCIENCES: Davis operates on a quarter system, with each quarter separated into two segments by a midterm week for study and examinations. The two-year pre-clinical program has a heavy clinical emphasis—more than 60 percent of courses are taught by physicians. The more typical basic science courses are taught primarily in the first year. The fall-quarter courses are Anatomy and Biochemistry. Winter-quarter courses are Histology, Biochemistry, and Physiology. Spring-quarter courses are Immunology, Endocrinology, and Neurobiology. Throughout the first year, patient communication, physical examination, and history-taking are taught in Introduction to Patient Evaluation and in the first-quarter course, Psychiatry. The six-week summer quarter is a transition between basic and clinical sciences with a continuation of the Pathology program initiated in the spring quarter, Human Reproduction, and Dermatology. Clinician-based courses in the second year include Hematology/Oncology, Musculoskeletal System, Cardiovascular Medicine, Pulmonary Medicine, Neurology, Clinical Psychiatry, Nephrology, Gastrointestinal System, Nutrition, and Clinical Endocrinology. Physical Diagnosis also continues throughout the entire second year. During the first two years, the students are in class approximately 30 hours per week, with an approximately equal distribution between lecture, student-centered discussion, and laboratory. The pre-clinical courses are taught in Tupper Hall, central to the UC Davis campus. The Health Science Library is adjacent to the complex, houses 142,000 volumes, and is fully computerized. The resources for the curriculum are provided by the Office of Curricular Support. Academic support for individual students is provided by the Office of Student Learning and Educational Resources (OSLER). An A–F grading system is used. Passing the USMLE Step 1 is a requirement for promotion to year three. In the last three years, the passing rate has been 100 percent. In addition to the formal courses, students gain clinical experience from volunteering in clinics such as Asian Clinic, Clinica Tepati, and Imani Clinic.

CLINICAL TRAINING: Third-year required clerkships are: Surgery (8 weeks); Medicine (8 weeks); Pediatrics (8 weeks); Ob/Gyn (8 weeks); Psychiatry (8 weeks); and Primary Care Plus (8 weeks), which includes four weeks in a family-practice setting and introduces primary care components of certain specialties. Required fourth-year clerkships are: Emergency Medicine (4 weeks); Physical Medicine and Rehabilitation (2 weeks); Ophthalmology (2 weeks); Neurology (2 weeks); and Otolaryngology (2 weeks). A two-week course that discusses the legal, ethical, and economic issues related to medicine is also required. Most of the fourth year is reserved for Selectives, chosen by the student within the directives of an oversight committee and Electives, which are unrestricted. Required clerkships take place at UC Davis Medical Center, in Sacramento (523 beds), and at Kaiser Permanente Hospital, David Grant Hospital (Travis Air Force Base), Sutter Hospital, Highland General (Oakland), and at community physician sites. Other clinical facilities include a new Shriners Hospital opened on the Sacramento campus to provide care to children with orthopedic and other disorders, an expanded hospital, the creation of the Ellison Ambulatory Care Center and the establishment of the Mather VA Hospital. Among these sites, students serve a diverse patient population. Selectives may be taken at any LCME-accredited medical school. Overseas clinical activities may be taken as electives with programs organized by the Departments of Family Practice and Epidemiology and Preventive Medicine, and through individual student efforts. Students must take the USMLE Step 2 in order to graduate.

Students

All but a few students in each class are California residents. Typically, Davis is among the top 10 schools nationwide in terms of its percentage of underrepresented minorities. There is also significant diversity in the age of incoming students, the average being 25 or 26. Class size is 93.

STUDENT LIFE: Although students live both on and off campus, student life is focused around the school. Recreational facilities on campus include the Recreation Hall, two swimming pools, a craft center, an equestrian center, a bowling alley, and tennis, handball, racquetball, volleyball, and basketball courts. The intramural program is popular with medical students. Student organizations, focused on professional and recreational interests and ethnic backgrounds, offer support and social opportunities to students. On-campus housing options include a residence hall with a dining room; one- and two-bedroom units; and student family housing, for married students. The Housing Listing Service assists students searching for off-campus accommodations.

GRADUATES: About 60 percent of graduates enter primary care fields. UC Davis Medical Center has at least 20 residency programs. Davis graduates are successful at obtaining residency positions in prestigious programs all over the country.

Admissions

REQUIREMENTS: The following courses must be completed prior to matriculation: English (1 year); Biology with lab (1 year); Chemistry with lab (1 year); Organic Chemistry (1 year); Physics (1 year); and Math (up to Differential Calculus). The MCAT is required and should have been taken within the past three years. For those who have repeated the MCAT, the best scores are considered.

SUGGESTIONS: Additional helpful courses are Biochemistry, Genetics, and Embryology. For students who have been out of school for a period of time, some recent course work is recommended. While no activities or qualities are specified, successful applicants demonstrate interpersonal skills, leadership potential, and the ability to work with diverse populations.

PROCESS: About 4,000 applicants, or roughly 50 percent of AMCAS applicants, receive secondaries. Secondary applications must be returned within a month. Only 500 applicants are interviewed, with interviews held from October through April. Interviews consist of two one-hour sessions with faculty members and/or medical students. About one-third of those interviewed are accepted on a rolling basis. Others are rejected or put on a wait list that is split into thirds, depending on the candidate's prospect for admission. Wait-listed candidates are not advised to send supplementary material.

Costs

The estimated cost of books for the first year is $2,016. Room, board, and additional living expenses range from $10,338 to $14,328. This includes a budget allocation for maintaining a car.

FINANCIAL AID: UC Davis offers grants and loans to students with financial need, as determined by the FAFSA process. Merit-based scholarships and awards aimed at students from disadvantaged backgrounds are also available. Parental financial disclosure is required for some forms of need-based assistance.

UNIVERSITY OF CALIFORNIA, DAVIS

STUDENT BODY

Type	Public
*Enrollment	406
*% male/female	50/50
*% underrepresented minorities	12
# applied (total/out)	9,231/NR
% interviewed (total/out)	10/NR
% accepted (total/out)	5/NR
% enrolled (total/out)	45/NR
Average age	25

ADMISSIONS

Average GPA and MCAT Scores

Overall GPA	3.5	Science GPA	3.50
MCAT Bio	11.44	MCAT Phys	11.25
MCAT Verbal	11.00	MCAT Essay	Q–R

Score Release Policy

Students have the right to withhold scores. There is no effect on the application if a student chooses this option.

Application Information

Regular application	11/1
Regular notification	10/15 until filled
†Transfers accepted?	Yes
Admissions may be deferred?	Yes
AMCAS application accepted?	Yes
Interview required?	Yes
Application fee	$40

COSTS AND AID

Tuition & Fees

Tuition (in/out)	$0/$9,384
Cost of books	$2,016
Fees	$9,900

Financial Aid

% students receiving aid	90
Average grant	$5,723
Average loan	$11,749
Average debt	$66,000

†Does not accept transfers from foreign schools

*Figures based on total enrollment

University of California, Irvine

COLLEGE OF MEDICINE

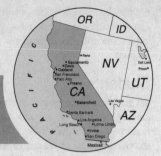

Medical Education Building 802, Irvine, CA 92697
Admission: 949-824-5388 • Fax: 949-824-2485
Email: pharvey1@uci.edu • Internet: www.com.uci.edu

The University of California Irvine (UCI) College of Medicine is located in Orange County, just an hour from Los Angeles and a few minutes from beautiful Southern California beaches. With only 92 students per class, UCI is able to provide personal attention to its students. Irvine is a public school, offering California residents an excellent medical education at an affordable price. The College of Medicine is renowned for its long-time emphasis on primary care, its innovative use of surrogate patients as a component of clinical instruction, and for its growth as a research center.

Academics

Four or five students each year enter the M.S.T.P. program, leading to a Ph.D. along with an M.D. The Ph.D. may be earned in a number of fields, including: Anatomy, Biochemistry, Biophysics, Microbiology, and Molecular Biology. For those who meet requirements, a joint M.B.A./M.D. program can be pursued in conjunction with UCI's Graduate School of Management. Most students follow a four-year curriculum, throughout which a course called Patient-Doctor integrates clinical, social, and basic science concepts.

BASIC SCIENCES: Irvine uses a quarter system. For the duration of year one, the course Patient-Doctor gives students an opportunity for interaction with real patients in a clinical setting and with simulated patients in a closely monitored learning environment. During the first quarter of year one, students also take Anatomy, Biochemistry, and Medical Genetics, all taught primarily in a lecture/lab format. During the second and third quarters, lecture/lab courses are the following: Histology, Neuroscience, Physiology, and Microbiology. The Patient-Doctor course continues throughout year two, using a case-based system to integrate basic science and other concepts such as ethical and statistical approaches to medicine. Second-year first-quarter courses are the following: Clinical Pathology, Pathology, and Pharmacology. The final quarter of year two serves as a transition into clinical studies. During this period, students focus on just one course—Mechanisms of Disease—in addition to Patient-Doctor. Tutorial programs, academic monitoring, and study-skills workshops promote student success in the basic sciences. The Medical Center Library (MCL) is located at the UCI Medical Center and meets the research, education, and patient care needs of the Medical Center staff and the UCI College of Medicine. The College of Medicine is fully computerized, with an internal electronic informational network. Students are evaluated with Honors, Pass, or Fail. The USMLE Step 1 is required for promotion to year three.

CLINICAL TRAINING: Patient contact begins when students learn interviewing techniques during the first year. Surrogate patients are employed, throughout the four years, to enhance interactive experience. During the third and fourth years, the Patient-Doctor course continues, teaching students to apply basic science concepts to clinical situations. Required clerkships begin in year three and include: Medicine (10 weeks); Ob/Gyn (9 weeks); Pediatrics (8 weeks); Psychiatry (8 weeks); and Surgery (10 weeks). The primary care requirement is satisfied through a year-long clerkship in which students work one half-day each week in a primary care physician's office. Year four rotations are Intensive Care Unit (4 weeks); Rehabilitation (4 weeks); Neuroscience (4 weeks); and Radiology (3 weeks). Fourth-year students choose from Surgical Selectives (4 weeks); Medically Related Electives (4 weeks); Surgically Related Electives (3 weeks); Senior Sub Internships (4 weeks) and Free Electives (7 weeks). The primary training sites are: UCI Medical Center in the City of Orange (462 beds), which includes several specialized clinical and research centers; the Veterans Administration Medical Center in Long Beach; and the College of Medicine's affiliated hospitals and clinics. Affiliates are located in Orange, Los Angeles, and San Bernardino counties, serving both rural and urban communities. During the clinical years, narrative evaluations supplement the Honors/Pass/Fail grading system. Passing the USMLE Step 2 is a requirement for graduation.

Students

About 5 percent of students are underrepresented minorities. Typically, the average age of entering classes is about 25, with a range in age from 20 to 30. Virtually all students are Californians, although many earn their undergraduate degrees from schools around the country.

STUDENT LIFE: UCI has many student-interest groups, including those that provide support to minority students and to students with children. Other groups, such as Students Teaching AIDS to Children, which organizes educational sessions in schools, are geared toward volunteer and community activities. Medical students have access to resources of the greater University, including cultural events, intramural athletics, and all facilities. On-campus, graduate-student housing is affordable, comfortable, and allows medical students to interact with students from other departments. Residence halls, apartments, and residential communities, that feature living spaces of all sizes, are available. The city of Irvine and nearby communities, such as Newport Beach, provide recreational opportunities and attractive housing options.

GRADUATES: A large proportion of graduates enter post-graduate programs at UCI, which has one of the nation's largest residency programs in primary care disciplines and internal medicine. Most graduates enter programs in California, but seniors have been successful in obtaining residencies all over the country. Of the 1997 graduating class, 69 percent entered primary care fields.

Admissions

REQUIREMENTS: Preference is given to California residents, with no more than one or two out-of-state candidates admitted in a given year. The following must be completed prior to matriculation: Chemistry (one year); Organic Chemistry (one year); Physics (one year); Biology (1.5 years); Calculus (1 quarter); and Biochemistry (1 semester or two quarters). The MCAT is required, and scores should be no more than three years old. For those who have retaken the exam, the most recent set of scores is considered.

SUGGESTIONS: A well-rounded liberal arts background is recommended, including courses in English, Humanities, and Social Sciences disciplines. Certain courses are considered to be particularly useful: Genetics, Cell Biology, Vertebrate Embryology, Physical Chemistry, and Spanish. For applicants who graduated college several years ago, some recent course work is advised. Involvement in clinical or research activities is important for all applicants. The Admissions Committee looks for qualities that are valuable in a physician, such as intellectual and emotional capabilities, dedication, and sensitivity.

PROCESS: About one-third of AMCAS applicants receive a secondary application. Of those returning secondaries, about one-third are interviewed. Interviews take place once a month, from October through April. The interview consists of two one-hour sessions, one with a faculty member and one with a student. Applicants are accepted on a rolling basis following interviews, to fill a class of 92. Others are put in a hold category, and either accepted or wait-listed later in the year. Wait-listed candidates may send supplementary information about course work or activities.

Costs

In addition to fees, the cost of living for a single student is estimated at $11,000 per year. This allows for on-campus housing and car ownership.

FINANCIAL AID: The FAFSA form is used to determine a student's financial need. Information on parents' financial resources is used to determine eligibility for certain federal programs, but is not generally used by UCI in making its awards. Institutional and private loans and scholarships are granted on the basis of need, academic merit, and other specialized criteria such as medical field of interest or ethnicity.

UNIVERSITY OF CALIFORNIA, IRVINE

STUDENT BODY

Type	Public
*Enrollment	396
*% male/female	56/44
*% underrepresented minorities	5
# applied (total/out)	3,931/386
% interviewed (total/out)	10/1
% accepted (total/out)	5/0
% enrolled (total/out)	44/0
Average age	25

ADMISSIONS

Average GPA and MCAT Scores

Overall GPA	3.67	Science GPA	3.65
MCAT Bio	11.01	MCAT Phys	10.78
MCAT Verbal	9.49	MCAT Essay	O

Score Release Policy

The school has not responded to our inquiry regarding withheld MCAT scores. Therefore, we advise caution. Contact the Admissions Office before withholding any scores.

Application Information

Regular application	11/1
Regular notification	11/15 until filled
Transfers accepted?	No
Admissions may be deferred?	Yes
AMCAS application accepted?	Yes
Interview required?	Yes
Application fee	$40

COSTS AND AID

Tuition & Fees

Tuition (in/out)	$0/$9,384
Cost of books	$3,200
Fees	$10,630

Financial Aid

% students receiving aid	87
Average grant	$2,900
Average loan	$13,700
Average debt	NR

*Figures based on total enrollment

UNIVERSITY OF CALIFORNIA, LOS ANGELES

UCLA SCHOOL OF MEDICINE

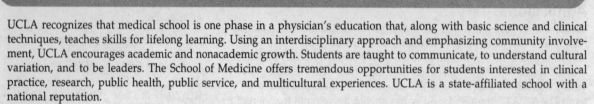

Office of Admissions, Box 957035, Los Angeles, CA 90095

Admission: 310-825-6081

Internet: www.medsch.ucla.edu/admiss

UCLA recognizes that medical school is one phase in a physician's education that, along with basic science and clinical techniques, teaches skills for lifelong learning. Using an interdisciplinary approach and emphasizing community involvement, UCLA encourages academic and nonacademic growth. Students are taught to communicate, to understand cultural variation, and to be leaders. The School of Medicine offers tremendous opportunities for students interested in clinical practice, research, public health, public service, and multicultural experiences. UCLA is a state-affiliated school with a national reputation.

Academics

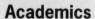

Each year, 10 students are admitted to an Extended Curriculum Program, which spreads the first two years of the standard curriculum over three years, creating opportunities for special projects or supplemental instruction. In each class, as many as 24 students who are interested in practicing in underserved communities spend their first two years at UCLA School of Medicine, and then complete clinical requirements at Drew University facilities. Drew University is a predominantly African American medical institution. Several joint-degree programs are offered to medical students, including an M.D./M.P.H. with the School of Public Health, an M.D./M.B.A. with the School of Management, and an M.S.T.P.-sponsored M.D./Ph.D. All entering students are required to purchase a computer because both the basic science and clinical curriculum emphasize its applications.

BASIC SCIENCES: During the first two years, students are in scheduled sessions for about 26 hours per week. In addition to required courses, Selectives give students an opportunity to explore topics of interest such as health care reform, addiction, and AIDS. Year-one courses are the following: Micro-Anatomy and Cell Biology; Topics in Physiology; Biological Chemistry; Anatomy; Organ System Physiology; Basic Neurology; Biomathematics; Doctoring I; and Clinical Applications of Basic Sciences (CAB.S.). Doctoring I is the beginning of the Doctoring Curriculum, which uses a case-based approach and addresses the interdisciplinary issues that pertain to practicing medicine. In this course, the cultural, ethical, legal, economic, and social perspectives on medicine are considered. In CAB.S., students participate in community-based, health education, or health care projects and learn to apply basic science concepts to real-life clinical problems. Year-two courses are the following: Microbiology; Pathology; Pharmacology; Pathophysiology; Psychopathology; Doctoring II; Genetics; and Clinical Fundamentals, which covers physical diagnosis and takes place largely at clinical sites. Both University-sponsored and student-initiated study and tutorial groups are available. Most classes are taught in the Health Sciences Building, a large structure on the UCLA campus in Westwood. The Biomedical Library is nearby and serves faculty, students, and the community with a collection of 500,000 volumes and 6,000 current journals. Grading is Pass/Fail, with written citations for outstanding achievement. Promotion to year three requires a passing score on the USMLE Step 1.

CLINICAL TRAINING: Outside of traditional clerkships, students gain experience with patients in Doctoring and through the extensive volunteer opportunities. Some students identify volunteer opportunities with the assistance of the Community Service Compendium, a list of community outreach sites. Formal clinical training takes place during the third and fourth years, which are treated as a continuum. Fifty-seven weeks of the third and fourth years are reserved for the following required rotations: Medicine (12 weeks); Surgery (12 weeks); Pediatrics (6 weeks); Ob/Gyn (6 weeks); Psychiatry (6 weeks); Family Medicine (6 weeks); Radiology (4 weeks); Neurology (2 weeks); and Ophthalmology (2 weeks). Clerkships take place primarily at the University Hospital (517 beds). Other affiliated sites are Harbor General (800 beds); Cedars-Sinai; Kaiser Sunset; Kaiser West LA; Kern Medical Center (Bakersfield); King/Drew Medical Center; Olive View-UCLA Medical Center (Sylmar); Sepulveda Veterans Affairs; St. Mary Medical Center (Long Beach); and West LA Veterans Affairs Medical Center. Doctoring III is taken throughout the years, occupying students for one full day every other week. This segment of the course takes students to community-based medical sites and uses a small-group format to discuss various patient problems. Twenty-seven weeks remain for electives. Some of the elective requirement may be fulfilled around the country or overseas. Grading is Pass/Fail supplemented with written evaluations. The USMLE Step 2 is required for graduation.

Students

The students reflect the multicultural population of Los Angeles, with underrepresented minorities accounting for one-third of the student body. In entering classes, the average age is 22, and there are usually no more than a few students over 28 years old. Eighty-five percent of the students are California residents. Class size is 145.

STUDENT LIFE: In addition to the beaches and beautiful weather of Southern California and Los Angeles, the UCLA campus itself offers excellent athletic facilities and plenty of entertainment. Student-led groups and activities within the medical school are numerous, ranging from the Iranian/American Medical Organization, to the Salvation Army Outreach Clinic. The medical school also sponsors activities that encourage cohesion between faculty and students. Although residence halls and married-student housing are available, most medical students opt to live off campus.

GRADUATES: Graduates are well-prepared for careers in primary care, more specialized clinical fields, and research. About half of the graduates enter primary care fields, which is roughly the current national average. Many enter residencies at UCLA or affiliated hospitals.

Admissions

REQUIREMENTS: Admissions requirements are: English (one year); college Math (one year, to include calculus and statistics); Physics (one year); Chemistry (two years, including inorganic and organic); and Biology (one year). Science courses must have associated labs, and AP credits are not counted. The MCAT is required, and scores must be no more than three years old. Generally, if a student has retaken the exam, the best set of scores is used.

SUGGESTIONS: Courses in Humanities and Social Sciences, as well as Spanish and Computer Skills are highly recommended. Undergraduate courses that overlap with those in the medical school curriculum, such as Anatomy, are not recommended. For applicants who graduated college several years ago, recent course work is expected. The April, rather than August, MCAT is advised. Extracurricular activities that are medically related, or that involve research or patient contact, are useful. UCLA is unusual among state-affiliated medical schools in California in that it welcomes applications from well-qualified, out-of-state residents.

PROCESS: Typically, 55 percent of AMCAS applicants are asked to submit supplementary information. Of those returning secondaries, about 20 percent are invited for interviews. Interviews take place from November through May and consist of one or two sessions with faculty members and/or medical students. Notification begins in January and continues until enough offers have been made to fill the class. About 25 percent of interviewees are accepted, and another group is wait-listed. Wait-listed candidates may send additional information about academic or extracurricular achievements. The UCLA/UC Riverside Biomedical Sciences Program allows 24 admitted students to obtain both the B.S. and M.D. degrees in 7 years. In this program, students enter UCLA School of Medicine after completing 3 years of undergraduate preparation at UC Riverside.

Costs

The anticipated student budget ranges from $12,000–$15,000. These figures assume shared housing and car ownership. First-year students are required to have a computer, the cost of which is figured into the student budget.

FINANCIAL AID: Most assistance is based on financial need, as determined by the FAFSA form and Needs Access Diskette. Parental financial information is required for some need-based assistance. A few merit-based Regents Scholarships are also offered.

UNIVERSITY OF CALIFORNIA, LOS ANGELES

STUDENT BODY

Type	Public
*Enrollment	674
*% male/female	58/42
*% underrepresented minorities	30
# applied (total/out)	5,244/1,733
% interviewed (total/out)	12/3
% accepted (total/out)	NR/NR
% enrolled (total/out)	21/10

ADMISSIONS

Average GPA and MCAT Scores

Overall GPA	NR	Science GPA	3.64
MCAT Bio	NR	MCAT Phys	NR
MCAT Verbal	NR	MCAT Essay	NR

Score Release Policy

There is no problem if a student chooses to withhold scores; the Admissions Committee tries to give applicants "the benefit of the doubt."

Application Information

Regular application	11/1
Regular notification	1/15–8/1
Admissions may be deferred?	Yes
AMCAS application accepted?	Yes
Interview required?	No
Application fee	$40

COSTS AND AID

Tuition & Fees

Tuition (in/out)	$0/$9,993
Cost of books	NR
Fees	$9,938

Financial Aid

% students receiving aid	NR
Average grant	NR
Average loan	NR
Average debt	NR

*Figures based on total enrollment

University of California, San Diego

SCHOOL OF MEDICINE

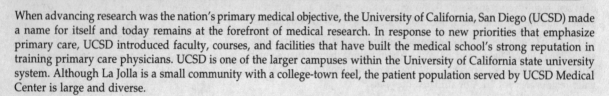

9500 Gilman Drive, La Jolla, CA 92093

Admission: 619-534-3880 • Fax: 619-534-5282

Internet: www.medicine.ucsd.edu

When advancing research was the nation's primary medical objective, the University of California, San Diego (UCSD) made a name for itself and today remains at the forefront of medical research. In response to new priorities that emphasize primary care, UCSD introduced faculty, courses, and facilities that have built the medical school's strong reputation in training primary care physicians. UCSD is one of the larger campuses within the University of California state university system. Although La Jolla is a small community with a college-town feel, the patient population served by UCSD Medical Center is large and diverse.

Academics

In addition to fulfilling course requirements, students must complete an Independent Study Project to graduate. These projects allow students to explore and define their own interests, and to collaborate with faculty members who share these interests. The medical school benefits from the resources of other parts of UCSD. Joint M.D./ Ph.D. programs are possible with UCSD Graduate Departments in Biochemistry, Biomedical Engineering; Biophysics, Cell Biology, Genetics, Immunology, Microbiology, Molecular Biology, Neuroscience, Pathology, Pharmacology, and Physiology. Normally, these degrees are M.S.T.P. sponsored. Students can earn an M.P.H. in conjunction with nearby San Diego State University Graduate School of Public Health.

BASIC SCIENCES: The first two years are organized into quarters. Electives are an important supplement to basic science requirements and account for about 20 percent of scheduled course time. During the fall quarter of year one, Cell Biology and Biochemistry is the principal endeavor. This lecture course is referred to as a "block," which means that the material is covered intensely during one or two quarters. Students also begin a sequence in Social and Behavioral Sciences, taught mostly through small-group sessions. Winter-quarter courses are Physiology, Pharmacology, and Introduction to Clinical Medicine, which continues throughout the basic science curriculum and prepares students for third-year rotations. The spring-quarter courses are Neurology, Pharmacology, Reproductive Biology, Metabolism, and Endocrinology, all of which are taught primarily through lectures. Year two begins with Anatomy, Histology, Biostatistics, and a Social/Behavioral Science course on Health Care Systems. Winter quarter consists of Human Disease, Psychopathology, and Hematology. The second-year, spring-quarter curriculum is Human Disease, Neurology, and Lab Medicine. During the basic science years there are, on average, 34 scheduled hours per week. Instruction takes place in the modern Basic

Science Building, which is adjacent to the Biomedical Library (100,000 volumes). Computers with access to online informational services and curricular programs are available for student use in the library and in the School's Learning Resource Center. Grading uses an Honors/Pass/ Fail system. The USMLE Step 1 is required for promotion to year three.

CLINICAL TRAINING: Supervised patient contact begins in January of year one, in Introduction to Clinical Medicine. The physical examination is taught in conjunction with the study of individual organ systems in the first year, and together with the history, refined in the second basic science year. In addition, a simulated-patient program provides students the opportunity to improve their history-taking and physical-examination skills, as well as to obtain feedback from faculty mentors and view videotapes of their patient interaction. Required third-year rotations are Medicine (12 weeks); Neurology (4weeks); Ob/Gyn (6 weeks); Pediatrics (8 weeks); Psychiatry (6 weeks); Surgery (12 weeks); and Primary Care (one afternoon per week, all year). Students design their fourth-year curricula by selecting courses from within broad subject areas. Twelve weeks are selected from Direct Patient Care Clerkships, 4 weeks must be a Primary Care experience, 4 weeks Inpatient Training, and 4 weeks Outpatient Training. An additional 12 weeks of pure elective, clinical clerkships are also required. Clinical training takes place at large hospitals and small clinics including: UCSD Medical Centers (577 beds total); VA Hospital (606 beds); Navy Hospital (750 beds); Children's Hospital (154 beds); Kaiser Foundation Hospital (1,285 beds); Sharp Memorial Community Hospital (1,415 beds); Clinica De Salubridad de Campesinos; and the U.S. Public Health Service Outpatient Clinic. Electives may be taken from the various departments of UCSD, or may be carried out in conjunction with community organizations. Most students take advantage of additional clinical training opportunities through volunteer work, some of which takes them across the border in Mexico. The USMLE Step 2 is required for graduation. UCSD students do exceptionally well on both parts of the USMLE.

Students

Students are predominantly Californians. There is a wide age range among students, and it is very common for them to have taken a year or two off after college for research or other activities. About 60 percent of incoming students in a recent class were science majors. Class size is 122.

STUDENT LIFE: On-campus housing is convenient, attractive, and popular with students. Modern apartments of all sizes are available for single and married students and for those who have children or pets. Some students rely on bicycles or shuttle buses, while others own cars. UCSD's location affords many recreational possibilities. Year-round outdoor activities include swimming, surfing, biking, sailing, rollerblading, running, and walking. Other activities are the San Diego Symphony, the zoo, and the Padres professional baseball team. Medical student organizations and events also contribute to students' extracurricular lives.

GRADUATES: Of the graduating class of 1997, the most popular fields for post-graduate training were Internal Medicine (22 graduates); Family Medicine (18); Pediatrics (17); Ob/Gyn (11); Emergency Medicine (11); Surgery (8); Radiology (4); Otolaryngology (3); Dermatology (2); and Ophthalmology (2). Many entered programs in San Diego, Oakland, San Jose, Los Angeles, and other California locations.

Admissions

REQUIREMENTS: One year of Chemistry, Organic Chemistry, Biology, Physics, and Math are all required. Strong written and spoken English is a requirement, and the ability to communicate in a second language is preferred. The rigor of an applicant's undergraduate institution is considered in assessing GPA. The MCAT is required, and the spring exam is advised.

SUGGESTIONS: Breadth of academic experience is important. Extracurricular activities are also important, particularly those that involve some sort of medical exposure, community involvement, or leadership.

PROCESS: About 40 percent of applicants receive a secondary application. Of those returning secondaries, about 500 are interviewed. Interviews take place from October through May and consist of two one-hour sessions with faculty members. Following interviews, candidates are accepted, rejected, or put on hold for later notification. About half of those interviewed are eventually accepted. An extensive wait list is established.

Costs

Yearly living expenses, beyond the $10,000 student fee, are estimated to be $13,000. This budget allows for car ownership and either on- or off-campus housing. The average accrued debt for 1997 graduates who used loans was $53,000.

FINANCIAL AID: Most aid is based on financial need although some merit-based scholarships exist. Scholarships and school-sponsored loans attempt to meet the financial needs of students after they secure $8,500 in a subsidized, federal Stafford loan each year.

UNIVERSITY OF CALIFORNIA, SAN DIEGO

STUDENT BODY

Type	Public
*Enrollment	495
*% male/female	58/42
*% underrepresented minorities	9
# applied (total/out)	4,627/1,241
% interviewed	13/1
% accepted (total/out)	NR/NR
% enrolled (total/out)	21/NR
Average age	23

ADMISSIONS

Average GPA and MCAT Scores

Overall GPA	3.74	Science GPA	3.70
MCAT Bio	10.00	MCAT Phys	11.00
MCAT Verbal	11.00	MCAT Essay	NR

Score Release Policy

The Admissions Committee does not see withholding scores as a problem.

Application Information

Regular application	11/1
Regular notification	10/15 until filled
Transfers accepted?	No
Admissions may be deferred?	Yes
AMCAS application accepted?	Yes
Interview required?	Yes
Application fee	$40

COSTS AND AID

Tuition & Fees

Tuition (in/out)	$0/$9,384
Cost of books	$1,134
Fees	$10,324

Financial Aid

% students receiving aid	75
Average grant	NR
Average loan	NR
Average debt	$53,000

*Figures based on total enrollment

UNIVERSITY OF CALIFORNIA, SAN FRANCISCO

SCHOOL OF MEDICINE

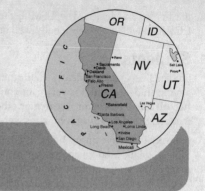

Admissions, C-200, Box 0408, San Francisco, CA 94143

Admission: 415-476-4044

Internet: www.som.ucsf.edu

The University of California, San Francisco (UCSF) is regarded as one of the best medical schools in the country, in part for the excellent research and clinical instruction it offers. Separating UCSF from schools of the same tier is its absolute dedication to community service. The patient population is urban, with a large contingent of native Spanish speakers and a relatively high prevalence of HIV. Clinical rotations also take students to underserved rural areas. The UCSF/Stanford merger will not affect the respective medical schools, but may enhance clinical opportunities for students.

Academics

While the majority of students earn an M.D. in four years, some devote an additional year to research activities. Twelve students each year enter a five-year program organized in collaboration with the School of Public Health at the University of California, Berkeley. These students earn a master's degree from Berkeley along with an M.D. from UCSF. Up to eight students enter the M.S.T.P. joint Ph.D./M.D. program yearly. Participants may earn a Ph.D. from the following UCSF departments: Anatomy, Biochemistry, Biophysics, Cell Biology, Developmental Biology, Endocrinology, Genetics, Immunology, Neuroscience, Pathology, Pharmaceutical Chemistry, and Physiology.

BASIC SCIENCES: The first two years are organized into quarters. Year-one, fall-quarter courses are Cell and Tissue Biology and Gross Anatomy. Winter courses are Metabolism, Head and Neck Anatomy, and Organ Physiology. Spring-quarter courses are Neuroscience, Endocrine and G.I. Physiology, Medical Genetics, and Epidemiology/Biostatistics. Throughout year one, students take Foundations of Patient Care. Year-two, fall-quarter curriculum is Immunology, Microbiology, and Reproduction, Growth, and Development. Winter is Introduction to Clinical Radiology. Spring is Introduction to Clinical Psychiatry and Parasitology. In addition, throughout year two, students take Pathology, Pharmacology, Introduction to Clinical Medicine, and Foundations of Patient Care. Lectures, labs, small-group discussions, and other scheduled sessions account for about 28 hours per week. For most lectures, students have access to detailed course outlines and notes so that class time can be devoted to listening and thinking rather than note-taking. Students have input into curriculum development through the Student-Faculty Liaison Committee. Grading is strictly Pass/Fail. The main library has 900,000 volumes subscribes to over 2,400 print journals, and 500 electronic journals. All major online informational services are available, and computers for student use are plentiful throughout campus. A passing score on USMLE

Step 1 is required for promotion to third year, and students must take Step 2 before graduation.

CLINICAL TRAINING: Patient contact begins during year one in Foundations of Patient Care. Clinical elements are gradually integrated into the basic science curriculum, allowing a smooth transition into the third year. Likewise, the clinical years include segments of classroom instruction that focus on basic science concepts. For example, fourth-year students take Mechanics of Disease, which uses lectures, case studies, and basic science principles to address illness. Required clerkships are Anesthesia (2 weeks); Family and Community Medicine (6 weeks); Medicine (8 weeks); Neurology (4 weeks); Ob/Gyn (6 weeks); Pediatrics (6 weeks); Psychiatry (6 weeks); Surgery (6 weeks;) and Surgical Specialties (4 weeks). Teaching sites are primarily in San Francisco, Oakland, and Fresno and include California Pacific Medical Center; Children's Hospital; Kaiser Foundation Hospitals; Mt. Zion Hospital and Medical Center of UCSF; San Francisco City Clinics; San Francisco General Hospital; Veterans Affairs Medical Center in San Francisco and Fresno; University Medical Center-Fresco; and Langly Porter Neuropsychiatric Institute. In between the third and fourth years, students take a course in Ethics. Year four is primarily elective study, which may entail research or international work in addition to traditional clinical rotations. Evaluation of students during years three and four uses an Honors/Pass/Fail system enhanced with written evaluations. Outside of clerkships, students gain clinical exposure through volunteer work at any number of UCSF-affiliated projects.

Students

Twenty percent of the student body are out-of-state residents. More than half are nonwhite, and more than 20 percent are underrepresented minorities, mostly African and Hispanic Americans. In a recent entering class, the age range among students was 20–39. Virtually all undergraduate majors are represented in the student body. Class size is 141.

STUDENT LIFE: University-owned housing appropriate for both married and single students is available. Many students take part in community programs, which provide not only an opportunity to contribute, but also a chance for student-student and student-faculty interaction in an extracurricular setting. Students have access to school athletic facilities and to many local, outdoor activities including running in Golden Gate Park, surfing at Ocean Beach, mountain biking in Marin County, and skiing around Lake Tahoe, four hours away by car.

GRADUATES: Of the graduating class of 1997, the following specialties were selected by the indicated number of students: Family Practice (16); Internal Medicine (16); Internal Medicine/Primary Care (13); Pediatrics (13); Emergency Medicine (13); Psychiatry (11); Ob/Gyn (10); Surgery (9); Orthopedic Surgery (6); Neurology (6); Opthalmology (4); Dermatology (4); Pediatrics/Primary Care (4); Medicine/Pediatrics (4); Transitional (3); Anesthesia (2); Neurosurgery (2); Radiology (2); Otolaryngology (2); and all others (5). In total, 49 percent entered residencies in fields classified as Primary Care. About one-third of graduates enter residency programs in UCSF-affiliated hospitals. Another third train at other sites in California.

Admissions

REQUIREMENTS: To be considered for admission, applicants must have taken: General Chemistry with lab (three quarters, equal to one year); Organic Chemistry (two quarters); Physics with lab (three quarters); and Biology with lab (four quarters). Applications are welcome from candidates who have taken time off between college and applying to medical school. The MCAT is required, and the spring MCAT is strongly advised. For those who retake the test, the most recent scores are considered. However, in most cases those who withhold scores from AMCAS are disqualified from the admissions process. MCAT scores must be no more than three years old. California residents are given preference.

SUGGESTIONS: Beyond requirements, applicants should have taken college-level Math, Humanities, and English courses. Upper-division Biology is also recommended. All extracurricular activities that reveal an applicant's interests and demonstrate his or her commitment strengthen the application. Some exposure to medical issues or to patient care is also valuable.

PROCESS: GPA, MCATs, residency, and the AMCAS applications are used to screen for secondary applications. The secondary application is straightforward and does not require additional essays. Applicants have one month from the date of receipt of the secondary application to the deadline for return. About 30 percent of applicants receive a secondary application and about one-third of those returning secondaries are invited to interview. There is also a "hold" category, which indicates that while the applicant is not in the top group, he or she may be interviewed as the year progresses. Interviews take place between September and March, and consist of two one-hour blind sessions each with a faculty member or one faculty member and one student. After offers have been made to fill the class, some remaining candidates are placed on a ranked wait list and may be offered a spot as late as August, depending on accepted students' matriculation rate.

Costs

Beyond tuition and fees, anticipated yearly expenses for a single student are about $14,000 per year. This presumes shared off-campus housing and use of public transportation.

FINANCIAL AID: With the exception of a handful of Regents Scholarships offered to all University of California medical schools, aid is entirely need based. Need is determined by the income and assets of the student and in some cases of his or her family.

UNIVERSITY OF CALIFORNIA, SAN FRANCISCO

STUDENT BODY

Type	Public
*Enrollment	626
*% male/female	40/60
*% underrepresented minorities	17
# applied (total/out)	5,508/2,654
% interviewed	11
% accepted (total/out)	23/69
% enrolled (total/out)	14/31

ADMISSIONS

Average GPA and MCAT Scores

Overall GPA	3.75	Science GPA	3.75
MCAT Bio	12.00	MCAT Phys	11.00
MCAT Verbal	11.00	MCAT Essay	O

Score Release Policy

The Admissions Committee prefers that all scores be released, but they only use the most recent MCAT. Students are often at a disadvantage if they withhold scores.

Application Information

Regular application	11/1
Regular notification	12/15 until filled
Transfers accepted?	No
Admissions may be deferred?	No/rarely
AMCAS application accepted?	Yes
Interview required?	Yes
Application fee	$40

COSTS AND AID

Tuition & Fees

Tuition (in/out)	$0/$8,984
Cost of books	NR
Fees	$9,940

Financial Aid

% students receiving aid	80
Average grant	NR
Average loan	NR
Average debt	$56,228

*Figures based on total enrollment

CASE WESTERN RESERVE UNIVERSITY
SCHOOL OF MEDICINE

10900 Euclid Avenue, Cleveland, OH 44106
Admission: 216-368-3450 • Fax: 216-368-4621
Internet: mediswww.cwru.edu

The School of Medicine is part of the greater institution, Case Western Reserve University, which offers undergraduate, graduate, and professional programs including a School of Management and a Law School. Medical students take advantage of other parts of the University through The Flexible Program, which encourages elective study. Although historically known for its research and still a major recipient of federal research funding, Case Western has earned a reputation for excellence in teaching and primary care training. Case Western is also known for the diversity of its student body of which at least 10 percent are over 30 years old. Curricular options encourage students to pursue primary care, another emphasis of the school. Case Western is located just outside of downtown Cleveland and benefits from the cultural and intellectual life of the city.

Academics

The curriculum is decidedly nontraditional, combining several approaches to learning and two distinct paths, each of which provides flexibility. All students participate in the Core Academic Program (CAP), which incorporates the Core Physician Development Program (CPDP), a case-based system. Patient Based Learning (PBL) is introduced in year one, required clerkships in year three, and the Flexible Program allows students to participate in pre-clinical and clinical electives throughout the four years. Students who elect the Primary Care Tract (PCT) have enhanced clinical opportunities early in the program and direct contact with primary care providers throughout medical school. Joint M.D./Ph.D. programs are offered in Physiology, Engineering, and Biophysics and in 13 divisions of Biomedical Sciences including Nutritional Sciences and Environmental Health. Approximately 10 students in each class are admitted as M.D./Ph.D. candidates. A B.A./M.D. is offered in conjunction with the undergraduate college, and approximately 10 students matriculate as part of this program yearly.

BASIC SCIENCES: During the first year, students are presented Cellular and Developmental Biology, Integrated Human Physiology, and the Cellular Basis of Disease by faculty teaching teams representing both basic science and clinical departments. Each course lasts two months and is followed by an exam. For the remainder of the first year and for the duration of year two, students cover basic sciences through study of the individual organ systems, and students retain the information with the help the case-study approach. With this integrated approach to learning, students attend class, and student note-taking collectives are not emphasized. Afternoons are generally free from scheduled courses, allowing for elective study or research. Computer facilities support classroom learning, and computers loaded with first- and second-year course material are available in the MicroComputer Lab. The Health Center Library houses 150,000 volumes. Grading is Pass/Fail. Students choose their own academic advisors and have a great deal of control over their own courses of study. The USMLE Steps 1 and 2 are required for graduation.

CLINICAL TRAINING: Students have ample opportunity for clinical training outside of traditional clerkships. Most students begin their clinical responsibilities during the first year when they are assigned to either a pregnant woman in the Family Clinic or a patient in the geriatric care program. For two years the student follows the patient and his or her development. Second-year students learn physical diagnosis and history-taking under the supervision of physician preceptors. In the third year, required rotations include Medicine, Ob/Gyn, Pediatrics, Psychiatry, Surgery, Neuroscience, and Family Medicine. Fourth year is devoted to clinical electives. Training takes place at affiliated teaching hospitals including the University Hospitals of Cleveland, Metro-Health Medical Center, Saint Luke's, VA Cleveland, Mount Sinai Medical Center, and the Henry Ford Health System. Some training takes place in clinics rather than in a traditional hospital setting. The patient population represents urban Cleveland and rural Ohio. The Primary Care Tract is a relatively new mechanism for encouraging and training primary care physicians that promotes ongoing student-physician mentorships and intensive primary-care clinical training. Grading during years three and four is pass/fail/honors.

Students

Case Western is partially supported by the State of Ohio and gives preference to in-state residents, which is reflected in its matriculates: 60 percent of students are Ohio residents. The student body is slightly more mature than average and is particularly diverse in terms of experience and background. Class size is about 135.

STUDENT LIFE: Although campus residence halls are available, most students choose to live off campus and most rely on cars for transportation to and from school. University-sponsored, married-student housing is unavailable. Student groups are involved in both community and social activities. The structure of the academic program allows time for extra-curricular activities, and students participate in both University and community events.

GRADUATES: Of the 140 graduates of a recent class, 52 went on to residency programs in Cleveland; another 5 remained in Ohio. The rest went to: California (7), Georgia (4), Illinois (5), Maryland (5), Michigan (6), New York (7), Pennsylvania (8), Texas (4), Washington (8), and other states (1–3). Specialties were: Family Medicine (22), Surgery (17), Pediatrics (13), Radiology (7), Ob/Gyn (9), Orthopedic Surgery (5), Psychiatry (5), Emergency Medicine (4), Anesthesiology (3), Neurology (3), Ophthalmology (3), Pathology (3), Urology (2), Transitional (2), Neurosurgery (2), Physical Medicine (1), and Plastic Surgery (1).

Admissions

REQUIREMENTS: One year of Biology, one of Physics, and two of Chemistry, which should include cover both organic and inorganic, are required. In addition, students should demonstrate writing ability through course work. Recent academic performance is more heavily weighted, and although many older students are admitted, most have taken some relevant courses within the past two years. The MCAT is required, and the most recent set of scores is considered. Due to the rolling admissions process, applicants are encouraged to submit materials as soon as possible.

SUGGESTIONS: Case offers no further recommendations for college courses, and accepts students of all undergraduate majors.

PROCESS: About half of those submitting AMCAS applications receive a secondary. Secondaries should be completed promptly and are due by December 15 at the latest. Less than one-third of those completing secondaries are interviewed, with interviews held from September to March. Students have a one-on-one interview with a faculty member that generally lasts one hour. Those interviewed are notified shortly afterward of their status: accept, reject, or wait list. The wait list is not ranked. About half of the students who are accepted decline the offer, freeing up spaces for wait-listed applicants. Wait-listed candidates may submit additional material and should indicate if Case Western is their top choice. All Case Western undergraduates are invited to interview at the Medical School.

Costs

The anticipated yearly cost of living is about $15,000. This figure presumes living off campus, but it does not account for car expenses.

FINANCIAL AID: Students are expected to borrow $8,500 in subsidized Stafford loan and $13,500 in unsubsidized loans before qualifying for institutional support, which is generally about 30 percent grant and 70 percent loan. Parental financial information is required. Case Western offers up to 15 merit scholarships of $20,000 per year to students demonstrating outstanding academic and personal achievement.

CASE WESTERN RESERVE UNIVERSITY

STUDENT BODY

Type	Private
*Enrollment	587
*% male/female	57/43
*% underrepresented minorities	14
# applied (total/out)	7,308/6,217
% interviewed (total/out)	14/8
% accepted (total/out)	NR/NR
% enrolled (total/out)	15/10

ADMISSIONS

Average GPA and MCAT Scores

Overall GPA	3.60	Science GPA	NR
MCAT Bio	10.6	MCAT Phys	10.6
MCAT Verbal	10.6	MCAT Essay	NR

Score Release Policy

The school has not responded to our inquiry regarding withheld MCAT scores. Therefore, we advise caution. Contact the Admissions Office before withholding any scores.

Application Information

Regular application	10/15
Regular notification	10/15 until filled
Early application	6/1–8/1
Early notification	10/1
Admissions may be deferred?	Yes
AMCAS application accepted?	Yes
Interview required?	No
Application fee	$60

COSTS AND AID

Tuition & Fees

Tuition	$28,600
Cost of books	NR
Fees	$890

Financial Aid

% students receiving aid	75
Average grant	NR
Average loan	NR
Average debt	NR

*Figures based on total enrollment

University of Chicago

PRITZKER SCHOOL OF MEDICINE

924 East 57th Street, BLSC 104, Chicago, IL 60637
Admission: 773-702-1937 • Fax: 773-702-2598
Internet: pritzker.bsd.uchicago.edu

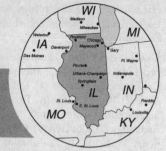

The Pritzker School of Medicine is the medical school at the University of Chicago, a private university in the city of Chicago. Pritzker is but one of the many impressive institutions/departments of the University, all of which share one campus. Pritzker values interdisciplinary studies, and medical students are encouraged to take advantage of the resources of the greater University. Although recognized as a premier research institution, the University of Chicago also puts a great deal of emphasis on teaching and developing clinical skills. As the nation's "most celebrated teacher of teachers," an unusually high number of Pritzker graduates go into academic medicine. Located in one of America's great cities, Pritzker is able to provide its students with intensive clinical exposure and a vibrant social life. Pritzker attracts students who enjoy research (one of the questions on the supplementary application asks specifically about research experience) and who seek a great deal of opportunity both in their academic and personal lives.

Academics

Pritzker offers a curriculum best characterized as "modified traditional." Although most pre-clinical topics are presented in lecture, case-based methods and clinical exposure supplement lectures. For example, as students study particular parts in Anatomy, they view afflictions of that body part in a clinical setting. About 20 percent of the students in each class earn a graduate degree in addition to the M.D. degree. Some of these students are M.S.T.P. participants; others are privately funded M.D./Ph.D. students, and still others earn a J.D. or an M.B.A. along with the M.D.

BASIC SCIENCES: Chicago follows a quarter system. Fall quarter, first-year medical students study Biochemistry and Molecular Biology; Human Morphology I; and Clinical Skills 1A, which introduces students to the patient interview. During the winter, first-year students study Molecular and Cell Biology, Cell and Organ Physiology, Human Morphology II, Doctor/Patient Relationships, and Clinical Skills 1B, which covers social issues related to medicine. Spring curriculum includes Organ Physiology, Neurobiology, Medical Genetics, Development and Psychopathology, and an opportunity for elective study. Second-year, fall-quarter curriculum includes: Immuno-Biology, Microbiology, Pharmacology and Cell Pathology. Winter quarter includes: Clinical Pathophysiology and Clinical Skills 2A, called Physical Diagnosis. The final quarter of pre-clinical studies includes Therapeutics, more clinical skills, Epidemiology, and Nutrition. Most students use a student-run note-taking co-op in which each participating student is responsible for providing notes on a lecture assigned to him or her. First- and second-year students spend their time in the new Biological Sciences Learning Center, which is both a center for instruction and research. Classrooms are equipped with audio/video technology, and excellent computer-based learning tools are available. The Knapp Center is a new medical research facility with modern laboratory space. The Crerar Library has one of the largest science collections in the country and houses almost one million volumes. Grading is Pass/Fail although students pay attention to their percentile rank on exams. Tutoring is available for students who are "deficient," or, in other words, are close to failure. The USMLE is not required for graduation although most students choose to take Step 1 after year two.

CLINICAL TRAINING: Students are introduced to clinical techniques and experiences during their first quarter at Prizker, with Clinical Skills 1A. Year three is composed of a series of clerkships with short breaks between rotations. Clerkships take place at the University of Chicago Hospitals and Health Systems and at Weiss Memorial Hospital. Recently, a new primary-care clerkship was developed and established at MacNeal Hospital. These hospitals serve a broad community, and students learn to treat a diverse patient population. Students rotate through the following departments: Internal Medicine (3 months); Ob/Gyn (2 months); Psychiatry (1 month); Surgery (3 months); Pediatrics (2 months); and Family Medicine (1 month), a new addition to the requirements. During the fourth year, students choose "selectives" from the following categories: Inpatient/Subinternship, Scientific Basis of Medical Practice, Neurology, and Anesthesia. The fourth year is also an opportunity for students to pursue individual research projects or to study overseas. The University of Chicago Medical facilities have expanded significantly during the past decade, suggesting a strong patient base and economic situation. Evaluation of clinical performance uses marks of Honors, High Pass, Pass, Low Pass, and Fail. Though the USMLE II is not required for graduation, it may be substituted for a comprehensive exam, which is otherwise required.

Students

Typically, Pritzker attracts research-oriented students. Underrepresented minorities have accounted for about 14 percent of the student body, and women about 50 percent. Class size is 104.

Student Life: The University of Chicago is located in Hyde Park, a diverse and interesting community; downtown Chicago is a 20-minute commute by car or by public transportation. Students are also active in curriculum development and have representatives on important administrative councils. Student volunteer organizations are involved in projects such as organizing and implementing health education into public schools. Medical students take part in university-wide activities such as intramural sports.

Graduates: During the past five years, the residency programs that attracted the most Pritzker graduates were: University of Chicago Hospital; UCSF; University of Michigan; Mass General; University of Washington; University of Penn; Brigham and Women's Boston; McGaw Medical Center; and UCLA. The following specialties were the most popular within the 2000 graduating class: Internal Medicine (24); Pediatrics (10); Surgery (5); Ob/Gyn (5); Dermatology (4); Ophthalmology (4); Family Practice (3); Orthopedic Surgery (4); Internal Medicine/Pediatrics (2); Anesthesiology (4); and Emergency Medicine (4). About 20 percent of Pritzker graduates ultimately serve as faculty members at universities.

Admissions

Requirements: One year of lecture plus lab is required in: Biology, General Chemistry, Organic Chemistry, and Physics. Biochemistry with lab may be substituted for one semester of organic chemistry. For applicants who graduated from college more than three years prior, recent science course work is important. The MCAT is required and should be no more than three years old. Although Pritzker is private, it seeks to matriculate 35 percent of the student body as Illinois residents.

Suggestions: Biochemistry is strongly recommended, as is significant course work in social sciences and humanities. The Admissions Committee is interested in what factors motivated applicants to pursue medicine and is also concerned with demonstrated problem-solving skills.

Process: Secondary applications are sent to all AMCAS applicants and should be returned as soon as possible, no later than January 1. About 20 percent of applicants returning secondaries are interviewed, with interviews held between October and April. Interviewees participate in three one-on-one sessions with faculty members and/or medical students. Of those interviewed, about one-third are accepted on a rolling basis, and the rest are placed on a wait list. Wait-listed candidates are encouraged to submit information that will strengthen their application and will indicate their interest in the school.

Costs

Living expenses are estimated at $14,000 per year, based on a budget which includes student fees, books, health insurance, and so forth. A car is not necessary.

Financial Aid: Parental and student assets and income are considered in determining financial need. Pritzker offers scholarships after a specified unit loan is assumed by the student. Many low-interest loans are available. There are no merit-based awards, but special assistance packages are available to students who are willing to commit to primary care specialties. Students in joint-degree programs are often funded either through federal or departmental sources.

UNIVERSITY OF CHICAGO

STUDENT BODY

Type	Private
*Enrollment	423
*% male/female	50/50
*% underrepresented minorities	14
# applied (total/out)	7,443/6,423
% interviewed (total/out)	8/7
% accepted (total/out)	3/3
% enrolled (total/out)	18/15
Average age	24

ADMISSIONS

Average GPA and MCAT Scores

Overall GPA	3.61	Science GPA	3.60
MCAT Bio	10.70	MCAT Phys	10.80
MCAT Verbal	10.10	MCAT Essay	Q

Score Release Policy

Scores should be withheld only in unusual circumstances. Explanation should accompany the application.

Application Information

Regular application	11/15
Regular notification	10/15 until filled
Early application	6/1–8/1
Early notification	10/1
Transfers accepted?	Yes
Admissions may be deferred?	Yes
AMCAS application accepted?	Yes
Interview required?	Yes
Application fee	$60

COSTS AND AID

Tuition & Fees

Tuition	$26,328
Cost of books	$882
Fees	$910

Financial Aid

% students receiving aid	86
Average grant	NR
Average loan	NR
Average debt	$89,563

*Figures based on total enrollment

UNIVERSITY OF CINCINNATI

COLLEGE OF MEDICINE

231 Bethesda Avenue, Rm E-251, M.S.B, Cincinnati, OH 45267-0552
Admission: 513-558-7314 • Fax: 513-558-1165
Internet: www.med.uc.edu

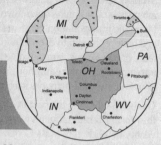

The University of Cincinnati Medical Center (UCMC) includes the colleges of Medicine, Nursing and Health, Pharmacy, Allied Health Sciences, Hoxworth Blood Center, and the Medical Center Libraries. As a state-supported institution, UCMC works to promote health among Ohio residents. Medical students enjoy early patient contact, an integrated curriculum, opportunities for research, and unusual options for training in primary care. For clinical exposure, Cincinnati provides experiences in a variety of clinical settings to allow students to learn first hand about diverse patient populations.

Academics

Most students follow a four-year curriculum leading to the M.D. degree. There is also a combined M.D./M.B.A. program with a five-year curriculum. Up to six positions a year are available in a combined M.D./Ph.D. program, the Physician Scientist Training Program (PSTP), which has a seven- to eight-year curriculum. The Ph.D. may be earned in one of the following disciplines: Cell and Molecular Biology; Developmental Biology; Environmental Health Sciences (includes clinical/genetic epidemiology); Molecular, Cellular, and Biochemical Pharmacology; Molecular and Cellular Physiology; Molecular Genetics, Biochemistry, and Microbiology; Neuroscience; and Pathobiology and Molecular Medicine. Medical students interested in shorter-term research projects may pursue them during the summer or as electives. Course grades are Honors/High Pass/Pass/Fail. Passing the USMLE Step 1 is a requirement for advancing to year three and passing Step 2 is a requirement for graduation.

BASIC SCIENCES: During the first and second years, courses are integrated around content blocks that foster critical thinking skills and problem solving. In both years, a major effort is made to limit lecture and laboratory time, to use more small group activities, and to ensure sufficient daily free time for active, independent learning. First-year classes are Gross Anatomy, Microscopic Anatomy, Biochemistry, Physiology, and Brain and Behavior I. Introduction to Clinical Practice I, also in the first year, includes interviewing, history taking, and basic physical examination skills as well as ethics, biopsychosocial issues, human sexuality, and death and loss, and provides each student with a one-on-one clinical experience in a physician's practice. Second-year courses are Pathology, Microbiology, Pharmacology, Brain and Behavior II, and Introduction to Clinical Practice II, which expands physical diagnosis and clinical skills training. An average of twenty contact hours per week and ample study time before each exam allow time for self-directed learning, group study, volunteering, and other activities in the basic science years. There continues to be a concerted effort to vertically integrate content blocks between the basic science and clinical science years. The Office of Students

Affairs Academic Support Programs provides tutoring services, academic counseling and training, and preparation seminars for the USMLE Step 1. Pre-clinical instruction takes place in the Medical Sciences Building, which is central to the Medical Center. The Health Sciences Library is also in the building and houses more than 350,000 books, journals, audiovisuals, software packages, and electronic resources. This includes more than 3,500 current journal subscriptions in print and electronic format. The library has more than 145 workstations (Macintosh and PC) with Internet access.

CLINICAL TRAINING: Third-year required clerkships are Internal Medicine (8 weeks); Surgery (8 weeks); Pediatrics (8 weeks); Obstetrics/Gynecology (8 weeks); Psychiatry (6 weeks); Family Medicine (4 weeks); Radiology (2 weeks); and two Specialty selectives (2 weeks each). During the fourth year, students complete an eight-week Internal Medicine acting internship, a four-week Neuroscience selective, and 24 weeks of electives, some of which must be in primary care fields. Most clinical training takes place at University Hospital, Veterans Administration Medical Center, Children's Hospital Medical Center, the Christ Hospital, the Good Samaritan Hospital, and the Jewish Hospital. Half of the elective credits may be earned at other institutions in the area, around the country, or abroad. One organized overseas program is the International Health Elective, which involves hands-on clinical experience in Honduras.

Students

Among students in the 1998 entering class, 83 percent are Ohio residents and 6 percent are from rural areas. Eight percent are minorities, and 14 percent were over 25 years of age at the time of application. Two percent of the class has a doctorate degree, and 10 percent have earned a master's degree. Seventy-four percent of students were science majors, and a total of 70 undergraduate institutions are represented. The 1998 entering class size was 165.

STUDENT LIFE: Medical students enjoy an overall cooperative environment at school. Student organizations are numerous and varied, and include the Family Practice Club, an anti-tobacco group called Doctors Ought to Care, an International Health Forum, a singing group, a support group for significant others, and local chapters of national medical student organizations. Medical students have access to athletic and other campus facilities. Cincinnati offers many attractions including theater, restaurants and bars, museums, parks, bookstores, and professional sporting events. University-owned apartments for single and married students are available on a limited basis.

GRADUATES: Of those who graduated in 1999, 30 percent entered residency programs in Cincinnati, 27 percent entered programs elsewhere in Ohio, and the remainder were successful in securing positions nationwide. The most prevalent fields for post-graduate study were Family Medicine (12.4%); Internal Medicine (all types, 36.4%); Pediatrics (16.1%); Emergency Medicine (5.8%); Surgery (5.1%); Ob/Gyn (8.8%); and Orthopedic Surgery (3.6%).

Admissions

REQUIREMENTS: The MCAT is required, and scores should be from within the past three years. Ohio residents are given preference. Although no courses are specified, applicants are expected to have the knowledge usually gained in a one year lecture and laboratory course in Biology, General Chemistry, Organic Chemistry, Physics, and Math. Applicants are expected to have an undergraduate preparation that provides insight into behavioral, social, and cultural issues. Academically, applicants are evaluated based on the following: GPA; MCAT scores; and undergrad, graduate, and post-bacc achievement. Applicants should demonstrate motivation, maturity, coping skills, leadership abilities, interpersonal skills, sensitivity and tolerance, acceptance of differences, and critical thinking.

PROCESS: All applicants who submit AMCAS applications are sent secondary applications. Approximately 600–650 applicants are invited to interview. Interviewees attend an informational program, eat lunch, go on a tour of campus, and sit in on presentations by faculty, the Director of Financial Aid, and the Assistant Dean of Admissions. Notification of the committee's decision occurs on a monthly basis, beginning on October 15th until May 15th. After that time, students are accepted from the alternate list as openings occur until the class is filled. Additional Programs: the College of Medicine has Dual Admissions Programs for exceptional high school seniors who know they want to pursue a career in medicine. These eight-year programs are in conjunction with John Caroll University, University of Dayton, Miami University, Xavier University, and the University of Cincinnati. There is also a nine-year Medicine and Engineering Dual Admissions Program (MEDA) that involves five years of undergraduate/graduate engineering studies at University of Cincinnati College of Engineering and four years of medical school. High school students who are interested in such programs should contact the admissions or pre-med office at the undergraduate colleges.

The University of Cincinnati College of Medicine and College of Business Administration have partnered to develop a joint M.D./M.B.A. degree program. The M.D./M.B.A. program is designed for highly qualified students who desire to complement standard medical training with a greater understanding of the economics, finance, marketing, and management of the health care system. Graduates of the combined degree program will have expanded career options, including management positions in major healthcare organizations.

Costs

The anticipated yearly cost of living for a single student is $11,500–$13,500. This budget supports off-campus housing and car maintenance and insurance.

FINANCIAL AID: Financial aid is awarded on the basis of financial need and/or scholastic or other special achievement. Participants in the PSTP receive complete financial support for tuition and living expenses.

UNIVERSITY OF CINCINNATI

STUDENT BODY

Type	Public
*Enrollment	635
* percent male/female	62/38
*% underrepresented minorities	10
# applied (total/out)	3,700/2,497
% interviewed (total/out)	18/7
% accepted (total/out)	60/53
% enrolled (total/out)	38/28
Average age	22

ADMISSIONS

Average GPA and MCAT Scores

Overall GPA	3.55	Science GPA	3.50
MCAT Bio	10.60	MCAT Phys	10.20
MCAT Verbal	9.70	MCAT Essay	NR

Score Release Policy

The school has not responded to our inquiry regarding withheld MCAT scores. Therefore, we advise caution. Contact the Admissions Office before withholding any scores.

Application Information

Regular application	11/15
Regular notification	10/15 until filled
Early application	6/1–8/1
Early notification	10/1
Transfers accepted?	Yes
Admissions may be deferred?	Yes
AMCAS application accepted?	Yes
Interview required?	Yes
Application fee	$25

COSTS AND AID

Tuition & Fees

Tuition (in/out)	$12,612/$22,500
Cost of books	$1,265
Fees	$561

Financial Aid

% students receiving aid	85
Average grant	$5,140
Average loan	$9,588
Average debt	$82,664

*Figures based on total enrollment

University of Colorado
SCHOOL OF MEDICINE

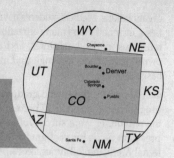

4200 East 9th Avenue, C-297, Denver, CO 80262
Admission: 303-315-7361 • Fax: 303-315-8494
Email: somadmin@uchsc.edu • Internet: www.uchsc.edu

According to a recent message from the Dean, the University of Colorado School of Medicine's primary objective is training excellent physicians. Over the past few years, as part of a Generalist Initiative, Colorado has adjusted its curriculum so that more graduates are better prepared to meet the statewide demand for primary care. The University of Colorado is a state school, focused on the needs of Colorado's largely rural population. However, as a major recipient of federal research funds, Colorado is also geared toward addressing national health priorities.

Academics

The School of Medicine is part of the University of Colorado Health Sciences Center, which includes schools of Dentistry, Nursing, Pharmacy, and Graduate Studies. A combined M.D./Ph.D. degree through the M.S.T.P. is possible in the following fields: Biochemistry, Biophysics, Cell Biology, Immunology, Molecular Biology, Microbiology, Pharmacology, and Physiology.

BASIC SCIENCES: The first two years are organized into quarters. Throughout year one, Microanatomy, Physiology, and Foundations of Doctoring are studied. Foundations of Doctoring, which establishes one-on-one mentoring relationships between students and local practicing physicians, is the first of three segments that together constitute the curricular element of the Generalist Initiative. In addition, during the fall, students take Biochemistry and Human Anatomy. Year one, winter-quarter courses are Genetics and Neurobiology. Spring courses are Biochemistry and Nutrition, Embryology, and Ethics. Year-long courses during year two are the following: Pathology, Pharmacology, Human Behavior, and Foundations of Doctoring. Immunology and Microbiology are also taken in the fall, and Neuroscience, Pathophysiology, and Epidemiology are taken in the winter. Students spend about 28 hours per week in a structured-learning environment. About 40 percent of this time is devoted to lecture, and another 40 percent to lab. Small-group sessions are also employed as an instructional technique. Academic tutoring and counseling are available to students through a student advocacy program. Grading is Honors/Pass/Fail. Students must pass the USMLE Step 1 to begin the clinical years.

CLINICAL TRAINING: Patient contact begins in year one, when students work closely with practicing physicians and gradually gain independent responsibility. Third-year, required clerkships consist of Medicine (12 weeks); Surgery (6 weeks); Family Medicine (6 weeks); Ob/Gyn (6 weeks); Neurology (4 weeks); Pediatrics (6 weeks); and Psychiatry (6 weeks). One afternoon each week is dedicated to the continuing primary care experience as the third segment of the Foundations of Doctoring sequence. During year four, students select from Surgical Specialties (6 weeks, including one week each of Anesthesiology, Ophthalmology, Orthopedics, Otolaryngology, and Urology) and from a wide range of general electives. Most clerkships take place at University Hospital; VA Medical Center; Denver Health Medical Center; Children's Hospital; and the National Jewish Center for Immunology and Respiratory Medicine. Electives and some required clerkships may be fulfilled at community hospitals and clinics around the state, or under the supervision of affiliated private physicians in the area. Denver is a rapidly growing city with a population of over 2 million. It is an international tourist destination, making the patient population more diverse than that associated with medical schools in other predominantly rural states. Evaluation during the clinical years uses an Honors/Pass/Fail system enhanced with narratives from professors. There are opportunities for clinical experiences outside of traditional rotations, generally through outreach activities and volunteer work. Students may volunteer at clinics that provide care to Denver's homeless population or may spend time working with low-income children in need of care. The Medical Student International Program is popular, granting students credit for up to 4 months of overseas study or work. Passing the USMLE Step 2 is required for graduation.

Students

At least 85 percent of students are Colorado residents. Science and nonscience majors are equally represented. Of the 1996 entering class, 15 percent are underrepresented minorities, most of whom are Hispanic Americans. With a mean age of 26 for entering students, there is clearly a wide age range within the student body. Class size is 132.

STUDENT LIFE: Denver is a comfortable, affordable, and student-friendly place to live. It is less than an hour from perhaps the best skiing in the country. During the summer, the hiking, swimming, climbing, and mountain biking are all outstanding. Single students live off campus in apartments and shared houses. Married students can find affordable family housing in various Denver neighborhoods. On-campus activities include student-run organizations and events having either a professional or social focus. The Office of Diversity provides support for minority students.

GRADUATES: The most popular residency programs of the 1999 graduating class were Internal Medicine (28 students); Family Medicine (22); Surgery (7); Pediatrics (13); Emergency Medicine (8); and Orthopedics (3). More than half of the graduates entered primary care fields. Graduates often stay in Denver for training. Other states popular for post-graduate training are Texas, Minnesota, and California.

Admissions

REQUIREMENTS: Required courses are College Mathematics (8 hours); Biology with lab (8 semester hours); Chemistry with lab (8 hours); Organic Chemistry with lab (8 hours); Physics with lab (8 hours); English Literature (6); and English Composition or Creative Writing (3 hours). Applicants must demonstrate mathematics competency at least through college level trigonometry, either with college courses or placement test results. The MCAT is required and, if retaken, the best scores are used.

SUGGESTIONS: In addition to required courses, a course in Biochemistry is recommended. For applicants who have been out of school for a significant period of time, recent course work is suggested. Personal qualities are valued a great deal, as are extracurricular activities that involve medical research or health-related experience. As part of the Generalist Initiative, applicants from rural backgrounds are encouraged to apply.

PROCESS: All AMCAS applicants receive secondary applications. Of Colorado residents completing secondaries, 75 percent are interviewed. Less than 20 percent of out-of-state applicants are interviewed. Interviews take place on campus from September through April and consist of two sessions, each with a member of the Admissions Committee. The Admissions Committee is made up of students, faculty, and community physicians. Notification occurs on a rolling basis. About one-quarter of Colorado residents who interview are accepted, and about one tenth of out of state interviewees are accepted. A wait list is established, from which 20–40 students are usually taken. Wait-listed candidates are not encouraged to send supplementary material.

Costs

Beyond tuition, yearly living expenses are estimated to be $10,920 for a single student. This presumes living off campus and, most likely, owning a car.

FINANCIAL AID: Primarily, students rely on Federal student loans. The State and the University of Colorado also offer student support in the form of grants and loans. Almost all aid is based on financial need as determined by student and parental financial resources. The Colorado Health Professions Loan repayment Program assists graduates with debt in exchange for work in under-served areas.

UNIVERSITY OF COLORADO

STUDENT BODY

Type	Public
*Enrollment	525
*% male/female	54/46
*% underrepresented minorities	13
# applied (total/out)	2,454/1,624
% interviewed (total/out)	27/7
% accepted (total/out)	NR/NR
% enrolled (total/out)	20/10
Average age	26

ADMISSIONS

Average GPA and MCAT Scores

Overall GPA	3.60	Science GPA	3.60
MCAT Bio	9.9	MCAT Phys	9.9
MCAT Verbal	10.0	MCAT Essay	NR

Score Release Policy

The Admissions Committee uses only the highest score, so withholding scores brings no negative consequences; however, they caution that they may assume scores are even worse if withheld.

Application Information

Regular application	11/15
Regular notification	Rolling
Are transfers accepted?	NR
Admissions may be deferred?	Yes
AMCAS application accepted?	Yes
Interview required?	Yes
Application fee	$70

COSTS AND AID

Tuition & Fees

Tuition (in/out)	$11,182/$54,576
Cost of books	NR
Fees	$1,847

Financial Aid

% students receiving aid	NR
Average grant	NR
Average loan	NR
Average debt	NR

*Figures based on total enrollment

COLUMBIA UNIVERSITY

COLLEGE OF PHYSICIANS AND SURGEONS

630 West 168th Street, Rm 1-416, New York, NY 10032

Admission: 212-305-3595 • Fax: 212-305-3545

Email: PT8@columbia.edu

Internet: www.cpmcnet.columbia.edu/dept/ps/admissions

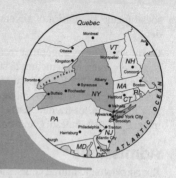

Columbia is a private, Ivy League institution with a strong reputation for both its undergraduate college and virtually all of its graduate and professional programs. Columbia's College of Physicians and Surgeons was the first medical school in North America to award a doctoral degree in medicine and continues to be a leader in the medical education field. Columbia's clinical facilities include an expansive network of hospitals and clinics that serves an unusually diverse patient population. This diversity contributes to the outstanding clinical education that medical students receive. Columbia is also a renowned medical research center.

Academics

The Columbia curriculum is multidisciplinary and integrated—it focuses on not only understanding the science, skills, and techniques of medicine, but also appreciating the art and ethics involved. Several joint-degree programs, such as the M.D./M.P.H. and M.D./M.B.A. are offered in conjunction with other schools and departments at Columbia. Qualified students interested in careers in scientific research may pursue a combined M.D./Ph.D., earning the doctorate in fields such as Anatomy, Biochemistry, Biophysics, Cell Biology, Genetics, Immunology, Microbiology, Molecular Biology, Neuroscience, Pathology, Pharmacology, and Physiology. Medical students are evaluated with an Honors/Pass/Fail system. Successful completion of Steps 1 and 2 of the USMLE are required for graduation.

BASIC SCIENCES: The first two years provides information and experiences essential for all physicians. The majority of instruction is conducted in lectures and lab, but small-group teaching is increasingly emphasized. Students spend approximately 25 hours per week in scheduled activity. The first year (42 weeks) includes Gross Anatomy, Neural Science, Clinical Practice and an integrated course that covers Biochemistry, Cell Biology, Genetics, Human Development, and Physiology. The majority of the second year (40 weeks) is devoted to a multidisciplinary course that examines the basic concepts of Immunology, Pathology, Microbiology, and Pharmacology. Physical Diagnosis, Basic Psychiatry, and Clinical Practice are also taught. Columbia has extensive laboratory, informational, and computer facilities that enhance classroom learning. The Augustus C. Long Health Sciences Library houses nearly 450,000 volumes and is one of the largest medical center libraries in the nation.

CLINICAL TRAINING: In the third year, students complete required rotations in the following: Medicine (10 weeks); Surgery (5 weeks); Pediatrics (5 weeks); Ob/Gyn (5 weeks); Primary Care (5 weeks); Psychiatry (5 weeks); Neurology (5 weeks); Anesthesiology/Dermatology (2

weeks); Orthopedics (2 weeks); Urology (2 weeks); Otolaryngology (1 week); and Ophthalmology (1 week). The fourth year consists of one- and two-month-long electives drawn from a large number of offerings and student-designed experiences. There are extensive opportunities for clinical electives abroad. Each student is also required to complete a "back-to-basic science" elective. These include one-month seminars in Advanced Pathophysiology, Clinical Pharmacology, or Clinical Pathology. Rotations are conducted at various medical centers and hospitals throughout the metropolitan area. Columbia-Presbyterian Medical Center, Harlem Hospital Center, Roosevelt Hospital, St. Luke's Hospital, and other institutions combine for a comprehensive clinical experience.

Students

Columbia attracts an extremely diverse, nationally represented student body. About 10 percent of students are underrepresented minorities. There is a wide age range among incoming students, with significant numbers of students in their late 20s and 30s.

STUDENT LIFE: Despite the rigorous schedule, student life abounds at Columbia. Medical students have access to the recreational and athletic facilities of Columbia University and to university-sponsored cultural events. The P&S Club, the oldest student organization of its kind at any medical school in America, provides a variety of extracurricular activities. Students have opportunities in the fine arts, athletics, and service-oriented projects. In addition, Manhattan offers unparalleled access to museums, concerts, and every imaginable type of dining. Most students live in on-campus housing, which helps make New York affordable. Both residential halls and apartments buildings are available. Newly accepted married students are guaranteed married-student housing.

GRADUATES: Graduates gain acceptance to the most competitive residency programs in the nation. A Columbia education allows students to emphasize academic medicine, research, or primary care.

Admissions

REQUIREMENTS: One year each of English, Biology, Physics, Chemistry, and Organic Chemistry are required for admission along with the MCAT. For those students who have taken the MCAT more than once, the most recent scores are weighed most heavily. Thus, there is no advantage in withholding scores. Columbia does not admit students on a rolling basis. Therefore, submitting MCAT scores from the fall of the admission year does not place applicants at a disadvantage.

SUGGESTIONS: The Admissions Committee is interested in the depth and breadth of an applicant's extracurricular experiences. Community service, artistic activities, athletics and medically related experiences are all valuable. It is valuable to denote that Columbia is an applicant's first choice for medical school, particularly for those who have been placed on the wait list.

PROCESS: Columbia does not participate in AMCAS. Rather, applications should be requested from the address above early in the summer. Between Labor Day and early March, approximately 25 percent of applicants are invited for an interview. The interview day consists of one session with a faculty member who is a member of the Admissions Committee. Applicants also have lunch and tour the facilities with a current medical student. About 15 percent of interviewed applicants are accepted, with notification occurring in February and March. A wait list is also created at this time. Wait-listed applicants may send additional information to update their files.

Costs

The anticipated yearly budget for a single student is about $16,000. This assumes on-campus housing and use of public transportation. Although New York can be an expensive city, student discounts are often available for theater, museums, and other attractions.

FINANCIAL AID: Parental resources are considered in determining financial need. Columbia offers a variety of university-based grants and loans in addition to facilitating federal, state, and outside loan programs.

COLUMBIA UNIVERSITY

STUDENT BODY

Type	Private
*Enrollment	631
*% male/female	56/44
*% underrepresented minorities	10
# applied (total/out)	3,727/2,846
% interviewed (total/out)	33/35
% accepted (total/out)	8/8
% enrolled (total/out)	49/49
Average age	24

ADMISSIONS

Average GPA and MCAT Scores

Overall GPA	NR	Science GPA	NR
MCAT Bio	11.86	MCAT Phys	12.09
MCAT Verbal	11.09	MCAT Essay	Q–R

Score Release Policy

The school has not responded to our inquiry regarding withheld MCAT scores. Therefore, we advise caution. Contact the Admissions Office before withholding any scores.

Application Information

Regular application	10/15
Regular notification	2/1–varies
Transfers accepted?	Yes
Admissions may be deferred?	Yes
AMCAS application accepted?	No
Interview required?	Yes
Application fee	$75

COSTS AND AID

Tuition & Fees

Tuition	$29,548
Cost of books	$1,716
Fees	NR

Financial Aid

% students receiving aid	79
Average grant	NR
Average loan	NR
Average debt	$72,000

*Figures based on total enrollment

UNIVERSITY OF CONNECTICUT

SCHOOL OF MEDICINE

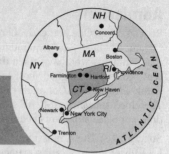

263 Farmington Avenue, Farmington, CT 06030
Admission: 203-679-3874 • Fax: 203-679-1282
Email: sanford@nso1.uchc.edu • Internet: www.uchc.edu

With significant input from medical students, the University of Connecticut revised its curriculum. The curriculum is designed to better prepare professional men and women to practice medicine in a health care system that is evolving at an accelerated rate and to empower them to formulate creative and courageous solutions to health care problems and issues. The primary goal of the curriculum is to develop in all students a fund of knowledge, skills, and attitudes that will enable them to pursue the postgraduate training necessary for their chosen career. The curriculum is dedicated to equipping students with the "career competencies" that will enable them to provide high-quality, cost-effective clinical care. Students are the focus at the School of Medicine, as demonstrated by its admissions brochure, much of which is in the words of students themselves. Humanistic medicine is also a priority, and Connecticut may be the only medical school that requires a certain number of community-service hours for graduation. The university is situated on 162 acres in an attractive part of the state, convenient to Hartford and to rural areas with genuine New England appeal.

Academics

In addition to the required courses, about 70 percent of students take part in a research project while in school. Grading is strictly Pass/Fall, based on the notion that, "each student is at the top of the class with regard to some important feature of skill or ability." A combined-degree program leading to both an M.D. and a Ph.D. is pursued by about four students each year in conjunction with the following Graduate Programs: Cell Biology, Developmental Biology, Immunology, Molecular Biology and Biochemistry, Neuroscience, Oral Biology, and Cellular and Molecular Pharmacology. It is also possible for medical students to earn a master's in Public Health from the University of Connecticut's Graduate Program in Public Health.

BASIC SCIENCES: The first two years cover the basic sciences, introduce clinical studies, and integrate behavioral and social aspects of medicine and health care. Instruction uses lectures, labs, case conferences, and problem-based learning. First-year courses are Human Systems, which is composed of: Human Biology; Organ Systems I (Neuroscience, Anatomy of the head and neck); Organ Systems II (Cardiovascular, Respiratory and Renal Systems, Anatomy of the thorax and abdomen); and Organ System III (Gastrointestinal, Endocrine and Reproductive, Genetics and Anatomy of the pelvis); Electives; Correlated Medical Problem Solving; and Principles of Clinical Medicine, which teaches history-taking, the physical examination, and general concepts related to clinical care. Second-year courses are Human Development and Health, which encompasses ethical, social, and legal issues; Mechanisms of Disease, which includes concepts related to Pathology; Pharmacology; Infectious Disease; Homeostasis; Oncology; Metabolism; Nervous System; Reproductive System; and Skin, Connective Tissue, and Joints; Correlated Medical Problem Solving; and Clinical Medicine. Facilities include modern lecture halls, class-rooms for small-group discussions, the Lyman Maynard Stowe Library, and computer resources. Passing the USMLE Step 1 is a requirement for promotion to year three.

CLINICAL TRAINING: The third year is organized into two segments, one that involves clinical training in ambulatory settings, and the other that takes place in hospitals. The ambulatory experience is composed of the following clerkships: General Internal Medicine (7 weeks); Pediatrics (5 weeks); Psychiatry (2 weeks); Family Medicine (7 weeks); Ob/Gyn (4 weeks); and Subspecialties (3 weeks). The Hospital, or Inpatient, segment includes rotations in Medicine (4 weeks); Surgery (4 weeks); Pediatrics (2 weeks); Psychiatry (2 weeks); Obstetrics (2 weeks); and Beginning to End (2 weeks), in which students follow patients from their admittance to each diagnosis/service area that they visit in the hospital. The fourth year includes 20 weeks of electives, which may be taken at local or distant sites. Other fourth-year requirements are Advanced Inpatient Experience (4 weeks); Critical Care Experience (4 weeks); Emergency/Urgent Experience (4 weeks); and Selectives, in which students choose from rotations in research, community health, or education-related fields. Each student is paired with a faculty member of his or her choice to assist in scheduling electives and in selecting post-graduate training programs. Clinical training takes place at the University Hospital (232 beds) and at about 10 affiliated hospitals in the area. Some students gain clinical experience overseas, by participating in projects in Latin America, Asia, or Africa. Passing the USMLE Step 2 is a requirement for graduation.

Students

Underrepresented minorities, mostly African American, comprise about 10 percent of the student body. The average age of incoming students is typically about 24, with ages ranging from 21 to late 30s. About 90 percent of the students are Connecticut residents, and about 10 percent graduated from the University of Connecticut undergraduate college. Approximately 80 percent of students majored in a scientific discipline in college. Class size is about 82. Dental students participate in some of the basic sciences classes.

STUDENT LIFE: Life outside the classroom includes theater, concerts, and restaurants in Hartford; organized team sports on campus; and numerous clubs and groups related to professional or extracurricular interests. The Office of Minority Affairs provides support services throughout the academic year to minority medical students. Community-service activities, such as volunteering at homeless shelters, bring students together around important projects. Facilities such as golf courses, ski slopes, and public parks are accessible to the campus. On-campus housing is not available. Students live off campus in communities surrounding the university.

GRADUATES: Of the class that graduated in 1995, the breakdown of the most prevalent specialty choices was Internal Medicine (17%); Preliminary Medicine (13%); Family Practice (12%); Pediatrics (10%); Psychiatry (6%); Ob/Gyn (5%); Radiology (4%); Surgery (3%); Emergency Medicine (2%); Orthopedics (2%); and Urology (2%). About 20 percent of graduates entered residency programs at the University of Connecticut Health Center. Other popular destinations were Massachusetts, New York, Rhode Island, and Washington, D.C.

Admissions

REQUIREMENTS: Requirements are one year of Chemistry, Organic Chemistry, Physics, and Biology. The MCAT is required and should be no more than three years old.

SUGGESTIONS: A broad and in-depth liberal arts education that includes English, Math, Foreign Language, Literature, History, Art, and Political Science is advised. The Admissions Committee looks very seriously at the nonacademic traits of applicants, such as their character and motivation.

PROCESS: All AMCAS applicants are sent secondary applications. About 60 percent of Connecticut applicants, and about 10 percent of out-of-state applicants are interviewed. Interviews are held from August through April and consist of two one-hour sessions with faculty, administrators, or students. Lunch and a campus tour with medical students are provided. Some candidates are accepted shortly after their interview, while others are notified later in the year. A wait list is established in the spring. Wait-listed candidates may send supplementary information, such as transcripts.

Costs

Beyond tuition, the standard budget for a single student is about $16,000. This includes fees, books, supplies, and living expenses. Most students own a car.

FINANCIAL AID: Financial aid is awarded on the basis of need, in the form of grants and loans. Need is determined by the FAFSA application and institutional forms. In 1996–1997, approximately 80 percent of the students borrowed from the Stafford Loan Program, and 30 percent received need-based aid from the school.

UNIVERSITY OF CONNECTICUT

STUDENT BODY

Type	Public
*Enrollment	337
*% male/female	50/50
*% underrepresented minorities	10
# applied (total/out)	2,220/1,882
% interviewed (total/out)	60/10
% accepted (total/out)	7/3
% enrolled (total/out)	50/22
Average age	24

ADMISSIONS

Average GPA and MCAT Scores

Overall GPA	3.56	Science GPA	3.52
MCAT Bio	10.00	MCAT Phys	10.00
MCAT Verbal	10.00	MCAT Essay	P

Score Release Policy
The Admissions Committee would prefer to look at all scores; however, they stress that scores are only a small part of the admissions process.

Application Information

Regular application	12/15
Regular notification	10/15 until filled
Early application	6/1–8/1
Early notification	10/1
Transfers accepted?	Yes
Admissions may be deferred?	Yes
AMCAS application accepted?	Yes
Interview required?	Yes
Application fee	$60

COSTS AND AID

Tuition & Fees

Tuition (in/out)	$9,100/$20,700
Cost of books	$1,430
Fees	$3,725

Financial Aid

% students receiving aid	80
Average grant	NR
Average loan	NR
Average debt	NR

*Figures based on total enrollment

CORNELL UNIVERSITY
MEDICAL COLLEGE

445 East 69th Street, New York, NY 10021

Admission: 212-746-1067

Internet: www.med.cornell.edu

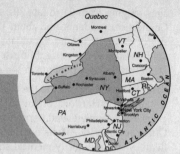

Cornell University Medical College is situated in an attractive, Upper East Side neighborhood of Manhattan, far from the main campus of Cornell in upstate New York. New York City generates one of the most diverse patient populations, offering intense clinical exposure to medical students. Cornell is known for outstanding research and, as a result of its association with some of the best hospitals in the city, also provides outstanding clinical instruction. Cornell emphasizes the idea that science underlies good medicine, and that research and patient care are linked. Four years ago, Cornell exchanged its traditional, lecture-based curriculum for an almost entirely case-based approach that has been extremely successful. Cornell is a private, Ivy League school with a nationally representative student body.

Academics

The newly revised curriculum strives to limit the time students spend in lectures, thereby promoting independent and interactive learning and research. The curriculum integrates basic and clinical sciences, utilizes problem-based learning, includes principles of public health, and encourages student research efforts. Joint M.D./Ph.D. programs can be pursued in conjunction with the Veill Graduate School of Medical Sciences, Rockefeller University, and the Sloan-Kettering Institute in the following fields: Biochemistry, Cell Biology, Immunology, Molecular Biology and Genetics; Molecular Pharmacology, Neuroscience, Physiology; and Microbiology. Twelve students per year enter joint programs.

BASIC SCIENCES: The curriculum was completely revised in 1996 and has been both highly successful and widely emulated. The first and second years of study consist of six basic science courses and Medicine, Patients, and Society. In the first year, the basic science courses are Molecules to Cells, Gene Structure and Expression, Human Structure and Function, and Host Defenses. In the second year, they are Brain and Mind and Basis of Disease. The core basic science courses are sequential, integrated, interdisciplinary block courses that employ problem-based learning (PBL) in small groups. PBL emphasizes active learning and requires the student first to identify issues needed to solve a medical problem, then to seek out the information needed to solve the problem, and then to reconvene in small groups with the faculty to apply the information learned. Lectures are few and emphasize the conceptual framework of a field. Anatomic dissection and experimental laboratories complete the learning experience. The course Medicine, Patients, and Society approaches the doctor-patient relationship from both the conceptual and practical perspectives. For one day each week throughout each year, students spend the morning in seminar and the afternoon in physicians' offices. Areas treated include medical interviewing, physical diagnosis, human behavior in illness, medical ethics, public health, biostatistics, clinical epidemiology, and others. Thus, students learn these vital topics in a patient-centered context. The evaluation system uses an Honor/Pass/Fail scale.

CLINICAL TRAINING: Upon completion of the second year and after taking the USMLE Step 1, students take three Introductory Clinical Courses: Clinical Pharmacology, Anesthesia, and the Introductory Clerkship. The third year is dedicated to clinical learning and emphasizes the core clerkships, including Medicine, Surgery, Pediatrics, Obstetrics-Gynecology, Psychiatry, Neurology, and Primary Care. In these courses, students are assigned to clinical inpatient and outpatient services at New York-Presbyterian Medical Center and throughout the network of clinical affiliates. Clinical affiliates include the Hospital for Special Surgery, a leader in the fields of orthopedics, rheumatology, and sports medicine; Memorial Sloan-Kettering Cancer Center, one the premier facilities in the world devoted to the study and treatment of cancer; The New York Methodist Hospital; and others throughout the city. Students are integral members of the health care team and actively care for patients, under the supervision of the faculty. The fourth year centers on completion of clinical requirements, a subinternship, and electives. While electives can be taken at any time in the third of fourth years, most students focus on three major types of electives in the fourth year: clinical electives, often in subspecialty areas; research; and international electives. Each year approximately half of the fourth-year class spends time abroad, typically in Cornell-funded programs that combine clinical care and research in the third world: South America, the Caribbean, Africa, and Asia. In the month before graduation, eight weeks of advanced basic science allow students to study leading-edge biomedical science in depth.

Students

In a typical class, students graduated from over 45 different undergraduate institutions. Cornell is particularly well represented. African and Hispanic Americans account for 20 percent of the student body. Class size is 101.

STUDENT LIFE: Despite the urban environment, students are cohesive and student life is apparent around the Medical College. Ninety-five percent of students live within three blocks of campus, generally in college-owned dorms or apartments. The rent is very inexpensive for New York, meaning that students have a bit more cash with which to enjoy the city. In the residence halls, there are athletic facilities for student use. Student organizations, including those that support women and minority students, are active. Parks, including Central Park, are accessible, as are countless museums, theaters, shops, and restaurants. Students do not own cars.

GRADUATES: Graduates gain acceptance to the nation's top residency programs in primary care and in specialized fields. Many stay in New York City for post-graduate training.

Admissions

REQUIREMENTS: Cornell requires 24 semester credit hours in science courses, including Biology, General Chemistry, Organic Chemistry, and Physics. In addition, six semester hours of English are required. The science GPA is given considerable weight. The MCAT is required and is used to assist the Admissions Committee in assessing the GPAs of applicants who typically come from a wide range of undergraduate backgrounds. If an applicant has repeated the MCAT, the best score is considered.

SUGGESTIONS: Beyond required courses, Cornell recommends two additional terms of Biology for nonscience majors. For students who graduated college several years ago, recent science course work is suggested. The Medical College is interested in the extracurricular activities of applicants, particularly if they demonstrate commitment and dedication. Some exposure to the field of medicine is also desirable. Biomedical research is recommended.

PROCESS: All AMCAS applicants receive secondary applications. About 13 percent of applicants who complete secondaries are invited to interview, and about 10 percent of those who interview are offered a place in the first-year class. Interviews are held from October through February and consist of two 45-minute sessions, each with a member of the Admissions Committee. Decisions are announced after March 15. For a wait-listed candidate, submitting supplemental material can serve to strengthen his or her application and is also helpful in that it indicates interest in attending Cornell.

Costs

Beyond tuition and fees, the estimated yearly budget for a single student is $15,000. This presumes living in Medical School housing and using public transportation.

FINANCIAL AID: All aid is based on financial need, as determined by the student's and the parents' resources. Before receiving grants and favorable loans, students are expected to secure a federal student loan of $8,500 per year.

CORNELL UNIVERSITY

STUDENT BODY

Type	Private
*Enrollment	416
*% male/female	46/54
*% underrepresented minorities	18
# applied (total/out)	6,782/5,381
% interviewed (total/out)	13/10
% accepted (total/out)	NR/NR
% enrolled (total/out)	9/7

ADMISSIONS

Average GPA and MCAT Scores

Overall GPA	3.64	Science GPA	3.66
MCAT Bio	11.40	MCAT Phys	11.40
MCAT Verbal	10.40	MCAT Essay	NR

Score Release Policy

The school has not responded to our inquiry regarding withheld MCAT scores. Therefore, we advise caution. Contact the Admissions Office before withholding any scores.

Application Information

Regular application	10/15
Regular notification	10/15 until filled
Early application	6/1–8/1
Early notification	10/1
Admissions may be deferred?	Yes
AMCAS application accepted?	Yes
Interview required?	Yes
Application fee	$75

COSTS AND AID

Tuition & Fees

Tuition	$27,000
Cost of books	NR
Fees	$640

Financial Aid

% students receiving aid	80
Average grant	NR
Average loan	NR
Average debt	NR

*Figures based on total enrollment

CREIGHTON UNIVERSITY

SCHOOL OF MEDICINE

2500 California Plaza, Omaha, NE 68178
Admission: 402-280-2799 • Fax: 402-280-1241
Email: medschadm@creighton.edu
Internet: medicine.creighton.edu/medschool/admissions/default.html

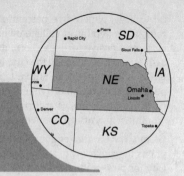

Creighton is a private, Jesuit university that features schools of Medicine, Dentistry, Pharmacy, Allied Health Professions, Nursing, Business, Law, Graduate Studies, and Arts and Sciences. Creighton is known for its emphasis on community service, and this is reflected in the priorities of the School of Medicine. Creighton promotes lifelong learning skills, problem solving, and primary care. The school's curriculum has evolved to respond to the technological, informational, ethical, economic, and social concerns of the 21st century.

Academics

The educational program is divided into four years based on: (1) biomedical fundamentals; (2) organ- and disease-based concepts; (3) clinical clerkships; and (4) continued patient care. Students may apply to Ph.D. programs in Anatomy, Biochemistry, Immunology, Pathology, and Physiology and pursue the degree jointly with the M.D. The grading system at Creighton uses Honors/Pass/Fail supplemented with written, narrative evaluations. Students are not ranked against their peers.

BASIC SCIENCES: In some cases, basic sciences are taught using the traditional lecture/lab format and in others, small groups and case-based learning is used. First- and second-year students are in scheduled sessions of some sort for about 25 hours per week. First-year courses, comprising the first unit, are Molecular and Cell Biology, Anatomy, Pharmacology, Microbiology, Host Defense, Neuroscience, and Patient and Society I. The Patient and Society I course includes ethics, behavioral science, and actual practice in patient care. Many students use the summer between years one and two for funded research projects. The second component, organized by organ- and disease-based concepts, occurs during year two. Concepts or systems are Cardiovascular; Respiratory; Renal-Urinary; Hematology/Oncology; Gastrointestinal; Muscular/Skeletal; Endocrinology; Reproductive; Special Sense; Psychiatry; Pediatrics/Aging; Infectious Disease; and Miscellaneous Topics. Throughout year two, students take Patient and Society II, in which they are exposed to health policy, public health, and behavioral science issues. During years one and two, students also participate in clinical activities related to the patient physical and examination. Tutoring and review sessions for the USMLE Step 1 are provided. Creighton's Bio-Information Center houses 200,000 books and maintains audio-visual collections, computer teaching laboratories, and computerized literature search facilities. Passing the USMLE Step 1 is a requirement for progression to year three. Students at Creighton will benefit from the new on-site computer testing facility, which is one of three in the nation.

CLINICAL TRAINING: Second-year students take part in a longitudinal care clerkship, which demands one half-day per week throughout the years. This allows students to develop longer-term relationships with mentors and patients. Third-year, core clerkships are Primary Care (8 weeks, encompassing Internal Medicine, and Family Practice); Inpatient General Medicine (8 weeks); Psychiatry with Integrated Neurology (8 weeks); Surgery (8 weeks); Pediatrics (8 weeks); and Ob/Gyn (8 weeks). Fourth-year guidelines require that students select two out of five Medicine clerkships, one of which must be critical care; one Surgery clerkship; one subinternship in any specialty; and one advanced basic science elective. The remaining 16 weeks are reserved for electives. Saint Joseph Hospital (404 beds) is the primary teaching hospital. Other sites for clinical training include Omaha Children's Hospital; Omaha Veterans Medical Center; Bergen Mercy Medical Center; and Clarkson Medical center. Additional training sites are expected to result from a recent affiliation with the Alegent Health System. During the summer, Creighton students have the opportunity to gain clinical experience through volunteer efforts in medical settings in the Dominican Republic, or in communities closer to home. The USMLE Step 2 is encouraged, but not required for graduation.

Students

Among the 115 students in a recent class, California, Minnesota, and Nebraska accounted for 37 percent of the students' home states, though 28 states and three foreign countries were represented. Sixty-four colleges were represented, with about 30 percent of the class having graduated from Creighton—either with an undergraduate or a graduate degree. About 84 percent of the students were science majors. The age range was 21 to 37, with an average of 23. Of the entire class, 50 percent are women, 6 percent are members of underrepresented minority groups (mostly Hispanic and African American), 10 percent are married, and 6 percent have at least one parent who is an M.D. alumnus/alumna of Creighton.

STUDENT LIFE: The student body is cohesive and supportive, as evidenced by a student-published Wellness Letter that offers tips and shares experiences on issues such as exercise, nutrition, mental health, relationships, and spirituality. Through clubs, organizations, and extensive volunteer opportunities, students associate with each other outside of an academic setting. The School of Medicine is part of the main campus of Creighton, allowing medical students to take advantage of programs and facilities of the greater University, and to integrate with students from other programs. The Physical Fitness Center, the Student Center, and graduate student housing are all convenient to the School of Medicine. Omaha is a comfortable, friendly, and inexpensive city, allowing students to meet their own lifestyle needs. Affordable off-campus housing is widely available.

GRADUATES: Over the last three years an average of 52 percent of the graduates enter primary care specialties, defined as Internal Medicine, Family Practice, or Pediatrics. This is well above the national average of 48 percent. Creighton alumni are found in every state, but are more numerous in the Midwest and Western regions.

Admissions

REQUIREMENTS: Requirements are Biology (8 semester hours); Chemistry (8 hours); Organic Chemistry (8 hours); Physics (8 hours); and English (6 hours). The MCAT is required, and scores must be from within the past three years. For applicants who have retaken the exam, the best set of scores is considered.

SUGGESTIONS: No particular courses or majors are recommended beyond requirements, but advanced courses including Biochemistry and/or Molecular Biology are a plus. Studying overseas is encouraged, as are volunteer and community activities that demonstrate motivation and character. In the past, ten positions were reserved for Wyoming residents. This arrangement has been discontinued.

PROCESS: All AMCAS applicants receive a secondary application, and about 15 percent of those returning secondaries are invited to interview. Interviews are held from September through the spring and consist of one 30-minute session with a faculty or alumnus member of the admissions committee, and one session with a medical student who is usually a committee member. A tour of the campus and lunch with current medical students are also provided. About half the interviewed candidates are initially offered a place in the class, with notification occurring on a rolling basis. Wait-listed candidates may send supplementary information, such as grades and updates on extracurricular activities.

Costs

Beyond tuition, total yearly expenses are about $12,000. This budget allows for either on- or off-campus living.

FINANCIAL AID: Students must file a FAFSA form, which assists the Financial Aid office in determining need. Most institutional aid is need-based, and most is in the form of loans. Some need-based grants, and some scholarships based on criteria beyond financial need are available.

CREIGHTON UNIVERSITY

STUDENT BODY

Type	Private
*Enrollment	450
*% male/female	57/43
*% underrepresented minorities	19
# applied (total/out)	4,669/4,434
% interviewed (total/out)	13/12
% accepted (total/out)	6/5
% enrolled (total/out)	2/2
Average age	24

ADMISSIONS

Average GPA and MCAT Scores

Overall GPA	3.73	Science GPA	3.71
MCAT Bio	10.00	MCAT Phys	9.90
MCAT Verbal	9.90	MCAT Essay	Q

Score Release Policy

The Admissions Committee advises students to release scores regardless of circumstances. Progress is taken into great consideration.

Application Information

Regular application	12/1
Regular notification	10/1 until filled
Early application	Yes
Early notification	10/1
Transfers accepted?	Yes
Admissions may be deferred?	No
AMCAS application accepted?	Yes
Interview required?	Yes
Application fee	$65

COSTS AND AID

Tuition & Fees

Tuition	$28,010
Cost of books	$1,835
Fees	$566

Financial Aid

% students receiving aid	82
Average grant	$20,000
Average loan	$40,431
Average debt	$125,794

*Figures based on total enrollment

DARTMOUTH MEDICAL SCHOOL

7020 Remsen, Room 306, Hanover, NH 03755
Admission: 603-650-1505 • Fax: 603-650-1614
Internet: www.dartmouth.edu/dms

Dartmouth Medical School (DMS) is a private, Ivy League institution known for excellent teaching, friendly students, a relaxed atmosphere, and beautiful surroundings. Dartmouth is also an important medical research center, with an approximate $59 million annually for sponsored research activities. Nationally, DMS ranks in the top fifth of medical schools in terms of extramural research funding on a "per faculty member" basis. Dartmouth's three medical centers, located in Hanover and Lebanon, NH, and White River Junction, VT, serve as comprehensive teaching hospitals and are among the few rurally based academic hospitals in the country. They are also among the most important health care facilities in the region that encompasses New Hampshire, Vermont, and Maine. Dartmouth's New Directions curriculum is highly integrated and includes interdisciplinary courses and problem-based learning. Dartmouth is relatively small, with only 75 students per entering class. This allows for personal attention and encourages faculty-student interaction.

Academics

Through representation on important committees, students have input into the Medical School's curriculum and administrative policies. Fifteen students in each entering class are part of the Brown/Dartmouth Program in Medical Education, meaning that they spend their first two years at Dartmouth and their second two years at Brown. A joint M.D./M.B.A. is offered in conjunction with the Tuck School of Business at Dartmouth, and joint M.D./Ph.D. programs may be pursued in Molecular and Cellular Biology (Biochemistry, Biological Sciences, and Microbiology/Immunology), Physiology, Pharmacology/Toxicology, Psychology, Physics, Chemistry, Mathematics, Engineering, Computer Science, Earth Science, Environmental Science, and the Evaluative Clinical Sciences. Grading is Honors/Pass/Fail for the first two years and High Honors/Honors/Pass/Fail for the second two years.

BASIC SCIENCES: The revised curriculum emphasizes seminars, small-group sessions, tutorials, problem-based learning, and computer-assisted instruction. During the first two years, in the Longitudinal Clinical Experience course, students learn about community medicine through partnerships with practicing physicians who are also faculty members. Other first-year courses are: Anatomy; Microscopic Anatomy; Physiology; Biochemistry; Microbiology; Pathology; Neuroscience; Genetics; Immunology; Physiology; Epidemiology; and Biostatistics. The second year curriculum includes: Cardiology; Respiration; Hematology; Neurology; Psychiatry; Oncology; Reproduction; Endocrinology; Gastroenterology; Dermatology; CT and Bone; Urinary System; Infectious Diseases; and Nutrition. Tutoring is available through the Student Affairs Office, often by other qualified students. The Big Sib program pairs upperclass medical students with incoming students so that new students have a source of information about academics and other elements of life at Dartmouth. The Dana Biomedical Library at the Hanover campus and the Matthews-Fuller Health Sciences Library at the Lebanon campus together support Dartmouth's

health and life sciences, educational, research, and clinical programs. The combined collections contain more than 235,000 volumes.

CLINICAL TRAINING: Required third-year rotations are: Inpatient Medicine and Psychiatry (16 weeks); Ambulatory Family Medicine, Ambulatory Medicine, and Ambulatory Pediatrics (16 weeks); and Inpatient Surgery, Inpatient Ob/Gyn, and Inpatient Pediatrics (16 weeks). Fourth-year requirements are: Neurology (4 weeks); Women's Health (4 weeks); Subinternship (4 weeks); and an interdisciplinary block (8 weeks). The remainder of the year is reserved for electives. Clinical training takes place at a number of facilities including the Dartmouth-Hitchcock Medical Center (396 beds), the Community Health Center in Lebanon and the Veterans Affairs Hospital in Vermont, the site of over 70,000 outpatient visits a year. Research facilities include the Norris Cotton Cancer Center, one of only 35 comprehensive cancer centers recognized nationally by the National Cancer Institute. Other notable academic centers are the C. Everett Koop Institute at Dartmouth and the Center for the Evaluative Clinical Sciences. Additional regional affiliates used for teaching are the New Hampshire Hospital (Psychiatric), the Brattleboro Retreat (Psychiatric), and the Family Medical Institute, which is the site of the Maine-Dartmouth Family Practice Residency program. Through special arrangements, medical students also have the opportunity to rotate to clinical sites in Miami, Florida; Tuba City, Arizona; Hartford, Connecticut; Cooperstown, New York; and Napier, New Zealand. Students may also arrange to fulfill elective requirements at other suitable locations around the country and overseas.

Students

Dartmouth attracts a nationally represented student body. The average age of entering students is usually 24, and about one-quarter of each entering class took several years off between college and medical school. Underrepresented minorities account for about 12 percent of the student body.

STUDENT LIFE: The medical school benefits from the educational, recreational, and cultural facilities of the main campus. The Hopkins Center shows high-quality films year-round and attracts both local and national performing arts groups. Students and the greater community both enjoy Dartmouth's Hood Museum of Art. Mountains and rivers surround the campus, which also has its own ski hill, golf course, and, during winter, a frozen pond for skating. Facilities for indoor athletic activities include Berry Sports Center, with squash and racquetball courts, Alumni Gym, with an indoor track and two pools, and Thompson Arena for skating and hockey. Many medical students are involved in community service activities such as peer counseling for teenagers or volunteering with the Vermont Handicapped Ski and Sports Association. Other organized activities revolve around medical student, or campus-wide organizations and interest groups. On-campus housing is available for married students, although most students opt to live off campus. Some live in Hanover, and either walk or ride a bike to class. Others live in neighboring New England towns and drive to school.

GRADUATES: Graduates are successful in securing residencies in all medical fields, at locations all across the country. Ninety percent of the class of 2000 secured positions in their first-, second-, or third-choice programs. Seventy-three percent secured places in their first-choice program. Dartmouth-Hitchcock Medical Center offers 15 post-graduate training programs and a variety of fellowships.

Admissions

REQUIREMENTS: In addition to the standard science requirements, three semester hours of Calculus are required. Strong spoken and written English are also requirements. The MCAT is effectively required and must be no more than three years old.

SUGGESTIONS: No additional courses are advised, and no particular majors are favored. Applicants should demonstrate motivation and interest in their chosen major, possibly through relevant research. Extracurricular activities, such as medically-related experiences or community service, are also important.

PROCESS: All AMCAS applicants receive a secondary application, which is due on December 31. About 500 applicants are invited to interview from a pool of over 6,000. Interviews take place between October and April. Students applying for the Brown/Dartmouth Program in Medical Education apply to Dartmouth and interview in Hanover. After the interview, candidates indicate their preference, and the files of those who select Brown/Dartmouth Program in Medical Education are sent to the Brown Admissions Committee for simultaneous review. Notification occurs on a rolling basis, beginning after January 1. About 30 percent of interviewees are accepted, and a number are put on a wait list. Wait-listed candidates may send supplementary materials to update their records or demonstrate interest in Dartmouth. Dartmouth has a special arrangement with Bryn Mawr post-baccalaureate program through which a few students are admitted each year.

Costs

The estimated first-year student cost covering rent, food, and miscellaneous expenses for a ten-month period, is $9,800.

FINANCIAL AID: Need is determined by FAFSA, the Needs Access Diskette, and institutional forms. The base loan for incoming students is $17,800. Financial need beyond this amount will be met by scholarship dollars.

DARTMOUTH MEDICAL SCHOOL

STUDENT BODY

Type	Private
*Enrollment	274
*% male/female	50/50
*% underrepresented minorities	12
# applied (total/out)	6,226/6,158
% interviewed (total/out)	10/10
% accepted (total/out)	NR/NR
% enrolled (total/out)	NR/NR

ADMISSIONS

Average GPA and MCAT Scores

Overall GPA	3.50	Science GPA	3.6
MCAT Bio	10.00	MCAT Phys	10.00
MCAT Verbal	10.00	MCAT Essay	NR

Score Release Policy

The Admissions Office says that withholding scores is not recommended.

Application Information

Regular application	11/1
Regular notification	1/1 until filled
Admissions may be deferred?	Yes
AMCAS application accepted?	Yes
Interview required?	Yes
Application fee	$60

COSTS AND AID

Tuition & Fees

Tuition	$27,300
Cost of books	NR
Fees	$1,555

Financial Aid

% students receiving aid	80
Average grant	NR
Average loan	NR
Average debt	NR

*Figures based on total enrollment

DUKE UNIVERSITY
SCHOOL OF MEDICINE

PO Box 3710, Durham, NC 27710
Admission: 919-684-2985 • Fax: 919-684-8893
Internet: www.mc.duke.edu/depts/som

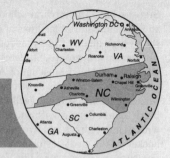

In addition to its reputation as one of the top medical schools in the country, Duke is known for generous financial aid, and for its curriculum, which introduces clinical rotations in year two instead of year three. Duke, one of the country's top research institutions, also offers a Primary Care Physician Program, which provides primary care mentors and special curricular options for those interested in careers as generalist physicians. Duke attracts a nationally represented student body, and prepares them for leadership roles in careers as practicing physicians, researchers, and academics. The school offers unparalleled flexibility and autonomy to its students.

Academics

By condensing the basic sciences into the first year, and scheduling required clinical clerkships for the second year, Duke allows medical students additional opportunities for research, clinical, or other enriching experiences during their third year. Those who are particularly interested in research may apply for joint M.D./Ph.D. programs in fields such as Anatomy, Biochemistry, Biomedical Engineering, Cell Biology, Genetics, Immunology, Microbiology, Molecular Biology, Neuroscience, Pathology, Pharmacology, and Physiology. Other joint degree programs are the M.D./J.D., M.D./M.B.A., M.D./ M.P.H., M.D./M.P.P., and the Medical Historian Program, which leads to an M.D. and either an M.A. or Ph.D. in History. In most courses, medical students are evaluated by the grades Pass with Honors, Pass, Incomplete, or Fail. The USMLE is not required for graduation, though most students opt to take it, and virtually all pass each section with scores in the 90th percentile or higher.

BASIC SCIENCES: A new Introduction to Critical Care course meets weekly during the first and second years, and integrates clinical and basic science concepts. Each week during the first year, Practice alternates between the classroom, where students meet in small groups, and the clinics, so that shortly after lessons are learned, they are applied. Computers are issued to all students to be used in the Practice course for informational and instructional purposes. Also, part of the course is an intensive three-week "Preparation for Year II" segment, which prepares students for clinical rotations. Other first-year courses, taught primarily in a lecture/lab format, are organized into five blocks, so that no more than three subjects are tackled at a time. Courses are Biochemistry, Cell Biology, Genetics, Gross Anatomy, Microanatomy, Physiology, Neurobiology, Microbiology, Immunology, Pathology I, Pharmacology, and Pathology II. In total, first-year students are in class or scheduled sessions for approximately 30 hours per week. Classes are held in buildings central to the medical complex. The Medical Center Library houses 276,000 books, including a renowned medical history collection. The Medical Library Education Center has electronic classroom and multimedia areas. Basic science concepts are reinforced during clinical rotations in year two.

CLINICAL TRAINING: Preparation for and exposure to clinical medicine begins during the first year, as part of the Introduction to Critical Care course. The year-long preparation for clinical clerkships provides students with significant experience in clinical settings before the beginning of their formal clerkships in year two. Clerkship requirements are fulfilled in the second year. They are: Medicine (8 weeks); Ob/Gyn (8 weeks); Pediatrics (8 weeks); Psychiatry (6 weeks); Cost-Effective Care (2 weeks); Surgery (8 weeks); and Family Medicine (8 weeks, or Neurology and Family Medicine, 4 weeks each). Clinical training takes place at Duke Hospital (1,124 beds), Durham Veterans Affairs Medical Center (455 beds), Lenox Baker Children's Hospital, Durham Regional Hospital (451 beds), and at multiple affiliated hospitals and clinics. The third year is spent in research as part of an independent scholarship project, which may be in Behavioral Neuroscience; Biomedical Engineering; Biometry; Biophysics; Cancer Biology; Cardiovascular Studies; Cell and Regulatory Biology; Epidemiology Health Services and Health Policy; Immunology; Infectious Diseases; Neurobiology; Ophthalmology and Visual Studies; and Pathology. Third-year students may design a year of mentored research at Duke or at approved extramural sites, e.g. NIH, or students may begin the dual-degree curricula. During their fourth year, students complete clinical training through elective clerkships. There are more than 150 electives offered at Duke. In addition, students may spend up to two months in rotations at other institutions.

Students

In the most recent class, 22 percent of the students are underrepresented minorities, most of whom are African American. Women account for 49 percent of the class, and the average age is 22, with an age range of 19–42. Forty-three undergraduate institutions are represented, the top six being Duke, Harvard, North Carolina State, Johns

Hopkins, UNC at Chapel Hill, and Yale. Twenty-eight states are represented, and the top five are North Carolina, California, New York, Ohio, and Virginia. Class size is 100.

STUDENT LIFE: Students, faculty, and administrators come together for events that promote a sense of community, congeniality, and friendship within the medical school. For example, the Dean hosts five "Dean's Desserts" for medical students to interact with teaching, research, and clinical faculty during the year. Organizations based on volunteer work, professional goals, or extracurricular interests are numerous. Medical students have access to all of Duke's athletic and recreational facilities. Durham is popular with students, offering parks, shopping districts, restaurants, and museums. Mountains and beaches are just a few hours away. Convenient campus-owned apartments, some of which have athletic facilities, are available on a limited basis. Social events sponsored by various medical school-based organizations provide opportunities for students to interact together. A fitness facility located with the major hospital complex for medial students and house staff only has recently opened.

GRADUATES: Graduates enter top residency programs, in primary and specialty fields. Most students get their top choice for residency appointment.

Admissions

REQUIREMENTS: Prerequisites are one year each of English, Inorganic Chemistry, Organic Chemistry, Physics, Biology, and Calculus. The MCAT is required, and scores must be from within the past four years. If the exam has been taken on multiple occasions, the most recent set of scores is generally considered. For those who have taken time off after college, science work must have been completed not more than seven years before matriculation at Duke.

SUGGESTIONS: An introductory course in Biochemistry is recommended. The character, motivation, and dedication of applicants is considered along with academic merits. Extracurricular activities, particularly those that are medically related, community service, volunteer experience, research exposure, and work experience are all considered in admission.

PROCESS: About 60 percent of AMCAS applicants receive secondary applications. Of those returning secondaries, about 30 percent are interviewed. Interviews are conducted from September through February, and consist of two half-hour sessions with members of the Admissions Committee. On interview day, students also receive a campus tour, and have the opportunity to eat lunch and speak with students. About one-third of interviewees will be considered for admission.

Costs

Total cost is all-inclusive of tuition, housing, utilities, board, books, fees, supplies, and computer fee. For 1998–99, the first-year cost of education is $44,960 for the twelve-month program. Each year's living expenses are prorated based on the number of months of full-time enrollment.

FINANCIAL AID: Financial aid is the vehicle by which many of our students pay for their education. By use of student and parental information, Duke is able to award generous aid packages that typically include institutional grants as well as loans. There are merit-based scholarships for entering students as well as rising fourth-year medical students.

DUKE UNIVERSITY

STUDENT BODY

Type	Private
*Enrollment	401
*% male/female	51/49
*% underrepresented minorities	22
# applied (total/out)	6,049/5,764
% interviewed	18
% accepted (total/out)	NR/NR
% enrolled (total/out)	12/NR
Average Age	22

ADMISSIONS

Average GPA and MCAT Scores

Overall GPA	NR	Science GPA	NR
MCAT Bio	NR	MCAT Phys	NR
MCAT Verbal	NR	MCAT Essay	NR

Score Release Policy
The school must have MCAT scores, but students may withhold scores without having it affect their status.

Application Information

Regular application	11/1
Regular notification	2/26
Transfers accepted?	No
Admissions may be deferred?	Yes
AMCAS application accepted?	Yes
Interview required?	Yes
Application fee	$65

COSTS AND AID

Tuition & Fees

Tuition	$26,700
Cost of books	$1,265
Fees	$2,479

Financial Aid

% students receiving aid	80
Average grant	NR
Average loan	NR
Average debt	NR

*Figures based on total enrollment

EAST CAROLINA UNIVERSITY

BRODY SCHOOL OF MEDICINE

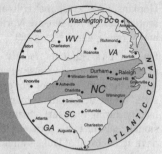

Brody AD52, Moye Boulevard, Greenville, NC 27858
Admission: 252-816-2202 • Fax: 252-816-1926
Internet: www.med.ecu.edu/deptmenu.htm

East Carolina University is part of the University of North Carolina educational system, and enrolls approximately 18,000 students in a full range of graduate and undergraduate programs. The Brody School of Medicine at East Carolina is concerned with educating skillful and caring physicians, and fostering better health among North Carolinians. In response to the state's demand for primary care providers, the School of Medicine emphasizes the training of generalist physicians. Greenville offers both a university community and the advantages of a small city with its own culture and character.

Academics

All first- and second-year students are paired with community physician mentors, and have the opportunity for ongoing patient contact and exposure to primary health care settings. Grading uses A, B, C and F. In addition, Honors may be awarded in some instances. Passing the USMLE Step 1 is a requirement for promotion to year three, and passing the USMLE Step 2 is a requirement for graduation. Joint Ph.D./M.D. programs can be arranged on a case-by-case basis.

BASIC SCIENCES: During the first two years, students spend about 28 hours per week in classes, most of which are taught in a lecture/lab format. Small group discussions, problem-based learning, and an introduction to clinical medicine are also part of the basic science curriculum. First-year courses are Microbiology and Immunology; Biochemistry; Behavioral Science; Primary Care Preceptorship; Genetics; Gross Anatomy; Histology; Embryology; Neurobiology; Ethical and Social Issues in Medicine; Physiology; and Clinical Skills I. Second-year courses are Introduction to Medicine; Primary Care Preceptorship; Psychopathology and Human Sexuality; Introduction to Child Development; Pathogenic Microbiology; Pathology; Pharmacology; Ethical Social Issues in Medicine; Clinical Skills II and Clinical Aspects of Lifestyle Abuse, which addresses behavioral aspects of health maintenance both for patients and physicians. The Academic Support and Counseling Center assists students in a variety of ways, including enrichment sessions and tutorials. Most classes take place in the Brody Medical Sciences Building, a modern facility that has classrooms with computer and video technology, large laboratories, auditoriums, and a clinical Outpatient Center. The presence of a clinical facility in this classroom structure suggests the importance of integrating basic and clinical sciences at East Carolina. Another building used frequently by first- and second-year students is the W.E. Laupus Health Sciences Library, which has 52,900 volumes and 1,550 subscriptions in addition to computer and audiovisual learning aids.

CLINICAL TRAINING: Required clerkships are Family Medicine (8 weeks); Internal Medicine (8 weeks); Ob/Gyn (8 weeks); Pediatrics (8 weeks); Psychiatry (8 weeks); and Surgery (8 weeks). At least 10 of these 48 weeks are spent in an ambulatory setting. Fourth-year students make selections from specified categories: Primary Care Experiences (2 months); Surgical Selectives (1 month); Medicine Selectives (1 month); Transition to Residency (1 month); and Electives (4 months). Clinical training takes place at sites throughout Eastern North Carolina, with the cooperation of the School's extended faculty members, some of whom practice in remote, rural areas. Training also takes place at: the Developmental Evaluation Clinic; Eastern Carolina Family Practice Center; Pitt County Memorial Hospital (731 beds); specialized research institutes; and at rural affiliated hospitals throughout the state.

Students

Virtually all students are North Carolina residents, many of whom attended college outside of the state. More than 20 percent of students are underrepresented minorities, mostly African Americans. Almost half of entering students have taken some time off between undergraduate and medical school. In a recent entering class, the mean age at matriculation was 26. Class size is 72.

STUDENT LIFE: The University has an active student union, and facilities such as student lounges, theaters, concert halls, museums, and an athletic center. Medical students are integrated into the greater campus community, but also have a cohesive social life among themselves. Medical student groups are organized around volunteer efforts, professional interests, support groups, and religious affiliations, among other themes. Examples are the Generalist Physicians in Training Interest Group, the Medical Student Council, Peer Counseling, the Christian Medical/ Dental Fellowship, and the Greenville Community Shelter Clinic. Greenville is known for its gentle climate and low cost of living, both assets for medical students. There are plenty of housing options, both on and off campus, for married or single students.

GRADUATES: The goal of the Generalist Physician Initiative is that at least half of medical school graduates enter primary care fields. There are at least 12 residency programs and several fellowship programs offered at Pitt County

Memorial Hospital, with the majority of positions in Internal Medicine, Family Medicine, and Emergency Medicine.

Admissions

REQUIREMENTS: One year each of Physics, Biology, General Chemistry, Organic Chemistry, and English are all required. Laboratories, are required with all science courses. The MCAT is required and must be no more than three years old. For those who have retaken the exam, the most recent set of scores is generally considered. State residency, or close affiliation with the state, is a requirement for admission.

SUGGESTIONS: Beyond required courses, students are advised to take Humanities and Social Science courses, and an additional year of English. Taking classes that are part of the medical school curriculum is not recommended. Extracurricular activities that involve exposure to the medical practice are important. The Admissions Committee looks for applicants who are likely to contribute to meeting the health care needs of North Carolina.

PROCESS: All AMCAS applicants who are state residents (or who demonstrate strong ties to the state) are sent secondary applications. About 60 percent of those returning secondaries are interviewed, with interviews taking place between August and April. The interview consists of two 30–60-minute sessions with faculty or student members of the committee. On interview day, applicants have an opportunity to meet with students and to tour the campus. About 15 percent of interviewed candidates are accepted, while others are rejected or wait-listed. Candidates awaiting a decision may send additional information to enhance their files.

Costs

In addition to tuition, which is remarkably low, the anticipated cost of living for a single student is $1,000 monthly. This budget allows for either on- or off-campus housing. Most students own cars.

FINANCIAL AID: Most aid is through federal loan programs and is need-based, with need determined by the FAFSA form. Through the Brody Scholarship program, three merit-based full scholarships are awarded each year to students with leadership potential and a sincere interest in primary care. Other private loan/scholarship programs geared toward promoting primary care physicians are also available.

EAST CAROLINA UNIVERSITY

STUDENT BODY

Type	Public
*Enrollment	307
*% male/female	50/50
*% underrepresented minorities	24
# applied (total/out)	1,377/638
% interviewed (total/out)	37/0
% accepted (total/out)	8/0
% enrolled (total/out)	65/0
Average age	25

ADMISSIONS

Average GPA and MCAT Scores

Overall GPA	3.50	Science GPA	3.45
MCAT Bio	9.2	MCAT Phys	8.8
MCAT Verbal	9.4	MCAT Essay	P

Score Release Policy

At least one set of recent MCAT scores are required, but students may withold scores from earlier exams if desired.

Application Information

Regular application	11/15
Regular notification	10/15 to matriculation
Early application	6/1–8/1
Early notification	10/1
Transfers accepted?	No
Admissions may be deferred?	No
AMCAS application accepted?	Yes
Interview required?	Yes
Application fee	$50

COSTS AND AID

Tuition & Fees

Tuition (in/out)	$2,280/$21,962
Cost of books	$1,500
Fees	$1,006

Financial Aid

% students receiving aid	83
Average grant	$5,923
Average loan	$14,058
Average debt	$51,047

*Figures based on total enrollment

EAST TENNESSEE STATE UNIVERSITY

JAMES H. QUILLEN COLLEGE OF MEDICINE

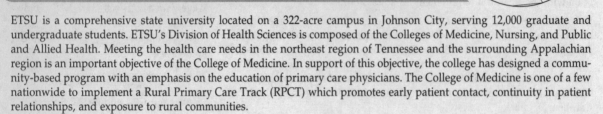

PO Box 70580, Johnson City, TN 37614
Admission: 423-439-4753 • Fax: 423-439-8206
Email: sacom@etsu.edu

ETSU is a comprehensive state university located on a 322-acre campus in Johnson City, serving 12,000 graduate and undergraduate students. ETSU's Division of Health Sciences is composed of the Colleges of Medicine, Nursing, and Public and Allied Health. Meeting the health care needs in the northeast region of Tennessee and the surrounding Appalachian region is an important objective of the College of Medicine. In support of this objective, the college has designed a community-based program with an emphasis on the education of primary care physicians. The College of Medicine is one of a few nationwide to implement a Rural Primary Care Track (RPCT) which promotes early patient contact, continuity in patient relationships, and exposure to rural communities.

Academics

Joint M.D./Ph.D. programs are offered through the School of Graduate Studies in Anatomy, Biochemistry, Cell Biology, Microbiology, Pharmacology, and Physiology. Most students earn an M.D. in four years, through either the traditional track, or the RPCT.

BASIC SCIENCES: With the exception of clinical work, basic science courses are taught primarily in a lecture/lab format. Students are in scheduled sessions for about 24 hours per week. First-year courses for all students are Anatomy, Biochemistry, Biostatistics, Neurobiology, Cell Biology, and Physiology. Traditional track students also take Practicing Medicine and Nutrition while RPCT students take Introduction to Rural Medicine, Communication for Health Professionals, Rural and Community Health Systems, and Health Assessment/Examination. Patient contact begins in Practicing Medicine for traditional track students and as part of weekly visits to rural health providers for RPCT students. The second-year curriculum for all students is Genetics, Microbiology, Immunology, Pathology, Psychiatry, and Pharmacology. Traditional track students take Clinical Skills and Practicing Medicine while RPCT students take Rural Health Needs, Health Assessment, RPCT practicing Medicine, and Patient/Client Assessment. Instructional facilities are located in several modern buildings on the main University campus, and on the grounds of the Mountain Home Veterans Affairs facility which also houses the Medical Library. The Library has almost 100,000 volumes, several online medical databases, educational software programs, computerized access to the University library system, computers for student use, and rooms for audiovisual study, reading, and conferences. Evaluation uses an A–F grading system. Students must pass Step 1 of the USMLE for promotion to year three.

CLINICAL TRAINING: Third-year required rotations for traditional track students are Family Medicine (8 weeks); Ob/Gyn (8 weeks); Pediatrics (8 weeks); Psychiatry (8 weeks); Internal Medicine (8 weeks); and Surgery (8 weeks). RPCT students take part in shorter rotations in the same specialties, and are required to complete a 16-week primary care clerkship in a rural area. During the fourth year, all students complete a minimum of 16 weeks of electives. RPCT students have additional rural, primary care requirements, and traditional tract students must take Internal Medicine and Senior Surgery. Clinical training takes place in three cities, Bristol, Kingsport, and Johnson City, and in neighboring rural towns. Affiliated hospitals are The Johnson City Medical Center; VA Medical Center; Woodridge Psychiatric Hospital; Johnson City Specialty Hospital; Northside Hospital; The Holston Valley Hospital; Indian Path Medical Center; Bristol Regional Medical Center; Johnson County Hospital; and Hawkins County Hospital. In total, these hospitals provide 3,000 patient beds. Evaluation uses an A–F grading system, and the USMLE Step 2 is required for graduation.

Students

Almost all students are from Tennessee or the immediately surrounding areas. Most students went to college in Tennessee, although undergraduate institutions from around the country are represented in the medical student body. About 15 percent of students are underrepresented minorities, most of them African American. Class size is 60.

STUDENT LIFE: Medical students take advantage of the extracurricular opportunities at ETSU, such as its theater, films, intramural sports, and athletic and recreational facilities. Campus housing is encouraged as a way of promoting friendship and a sense of community among students. Options include residence halls, efficiency apartments, and larger units suitable for couples or parents. As an urban area, Johnson City offers many services and attractions.

GRADUATES: Of the 56 students that graduated and entered residency programs in 1997, 16 chose Family Practice, 10 chose Internal Medicine, eight chose Surgery, four chose Medicine/Pediatrics, three chose Pediatrics, two each chose Ophthalmology, Ob/Gyn, Psychiatry, Radiology, and Orthopedic Surgery, and one each chose Dermatology, Emergency Medicine, Neurology, and Urology. A few Seniors each year enter the Accelerated Residency

Training Program (ARTP), which combines the final year of medical school with the first year of residency in Family or Internal Medicine.

Admissions

REQUIREMENTS: Applicants must complete Chemistry (8 semester hours); Organic Chemistry (8 hours); Physics (8 hours); Biology (8 hours); and Communication Skills/English (9 hours). An additional 49 hours of course work in liberal arts disciplines is required. The MCAT is required and should be no more than two years old. The April MCAT is advised as the August exam will delay application processing.

SUGGESTIONS: Other recommended courses are Comparative Vertebrate Anatomy, Histology, Mammalian Anatomy, Advanced Mathematics, Statistics, Biochemistry, Microbiology, Public Speaking, History, Economics, Philosophy, Psychology, Social Science, and Foreign Languages. For those who have been out of school for a significant period of time, recent course work is helpful. The Admissions Committee looks for traits and experiences that are consistent with primary care practice. Admissions is particularly competitive for out-of-state residents, and with the exception of applicants from the contiguous Appalachian region who are interested in primary care, out-of-state applicants must have extremely strong qualifications to be considered.

PROCESS: About one-third of AMCAS applicants are sent secondary applications. Of those submitting secondaries, the majority of Tennessee residents and about 10 percent of out-of-state residents are invited to interview between September and March. Applicants receive two one-hour interviews with faculty, medical students, administrators, or community members. Of interviewed candidates, about 40 percent of Tennessee residents and 10 percent of out-of-state residents are accepted on a rolling basis. Others are either rejected or wait-listed. Generally, only a few students are accepted off of the wait list. Undergraduate students at ETSU may apply for a Pre-medical/Medical program at the end of their Freshman year that leads them through a well-rounded undergraduate curriculum and into the College of Medicine.

Costs

Not including tuition, yearly cost-of-living expenses for a single student range from $11,000–$15,000, depending on whether campus housing is used. This type of budget includes all expenses and allows for car ownership.

FINANCIAL AID: Most financial aid is in the form of loans, from either federal or institutional sources. Grants are available for those with the most financial need, and some are specifically for minority students. Merit scholarships are awarded. The Practice Scholars Program is a tuition assistance program offered by hospitals to a limited number of students which provides a stipend during medical school in exchange for a commitment to practice in the community of the hospital.

EAST TENNESSEE STATE UNIVERSITY

STUDENT BODY

Type	Public
*Enrollment	237
*% male/female	56/44
*% underrepresented minorities	12
# applied (total/out)	1,464/895
% interviewed (total/out)	18/5
% accepted (total/out)	NR/NR
% enrolled (total/out)	6/2

ADMISSIONS

Average GPA and MCAT Scores

Overall GPA	3.49	Science GPA	3.42
MCAT Bio	9.30	MCAT Phys	8.90
MCAT Verbal	9.60	MCAT Essay	NR

Score Release Policy

The MCAT is required, but the school will allow students to withhold scores in certain circumstances.

Application Information

Regular application	12/1
Regular notification	10/15 until filled
Early application	6/1–8/1
Early notification	10/1
Admissions may be deferred?	Yes
AMCAS application accepted?	Yes
Interview required?	No
Application fee	$25

COSTS AND AID

Tuition & Fees

Tuition (in/out)	$11,000/$28,000
Cost of books	NR
Fees	$780

Financial Aid

% students receiving aid	NR
Average grant	NR
Average loan	NR
Average debt	NR

*Figures based on total enrollment

EASTERN VIRGINIA MEDICAL SCHOOL
OF THE MEDICAL COLLEGE OF HAMPTON ROADS

721 Fairfax Avenue, Norfolk, VA 23507
Admission: 757-446-5812 • Fax: 757-446-5896
Internet: www.evms.edu

Eastern Virginia Medical School (EVMS) was founded to help meet the health care needs of the population of a region of the state encompassing Norfolk, Virginia Beach, Portsmouth, Chesapeake, Suffolk, Newport News, and Hampton. EVMS is referred to as the "school without walls" because its clinical facilities include more than 30 different health care institutions located throughout the region. Students train in large hospitals, small clinics, and private offices and benefit from the diverse patient population that this exposure affords. EVMS is known for its emphasis on training caring and humanistic physicians.

Academics

The curriculum is designed to help students master both the science of medicine and the art of clinical problem solving. A combined M.D./Ph.D. program is available for qualified students, leading to the doctorate degree in one of the biomedical science fields. For medical students interested in medical research, summer research projects are available. Medical students are evaluated with Honors, High Pass, Pass, and Fail.

BASIC SCIENCES: The first two years are devoted to basic sciences that are fundamental to the practice of medicine. Students also learn the clinical skills of physical diagnosis and interviewing. Throughout the first two years, students are in class or other scheduled sessions for about 25 hours per week. Lectures, labs, and small-group discussions are the instructional modalities used. First-year courses are the following: Biochemistry; Gross Anatomy; Histology; Human Development; Introduction to the Patient/Longitudinal Generalist Mentorship; Medical Ethics; Medical Molecular and Cellular Biology; Neuroscience; Physiology; and The Doctor, The Patient. Second-year courses are the following: Biostatistics; Epidemiology; Introduction to the Patient/Longitudinal Mentorship; Medical Ethics; Microbiology/Immunology; Pathology; Pathophysiology; Pharmacology; and Psychopathology.

CLINICAL TRAINING: Required third-year clerkships are: Family Medicine (6 weeks); Internal Medicine (12 weeks); Ob/Gyn (8 weeks); Pediatrics (8 weeks); Psychiatry (6 weeks); and Surgery (8 weeks). Fourth-year required clerkships include four weeks of Surgical Specialties, two weeks of Geriatrics, one week of Substance Abuse, and 25 weeks of electives, which may be selected from basic science and clinical offerings. For clinical training, students have access to a wide range of facilities including the East Coast's largest naval hospital, full-service community hospitals, interdisciplinary primary care centers, one of the largest Level I shock trauma centers in the state, private hospitals, a prestigious children's hospital, and clinics built for the medically underserved.

Students

At least 70 percent of students are Virginia residents. The student body has a number of older or "nontraditional" students, and the average age of incoming students is often around 26. Underrepresented minorities account for approximately 7 percent of the student body. Class size is 105.

STUDENT LIFE: EVMS supports students' non-academic lives and puts significant resources into the well-being of its students. Each fall, students and faculty members convene at a nearby resort for the orientation retreat sponsored by the school's Human Values in Medicine Program. The retreat provides a relaxed and informal atmosphere and allows incoming students the chance to interact before classes begin. Throughout the year, students are involved in a number of organizations and events, including ongoing community-service projects and a monthly Friday-night social hour. In general, the school's location in the Hampton Roads area is ideal for medical students, offering urban conveniences, the friendliness of a small town, and the attractions of a beach community. Most medical students live in the section of Norfolk near the medical school known as Ghent, a beautiful neighborhood of tree-lined streets and Victorian houses. EVMS also owns and operates an apartment complex near the school that offers housing for both married and single students. Washington, D.C., with its many attractions and recreational opportunities, is only a four-hour drive.

GRADUATES: From 20 percent to 25 percent of graduates are accepted into one of the many residency programs sponsored by the Eastern Virginia Graduate School. Other graduating students are successful in securing residency positions at institutions throughout the state and at locations around the country.

Admissions

REQUIREMENTS: Required courses are one year each of Biology, Chemistry, Organic Chemistry, and Physics all with associated labs. Applicants are expected to have a B or better in these courses. The MCAT is required, and scores should be from no more than two years prior to the date of application. For applicants who have retaken the exam, the best set of scores is weighed most heavily. Thus, there is no advantage in withholding scores.

SUGGESTIONS: In addition to academic transcripts, an applicant's experiences and background are examined. Personal characteristics are evaluated during the interviews, and honesty and spontaneity are considered essential qualities. Interviewers are interested in an applicant's concept of a physician's role, motivation, sensitivity to the needs of others, and communication skills.

PROCESS: After an initial screening of academic credentials, state residency, and other factors, about 50 percent of AMCAS applicants are sent secondary applications. A slightly larger percentage of state-resident applicants are asked to submit secondaries. Of those returning secondaries, about one-third are interviewed between September and March. Interviews consist of one session with a small panel of faculty members and medical students. On interview day, candidates also have the opportunity to meet with current students, tour the campus, and attend group information presentations. About one-third of interviewed candidates are accepted on a rolling basis. Alternate paths to admission are possible for students at schools that have special arrangements with EVMS. These are Old Dominion University, The College of William and Mary, Norfolk State University, Hampton University, and Hampden-Sydney College.

Costs

Living expenses vary, but average $1,100 a month. Books and equipment costs are approximately $1,500.

FINANCIAL AID: Scholarships averaging $2,700 are available for bona fide Virginia residents. Scholarships and interest-free loans during enrollment are awarded based on demonstrated financial need. Primary care funds are available for those who will commit to a primary care residency and practice.

EASTERN VIRGINIA MEDICAL SCHOOL

STUDENT BODY

Type	Private
*Enrollment	406
*% male/female	57/43
*% underrepresented minorities	7
# applied (total/out)	4,681/3,811
% interviewed (total/out)	11/6
% accepted (total/out)	NR/NR
% enrolled (total/out)	17/8
Average age	26

ADMISSIONS

Average GPA and MCAT Scores

Overall GPA	3.5	Science GPA	3.5
MCAT Bio	10.00	MCAT Phys	10.00
MCAT Verbal	10.00	MCAT Essay	NR

Score Release Policy

The school has not responded to our inquiry regarding withheld MCAT scores. Therefore, we advise caution. Contact the Admissions Office before withholding any scores.

Application Information

Regular application	11/15
Regular notification	10/15 until filled
Early application	6/1–8/1
Early notification	10/1
Transfers accepted?	Yes
Admissions may be deferred?	Yes
AMCAS application accepted?	Yes
Interview required?	Yes
Application fee	$85

COSTS AND AID

Tuition & Fees

Tuition (in/out)	$15,000/$27,500
Cost of books	$1,500
Fees	$1,291

Financial Aid

% students receiving aid	90
Average grant	$2,700
Average loan	$25,000
Average debt	$88,876

*Figures based on total enrollment

EMORY UNIVERSITY
SCHOOL OF MEDICINE

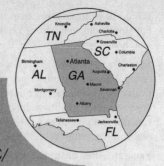

Medical School Admissions, Room 303

Woodruff Health Sciences Center, Administration Building

Atlanta, GA 30322-4510 • Admission: 404-727-5660 • Fax: 404-727-5456

Email: medschadmiss@medadm.emory.edu • Internet: www.emory.edu/WHSC/

Emory University School of Medicine is a private school that enjoys a national reputation for the medical education it provides, the biomedical research it conducts, and the outstanding clinical care it provides. Located in the suburbs of Atlanta on the University's main campus, the medical school offers rigorous basic-science education, clinical and research opportunities. The National Centers for Disease Control (CDC) is only a few blocks away. In addition, the medical school conducts most of its clinical instruction at Grady Memorial Hospital, Atlanta's busiest public hospital, which gives students wide exposure to a diverse patient population.

Academics

The four-year medical curriculum consists of two years of basic-science instruction, followed by two years of clinical rotations. Emory offers various joint-degree programs that allow qualified students to explore interdisciplinary aspects of medicine. Students may enter a combined M.D./M.P.H. program organized with the School of Public Health. In conjunction with the graduate school, medical students may earn the Ph.D. degree concurrently with the M.D. Fields of study for the doctorate degree are Biochemistry; Biomedical Engineering; Biophysics; Cell and Developmental Biology; Genetics; Immunology; Microbiology; Molecular Pathogenesis; Pharmacology; Physiology; Molecular Genetics; Neuroscience; and Nutrition and Health Science. Both Steps of the USMLE are required for graduation.

BASIC SCIENCES: The basic-science portion of the curriculum is comprehensive and intensive, with an instructional methodology that relies on lectures, small-group problem-based learning sessions, and labs. Introductory clinical experiences, discussions about the doctor-patient relationship and medical decision making, and the behavioral aspects of medicine are integrated with basic-science concepts during the first and second years. First-year (10 months) courses are Anatomy, Embryology, Biochemistry, Neurobiology, Physiology, Histology, and Genetics. Students attend class or other scheduled sessions for about 25 hours per week. The second year (10 months) includes courses in Immunology, Pathology, Behavioral Science, Clincal Methods, Human Values and Ethics, Pharmacology, and Pathophysiology. During the pre-clinical years, students are evaluated with a letter grade.

CLINICAL TRAINING: The third and fourth years consist of 19 months of required clerkships: Ob/Gyn (8 weeks), Medicine (12 weeks), Pediatrics (8 weeks), Psychiatry (6 weeks), Radiology (3 weeks) or Dermatology (2 weeks), Surgery (8 weeks), Family Medicine (4 weeks), Neurology (4 weeks), and Anesthesiology (2 weeks). Students also spend two hours every other week discussing ethical issues specific to patient care. The fourth year includes periods reserved for elective study in a wide variety of areas. Most of the clinical instruction takes place at Grady Memorial Hospital, an enormous public hospital in downtown Atlanta. Students are evaluated with satisfactory/unsatisfactory for fall semester with final letter grade following spring semester. Elective courses are graded satisfactory/unsatisfactory.

Students

About 50 percent of students are Georgia residents. Although Emory attracts students from all regions of the country, the southern states are particularly well represented. Of the 110 students in a class, approximately 25 percent completed their undergraduate studies at Emory. About 15 percent of students are underrepresented minorities, most of whom are African American. Typically, about one-third of entering students are somewhat older, having taken time off between college and medical school.

STUDENT LIFE: Students have access to the organizations, events, and facilities of both the medical and undergraduate schools. As a release from studying, students use the athletic center, which is modern and comprehensive. Students also participate in intramural sports. Medical students organize community service projects, which serve to integrate students into the greater community and often provide additional clinical exposure. Atlanta is an excellent city for students as it is affordable and offers many cultural, recreational, and entertainment opportunities. Emory owns a variety of student housing options. However, most choose to live off campus, where apartments are plentiful and affordable.

GRADUATES: Emory students consistently score well above the national average on the USMLE Step 1. This is one factor that contributes to their success in residency placement. Many students enter primary care, but large numbers also go into academic medicine.

Admissions

REQUIREMENTS: In addition to the traditional requirements of one year each of Biology, Chemistry, Physics, and Organic Chemistry, Emory also requires six semester hours of English and 18 semester hours of Humanities and Behavioral/Social Science course work. The MCAT is required and scores must be from the new version of the exam. For applicants who have retaken the exam, the best set of scores is typically weighed most heavily. Emory operates a rolling admissions process, making it beneficial to submit MCAT scores and application material early in the summer.

SUGGESTIONS: About half of the positions in each class are reserved for residents of Georgia, giving in-state applicants an advantage in the admissions process. Residents of other southeastern states are also given some preference in admissions. In addition to required courses, Genetics and Biochemistry are both strongly recommended. It is also important that students have hospital or other medical experience.

PROCESS: All AMCAS applicants are sent supplemental applications. Of the nearly 6,800 applicants who return supplementals, approximately 800 are invited to interview between October and March. Emory conducts group interviews that involve three applicants and two faculty members and a current medical student. An additional one-on-one interview is conducted with a faculty member. On interview day, candidates also have the opportunity to meet the Dean of Admissions, to tour the campus, and to have lunch with a third- or fourth-year student. Following the interview, accepted students are notified on a monthly basis. Students placed on the alternate list are encouraged to submit new information to update their files.

Costs

The expected yearly budget for a single student is about $15,000. This allows for off-campus housing and car maintenance.

FINANCIAL AID: Need-based federal and institutional loans are available, with financial need determined by parents' and students' assets. In addition, Emory offers various scholarships awarded on the basis of merit or other special criteria. Several full scholarships are available each year.

EMORY UNIVERSITY

STUDENT BODY

Type	Private
*Enrollment	455
*% male/female	59/41
*% underrepresented minorities	30
# applied (total/out)	7,420/6,744
% interviewed (total/out)	10/8
% accepted (total/out)	4/64
*% enrolled (total/out)	42/NR

ADMISSIONS

Average GPA and MCAT Scores

Overall GPA	3.69	Science GPA	3.68
MCAT Bio	10.5	MCAT Phys	10.6
MCAT Verbal	9.8	MCAT Essay	P

Score Release Policy

Generally, it is not advisable to withhold the release of scores.

Application Information

Regular application	10/15
Regular notification	10/15–mid March
Admissions may be deferred?	Yes
AMCAS application accepted?	Yes
Interview required?	Yes
Application fee	$60

COSTS AND AID

Tuition & Fees

Tuition	$25,770
Cost of books	$2,275
Fees	$402

Financial Aid

% students receiving aid	79
Average grant	NR
Average loan	NR
Average debt	$70,068

*Figures based on total enrollment

Finch University of Health Sciences

CHICAGO MEDICAL SCHOOL

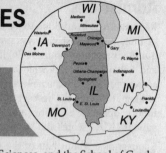

3333 Green Bay Road, North Chicago, IL 60064

Admission: 847-578-3206/3207

Email: jonesk@mis.finchcms.edu • Internet: www.finchcms.edu

Finch University encompasses The Chicago Medical School, the School of Related Health Sciences, and the School of Graduate and Postdoctoral Studies. Located on 92 acres of land 40 miles north of Chicago, Finch offers its students the diverse patient population of an urban area, along with the advantages of a self-contained campus and student life. The school is dedicated to encouraging and educating students to become competent, responsible, and concerned physicians.

Academics

Though most students earn an M.D. in four years, arrangements may be made to extend the first two years into three. A few students each year enter joint M.D./M.S. or M.D./Ph.D. programs in the following fields: Anatomy, Biochemistry, Cell Biology, Immunology, Microbiology, Molecular and Cell Sciences, Neuroscience, Pathology, Physiology, and Pharmacology. A joint degree program leading to an M.S. in the fields of Clinical Immunology or Pathology is also offered. Grading for medical students uses an A–F scale, with the exception of some electives, which are Pass/Fail.

BASIC SCIENCES: First-year required courses are: Genetics, Biostatistics/Epidemiology, Molecular Cell Biology, Medical Ethics, Anatomy, Embryology, Histology, Physiology, Biochemistry, Neuroscience, and Introduction to Clinical Medicine. Courses are taught using primarily a lecture/lab format, and students are in class for about 23 hours per week. Second-year courses are Clinical Neuroscience, Pathology, Introduction to Clinical Medicine, Microbiology, Pharmacology, Electives, and Preventive Medicine. Tutoring is available to students on an as-needed basis. Classes are held in a modern building reserved for basic-science instruction, research, and administration. Students also spend time in the Learning Resource Center, which houses the Boxer University Library, among other academic resources. The Library contains 92,966 volumes, 1,100 current subscriptions, a complete audiovisual center, and three computer labs with Internet access, databases, academic software programs, and computer-based exams. Students must pass the USMLE Step 1 in order to progress to year three.

CLINICAL TRAINING: Required third-year clerkships are: Medicine Core (2 weeks), Medicine (8 weeks), Surgery (8 weeks), Pediatrics (6 weeks), Ob/Gyn (6 weeks), Psychiatry (6 weeks), Ambulatory Care (3 weeks), Family Medicine (4 weeks), Emergency Medicine (4 weeks), and Neurology (3 weeks). The fourth year is reserved for Electives (14 weeks), Internal Selectives (14 weeks), a Primary Care Block (4 weeks), and a Subinternship in Medicine (4 weeks). There is a great deal of flexibility in terms of fulfilling elective requirements. However, no more than half of elective credits may be earned in a single field. Clinical

training takes place at Cook County Hospital (1,418 beds), Hines Veterans Affairs Medical Center (1,383 beds), Illinois Masonic Medical Center (530 beds), Lutheran General Hospital, Mount Sinai Hospital (469 beds), North Chicago Veterans Affairs Medical Center, Norwalk Hospital (in Norwalk, Connecticut), Swedish Covenant Hospital (340 beds), and Henry Ford Hospital in Detroit, Michigan (903 beds).

Students

Underrepresented minorities, mostly African American students, account for about 11 percent of the student body. Of the class entering in 1997, 35 percent were in-state residents. The average age was 25, with a range in age of 20–56. The entering class size in 1998 was 180.

STUDENT LIFE: Most first- and second-year students live in the vicinity of campus and drive to school. Often, third- and fourth-year students elect to live in Chicago, where they are closer to clinical training sites. Public transportation from downtown Chicago to campus facilitates such living arrangements. Finch offers no university-owned housing. Chicago is one of the largest and most culturally rich cities in the country, providing a wealth of entertainment, museums, theater, restaurants, nightlife, indoor and outdoor athletic activities, and spectator sporting events. The city provides distraction for medical students when they need it. Students have a voice in school administrative affairs through the University Student Council and through participation on various boards and committees. The Chicago Medical School has chapters of most national medical student associations and has special interest clubs and organizations based on recreational activities, professional interests, and ethnic/social background.

GRADUATES: Of the 1998 graduating class, the most popular specialty choices were Internal Medicine (22%), Family Practice (17%), Surgery (7%), Transitional (11%), Emergency Medicine (12%), Ob/Gyn (9%), and Pediatrics (11%).

Admissions

REQUIREMENTS: One year of Biology, Chemistry, Organic Chemistry, and Physics, all with labs, are required. The MCAT is required and must be no more than three years old at time of matriculation. For those who have retaken the exam, the best set of scores is used.

SUGGESTIONS: In addition to requirements, courses in math, social sciences, English, and the arts are recommended. A solid preparation in science, accompanied by a broad background in the liberal arts, is recommended. The Admissions Committee also puts strong emphasis on other non-academic factors, such as an applicant's motivation, character, personality, experience, and achievements.

PROCESS: All AMCAS applicants receive secondary applications. Typically, about 5 percent of applicants are interviewed. Interviews take place from October through May and consist of two sessions with faculty, administrators, and/or medical students. Notification of acceptance begins in November and is an ongoing process until the class is filled. Candidates awaiting a decision may submit supplemental information about course work, activities, or new MCAT scores.

Costs

The 1998 tuition was $32,270, which is subject to change.

FINANCIAL AID: All aid is need-based, with need determined by the FAFSA. Most assistance is in the form of loans. The average award of institutional funds for full-need students is $2,500. In addition to federal loan programs, the State of Illinois offers scholarships to medical students who agree to practice primary care medicine in areas of the state that have physician shortages.

FINCH UNIVERSITY OF HEALTH SCIENCES

STUDENT BODY

Type	Private
*Enrollment	761
*% male/female	60/40
*% underrepresented minorities	12
# applied (total/out)	10,102/8,790
Interviewed (total/out)	536/381
accepted (total/out)	240/165
enrolled (total/out)	180/117
Average age	25

ADMISSIONS

Average GPA and MCAT Scores

Overall GPA	3.23	Science GPA	3.14
MCAT Bio	10.00	MCAT Phys	9.00
MCAT Verbal	9.00	MCAT Essay	NR

Score Release Policy

It is up to the applicants whether they want their scores released or not. But, if no scores are submitted, application will not be considered.

Application Information

Regular application	11/15
Regular notification	10/15 until filled
Early application	6/1–8/1
Early notification	10/1
Transfers accepted?	Yes
Admissions may be deferred?	Yes
AMCAS application accepted?	Yes
Interview required?	Yes
Application fee	$65

COSTS AND AID

Tuition & Fees

Tuition	$32,270
Cost of books	$1,773
Fees	$300

Financial Aid

% students receiving aid	87
Average grant	NR
Average loan	NR
Average debt	$135,133

*Figures based on total enrollment

University of Florida

COLLEGE OF MEDICINE

Box 100216, Gainesville, FL 32610
Admission: 352-392-4569 • Fax: 352-846-0622
Internet: www.med.ufl.edu

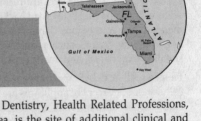

At the Gainsville campus, the College of Medicine is joined by the Colleges of Dentistry, Health Related Professions, Nursing, Pharmacy, and Veterinary Medicine. Jackson, Florida, a more urban area, is the site of additional clinical and instructional facilities. University of Florida students benefit from clinical facilities that range from small community health centers to hospitals that are ranked among the best in the country. A hallmark of the curriculum is early patient contact through mentorships with practicing physicians in rural or inner city environments.

Academics

Students may pursue their own interests with specialized institutes and centers, such as the Health Policy Institute, the Center for Mammalian Genetics, and the Brain and Cancer Institutes. A few students each year enter into a joint M.D./Ph.D. program offered in Anatomy, Biochemistry, Biomedical Engineering, Cell Biology, Genetics, Immunology, Microbiology, Molecular Biology, Neuroscience, Pathology, Pharmacology, and Physiology. Students with an interest in public health are encouraged to pursue the M.P.H. degree in conjunction with other academic institutions. Grading uses an A–F scale, and a ranking system. Both steps of the USMLE are required for graduation.

BASIC SCIENCES: Instructional methods include lectures, labs, and small-group sessions that together occupy 25 hours per week or less. First-year basic science courses are Biochemistry; Anatomy; Radiology; Genetics; Cell and Tissue Biology; Physiology; and Neuroscience. Integrated into basic sciences are behavioral sciences, ethical issues, and clinical training. Examples of first-year courses in these areas are Essentials of Patient Care, Keeping Families Healthy, Human Behavior, and the Preceptor Program. Students in the PIMS. program receive additional clinical exposure during their first year through a preceptorship within a Family Practice residency program. Second-year courses are Pathology; Oncology; Physical Diagnosis; Clinical Diagnosis; Pharmacology; Clinical Radiology; Social and Ethical Issues in Medical Practice; Public Health; and Microbiology. Classrooms, labs, and the library are in one complex. A satellite library also operates in Jacksonville.

CLINICAL TRAINING: Required third-year rotations are Medicine (8 weeks); Neurology (2 weeks); Psychiatry (6 weeks); Surgery (8 weeks); Ob/Gyn (6 weeks); Pediatrics (8 weeks); and Interdisciplinary Generalist Clerkships (10 weeks). Fourth-year clerkships are Advanced Surgery (4 weeks); Advanced Medicine, Pediatrics, or Family Medicine (4 weeks); Clinical Pharmacology (4 weeks); and Electives (28 weeks). The primary teaching hospitals are Shands Hospital (576 beds), the Gainesville Veterans Affairs Medical Center (403 beds), and the University Medical Center (528 beds). Training also takes place at outpatient clinics in nearby communities, and at clinical research facilities. Educational affiliations have been established in Tallahassee, Pensacola, Jacksonville, Leesburg, Broward County, and Orlando. With approval, up to three months of elective credits may be earned at other institutions around the country and overseas. Outside of formal rotations, students gain clinical experience through outreach projects such as Camps for Sick Kids and Care for the Homeless.

Students

About 95 percent of the students are Florida residents. Underrepresented minorities account for 6 percent of the student body, and students who have taken time off after college make up at least one-quarter of each entering class. Class size is 85.

STUDENT LIFE: Popular extracurricular activities include viewing intercollegiate sports, taking part in outdoor activities made possible by the year-round temperate climate, and occasionally going out at night to restaurants, clubs, and theaters. The University has an active student union with a theater, pool tables, a bowling alley, and a cafeteria. Athletic facilities are expansive and are well-used by medical students. Outside of the classroom, students get to know each other through involvement with organizations and projects. A few examples of the numerous medical student organizations are Physicians for Social Responsibility, the Christian Medical and Dental Group, and the Family Practice Student Organization. Service projects, such as the School of Medicine Outreach to Rural Students (S.M.O.R.S) and the EqualAccess Clinic improve students' interactive skills, and give them the opportunity to contribute to their community. On-campus housing for single and married students is available.

GRADUATES: There are about 6,500 graduates of the College of Medicine, a number of whom are renowned for important contributions made in their respective fields. At University of Florida-affiliated hospitals there are 56 post-graduate programs. Many of the positions in these programs are filled by graduates of the College of Medicine.

Admissions

REQUIREMENTS: Requirements are Chemistry (8 hours); Organic Chemistry (4 hours); Biochemistry (4 hours); Biology (8 hours); and Physics (8 hours). The MCAT is required and scores must be no more than two years old. Generally, the best set of scores is looked at most closely.

SUGGESTIONS: Early submission, preferably by June, of the AMCAS application is advised. No undergraduate major is preferred and, science and nonscience majors are considered equally. Course work in Statistics, Biochemistry, Genetics, and Microbiology is useful. Though there is no math requirement; there is an assumption that math up through Calculus was taken as an undergraduate prerequisite for Chemistry. Extracurricular activities, including volunteer and medically related experiences, are important.

PROCESS: Typically, the college receives 2,000 AMCAS applications for 73 available spaces. About half of Florida AMCAS applicants receive secondary applications, and about one-third of those returning secondaries are invited to interview. Interviews are held on Fridays, from September through March, and consist of two sessions with faculty members. On interview day, candidates also receive lunch and tours. Notification occurs on a rolling basis, and applicants are either accepted, rejected, or put on hold for a later decision. In April, a wait list is established. Additional material, and updates on course work, may be submitted by wait-listed candidates. There are two routes of admission to the College of Medicine: Junior Honors (12 places); and regular admissions (73 places). To apply for the Junior Honors program, students apply directly to the College of Medicine during their sophomore year of college. If accepted to the program, they complete a special series of seminars at the University of Florida during their junior year and begin medical school after the completion of their junior year. For Junior Honors, call (352)-392-4569.

Costs

In addition to tuition, the anticipated yearly expenditures for a single student are about $12,000 per year. This assumes either on- or off-campus living and car ownership.

FINANCIAL AID: Private and institutional scholarships are available based on merit and financial need. Federally sponsored loans and a university need-based loan program are also available. Financial need is established through the FAFSA and supplementary forms.

UNIVERSITY OF FLORIDA

STUDENT BODY

Type	Public
*Enrollment	472
*% male/female	54/46
*% underrepresented minorities	6
# applied (total/out)	2,047/994
% interviewed (total/out)	14/3
% accepted (total/out)	NR/NR
% enrolled (total/out)	29/10

ADMISSIONS

Average GPA and MCAT Scores

Overall GPA	3.72	Science GPA	NR
MCAT Bio	9.00	MCAT Phys	9.00
MCAT Verbal	9.00	MCAT Essay	NR

Score Release Policy

The Admissions Committee looks at the student's highest score. It doesn't necessarily hurt the application to withhold scores.

Application Information

Regular application	12/1
Regular notification	10/15 until filled
Admissions may be deferred?	Yes
AMCAS application accepted?	Yes
Interview required?	Yes
Application fee	$0

COSTS AND AID

Tuition & Fees

Tuition (in/out)	$9,233/$26,033
Cost of books	NR
Fees (total/out)	$1,299/$2,139

Financial Aid

% students receiving aid	NR
Average grant	NR
Average loan	NR
Average debt	NR

*Figures based on total enrollment

GEORGE WASHINGTON UNIVERSITY
SCHOOL OF MEDICINE AND HEALTH SCIENCES

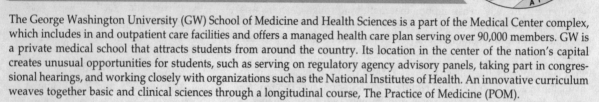

2300 Eye Street, NW, Washington, D.C. 20037

Admission: 202-994-3506

Email: medadmit@gwis2.circ.gwu.edu • Internet: www.gwumc.edu/edu/admis

The George Washington University (GW) School of Medicine and Health Sciences is a part of the Medical Center complex, which includes in and outpatient care facilities and offers a managed health care plan serving over 90,000 members. GW is a private medical school that attracts students from around the country. Its location in the center of the nation's capital creates unusual opportunities for students, such as serving on regulatory agency advisory panels, taking part in congressional hearings, and working closely with organizations such as the National Institutes of Health. An innovative curriculum weaves together basic and clinical sciences through a longitudinal course, The Practice of Medicine (POM).

Academics

The school offers several combined degree programs, including an M.D./M.P.H. program offered in conjunction with the GW School of Public Health and Health Services. Qualified students may enter a program leading to the M.D. and a graduate degree in engineering. Joint M.D./Ph.D. programs in the following fields are possible: Anatomy, Biochemistry, Cell Biology, Genetics, Immunology, Microbiology, Neuroscience, Pathology, Pharmacology, and Physiology.

BASIC SCIENCES: Three segments of the POM course occur during the first two years. One segment uses a small-group format; introduces clinical assessment skills; and discusses ethical, legal, and social issues involved in health care. Another segment is the primary care apprenticeship in which students work one-on-one with an assigned physician. In the third segment, problem-based learning serves to integrate clinical and basic science concepts around documented case studies. First-year courses, taught primarily through lectures and labs, are the following: Cells and Tissues, Gross Anatomy, Biochemistry, Micro Anatomy, Physiology, Neurobiology, and Immunology. Students are in scheduled classes for about 28 hours per week during the first year. The second-year curriculum is organized by organ systems: Infectious Disease, Cardiology, Hematology, Pulmonary, Endocrinology, Reproduction, Renal, Gastroenterology, Neurology, Rheumatology, and Human Sexuality. Each unit uses an interdisciplinary approach, including concepts of Pathology, Microbiology, and Pharmacology. Throughout the second year, students are in class for about 22 hours per week. Students may apply for research fellowships offered during the summer between years one and two. Basic science instruction takes place in a modern building, Ross Hall, that is close to the Health Sciences Library, which houses 100,000 volumes and has an extensive audiovisual study center and microcomputer lab. Passing the USMLE Step 1 is a requirement for promotion to year three.

CLINICAL TRAINING: Patient contact actually begins in year one, in POM. Formal rotations begin in year three with the following required clerkships: Medicine (8 weeks); Surgery (8 weeks); Ob/Gyn (8 weeks); Pediatrics (8 weeks);

Psychiatry (8 weeks); Primary Care (6 weeks); and the fourth segment of POM, which occupies one afternoon per week and reinforces basic science concepts of evidence-based medicine, medical decision-making, and ethics. The fourth year begins in July, and must include: an acting internship; two weeks of Anesthesiology, Emergency Medicine, and Neuroscience; four weeks to be selected among certain Surgical specialties; a course in medical decision-making; and continuation of POM from year three. The remaining 20 weeks are reserved for elective study at affiliated hospitals or elsewhere around the country or abroad. Evaluation during all four years uses an Honors/Pass/Conditional/Fail scale, and the USMLE Step 2 must be passed in order to graduate. Required clerkships take place at the University Hospital and affiliated organizations, which together feature comprehensive services including intensive care, emergency room treatment, and outpatient care to HMO members. GW, in partnership with Universal Health Services, Inc., is in the process of building a new, state-of-the-art replacement hospital, the first new hospital in the District of Columbia in more than 20 years.

Students

The class that entered in 1999 came from 68 different undergraduate institutions. About 58 percent were science majors in college, and almost 23 percent had graduate degrees. Approximately 14 percent of the student body are under-represented minorities, most of whom are African American. The average age of incoming students was 24, with a range in age from 20 to 51 years old. Class size is 151.

STUDENT LIFE: On-campus facilities include a theater, lounges and meeting rooms, study rooms, gyms, a swimming pool, a new wellness center, and several dining areas. Numerous organizations exist, among them student groups providing support to minority and older students. GW is within walking distance of downtown D.C.; the Smithsonian Museums; lively neighborhoods such as Georgetown; and Rock Creek Park, used by runners, bikers, and skaters. The campus has its own Metro stop, making it accessible to the city and surrounding areas. Students live off campus, either in the neighborhood around the school, which is among the more desirable parts of the city, or in Metro-accessible areas.

GRADUATES: In the 1999 graduating class, 47 percent of the students chose primary care specialties. Fifty-six percent of students matched to their first choice or residency program, while 84 percent matched to one of their top three choices. A significant proportion of graduates enter residencies at GW Hospital, which has about 15 post-graduate programs.

Admissions

REQUIREMENTS: Requirements are: Biology (8 semester hours); Chemistry (8 hours); Organic Chemistry (8 hours); Physics (8 hours); and English (6 hours). The MCAT is required and should be no more than three years old. For those who have retaken the test, all sets of scores are considered. Test scores, GPA, and the strength of an applicant's undergraduate institution are all academic factors that GW weighs. High School seniors may apply to a seven-year, joint B.A./M.D. program organized with GW's undergraduate college.

SUGGESTIONS: Beyond required courses, undergraduate records should demonstrate interest and achievement in an area of concentration. No specific courses are advised. An applicant's nonacademic activities, particularly those that are medically related, are carefully reviewed.

PROCESS: All AMCAS applicants receive secondary applications. Of those returning secondaries, 1,000 applicants, or about 10 percent of the pool, are interviewed. Others are either rejected or put on hold for later consideration. Interviews are conducted from September through March and consist of one or two half-hour meetings with faculty and/or students. Candidates are notified within six weeks of the interview. Another group is wait-listed. Those on the wait list may send supplementary information to strengthen their files.

Costs

Cost-of-living expenses vary a great deal, depending mainly on the student's housing situation. A budget of $12,000 is possible for shared housing in lower rent areas. Car ownership is not necessary in D.C., but is practical in the surrounding suburban areas.

FINANCIAL AID: With the exception of a few merit scholarships awarded each year, financial aid is need-based. During the 1999–2000 year, institutional aid helped meet the financial need of 17 percent of our students. The remainder was met through federal and private loans and private scholarships.

GEORGE WASHINGTON UNIVERSITY

STUDENT BODY

Type	Private
*Enrollment	631
*% male/female	52/48
*% underrepresented minorities	21
# applied (total/out)	9,672/9,626
% interviewed (total/out)	1/1
% accepted (total/out)	NR/NR
% enrolled (total/out)	15/15
Average age	24

ADMISSIONS

Average GPA and MCAT Scores

Overall GPA	3.57	Science GPA	3.50
MCAT Bio	10.00	MCAT Phys	10.00
MCAT Verbal	9.00	MCAT Essay	P

Score Release Policy
Review on a case-by-case basis.

Application Information

Regular application	12/1
Regular notification	10/15 until filled
Early application	6/1–8/1
Early notification	10/1
Transfers accepted?	Yes
Admissions may be deferred?	Yes
AMCAS application accepted?	Yes
Interview required?	Yes
Application fee	$80

COSTS AND AID

Tuition & Fees

Tuition	$33,800
Cost of books	$890
Fees	$1,035

Financial Aid

% students receiving aid	
Average grant	$6,430
Average loan	$30,990
Average debt	$118,142

*Figures based on total enrollment

GEORGETOWN UNIVERSITY

SCHOOL OF MEDICINE

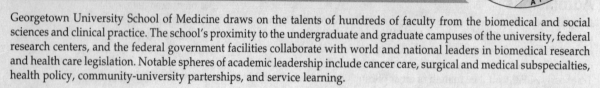

3900 Reservoir Road, NW, Washington, D.C. 20007

Admission: 202-687-1154

Internet: www.dml.georgetown.edu/schmed

Georgetown University School of Medicine draws on the talents of hundreds of faculty from the biomedical and social sciences and clinical practice. The school's proximity to the undergraduate and graduate campuses of the university, federal research centers, and the federal government facilities collaborate with world and national leaders in biomedical research and health care legislation. Notable spheres of academic leadership include cancer care, surgical and medical subspecialties, health policy, community-university parterships, and service learning.

Academics

While most students earn the M.D. through a four-year program, some extend their studies over five years in order to take part in year-long research projects between their second and third years. Others participate in combined degree programs leading to the M.D. and the Ph.D. in Cell Biology, Biochemistry, Molecular Biology, Microbiology and Immunology, Pathology, Pharmacology, Physiology, Biophysics, Neuroscience, Tumor Biology, Bioethics, or other disciplines. The proximity of the National Institute of Health facilitates student involvement in important research projects, either during summers or year-long periods. Medical students are evaluated with grades of Honors, High Pass, Pass, and Fail, with the exception of elective courses, which are usually taken as Satisfactory/Unsatisfactory. Passing Step 1 of the USMLE is a requirement for promotion to year three, and passing Step 2 is a graduation requirement.

BASIC SCIENCES: The first two years focus on basic science instruction, but also incorporate interdisciplinary courses; principles of patient care; problem-based learning modules; and ethical, social, economic, and religious aspects of health care. Lectures, labs, and small-group discussions are the teaching methods used, with students in scheduled sessions for about 22 hours per week. A student-run note taking service assists with the volume of material presented during the first two years. First-year courses are Medical Data and Reasoning; Gross Anatomy; Microscopic Anatomy; Biochemistry; Biostatistics and Epidemiology; Embryology; Endocrinology; Ambulatory Care; Neurobiology; Physiology; Introduction to Health Care; and Introduction to the Patient. Second-year courses are Pharmacology; Pathology; Microbiology and Immunology; Clinical Problem Solving; Physical Diagnosis; Psychiatry; and Ambulatory Care. Also during the second year, two hours each week are reserved for elective courses, some of which may be taken at Georgetown's main campus. Basic science instruction takes place in several science/research buildings that are part of the medical center complex. The Dahlgren Memorial Library houses over 177,000 volumes and subscribes to over 1,800 journals. Within the library is the Biomedical Academic Computer Center (BACC) with a variety of audiovisual, computer, and educational services. Students have access to the Internet, e-mail, medical software, and databases.

CLINICAL TRAINING: Third-year required rotations are Medicine (12 weeks), Surgery (12 weeks), Pediatrics (6 weeks), Ob/Gyn (6 weeks), Neurology (4 weeks), Psychiatry (4 weeks), and Family Medicine (4 weeks). Fourth-year requirements are Medicine (6 weeks), Surgery (6 weeks), Emergency Medicine (4 weeks), Selectives (20 weeks), and Electives (20 weeks). Medical students train at the Georgetown University Hospital (407 beds) and at nine other affiliated federal and community hospitals in the Washington, D.C., metropolitan area. Electives may be taken abroad through Georgetown's International Programs or through individually arranged clerkships. Examples of possible training sites are the Bahamas, Colombia, and the Dominican Republic.

Students

Virtually all states are represented in the student body. Among students in the 1997 entering class, 49 percent majored in Biological Sciences, 24 percent in Physical Sciences, 18 percent in Social Sciences, and 9 percent in various Humanities or other disciplines. Approximately 11 percent of students are underrepresented minorities. Class size is 165.

STUDENT LIFE: Though Georgetown is a Jesuit institution, the school encourages students of all denominations to express their spirituality. In addition to religious organizations, student groups focused on professional interests and community service are active. Outside of the classroom, students socialize at organized events and informally in common areas such as the new Student Lounge in the Preclinical Science Building. Medical students take advantage of the Yates Memorial Field House, which is conveniently located behind the Library. It has a pool, track, squash and tennis courts, a fitness center, and other athletic facilities. At the Leavey Center, students enjoy performing arts, shops, services, and restaurants. Washington, D.C. has vast cultural and recreational opportunities. Admission to the Smithsonian museums is free; restaurants abound; Rock Creek Park offers running and biking trails, and the city's attractions are all accessible on the metro system. A free shuttle between the Medical Center and nearby metro stations is provided. Baltimore, Philadelphia, and New York are easily reached by train, and the Appalachian Mountains and the Atlantic coast are within a few hours drive. All students live off campus, within walking or biking distance of campus.

GRADUATES: Graduates are successful in securing residency positions at institutions throughout the country.

Admissions

REQUIREMENTS: Prerequisites are one year each of Chemistry, Organic Chemistry, Biology, Physics, English, and Math. One semester of Biochemistry may be substituted for one semester of Organic Chemistry. Science courses should include associated labs. The MCAT is required, and scores should be from within the past three years. All sets of scores are considered.

SUGGESTIONS: Recommended courses include Biochemistry, Computer Science, Cellular Physiology, Genetics, Embryology, Biostatistics, Quantitative Analysis, and Physical Chemistry. Applications are not processed until MCAT scores are received. Thus, the April MCAT is preferable to the August exam. The Committee on Admissions considers character, maturity, and motivation along with academic achievement.

PROCESS: All AMCAS applicants are sent secondary applications. Of those returning secondaries, about 15 percent are interviewed between September and May. Interviews consist of one session with a faculty member or senior medical student. Also on interview day, candidates have lunch with medical students, tour the campus, and attend informational meetings. About 20 percent of interviewees are accepted. Notification begins after October 15 and continues on a rolling basis. A few highly qualified Georgetown undergraduates may be accepted to the School of Medicine during their sophomore year without MCAT scores.

Costs

The anticipated yearly cost of living for a single student is about $15,500. This budget allows for off-campus housing and use of public transportation. Car maintenance is accounted for in the budget of third- and fourth-year students.

FINANCIAL AID: Financial aid is primarily in the form of loans and is awarded on the basis of need. Parental financial disclosure is required for most forms of assistance.

GEORGETOWN UNIVERSITY

STUDENT BODY

Type	Private
*Enrollment	699
*% male/female	56/44
*% underrepresented minorities	26
# applied (total/out)	8,796/8,748
% interviewed (total/out)	12/12
% accepted (total/out)	4/4
% enrolled (total/out)	50/98
Average age	22.6

ADMISSIONS

Average GPA and MCAT Scores

Overall GPA	3.59	Science GPA	3.56
MCAT Bio	10.50	MCAT Phys	10.40
MCAT Verbal	10.00	MCAT Essay	NR

Score Release Policy

The Admissions Office says that regardless of whether they withhold scores, students must have MCAT in order to be eligible for admission.

Application Information

Regular application	11/1
Regular notification	10/15 until filled
Transfers accepted?	Yes
Admissions may be deferred?	Yes
AMCAS application accepted?	Yes
Interview required?	Yes
Application fee	$90

COSTS AND AID

Tuition & Fees

Tuition	$28,650
Cost of books	$1,461
Fees	$0

Financial Aid

% students receiving aid	80
Average grant	$4,915
Average loan	$5,000
Average debt	$120,000

*Figures based on total enrollment

MEDICAL COLLEGE OF GEORGIA

SCHOOL OF MEDICINE

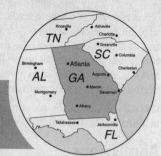

Augusta, GA 30912

Admission: 706-721-3186 • Fax: 706-721-0959

Email: sclmed.stdadmin@mail.mcg.edu • Internet: www.mcg.edu

The Medical College of Georgia is part of the University System of Georgia, which encompasses 33 institutions. The Medical College serves as the primary health-related academic center for the state, and includes Schools of Medicine, Allied Health Sciences, Dentistry, Graduate Studies, and Nursing. The campus is located in Augusta, a medium-sized city that is close to both the Appalachian Mountains and the Atlantic Ocean. The location allows medical students to gain experience treating both urban and rural patient populations. Georgia has the most comprehensive statewide telemedicine systems in the country, bringing specialty care and health education to remote, often underserved areas. Half of the practicing physicians in Georgia graduated from the Medical College of Georgia.

Academics

The School emphasizes early patient contact, uses problem-based learning, and strives to educate physicians who will help meet the health care needs of Georgians. Students and applicants interested in earning both an M.D. and a Ph.D. may apply to combined degree programs arranged with the School of Graduate Studies or with departments of the University of Georgia, Georgia Institute of Technology, or Georgia State University. Areas of doctorate study include, but are not limited to, Biochemistry, Anatomy, Biomedical Engineering, Biophysics, Cell Biology, Genetics, Immunology, Microbiology, Molecular Biology, Neuroscience, Pharmacology, and Physiology.

BASIC SCIENCES: During their first year, students take the following courses, which are primarily taught using lectures and labs: Biochemistry, Cell Biology, Gross Anatomy, Neuroscience, Physiology, and Psychiatry. Other courses are taught in small groups: Health Promotion; Patient-Doctor; Medical Ethics; and Problem-Based Learning, which applies topics covered in other classes to case studies. The second-year curriculum also uses both lecture and small-group and integrates concepts through case studies. Courses are Medical Microbiology, Ophthalmology, Pathology, Pharmacology, Physical Diagnosis, Problem-Based Learning, Problem Solving, and Reproduction. On average, students are in scheduled classes for 26 hours per week during the first two years. Classes are held in the modern Research and Education Building. Each student is advised to purchase a computer that is capable of using relevant educational software. The Greenblatt Library consists of approximately 185,000 volumes, 1,200 journal titles, and offers MEDLINE and other electronic informational systems. Audiovisual learning aids are used in class and are available at the library. Grading is A–F, with a C constituting a passing grade. Passing the USMLE Step 1 is a requirement for promotion to year three.

CLINICAL TRAINING: Patient contact begins in Patient-Doctor during year one and continues in Physical Diagnosis in year two. Year three consists of required core clerkships: Internal Medicine (12 weeks); Pediatrics (6 weeks); Family Medicine (6 weeks); Ob/Gyn (6 weeks); Surgery (6 weeks); Psychiatry (6 weeks); and Neuroscience (4 weeks). Core clerkships take place primarily at the Medical College of Georgia Hospital and Clinics (520 beds), which include separate Pediatric and Trauma units. Students may rotate to affiliated community hospitals for part of the core curriculum. During year four, students must complete an Emergency Medicine clerkship (4 weeks) in addition to a rotation in one of the following: Medicine, Family Medicine, or Pediatrics. The remainder of the fourth year is for elective study, which can include both clinical and research courses. The Medical College of Georgia is concerned with the health of the entire state, and is developing innovative outreach techniques by using, among other methods, cable television. The faculty are involved in 134 outreach clinics in 35 rural and 10 metropolitan counties. Students may participate in outreach efforts and, with permission, may rotate to alternative clinical sites. Evaluation during the clinical years uses an A–F scale. Passing the USMLE Step 2 is a requirement for graduation.

Students

At least 95 percent of students are Georgia residents. Underrepresented minorities account for about 5 percent of the student body. About one-quarter of each class took time off after college, and there is a wide age range within the student body. Class size is 180.

STUDENT LIFE: The campus is close to downtown Augusta, the second-largest metropolitan area in Georgia. Augusta offers a wide range of activities including museums, theater, restaurants, music, shopping, sailing, and golf. Students are cohesive, brought together by popular on-campus housing and student groups. Students are involved in organizations focused on professional, social, athletic, and community service activities. Many on-campus housing options are available, including residence halls, one- or two-bedroom apartments, and family housing.

GRADUATES: In the past, the majority of graduates have selected specialized fields. As part of their Generalist Initiative, the Medical College encourages students to explore primary care. The goal of the Initiative is for at least half of the graduates to enter residencies in Family Practice, Internal Medicine, or Pediatrics. Many students remain in Augusta for their post-graduate study while others enter programs elsewhere in the state and the nation.

Admissions

REQUIREMENTS: Undergraduate preparation must include: Biology with lab (1 year); Chemistry with lab (1 year); Organic Chemistry with lab (1 semester); additional upper-level Chemistry (1 semester); Physics with lab (1 year); and English (1 year). Transcripts should have grades; Pass/Fail courses are not advised. The MCAT is required and must be no more than three years old. Generally, the most recent set of scores is considered.

SUGGESTIONS: The April, rather than August, MCAT is strongly advised. For students who have taken time off after college, recent course work is recommended. Experience that involves patient contact is valuable. In addition to academic strength and general personal qualities, the Admissions Committee looks for an individual's potential for meeting the health care needs of Georgia.

PROCESS: All Georgia residents who submit AMCAS application are sent secondary applications, while only selected out-of-state residents receive secondaries. About half of in-state residents and less than 5 percent of out of state residents are interviewed. Interviews consist of two one-hour sessions, with faculty, administrators, or students who may or may not be members of the Admissions Committee. Interviews take place from October through March. Notification is rolling, but some candidates may be put on hold and notified later in the spring. After enough offers have been made to fill the class, a wait list is established from which about 30 candidates are usually admitted.

Costs

In addition to the matriculation fee, yearly living expenses range from $11,500 to $14,000, depending on whether the student lives on or off campus. This budget allows for car ownership.

FINANCIAL AID: Students apply for federal student loans through FAFSA. Institutional loans and grants are available to students with financial need, as determined by FAFSA and additional financial aid forms. Parental financial disclosure is required for all need-based assistance. A number of specialized scholarships are available to qualifying students, and scholarships based solely on academic achievement are awarded by the School of Medicine Scholarship Committee. The state sponsors a loan-repayment program for graduates who agree to serve in underserved communities.

MEDICAL COLLEGE OF GEORGIA

STUDENT BODY

Type	Public
*Enrollment	721
*% male/female	69/31
*% underrepresented minorities	5
# applied (total/out)	1,632/716
% interviewed (total/out)	23/1
% accepted (total/out)	NR/NR
% enrolled (total/out)	40/4

ADMISSIONS

Average GPA and MCAT Scores

Overall GPA	NR	Science GPA	NR
MCAT Bio	9.90	MCAT Phys	9.50
MCAT Verbal	9.80	MCAT Essay	NR

Score Release Policy

The school has not responded to our inquiry regarding withheld MCAT scores. Therefore, we advise caution. Contact the Admissions Office before withholding any scores.

Application Information

Regular application	11/1
Regular notification	10/15 until filled
Early application	6/1–8/1
Early notification	10/1
Admissions may be deferred?	Yes
AMCAS application accepted?	Yes
Interview required?	Yes
Application fee	$0

COSTS AND AID

Tuition & Fees

Tuition (in/out)	$4,862/$19,488
Cost of books	NR
Fees	$483

Financial Aid

% students receiving aid	80
Average grant	NR
Average loan	NR
Average debt	$37,943

*Figures based on total enrollment

HARVARD MEDICAL SCHOOL

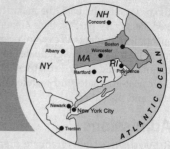

25 Shattuck Street, Boston, MA 02115
Admission: 617-432-1550 • Fax: 617-432-3307
Email: admissions_office@hms.harvard.edu
Internet: www.hms.harvard.edu

Case-based learning, a popular approach in law and business schools, was developed for medical schools at Harvard 12 years ago. This method has gained widespread acceptance and is gradually being implemented into the curricula of medical schools nationwide. At Harvard, impressive and diverse students are coupled with esteemed faculty in a structure that encourages intensive teacher-student interaction. Harvard focuses on imparting the skills for lifelong learning and with its tremendous resources, is able to accommodate the wide range of backgrounds and career goals of students.

Academics

Two distinct programs are available at Harvard—the New Pathway and the Health Science and Technology (HST) Program. All entering students are assigned to one of five Societies, organizational units used both to structure academic activities and to facilitate interaction among students and between faculty and students. Joint Degree opportunities include the M.S.T.P.; other M.D./Ph.D. programs designed in collaboration with science and nonscience graduate departments; the combined M.D./M.P.H.; and an M.D./M.P.P. with the Kennedy School of Government. More than half of the students take at least five years to complete their education in order to take full advantage of scholastic and research opportunities, some of which are actually off campus and perhaps overseas.

BASIC SCIENCES: Students in the first year of the New Pathway concentrate on Biomedical and Social Sciences. The year is divided into six sections: The Human Body, Chemistry and Biology of the Cell, Physiology, Pharmacology, Genetics, and Immunology. Students are also introduced to clinical medicine in their first year. Year two has four segments: Human Nervous System, Pathology, Human Systems I, and Human Systems II. Concepts of behavioral and community health are integrated into the basic science studies. During the first two years, lectures are scheduled for only one hour out of each day. Lectures are enhanced with tutorials and labs, but most learning takes place outside of the classroom environment. Students are responsible for addressing specific clinical challenges through independent and small-group research and analysis. Participants in HST also manage their own learning but pose questions to answer through research rather than answering questions that arise through case presentations. During the Fall Semester of year one, M.S.T. students take the following: Functional Human Anatomy, Human Pathology, Cellular and Molecular Immunology, Molecular Biology, and Genetics. During Spring Semester students take Endocrinology; Cardiovascular, Renal, and Respiratory Pathophysiology; and Research. Electives in Social and Clinical Medicine are taken throughout the year. During Year Two, Students take Neuroscience, Microbial Pathogenesis, Research, Reproductive Biology,

and Gastroenterology during the first semester and Pharmacology, Clinical Medicine, Hematology, and Psychopathology during the second semester. HST students complete a thesis as part of their requirements. Computers, loaded with curriculum-related software and linked with online data sources, are considered an important information management tool and are accessible in the Educational Center, the library, and the residence hall. The Countway Library of Medicine has one of the largest biomedical collections in the country. Grading is Satisfactory/Unsatisfactory for all courses. Passing Step 1 of the USMLE is required prior to graduation.

CLINICAL TRAINING: Patient contact begins in year one, when students learn to take histories and become familiar with basic elements of the physical exam. Formal clinical instruction begins in year three, when H.S.T. and New Pathway students join for required clerkships. These are Medicine (4 months); Neurology (1 month); Women's and Children's Health (3 months); Psychiatry (1 month); Radiology (1 month); and Surgery (3 months). Throughout years three and four, students take part in ongoing, part-time primary care training. Year four is composed mostly of electives, which can be clinical and/or research oriented. Elective credit may be earned from several departments at Harvard University or from MIT. Clinical training takes place at Harvard-affiliated hospitals, which are Beth Israel Medical Center; Brigham and Women's Hospital; Cambridge Hospital; The Center for Blood Research; The Children's Hospital; The Dana-Farber Cancer Institute; DVA Medical Center; Harvard Pilgrim Health Care; Joslin Diabetes Center; Judge Baker Children's Center; Mass. Eye and Ear; Mass. General; Mass. Mental Health Center; McLean Hospital; Mount Auburn Hospital; Schepens Eye Research; and Spaulding Rehab Hospital. Evaluation of student performance in clinical settings uses a High Honors/Honors/Satisfactory/Unsatisfactory scale. Narrative comments accompany these marks. In addition to formal rotations, students can gain experience in clinical environments through volunteer activities such as the Urban Health Project, which provides preventive and curative care to community health centers and underserved populations. Students must pass the USMLE Step 2 in order to graduate.

Students

About 75 percent of students were science majors in college. About 20 percent of the members of a typical class are underrepresented minorities, and about 30 percent took significant time off between college and medical school. Students are from all around the country. Class size is 165, of which 30 are H.S.T. and 135 are New Pathway participants.

STUDENT LIFE: The compact class schedule allows students to take part in activities of the Medical School, the greater University, and the city of Boston. About 50 percent of medical students live in Vanderbilt Hall, a renovated building adjacent to the Medical School. Married students live either off campus or in university-owned apartments. Students are active in organizations focused on topics ranging from support for various minority groups, to abortion rights, to soccer.

GRADUATES: Approximately half of each graduating class remains at Harvard for their residencies. The University of California at San Francisco also appears to be a popular choice. Of the 1997 graduating class, the most common specialty choices were Internal Medicine (34%); Pediatrics (13%); General Surgery (9%); and Orthopedic Surgery (7%).

Admissions

REQUIREMENTS: Requirements include one year of Biology with lab; Physics with lab; Expository Writing; and college-level Calculus. Two years of Chemistry are required, both of which should involve laboratory experience. For New Pathway applicants, at least 16 additional credit hours in nonscience courses are required. For HST applicants, Calculus through differential equations and Calculus-based Physics are required. The quality of an applicant's undergraduate institution is assessed in evaluating his or her GPA. The MCAT is required, and all scores are considered.

SUGGESTIONS: Unlike many schools with rolling admissions, decisions at Harvard are made after all interviews are complete. Thus, applicants submitting scores from the August MCAT are not penalized. There is no preference for particular undergraduate majors, but demonstration of academic excellence is expected. In addition, most successful applicants have impressive professional, volunteer, community service, or other extracurricular achievements.

PROCESS: In 1998 Harvard began to participate in AMCAS, a change of procedure from recent years. In the past, about 14 percent of applicants were interviewed. Interviews take place from September through January and consist of two one-hour sessions each with a member of the Admissions Committee. Decisions are made in late February, and all applicants are notified at once. A wait list is established at that time, but usually only a few candidates are ultimately accepted from the list.

Costs

In addition to tuition, yearly expenses are approximately $16,000. This presumes use of public transportation and either on-campus or shared off-campus housing.

FINANCIAL AID: Parental financial disclosure is required for almost all forms of aid. The family's resources are assessed, and if financial need is determined, a unit loan is granted for up to $20,000 per year. This loan is actually a package of federally funded student loans, and other low-interest loans. If need exists beyond the unit loan, Harvard grants scholarships to make up the difference.

HARVARD MEDICAL SCHOOL

STUDENT BODY

Type	Private
*Enrollment	744
*% male/female	53/47
*% underrepresented minorities	18
# applied (total/out)	6,017/NR
% interviewed (total/out)	17/NR
% accepted (total/out)	4/NR
% enrolled (total/out)	2.7/NR

ADMISSIONS

Average GPA and MCAT Scores

Overall GPA	3.8	Science GPA	NR
MCAT Bio	11.80	MCAT Phys	11.70
MCAT Verbal	10.50	MCAT Essay	NR

Score Release Policy

Students are required to submit all scores with application.

Application Information

Regular application	10/15
Regular notification	2/28
Admissions may be deferred?	Yes
AMCAS application accepted?	Yes
Interview required?	Yes
Application fee	$75

COSTS AND AID

Tuition & Fees

Tuition	$27,000
Cost of books	NR
Fees	$1,676

Financial Aid

% students receiving aid	70
Average grant	$14,650
Average loan	$20,000
Average debt	$85,000

*Figures based on total enrollment

UNIVERSITY OF HAWAII
JOHN A. BURNS SCHOOL OF MEDICINE

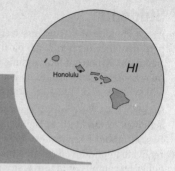

1960 East-West Road, Honolulu, HI 96822

Admission: 808-956-8300 • Fax: 808-956-9547

Email: nishikim@jabsom.biomed.hawaii.edu

Internet: medworld.biomed.hawaii.edu

The John Burns School of Medicine is part of the main campus of the University of Hawaii, located in Honolulu. As a state-supported institution, the emphasis at the School of Medicine is to train primary care physicians with the goal of improving health care in Hawaii and the Pacific area. As a result of its location and the multi-ethnic population it serves, the Medical School excels in areas of research such as communicable diseases and cross-cultural psychiatric issues. Instead of a university teaching hospital, several affiliated clinics and hospitals are used for training, giving students a first-hand understanding of community medicine and allowing them to develop strong mentor relationships with local physicians.

Academics

The School of Medicine, along with the Schools of Nursing, Public Health, and Social Work, comprise the College of Health Sciences and Social Welfare. A Master's or Ph.D. may be earned from the School of Public Health or from selected departments within the University of Hawaii, along with the M.D. Areas of study for joint degrees are Biochemistry, Biophysics, Genetics, Pharmacology, Physiology, Anatomy, Tropical Medicine, Biostatistics, and Interdisciplinary Studies.

BASIC SCIENCES: Instruction is entirely case-based and emphasizes self-directed learning and early clinical training. Throughout the first two years, students take Clinical Skills, which involves patient contact, and Community Medicine, an interdisciplinary course. Other subjects are organized into units, each one occupying three or four months. Unit 1 courses are Health and Illness and Introduction to Problem-based Learning. Unit 2 focuses on Cardiovascular, Respiratory, and Renal Problems. Unit 3 is Hematology, Endocrine, and Gastrointestinal Problems. During the summer following year one, students take part in a Primary Care Precept, which entails working with local physicians. Unit 4 is Locomoter, Neurologic, and Behavioral Problems. Unit 5 is Life Cycle Problems in Ob/Gyn, Pediatrics, Adolescents, and Geriatrics. The final three months of year two are used for a basic science review in preparation for the USMLE Step 1, which is required for promotion to year three. Scheduled classes during the first two years occupy about 20 hours per week, providing ample time for independent, self-directed study. Grading is Pass/Fail, and students are not ranked. The Biomedical Sciences Building, where basic sciences are taught, is equipped with laboratories, audiovisual computer centers, classrooms, and areas for group study and tutorials. The University Library System has the largest collection of information and research materials in the state, and includes the Hamilton Library (85,000 volumes), which serves the School of Medicine. The Library of the School of Public Health, the affiliated hospitals' libraries, and a private institution called the Hawaii Medical Library are additional resources.

CLINICAL TRAINING: Most students enter Block Rotations, referred to as Unit 6B. For these students, third-year clerkships are Surgery (7 weeks); Family Medicine (7 weeks); Ob/Gyn (7 weeks); Pediatrics (7 weeks); Psychiatry (7 weeks); and Internal Medicine (11 weeks). Two weeks are free during year three for an elective. As an alternative to the block system, Unit 6L is a longitudinal clerkship, giving selected students an opportunity to have ongoing contact with patients throughout the year. Year four, Unit 7, is reserved for electives, with the exception of one required rotation in Emergency Medicine (4 weeks). Unit 7IM is an optional fourth-year tract that prepares students for residencies in Internal Medicine. The final month of the four-year curriculum is used for a Senior Seminar, which provides an in-depth review of important topics. Grading is Honors/Credit/No Credit during the third year, and Pass/Fail during the fourth year. Students must pass the USMLE Step 2 to graduate. Training takes place at many sites including: Kapi'olani Medical Center for Women and Children; Kapi'olani Medical Center at Pali Momi; St. Francis Medical Centers; Queen's Medical Center; Tripler Army Medical Center; Hilo Family Medical Center; Milo Medical Center; Kuakini Medical Center; Shriners Hospital; Kaiser Medial Center; Wahiawa General Hospital; Sai'anae Coast Health Center; Kalihi-Palama Health Center; and the Rehabilitation Hospital of the Pacific.

Students

Hawaii's multi-ethnic population is reflected in the student body, made up of men and women of Caucasian, Chinese, Korean, Japanese, Hawaiian, Filipino, Samoan, Micronesian, and other ancestries. All but a few students per class are Hawaiian residents, most of whom completed their undergraduate training in Hawaii. Class size is 56.

STUDENT LIFE: Although the School of Medicine is relatively small and intimate, the University of Hawaii at Manoa enrolls 20,000 students. Medical students take part in campus activities but are integrated into the greater community of the city and the Island. Almost all students live off campus. Honolulu is a city with a population of almost 1 million. It is a major tourist center, offering beautiful beaches in addition to many cultural, recreational, and outdoor activities.

GRADUATES: Residency programs in Hawaii are popular with graduates and include the following specialties: Transitional; Internal Medicine; Ob/Gyn; Orthopedics; Pathology; Pediatrics; Psychiatry; Surgery; and Family Practice. Four percent of graduates are in the military service, and 1 percent are in full-time academic positions.

Admissions

REQUIREMENTS: The initial screening of applicants selects those who have very close ties to Hawaii and who are most likely to practice in Hawaii upon completion of post-graduate study. An exception is made for applicants from Wyoming and Montana, states without medical schools that have arrangements with the University of Hawaii. Undergraduate course requirements are Biology (12 semester units); Chemistry (4 units); Biochemistry (4 units); and Physics (8 units). All courses must include laboratory experience. The MCAT is required and must be no more than three years old. If the MCAT has been taken more than once, the most recent set of scores is used.

SUGGESTIONS: Additional courses in Biological and Social Science are advised, such as Immunology, Genetics, Microbiology, Anatomy, Physiology, Embryology, Psychology, and Sociology. Previous medical experience is important, as are personal qualities that suggest the applicant will become a humanistic physician. For those who have been out of school for a significant period of time, recent course work is recommended. Each year, a post-baccalaureate program selects 10 students whose applications were rejected from medical schools—though they are nonetheless promising—to participate in a year-long pre-medical training. If these students successfully complete training, they are offered a place in the School of Medicine.

PROCESS: About 15 to 20 percent of applicants are interviewed. Interviews are conducted from October through March and consist of two sessions with faculty members, practicing physicians, or members of the community. Of those interviewed, about 25 percent of in-state applicants and 5 percent of out-of-state residents are accepted. Most applicants are notified of the committee's decision in early April, though a few highly qualified applicants may hear earlier. A wait list is established at this time. Wait-listed candidates are not advised to send supplementary information.

Costs

Since the University of Hawaii is basically a commuter school, the cost of living varies a great deal from student to student. Rent is relatively high in the area, and most students own cars.

FINANCIAL AID: Most financial aid is need-based and is from federal sources. Other institutional and private assistance is need-based, merit-based, or granted on the basis of background or other special criteria.

UNIVERSITY OF HAWAII

STUDENT BODY

Type	Public
*Enrollment	230
*% male/female	53/47
*% underrepresented minorities	15
# applied (total/out)	1,098/867
% interviewed (total/out)	20/5
% accepted (total/out)	NR/NR
% enrolled (total/out)	24/16
Average age	24

ADMISSIONS

Average GPA and MCAT Scores

Overall GPA	3.43	Science GPA	3.49
MCAT Bio	9.88	MCAT Phys	9.12
MCAT Verbal	8.87	MCAT Essay	NR

Score Release Policy

The Admissions Committee does not penalize students who withhold scores, but they do caution that withholding scores "raises questions."

Application Information

Regular application	12/1
Regular notification	10/15
Early application	6/1–8/1
Early notification	10/1
Admissions may be deferred?	Yes
AMCAS application accepted?	Yes
Interview required?	Yes
Application fee	$50

COSTS AND AID

Tuition & Fees

Tuition (in/out)	$10,824/$24,528
Cost of books	$2,409
Fees	$107

Financial Aid

% students receiving aid	70
Average grant	NR
Average loan	NR
Average debt	NR

*Figures based on total enrollment

HOWARD UNIVERSITY
COLLEGE OF MEDICINE

520 W Street, NW, Washington, D.C. 20059
Admission: 202-806-6270 • Fax: 202-806-7934
Internet: www.med.howard.edu

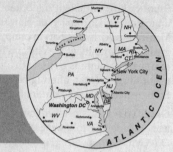

Howard University is a comprehensive, predominantly African American academic institution. It has 16 Schools and Colleges including several in health-related fields and occupies four campuses in and around Washington, D.C. Howard is a resource not only for its students, but also federal policymakers and the D.C. community as well. At the same time, the College of Medicine benefits from the resources of the area, such as the National Institutes of Health (NIH) and an expansive network of clinical-training sites that serve a large urban population. A fundamental objective of the College of Medicine is to train primary care physicians for underserved areas.

Academics

Although most students earn their M.D. in four years, some are given permission to complete requirements over a five-year period. The College of Medicine and the Graduate School of Arts and Sciences offer a joint M.D./Ph.D. program. The departments that award the Ph.D. are the following: Anatomy, Biochemistry, Biology, Chemistry, Genetics, Microbiology, Pharmacology, and Physiology.

BASIC SCIENCES: Basic sciences are presented primarily in a lecture/lab format. Students are in scheduled classes from 25 to 30 hours per week. First-year courses are: Anatomy; Biochemistry; Psychiatry; Histology; Microbiology; Immunology; Physiology; Neuroscience; Introduction to Patient Care, in which students visit clinics and interact with physicians; and Introduction to Psychodynamic Thinking, which discusses healthy and pathological mental mechanisms. Second-year courses are the following: Microbiology, Immunology, Pathology, Genetics, Physiology, Physical Diagnosis, Pathophysiology, Pharmacology, Psychopathology, and Epidemiology. Grading is Honors/Satisfactory and Unsatisfactory, and academic support services such as workshops, tutorials, and summer sessions are available. The USMLE Step 1 is required for promotion to year three. Instruction takes place in the Seeley G. Mudd Building, which features auditoriums, laboratories, and audiovisual and computer-assisted study areas. The Health Sciences Library has 260,000 volumes and journals, video equipment, and a computer linkage with the National Library of Medicine.

CLINICAL TRAINING: Patient contact begins in the first year, in Introduction to Patient Care. Throughout medical school, students have the opportunity to gain clinical experience by volunteering and participating in community outreach programs. Others gain research experience through work at NIH or other prominent institutions. Formal clinical training begins in year three (or year four for those in a five-year course of study), with the following required clerkships: Medicine (12 weeks); Surgery (8 weeks); Ob/Gyn (8 weeks); Pediatrics (8 weeks); Psychiatry (6 weeks); Rehabilitation and Neurological Disease (4 weeks); and Family Practice (4 weeks). For two hours per week, during one semester, third-year students attend lectures on ethical and legal issues in health care. Senior-year requirements are Medicine (4 weeks) and Surgery (4 weeks). In addition, students take 20–24 weeks of electives in four-week blocks. Evaluation of clinical performance uses Honors/Satisfactory/Unsatisfactory, and the USMLE Step 2 is required for graduation. Clinical training takes place largely at Howard University Hospital (300 beds). Other sites used are Howard University Cancer Center; Center for Sickle Cell Disease; Walter Reed Army and National Naval Medical Centers; D.C. General Hospital; St. Elizabeth's Hospital; VA Medical Center; Providence Hospital; Greater Southeast Community Hospital; Prince George's Hospital Center; Washington Hospital Center; and National Rehabilitation Hospital.

Students

About 60 percent of the students are African American, and about 10 percent are from African or Caribbean countries. An average of thirty states and several foreign countries are usually represented. From 10 percent to 20 percent of the students in each entering class attended Howard for undergraduate, pre-medical studies. About 20 percent of entrants are considered nontraditional, having taken time off between college and medical school and participated in some sort of post-baccalaureate pre-medical program. Class size is 110.

STUDENT LIFE: Medical students enjoy both an active campus life and involvement in the greater community. They may participate in Howard University activities, such as its radio and television stations, intramural athletic teams and events, conferences, and social or special-interest clubs. Washington, D.C., is a center for cultural, academic, recreational, and obviously, political activities. In addition to being an international city, D.C. has a strong local, predominantly African American community that is highly diverse. The College of Medicine is part of Howard's downtown campus, which is metro accessible and convenient to lively neighborhoods and interesting parts of the city such as the White House and Smithsonian

Museums. Housing for graduate students is available in modern, University-owned apartments. However, most students live off campus and either walk or take public transportation to school.

GRADUATES: About 25 percent of African American physicians practicing in the United States are Howard Alumni. Howard graduates secure post-graduate positions at institutions all over the country. Significant numbers enter one of the 16 residency programs at Howard University Hospital or at D.C. General Hospital, where they are also supervised by Howard faculty.

Admissions

REQUIREMENTS: Requirements are the following: Biology (8 hours); Chemistry (8 hours); Organic Chemistry (8 hours); Physics (8 hours); College Math (6 hours); and English (6 hours). The MCAT is required and must have been taken within the past three years.

SUGGESTIONS: Beyond required courses, Cell Biology, Biochemistry, and Developmental Biology or Embryology are recommended. For students who have taken time off after college, recent course work is helpful. The Admissions Committee values activities that demonstrate an interest in working with underserved communities.

PROCESS: All AMCAS applicants receive secondary applications. Of those submitting secondaries, about 10 percent are interviewed with faculty or administrators. Others are rejected, advised to retake the MCAT, or put in a hold category and considered for interview later in the year. Of those interviewed, 70 percent are accepted on a rolling basis, and the rest are either rejected or wait-listed. Wait-listed candidates may submit supplementary information and grades. A limited number of high school seniors are accepted into a combined B.S./M.D. program organized with Howard's College of Arts and Sciences that allows students to earn both degrees in a six-year period. Through an Early Entrance Program, a few students nationwide may be admitted to the College of Medicine after their college junior year.

Costs

Rent might range from $300 to $700 per month, depending on the type of housing and its location. The University offers full meal plans, for about $900 per semester. Car ownership is not necessary in D.C.

FINANCIAL AID: About 85 percent of students receive financial assistance, most of which is need-based. Students are expected to borrow $8,500 in subsidized federal loans prior to receiving need-based institutional aid. Merit scholarships are also available.

HOWARD UNIVERSITY

STUDENT BODY

Type	Private
*Enrollment	455
*% male/female	51/49
*% underrepresented minorities	60
# applied (total/out)	5,505/5,460
% interviewed (total/out)	10/10
% accepted (total/out)	NR/NR
% enrolled (total/out)	25/24

ADMISSIONS

Average GPA and MCAT Scores

Overall GPA	3.14	Science GPA	3.02
MCAT Bio	8.10	MCAT Phys	7.60
MCAT Verbal	7.90	MCAT Essay	NR

Score Release Policy

The school has not responded to our inquiry regarding withheld MCAT scores. Therefore, we advise caution. Contact the Admissions Office before withholding any scores.

Application Information

Regular application	12/15
Regular notification	10/15 until filled
Admissions may be deferred?	Yes
AMCAS application accepted?	Yes
Interview required?	No
Application fee	$45

COSTS AND AID

Tuition & Fees

Tuition	$16,460
Cost of books	NR
Fees	$888

Financial Aid

% students receiving aid	85
Average grant	NR
Average loan	NR
Average debt	$63,000

*Figures based on total enrollment

UNIVERSITY OF ILLINOIS AT CHICAGO

COLLEGE OF MEDICINE

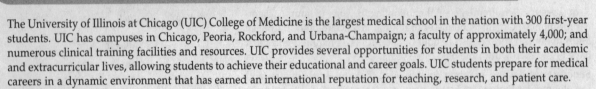

808 South Wood Street, Chicago, IL 60612-7302

Admission: 312-996-5635 • Fax: 312-996-6693

Internet: www.uic.edu/depts/mcam

Email: med-admit@mailbox.comd.vic.edu

The University of Illinois at Chicago (UIC) College of Medicine is the largest medical school in the nation with 300 first-year students. UIC has campuses in Chicago, Peoria, Rockford, and Urbana-Champaign; a faculty of approximately 4,000; and numerous clinical training facilities and resources. UIC provides several opportunities for students in both their academic and extracurricular lives, allowing students to achieve their educational and career goals. UIC students prepare for medical careers in a dynamic environment that has earned an international reputation for teaching, research, and patient care.

Academics

Students participate in one of two educational tracks: 175 students complete all four years in Chicago, while 125 spend their first year in Urbana-Champaign. After the first year in Urbana-Champaign, 50 students each complete years two, three, and four in Peoria or Rockford. The remaining 25 students in Urbana-Champaign participate in the Medical Scholars Program.

BASIC SCIENCES: The first and second years include the Principles of Anatomy, Behavioral Science, Biochemistry, Genetics, Histology, Immunology, Microbiology, Neuroscience, Pathology, Pathophysiology, Pharmacology, and Physiology. All students participate in a clinical medicine course. Lectures and labs are the predominant instructional modality.

CLINICAL TRAINING: Patient contact begins in the first year when students are assigned individual physician preceptors. Students sharpen their skills in diagnosis and treatment through problem solving sessions. In the third and fourth years, students focus on patient care with a series of clerkships supplemented by conferences and lectures. The 25 affiliated facilities range from rural ambulatory healthcare centers to major metropolitan hospitals. The diverse clinical experiences prepare UIC graduates to succeed within the nation's ever-changing health care system.

Required clerkships include: Family Medicine, Internal Medicine, Obstetrics/Gynecology, Pediatrics, Psychiatry, and Surgery. The elective phase provides students with the opportunity to identify special interest areas and to select educational experiences most relevant to their goals. The objective of the M.D./Ph.D. Program is to train students for careers in academic medicine and research. The Medical Scholars Program (M.S.P.), located on the Urbana-Champaign campus, permits students to integrate medicine with graduate studies in both science and nonscience fields. The Independent Study Program (ISP) allows students to design their own academic programs with advice from faculty. ISP students complete an in-depth study, usually involving the basic sciences or clinical medicine. The ISP program is offered on the Chicago, Peoria, and Rockford campuses. The Rural Medical Education Program (RMED) and Rural Illinois Medical Student Assistance Program (RIMSAP) recruit students who commit to practice in medically underserved areas of Illinois.

Students

UIC is one of the most ethnically diverse medical schools in the country. Students are assigned to a faculty member who serves as an advisor. The advisor's major role is to be available to the student throughout his or her medical education for academic and personal counseling. Research interests are widely diversified and range from basic molecular biology to patient-related clinical research.

STUDENT LIFE: Students in Chicago enjoy living in one of the country's most exciting cities. In Urbana-Champaign, students benefit from a large and exciting university community. Rockford and Peoria are mid-size cities offering all students basic urban amenities. Campus housing in Chicago includes three residence halls near the college. In Urbana-Champaign, university-certified housing includes campus and private residence halls, and university apartments for family housing. In Peoria and Rockford housing is easily accessible and reasonable.

GRADUATES: UIC students undertake career specialization and training in all disciplines. Most graduates who participate in the National Residency Matching Program receive one of their top three residency choices.

Admissions

REQUIREMENTS: Only those applicants who indicate plans to obtain a baccalaureate degree prior to enrollment will be considered for admission. Major fields may be in humanities, behavioral, biological, or physical sciences. All applicants must complete: Two semesters of Introductory Biology or the equivalent with laboratory. Two semesters of General Inorganic Chemistry or the equivalent with laboratory. Two semesters of Organic Chemistry with laboratory. (Introductory Biochemistry may substitute for one semester of Organic Chemistry.) Two semesters of General Physics or the equivalent. All applicants are expected to complete three semesters of Social Science courses with an emphasis in the behavioral sciences. In addition, candidates are expected to take at least one of the following courses: Advanced-level Biology, Biochemistry, Physiology, Mammalian Histology, Comparative Vertebrate Anatomy, or Molecular Genetics.

All applicants must take the MCAT no later than the fall of the year prior to enrollment and no more than three years prior to application. All applicants must complete an application to the AMCAS no later than December 31 of the year prior to enrollment. All applicants must be U.S. citizens or possess a permanent resident immigrant visa at the time of application through AMCAS. On receipt of the AMCAS application, eligible applicants will be sent a UIC Supplemental Application. Materials must be postmarked by February 15 of the year prior to enrollment.

A minimum of three academic letters of recommendation or one composite recommendation from a pre-professional committee must be postmarked by February 15 of the year prior to enrollment. If you are currently enrolled in a graduate or professional school, one of your three letters of recommendation must be from a faculty member at your graduate or professional school. It is advisable that letters of recommendation be sent from the institution at which the applicant had been most recently enrolled and must be completed on official university or business letterhead. Personal letters of recommendation are not acceptable.

SUGGESTIONS: At least 90 percent of UIC students are Illinois residents. Although Illinois residents are given preference, positions are open to highly qualified nonresidents. In addition to academic strength, experience and background are considered important factors in admissions decisions.

PROCESS: About one-third of AMCAS applicants are sent a UIC Supplementary Application. Of those returning supplementals, the most highly qualified are invited to interview between September and April. The interview is a requirement and will be arranged by the Office of Medical College Admissions. Interviews are granted by invitation only. Interviews are held on all four campuses, and the interview location does not determine the campus where matriculants may attend. The interview consists of one panel interview session. Candidates have the opportunity to meet faculty members and students, receive financial aid information, tour the campus, and learn more about the College of Medicine. Interviewed candidates are accepted on a batch system. Students not immediately accepted may be put on an alternate list.

Costs

The cost of a medical education at UIC is moderate in comparison with many other institutions.

FINANCIAL AID: The Office of Student Financial Aid participates in most state, federal and private financial aid programs available. Students who complete the FAFSA will be considered for most federal financial aid programs. In addition to administering state and federal aid programs, the OSFA awards grant and loan money bequeathed for this purpose. The OSFA publishes a listing of college-administered aid programs, including programs administered by outside agencies. Most assistance is in the form of long-term loans.

UNIVERSITY OF ILLINOIS AT CHICAGO

STUDENT BODY

Type	Public
*Enrollment	1,221
*% male/female	60/40
*% underrepresented minorities	20
# applied (total/out)	4,688/2,558
% interviewed (total/out)	18/4
% accepted (total/out)	NR/NR
% enrolled (total/out)	39/19

ADMISSIONS

Average GPA and MCAT Scores

Overall GPA	3.51	Science GPA	3.34
MCAT Bio	9.8	MCAT Phys	10.0
MCAT Verbal	9.6	MCAT Essay	NR

Score Release Policy

The Admissions Committee uses the highest set of scores; withholding scores will not affect the application.

Application Information

Regular application	12/31
Regular notification	10/15 until filled
Early application	6/1–8/1
Early notification	10/1
Admissions may be deferred?	Yes
AMCAS application accepted?	Yes
Interview required?	Yes
Application fee	$40

COSTS AND AID

Tuition & Fees

Tuition (in/out)	$16,294/$39,826
Cost of books	$1,280
Fees	$1,576

Financial Aid

% students receiving aid	NR
Average grant	NR
Average loan	NR
Average debt	NR

*Figures based on total enrollment

Indiana University

SCHOOL OF MEDICINE

1120 South Drive, Indianapolis, IN 46202

Admission: 317-274-3772

Internet: www.iupui.edu/it/medschl/home.html

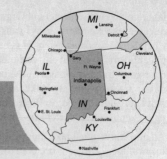

The Indiana University School of Medicine is a unique state medical school, structured to provide flexibility and choice to its students. Although based in Indianapolis, the School of Medicine is part of a network that uses nine campuses, giving students access to basic science and clinical training facilities in locations throughout the state. The School directs its resources towards training physicians to meet the medical demands of Indiana's population. The newly revised curriculum is highly interdisciplinary and reflects recent trends in health care delivery. Indiana is one of the largest medical schools in the country, with 280 students per class.

Academics

The School of Medicine in Indianapolis is part of the Indiana University (IU) Medical Center, which includes schools of Nursing, Dentistry, and Allied Health Sciences. The Medical Center complex occupies 85 acres and is situated one mile from downtown Indianapolis. In conjunction with the University Graduate School, The School of Medicine offers selected students an opportunity to pursue the M.S. or Ph.D. degrees along with an M.D. Through this program, degrees may be earned in Anatomy, Biochemistry, Biophysics, Genetics, Neurobiology, Microbiology, Pathology, Pharmacology, Physiology, Toxicology, and in Humanities and Social Studies disciplines.

BASIC SCIENCES: First-year students select one of the following nine locations for their pre-clinical studies: IU Bloomington; IU Indianapolis; Lafayette Center at Purdue; University of Notre Dame; Ball State University; Indiana State University; University of Evansville; Indiana University Northwest; and Fort Wayne Center for Medical Education at Purdue. While the curriculum is essentially the same at each campus, the methods of instruction may differ, with some programs relying more or less on case-based learning. At all schools, the "core" basic science courses are complemented by early clinical correlations. Throughout the first two years, scheduled classes account for 26-28 hours per week. At the Indianapolis campus, 80 percent of class time is devoted to lectures and labs, and 20 percent is used for small-group discussions. First-year courses are the following: Anatomy; Histology; Biochemistry; Physiology; Microbiology; Evidence-Based Medicine; Immunology; Patient/Doctor Relationship; and Concepts of Health and Disease, which teaches students how to apply basic science concepts to clinical problems. Year two courses are: Biostatistics; Pharmacology; Pathology; Clinical Medicine; Medical Genetics; and Neurobiology. With the exception of Clinical Medicine, during which students join medical teams in hospitals, second-year courses use lectures and labs as instructional techniques. The Medical Center offers all modern learning tools, including computers and audiovisual equipment. The Ruth Lilly Medical Library (200,000 volumes) is located in the Medical Research Building in Indianapolis and serves the Schools of Medicine and Nursing. All campuses have affiliated library systems, and all libraries are electronically linked. The libraries have access to 400 databases and online informational resources. Evaluation uses an Honors/High Pass/Pass/Fail system. Passing the USMLE Step 1 is a requirement for promotion to year three.

CLINICAL TRAINING: All students spend their third year at the Medical Center in Indianapolis, rotating through 11 hospitals in the Indianapolis area. The patient population is drawn from both urban and rural areas. Year three is largely composed of required rotations which are the following: Medicine (12 weeks); Surgery (8 weeks); Pediatrics (8 weeks); Ob/Gyn (6 weeks); Psychiatry (6 weeks); and Family Medicine (4 weeks). Required fourth-year clerkships are Surgical Subspecialties (8 weeks), Neurology (4 weeks), and Radiology (4 weeks). Year four is mostly dedicated to elective study, which may be pursued off campus, around the country, or overseas. Evaluation of clinical performance uses an Honors/High Pass/Pass/Fail system, augmented by narratives. Honors students generally take part in departmental research activities. Passing the USMLE Step 2 is a requirement for graduation.

Students

Typically, 95 percent of an entering class are Indiana residents. About 6 percent are underrepresented minorities, most of whom are African Americans. Approximately 5 percent of students are older than 30 at the time of matriculation.

STUDENT LIFE: Students are given a voice in school administration and curriculum development through an elected Student Government. Though student life differs from one campus to another, in general medical students benefit from the social and cultural offerings of a large university system. There is a wide range of lifestyles among students, with some living on campus in residence halls or apartments and others living off campus, perhaps with their families. Medical students have access to all campus recreational facilities and events.

GRADUATES: Slightly less than half of the 2000 graduating class entered residency programs in Indiana. Other popular locations for post-graduate training were Michigan, Ohio, and Illinois. The most common specialty choices were Family Medicine (16% of the class); Internal Medicine (11%); Pediatrics (11%); Surgery (10%); Radiology (9%); Ob/Gyn (8%); and Emergency Medicine (7%); and Anesthesia (7%). About 60% of graduates entered fields considered to be primary care.

Admissions

REQUIREMENTS: Required undergraduate courses are one year each of the following: Chemistry, Organic Chemistry, Biology, and Physics. All courses must include labs. Beyond GPA, the quality of an applicant's undergraduate course load is considered rather than the quantity of extra course hours. The MCAT is required, and must be no more than four years old. If an applicant has retaken the MCAT, the most recent score is considered.

SUGGESTIONS: Undergraduate course work in Social Sciences and Humanities is important. For applicants who have taken significant time off after college, some recent course work is useful. The April, rather than August MCAT is strongly recommended. Among out-of-state applicants, those with strong qualifications and some sort of ties to the state are the most likely to be admitted. The School aims to admit candidates who are likely to choose careers in primary care.

PROCESS: Almost all Indiana residents receive a secondary application, and about 93 percent of those returning secondaries are interviewed. Among out-of-state applicants, only highly qualified candidates are sent secondary applications, and about 10 percent are invited to interview. Interviews take place on Wednesdays, from September through February and are scheduled in the order in which completed applications are received. Interviews consist of a one-hour session with a team of faculty members. Notification occurs on a monthly basis, beginning in October. Applicants are either accepted, rejected, or deferred and re-evaluated later in the year. In the spring, a wait list is established. Wait-listed candidates may submit supplementary material if it adds new information to his or her file.

Costs

Beyond tuition and fees, cost of living varies depending on campus selection and lifestyle choices. The range for a single student is likely to be $7,000–$10,000 per year. This type of budget allows for either on- or off-campus housing and car ownership.

FINANCIAL AID: Depending on the source, aid is awarded on the basis of financial need, academic merit, or in some cases, a combination of the two. Some scholarships are directed at residents of particular counties, at individuals of particular ethnic groups, or at students headed toward a particular specialty. Most aid to incoming students is need-based and requires parental financial disclosure. To be considered for need-based aid, students must complete both federal and institutional forms.

INDIANA UNIVERSITY

STUDENT BODY

Type	Public
*Enrollment	1,118
*% male/female	61/39
*% underrepresented minorities	6
# applied (total/out)	2,135/1,491
% interviewed (total/out)	40/12
% accepted (total/out)	NR/NR
% enrolled (total/out)	32/9

ADMISSIONS

Average GPA and MCAT Scores

Overall GPA	3.68	Science GPA	3.64
MCAT Bio	10.00	MCAT Phys	9.70
MCAT Verbal	9.50	MCAT Essay	O

Score Release Policy
The school has not responded to our inquiry regarding withheld MCAT scores. Therefore, we advise caution. Contact the Admissions Office before withholding any scores.

Application Information

Regular application	12/15
Regular notification	10/15–varies
Early application	6/1–8/1
Early notification	10/1
Transfers accepted?	Yes
Admissions may be deferred?	Yes
AMCAS application accepted?	Yes
Interview required?	Yes
Application fee	$35

COSTS AND AID

Tuition & Fees

Tuition (in/out)	$13,245/$33,330
Cost of books	NR
Fees	$1,102

Financial Aid

% students receiving aid	NR
Average grant	NR
Average loan	NR
Average debt	NR

*Figures based on total enrollment

UNIVERSITY OF IOWA
COLLEGE OF MEDICINE

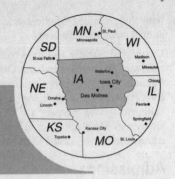

100 Medicine Administration Building, Iowa City, IA 52242
Admission: 319-335-8052 • Fax: 319-335-8049
Email: medical-admissions@uiowa.edu
Internet: www.medicine.uiowa.edu/osac/admiss.htm

The University of Iowa College of Medicine is part of the University Health Sciences Center, which also includes the Colleges of Dentistry, Nursing, Pharmacy, and Public Health. The College of Medicine is known for excellence in rural medicine and community care and is an important health care provider to Iowa's largely rural population. The curriculum was recently revised to emphasize problem-based and self-directed learning, clinical correlation, computer-based learning, small-group activities, and vertical integration of material.

Academics

Most students at Iowa follow a four-year course of study, leading to the M.D. About 5 percent of students are M.S.T.P. participants, earning a Ph.D. concurrently with the M.D. The doctorate degree may be earned in Anatomy, Biochemistry, Microbiology, Pharmacology, and Physiology and Biophysics, among other fields. Other joint-degree programs, such as those leading to a master's degree along with the M.D., are also possible. Medical students are evaluated with Honors/Pass/Fail for all courses except electives, which are Pass/Fail. Although the first two years are primarily devoted to basic sciences, introductory clinical training is also an important part of the curriculum. The second two years are devoted to clinical rotations.

BASIC SCIENCES: First-year courses are the following: Biochemistry; Cell Biology; Medical Genetics; Gross Anatomy; Development, Structure and Functions of Human Organ Systems; Neuroscience; Immunology; and Foundations of Clinical Practice, which continues through the second year. This course covers topics ranging from biomedical ethics and problem-based learning to behavioral medicine, human sexuality, continuity of care, and important clinical techniques such as history-taking, the physical examination, and the doctor-patient relationship. The course Structure and Functions of Human Organ Systems covers principles of Histology and Physiology and is organized around body/organ systems. After completing their first year, many students spend the summer working and learning in an Iowa community hospital or conducting medical research projects. Second-year courses are: Principles of Infectious Diseases; Health Law and Foundations of Clinical Practice; Pharmacology; Pathology; Clinical Therapeutics. Throughout the first two years, students are in lectures, discussions, labs, or tutorials for about 23 hours per week. Basic sciences are taught in the Medical Laboratories Building and the Basic Science Building. The Hardin Library holds over 200,000 volumes and nearly 3,000 periodicals and is used by students, faculty, and the medical community for research and studying. It also has a multimedia computer classroom and computer-based informational resources.

CLINICAL TRAINING: Third- and fourth-year required core clerkships are the following: Community-Based Primary Care (6 weeks); Family Practice (3 weeks); Internal Medicine (6 weeks); Ob/Gyn (6 weeks); Pediatrics (6 weeks); and Surgery (6 weeks). Subspecialty clerkships are Neurology (4 weeks); Psychiatry (4 weeks); two weeks of each of the following: Anesthesia; Dermatology; Ophthalmology; Orthopedics; Otolaryngology; Radiology; and week each of Urology, Electrocardiography; and Laboratory Medicine. Two advanced clerkships and at least 12 weeks of electives are also required. Clinical training takes place at the University Hospital (1,100 beds), the Veterans Affairs Hospital (440 beds), and various sites within the state.

Students

Each entering class has 157 students. About 70 percent of students are Iowa residents. Generally, about 30 undergraduate majors are represented in a class. Approximately 9 percent of students are underrepresented minorities. The majority of students entered medical school one year after college graduation.

STUDENT LIFE: Medical students are active in student organizations ranging from groups that support minorities to professional interest groups to a medical school band. As part of the greater University of Iowa, medical students enjoy its facilities, resources, and sponsored events, such as big ten football games. The campus is central to Iowa City and is convenient to restaurants, clubs, theaters, shopping areas, and parks. Though the city has a population of 60,000 people, it is relatively safe and has the feeling of a friendly small town. Just outside of the city are lakes, hiking areas, and other outdoor attractions. Urban centers such as Chicago, St. Louis, Minneapolis, Omaha, and Kansas City are within a five-hour drive. On campus housing options include coed medical fraternities with both single and double rooms, and university-owned family housing. Off-campus, reasonably priced apartments are available.

GRADUATES: Graduates are successful in entering residency programs of their choice. Iowa itself offers post-graduate training programs in about 15 fields.

Admissions

REQUIREMENTS: Prerequisites are one year each of Physics, Chemistry, Organic Chemistry, General Biology, one semester of Advanced Biology, and college-level Math. All science courses should include laboratory instruction. The MCAT is required, and scores must be from exams no earlier than April 1991 and no later than August 2000 for the 2001 entering class. All sets of scores are evaluated.

SUGGESTIONS: Though preference is given to Iowa residents, well-qualified nonresidents are also considered. Nonscience majors might benefit from additional science courses beyond requirements. Computer literacy, the ability to write well, strong verbal skills, and general decision-making capabilities are some of the skills sought in applicants. Also important are an applicant's personal characteristics, which are evaluated with the help of evaluation forms and interviews. Some medically related experience is important.

PROCESS: Iowa participates in the AMCAS process. Most who apply through AMCAS are sent secondary applications. About one-third of Iowa residents who apply are accepted. Of the nonresident applicant pool, about 6 percent are accepted. Applicants are notified on a rolling basis and are either accepted, rejected, or wait-listed. Usually, a significant number of wait-listed candidates are admitted later in the year. Wait-listed candidates are not encouraged to send additional information.

Costs

The estimated student budget is about $11,000 per year. This covers all expenses except tuition and fees for a single student. Most students own cars.

FINANCIAL AID: Financial assistance is provided on the basis of demonstrated need. Though most aid is in the form of loans, a limited number of grants (usually for about $1,200) are awarded each year to those with exceptional need.

UNIVERSITY OF IOWA

STUDENT BODY

Type	Public
*Enrollment	680
*% male/female	60/40
*% underrepresented minorities	9
# applied (total/out)	2,487/2,148
% interviewed (total/out)	19/11
% accepted (total/out)	11/6
% enrolled (total/out)	55/28

ADMISSIONS

Average GPA and MCAT Scores

Overall GPA	3.68	Science GPA	3.66
MCAT Bio	NR	MCAT Phys	10.00
MCAT Verbal	NR	MCAT Essay	P

Score Release Policy

The school has not responded to our inquiry regarding withheld MCAT scores. Therefore, we advise caution. Contact the Admissions office before withholding any scores.

Application Information

Regular application	11/1
Regular notification	10/15–rolling
Early application	6/1–8/1
Early notification	10/1
Admissions may be deferred?	Yes
AMCAS application accepted?	Yes
Interview required?	Yes
Application fee	$30

COSTS AND AID

Tuition & Fees

Tuition (in/out)	$10,264/$27,490
Cost of books	$2,450
Fees	$324

Financial Aid

% students receiving aid	NR
Average grant	NR
Average loan	NR
Average debt	NR

*Figures based on total enrollment

JEFFERSON MEDICAL COLLEGE
OF THOMAS JEFFERSON UNIVERSITY

1025 Walnut Street, Philadelphia, PA 19107
Admission: 215-955-6983 • Fax: 215-923-6939
Internet: www.tju.edu

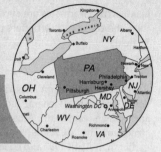

Thomas Jefferson University has three major educational components, Jefferson Medical College, The College of Health Professionals and College of Graduate Studies, and the expansive medical facilities of the University. The institution's principle mission is to provide outstanding education in health care fields. Jefferson is renowned for excellent teaching at the medical school and for high-quality medical care provided through its clinical institutions. Though the University itself occupies 13 acres, it is situated in central Philadelphia and is well-integrated into the urban community. Class size is relatively large, but Jefferson has enough resources to offer students individual attention.

Academics

Along with basic science and clinical training, Jefferson's curriculum emphasizes the social and public health issues related to medicine. The academic year is organized around "blocks," with the January block devoted to these nontraditional topics. Students with solid science backgrounds may pursue an M.D. and a Ph.D. in one of the departments of the College of Graduate Studies. These include: Biochemistry, Developmental Biology, Genetics, Immunology, Microbiology, Molecular Pharmacology, Pathology, Cell Biology, and Physiology. A joint M.D./M.B.A. degree is offered in conjunction with Widener University in Chester, Pennsylvania, as is a combined M.D./Masters in Hospital Administration. Pennsylvania State University and Jefferson Medical College allow students to pursue a combined B.S./M.D. program, which grants both degrees in a six-year period. Jefferson has special arrangements with the University of Pennsylvania's, Bryn Mawr's, and Columbia University's post-bacc programs through which highly qualified students may be admitted to Jefferson prior to completion of their pre-medical requirements. Upon arrival at Jefferson, all students are assigned a faculty advisor.

BASIC SCIENCES: Innovations in instructional techniques have reduced the time spent in lecture. To supplement lectures and labs, students participate in small group discussions. In the first year, Block One begins in September and continues through December. Courses include Biochemistry and Molecular Biology, Anatomy and The Doctor in Health and Illness, a course which asks students to apply their developing scientific knowledge to patient problems and to learn fundamental skills in patient interaction, history-taking, examination, and diagnosis. During Block Two, which occurs entirely in January, first-year students focus on Health Policy, Ethics, Biostatistics, and Genetics. Block Three, lasting from February through May, includes Physiology, Histology, and The Doctor in Health and Illness. Block 5, May-June, is reserved for Neuroscience. Year Two, Block One occurs in August and September and consists of Pathology, Microbiology, Pharmacology and elective study. Year Two, Block Two occurs in November and December and includes Physical Diag-

nosis and Introduction to Clinical Medicine. The January Block curriculum is Nutrition, Health of the Public, Law and Medicine, Physical Diagnosis and elective study. The final Block, lasting from February through May, includes Pathology, Electives, Clinical Medicine and Physical Diagnosis. Grades are on a percentile scale, and the passing score is determined for each course. Pre-clinical studies take place in the central Medical College building complex, which includes administrative offices, labs, lecture halls, common areas, and recreational facilities. The Samuel Parsons Scott Library includes 160,000 volumes, a Learning Resources Center and computer labs in addition to videos, slides, and supplemental learning materials. MEDLINE and other electronic data systems are available. The USMLE is required after completion of Year Two.

CLINICAL TRAINING: Patient contact officially begins in Year Two, with Introduction to Clinical Medicine. There are also ongoing opportunities for medical students interested in volunteer clinical experience or clinical research through summer programs and part-time jobs. Formally, the clinical portion of the curriculum begins in year three with required rotations. These are: Family Medicine (6 weeks); General Surgery (6 weeks); Internal Medicine (12 weeks); Pediatrics (6 weeks); Psychiatry and Human Behavior (6 weeks); and Ob/Gyn (6 weeks). Phase II of clinical rotations are selectives in which students choose specialties within broadly defined categories. Twelve weeks are also designated as purely elective. Training sites include: Alfred DuPont Institute (children's hospital); Bryn Mawr Hospital (383 beds); Bryn Mawr Rehabilitation Hospital; DuPont Hospital for Children; Geisinger Medical Center (in Danville, Pennsylvania, providing rural exposure); Lankenau Hospital (475 beds); Latrobe Hospital (280 beds, family medicine); Magee Rehabilitation Hospital; Mercy Hospital, Pittsburgh; The Medial Center of Delaware; Wills Eye Hospital; and West Jersey Health System. The patients come from several states and represent extremely diverse populations. Students are evaluated on a 1–5 scale, roughly analogous to A–F. The USMLE Step 2 is required for graduation.

Students

About 30 states are represented by the students within a class, mostly those of the eastern part of the country. About 40 percent of the students are Pennsylvania state residents. Underrepresented minorities make up about 6 percent of each class, the majority of whom are African American. Class size is 223. Approximately 25 percent of each class is over 25 years of age upon matriculation. In recent years, about 18 percent of matriculates have held advanced degrees.

STUDENT LIFE: Student organizations range from the Jefferson Karate Club to the Asian Professional Society. Medical fraternities are relatively popular and sponsor activities such as intramural sports. Beyond campus, the city of Philadelphia provides ample recreational and cultural possibilities and New York is just over an hour away. On-campus housing options include residence halls and apartments of all sizes; housing is guaranteed to first-year students. With Jefferson's central and urban location, a car is unnecessary.

GRADUATES: More than half of Jefferson graduates enter residency programs at University-affiliated hospitals around the nation. Jefferson graduates do very well in the residency-matching program, both in primary care and in more specialized fields.

Admissions

REQUIREMENTS: Required course work is one year of: Biology with lab; Chemistry with lab; Organic Chemistry with lab; and Physics with lab. The quality of an applicant's undergraduate institution is assessed and considered in evaluating GPA. The MCAT is required and an applicant's most recent score is used, along with grades, to determine if he or she will be interviewed.

SUGGESTIONS: Applicants should demonstrate problem-solving capability, success in a range of subjects, and some in-depth knowledge of one or a few subjects. Strong writing skills are also valued. Experience in a medical or research environment is important. State residents are given slight preference, as are children of alumni and applicants from programs that have special arrangements with Jefferson. Because the admissions process is rolling, applicants are advised to take the April MCAT and to submit all materials in a timely fashion.

PROCESS: All AMCAS applicants receive a secondary application. Interviews are conducted from September through March, and about 20 percent of the applicant pool is eventually interviewed. Interviews are one hour in length and are conducted by a member of the faculty or administration. About 113 of those who interview are accepted. Others are either rejected or wait-listed. When places become available later in the Spring, wait-listed applicants will be notified and offered positions. Indicating interest in Jefferson may help the prospects of wait-listed candidates.

Costs

The anticipated yearly budget, not including tuition, is $13,000. This includes all fees and expenses associated with school and general living.

FINANCIAL AID: Financial aid is granted solely on the basis of need, and parental resources are considered in determining a student's need. Institutional loans and grants are offered after a student has obtained the yearly maximum in subsidized and unsubsidized federal student loans. Jefferson alumni are among the many sources of scholarship funds. There are no merit-based scholarships, but some low-interest loans may be available to students who commit to entering primary care fields.

JEFFERSON MEDICAL COLLEGE OF THOMAS JEFFERSON UNIVERSITY

STUDENT BODY

Type	Private
*Enrollment	901
*% male/female	60/40
*% underrepresented minorities	6
# applied (total/out)	9,979/8,727
% interviewed (total/out)	10/7
% accepted (total/out)	NR/NR
% enrolled (total/out)	22/22
Average age	25

ADMISSIONS

Average GPA and MCAT Scores

Overall GPA	3.59	Science GPA	3.50
MCAT Bio	9.80	MCAT Phys	9.70
MCAT Verbal	9.70	MCAT Essay	NR

Score Release Policy

The school has not responded to our inquiry regarding withheld MCAT scores. Therefore, we advise caution. Contact the Admissions Office before withholding any scores.

Application Information

Regular application	11/15
Regular notification	10/15 until filled
Early application	6/1–8/1
Early notification	10/1
Transfers accepted?	Yes
Admissions may be deferred?	Yes
AMCAS application accepted?	Yes
Interview required?	Yes
Application fee	$65

COSTS AND AID

Tuition & Fees

Tuition	$25,235
Cost of books	NR
Fees	$0

Financial Aid

% students receiving aid	70
Average grant	$4,300
Average loan	$27,165
Average debt	NR

*Figures based on total enrollment

JOHNS HOPKINS UNIVERSITY
SCHOOL OF MEDICINE

720 Rutland Avenue, Baltimore, MD 21205

Admission: 410-955-3182

Internet: www.med.jhu.edu/admissions

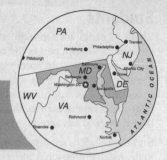

Exceptional students, dedicated faculty, abundant research opportunities, and impressive clinical facilities contribute to Johns Hopkins' reputation as one of the very best medical schools in the country. Hopkins prepares students for the career pathway of their choice, whether it be primary care, subspecialties, or academic medicine. Although Johns Hopkins University encompasses an undergraduate college and other strong graduate programs, some of which are located 50 miles away in Washington, D.C., it is the medical school and center that earns Hopkins international recognition.

Academics

In 1992 Hopkins implemented a revised curriculum that introduced case-based learning, exposure to clinical settings during the first year, and a Physicians and Society (P&S) course, which integrates social, economic, and ethical perspectives into the four-year basic and clinical science curriculum. Studies leading to both an M.D. and a Ph.D. or M.A./M.S. in the following fields are possible: Biochemistry, Cellular and Molecular Biology, Biological Chemistry, Biomedical Engineering, Biophysics, Biophysics/Molecular Biophysics, Cell Biology and Anatomy, Cellular and Molecular Medicine, History of Medicine, Genetics, History of Science, Medicine and Technology, Human Genetics and Molecular Biology, Immunology, Medical and Biological Illustration, Neuroscience, Pharmacology, Molecular Sciences, Physiology, and Public Health. The combined M.D./M.P.H. is particularly popular, which is not surprising given the excellent reputation of the School of Public Health.

BASIC SCIENCES: The first year is organized into four Blocks, all 10 weeks in length: Molecules and Cells (Block 1); Anatomy and Developmental Biology (Block 2); Neuroscience and Clinical Epidemiology (Block 3) and Organ Systems (Block 4). The P&S course is year-long as is Introduction to Clinical Medicine, in which students spend two days a month working with a private physician. During the first year, classes ends at 1:00 p.m. four days a week, giving students ample time to study. Many students take on research projects during the summer between their first and second years. Second-year students study Pathology, Pathophysiology, and Pharmacology, which are offered as year-long courses. All three courses are integrated and are organized around organ systems. Lectures, discussion, case-study, and labs are all important components of the basic science curriculum. With relatively few hours of scheduled lectures, students generally attend classes and do not rely on student note-taking cooperatives. Grading is A–F, with the majority of students receiving Bs. Grades of A are reserved for exceptional performance, and grades below C are rare. Faculty members, assigned to incoming students, both advise and monitor their progress. The Welch Medical Library and its three

affiliated sites own over 380,000 books and subscribe to about 3,000 journals. It provides resources that support instruction, such as extensive database and Internet tools. The USMLE is not used for grading or promotional purposes.

CLINICAL TRAINING: Facilities for clinical training include the Johns Hopkins Hospital complex, which is comprised of numerous affiliates, is housed in 37 buildings, and contains over 1,100 beds. In addition to serving the urban population of Baltimore and the surrounding areas, Johns Hopkins Hospitals attract patients from around the country and the world. Students are exposed to patient care at renowned institutions such as the Wilmer Eye Institute, Adolf Meyer Center for Psychiatry, Brady Urological Institute, Clayton Heart Center, Meyerhoff Center for Digestive Diseases, the Children's Center, Oncology Center, Halsted Surgical Service, and Osler Medical Service. Students are also encouraged to pursue clinical experiences away from Hopkins, and a significant number do so overseas. With faculty input, students determine the order of their required clerkships and electives. Requirements are the following: Medicine (9 weeks); Surgery (9 weeks); Pediatrics (9 weeks); Opthalmology (1 week); Psychiatry (4 weeks); Neurology (4 weeks); Ob/Gyn (6 weeks); Emergency Medicine (4 weeks); and Ambulatory Internal Medicine (3 weeks). Clinical instruction is generally carried out in small groups, and individual initiative is encouraged. Grading is A–F for required courses and pass/fail for electives. Through its subsidiaries, The Johns Hopkins Health Systems provides statewide healthcare services to individuals and health-plan participants. This integration into managed care operations, coupled with large federal research grants, suggest that the institution is financially stable.

Students

The diversity of the student body reflects the School's national reputation. A typical class has students from 35 different states and 70 or more colleges. As is the case with most top schools, half the entrants are women. Efforts are made to recruit ethnic minorities, and about 8 percent of the student body is African American. Class size is limited to 120.

STUDENT LIFE: For some, social life revolves around school, where students spend a great deal of time. Others, particularly those from the area or with families, have lives outside of the Medical School. Housing is available for single students or for married students living alone, in Reed Hall dorms adjacent to campus. However, most choose to live in apartments off campus. For those accustomed to New York or Washington, D.C., the housing situation in Baltimore is good. The Housing Office assists students in their apartment searches. Recreational facilities, including a full-size gym, are free to medical students and are located next to Reed Hall. Several medical societies exist, including a Women's Medical Alumni Association, which provides support for women students and physicians. There is also a Black Student Organization, which is active in both campus and community affairs.

GRADUATES: Graduates of Hopkins have their pick of residency programs, even those graduating with GPAs that are at the lower end of their class. About 50 percent of graduates enter Primary Care specialties; 20 percent ultimately enter academic medicine or work primarily in research.

Admissions

REQUIREMENTS: In addition to the typical requirement of one year each, Biology, Chemistry, Organic Chemistry, and Physics, one semester of Calculus (high school is acceptable), and 24 semester hours combined of humanities and social sciences are required. Johns Hopkins is one of the only medical schools that does not require the MCAT. Rather, students may submit the results of any standardized test. Hopkins is also among those medical schools that do not participate in AMCAS. The application is generally available in June or July, and applicants should complete it in a timely fashion.

SUGGESTIONS: Hopkins is concerned with both the academic and personal records of applicants and notes that intellectual progress through college is important. Extracurricular activities need not be medically related, but should demonstrate humanistic values and perseverance.

PROCESS: About 25 percent of applicants are invited for interviews, which occur between September and March, and about 25 percent of those interviewed are accepted on a rolling basis. Applicants are interviewed by Admissions Committee Members, and regional interviews may be arranged for applicants living a distance from Baltimore. At Admissions Committee meetings, decisions are made to admit, reject, or wait list applicants. In April, wait-listed candidates are notified of their positions on the list.

Costs

Yearly cost of living, in addition to tuition, is estimated at $17,000. This budget is realistic for students living on campus or off campus in shared housing. Cars are useful in the Baltimore area, though some students live without.

FINANCIAL AID: After securing $17,000 per year in loans, students' financial need is addressed through grants, which are financed by private scholarships. Most scholarships are need based. Applicants admitted to the M.D./Ph.D. program are also considered for M.S.T.P. awards. In addition, Predoctoral Research stipends are available for qualified students who engage in research while in school.

JOHNS HOPKINS UNIVERSITY

STUDENT BODY

Type	Private
*Enrollment	550
*% male/female	53/47
*% underrepresented minorities	10
# applied (total/out)	3,290/2,992
% interviewed (total/out)	19/17
% accepted (total/out)	NR/NR

ADMISSIONS

Average GPA and MCAT Scores

Overall GPA	NR	Science GPA	NR
MCAT Bio	NR	MCAT Phys	NR
MCAT Verbal	NR	MCAT Essay	NR

Score Release Policy

The MCAT is not required

Application Information

Regular application	11/1
Regular notification	11/1–3/31
Early application	7/1–8/15
Early notification	10/1
Transfers accepted?	Yes
Admissions may be deferred?	Yes
AMCAS application accepted?	No
Interview required?	Yes
Application fee	$60

COSTS AND AID

Tuition & Fees

Tuition	$24,500
Cost of books	$8,190
Fees	$2,608

Financial Aid

% students receiving aid	82
Average grant	$11,900
Average loan	$17,590
Averge debt	NR

*Figures based on total enrollment

UNIVERSITY OF KANSAS
SCHOOL OF MEDICINE

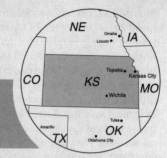

3901 Rainbow Boulevard, Kansas City, KS 66160
Admission: 913-588-5245 • Fax: 913-588-5259
Internet: www.kumc.edu/som/som.html

Although the School of Medicine at the University of Kansas was founded in 1889, it offers both a modern curriculum and modern facilities. Its mandate is to provide Kansas residents with an excellent medical education and to train health practitioners to serve the state's population. The Medical Center attracts patients from neighboring states who seek top-notch, often specialized treatments. The School of Medicine, together with the Schools of Allied Health, Graduate Studies, and Nursing, make up the University of Kansas Medical Center. The Medical Center is an integrated part of the University of Kansas, which enrolls more than 27,000 students. The main campus is in Lawerence, and the medical center is located in Kansas City, with a branch clinical campus in Wichita.

Academics

In comparison to many medical schools, clinical training at the University of Kansas emphasizes rural and primary health care. Joint M.D./Ph.D. degrees are offered in the following fields: Anatomy and Cell Biology; Biochemistry and Molecular Biology; Microbiology, Molecular Genetics and Toxicology; Pathology and Oncology; Pharmacology; and Physiology. A joint M.D./M.P.H. is also offered.

BASIC SCIENCES: Basic sciences are taught in Kansas City. The facilities are modern and fully equipped with learning tools such as computers and visual-aid equipment. The School of Medicine has recently implemented a systemic methodology for teaching basic sciences. Students take part in individual and small-group projects that require initiative and problem-solving skills. First-year students take Cell and Tissue Biology; Physiology; Biochemistry; Gross Anatomy; Neuroscience; and Introduction to Clinical Medicine. Second-year students take Microbiology; Pathology; Pharmacology; and Introduction to Clinical Medicine. Tutoring is available through the Learning Resources Counseling service. A student-operated note service, in which students share note-taking, covers regularly scheduled lectures. Students are evaluated using the following descriptions: Superior, High Satisfactory, Satisfactory, Low Satisfactory, and Unsatisfactory. These marks are translated into numeric scores to determine class rank. The USMLE is required upon completion of year two. The Dykes Library of the Health Sciences supports the educational and research demands of medical students, faculty, and the public. It contains 150,000 books and offers online informational services. In addition, the Clendening History of Medicine Library has one of the top five collections of rare medical books in the country.

CLINICAL TRAINING: Patient contact begins in year one, when students take part in weekly sessions with practicing physicians. Required clinical clerkships are Ambulatory Medicine/Geriatrics (6 weeks); Family Medicine (6 weeks); Ob/Gyn (6 weeks); Medicine (8 weeks); Pediatrics (6 weeks); Neuropsychiatry (8 weeks); and General Surgery (8 weeks). Year four is filled primarily with electives, from which there are many to choose including Preventive Medicine and the History of Medicine. Clinical training takes place both at the University of Kansas Hospital (464 beds), which houses nearly all the diagnostic and treatment facilities of the Medical Center, and at hospitals in Wichita. Included at the Medical Center in Kansas City are the Kansas Cancer Institute, the Burnett Burn Center, the Smith Mental Retardation Center, the Center on Aging, and the Center on Environmental and Occupational Health. Patients are drawn from Kansas, Missouri, Oklahoma, Arkansas, and Nebraska. The grading scale is the same for performance in clinical rotations as it for basic science courses. In addition to formal rotations, students gain clinical experience through volunteer activities, like the Mobile Medical Unit, which brings basic prevention and care to communities in need. Many students devote free summers to volunteer in medically related activities.

Students

About 95 percent of a typical class are Kansas residents, and most students have liberal arts backgrounds. In recent years, about 13 percent of the student body have been underrepresented minorities, mostly African and Hispanic Americans. Usually, almost a quarter of matriculates in a given year are older than 25 years of age. Class size is 175.

STUDENT LIFE: Beyond the medical school, which brings students together around academic and extracurricular activities, the greater university is the center of student life. The Kirmayer Fitness Center is a modern facility open to all medical students. Numerous organized activities enrich the lives of medical students. Activities such as Rural Health Weekends provide opportunities for interaction and contribution. Organizations such as the American Student's Association and the Community Outreach Project organize lectures and social occasions. All students live off campus.

GRADUATES: About 60 percent of graduates enter primary care fields, often Family Medicine. Graduates are successful in obtaining residency positions throughout the country. The medical school sponsors events and scholarships that encourage students and residents to consider practicing in Kansas.

Admissions

REQUIREMENTS: Required college courses are one year of Biology with lab; Chemistry with lab; Organic Chemistry with lab; Physics with lab, and one year of English. Evaluation of GPA is irrespective of where course work was completed. The MCAT is required, with the two most recent sets of scores considered. The August MCAT is acceptable.

SUGGESTIONS: Experience in a health care setting is valued, and the breadth of an applicant's undergraduate course work is important. Demonstrated interests in rural and primary care medicine are pluses. Out-of-state residents should have particularly strong qualifications. A few students each year are accepted from the University of Kansas Post-baccalaureate Program.

PROCESS: All Kansas residents are sent secondary applicants, while only about 10 percent of out-of-state applicants receive them. About 75 percent of Kansas residents and about 5 percent of out-of-state applicants are interviewed. Interviews are conducted in Kansas City, from October through January, and consist of two sessions each with two members of the interview panel. Approximately one-half of those interviewed are offered positions in the class and are notified on a rolling basis after the interview. The wait list is short, and wait-listed candidates are not encouraged to send supplementary material.

Costs

Excluding tuition and fees, the estimated student budget is $15,000 per year; this presumes car ownership.

FINANCIAL AID: In addition to federally funded loan programs, numerous private scholarships are offered based on need and merit. The Kansas Medical Student Loan Program grants scholarships covering yearly tuition and living expenses. For each year a student receives funding, he or she is obligated to practice medicine for one year within the State. National Medical Fellowships are awarded to minority students.

UNIVERSITY OF KANSAS

STUDENT BODY

Type	Public
*Enrollment	700
*% male/female	60/40
*% underrepresented minorities	13
# applied (total/out)	1,392/977
% interviewed (total/out)	27/5
% accepted (total/out)	15/4
% enrolled (total/out)	13/3
Average age	26

ADMISSIONS

Average GPA and MCAT Scores

Overall GPA	3.60	Science GPA	3.55
MCAT Bio	9.4	MCAT Phys	9.0
MCAT Verbal	9.2	MCAT Essay	O

Score Release Policy

The Admissions Committee has no position on withholding scores.

Application Information

Regular application	10/15
Regular notification	2/1–varies
Early application	6/1–8/1
Early notification	10/1
Transfers accepted?	Yes
Admissions may be deferred?	Yes
AMCAS application accepted?	Yes
Interview required?	Yes
Application fee for non-residents	$40

COSTS AND AID

Tuition & Fees

Tuition (in/out)	$10,100/$24,160
Cost of books	$2,100
Fees	$400

Financial Aid

% students receiving aid	85
Average grant	NR
Average loan	NR
Average debt	$65,000

*Figures based on total enrollment

UNIVERSITY OF KENTUCKY
COLLEGE OF MEDICINE

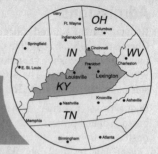

MN102 UKMC, 800 Rose Street, Lexington, KY 40536-0084
Admission: 859-323-6161 • Fax: 859-323-2076
Internet: www.comed.uky.edu/medicine

University of Kentucky (UK) College of Medicine primarily focuses on training physicians to be excellent caregivers. The faculty works closely with students, preparing them for a future of advancing technology while emphasizing humanistic values. In addition to affiliated hospitals, UK maintains a Rural Health Center and works with several Area Health Education Centers (AHEC) all of which serve as important clinical training facilities.

Academics

With support from the Robert Wood Johnson Foundation, the curriculum was recently revised and enhanced. It includes early patient contact and teaches lifelong learning skills, ethics, and computer-assisted learning along with traditional basic science and clinical techniques. The goal of the medical education program is to focus on principles and the organization of factual bodies of knowledge rather than on unconnected detail. Although most students complete a four-year curriculum, a few students each year enter a combined M.D./Ph.D. program. The doctorate may be earned in Anatomy, Biochemistry, Biophysics, Cell Biology, Genetics, Immunology, Microbiology, Molecular Biology, Neuroscience, Pharmacology, or Physiology. Medical students are evaluated with letter grades and, in some cases, with Pass/Fail. Passing Step 1 of the USMLE is a requirement for promotion to year three, and passing Step 2 is a graduation requirement.

BASIC SCIENCES: During the first and second years, students are in class or other scheduled sessions for about 24 hours per week. Lectures and tutorials are the primary instructional methods. Laboratories, hands-on clinical work, and conferences are also important parts of the curriculum. The first year is devoted to basic sciences and interdisciplinary perspectives. The year is organized into blocks, each of which contains one or two courses. First-year courses are Patients, Physicians, and Society; Introduction to the Medical Profession; Human Structure/Gross Anatomy; Human Structure/Histology; Healthy Human; Cellular Structure and Function/Biochemistry; Cellular Structure and Function/Genetics; Neuroscience; and Human Function. The second year is focused on the disease process and is also broken into blocks. These are Patients, Physicians, and Society II; Introduction to the Medical Profession II; Immunity, Infection, and Disease; and Mechanisms of Disease and Treatment, which covers Pathology and Pharmacology. Students spend most of their first two years in the Medical Science Building, which houses classrooms and laboratories. Computers are important educational tools, and all incoming students are required to have their own computers. The College of Medicine has a nationally recognized program of academic computing in medical education,

which provides a wide variety of services to enhance student learning. These educational support services are offered in facilities located in the College of Medicine, the Chandler Medical Center, and in the AHECs. The library, which contains more than 150,000 volumes, is also an important resource.

CLINICAL TRAINING: Third-year required clerkships are: Women's Maternal and Child Health (12 weeks); Clinical Neuroscience (8 weeks); Principles Of Primary Care (12 weeks); and Medical and Surgical Care (16 weeks). The fourth year is comprised of a one-month acting internship selected from medical specialties (family practice, internal medicine, pediatric, neurology, psychiatry, rehabilitation medicine), a one-month acting internship selected from surgical specialties (general, subspecialty, ob/gyn), a one-month emergency medicine clerkship, one month of a clinical pharmacology and anesthesiology clerkship, and one month of a primary care or rural medicine selective. In addition, 8 weeks of electives are required. Training takes place primarily at the University of Kentucky Hospital (473 beds), although a number of affiliated hospitals and clinics are also used.

Students

At least 90 percent of students are Kentucky residents. Approximately 6 percent of students are underrepresented minorities, most of whom are African American. Generally, about 25 percent of students in each class are "nontraditional," having pursued other careers or interests in between college and medical school.

STUDENT LIFE: Medical students enjoy extracurricular activities associated with the main university such as attending UK basketball games. Student groups provide additional extracurricular activities, including opportunities for involvement in community service projects. They also serve as a means of interacting outside of class. Women in Science and Medicine is a group, comprised primarily of faculty and administrators, focused on improving all aspects of life for women in medicine. Lexington is an attractive and safe city with affordable housing.

GRADUATES: Most graduates enter primary care fields, and a large number practice in Kentucky. The University of Kentucky has post-graduate training programs in more than 20 fields.

Admissions

REQUIREMENTS: One year each of Biology, General Chemistry, Organic Chemistry, Physics, and English are required. All science courses should include associated labs. The MCAT is required, and scores should be from within the past two years. For applicants who have taken the exam more than once, the most recent set of scores is weighed most heavily.

SUGGESTIONS: In addition to academic qualifications, UK seeks students who have the character, personality, values, and motivation for human service. Individual initiative and good judgment are important traits. Some medically related experience is important.

PROCESS: All AMCAS applicants who are Kentucky residents are sent secondary applications. Highly qualified nonresidents are also sent secondaries. About 50 percent of Kentucky residents and 5 percent of nonresidents who return secondary applications are invited to interview between September and April. On interview day, candidates also tour the campus, attend group informational sessions, and have the opportunity to meet informally with current students. About 45 percent of interviewed candidates are accepted on a rolling basis. Others are rejected or wait-listed. Wait-listed candidates may send additional information to update their files.

Costs

The estimated yearly cost of living for a single student is $15,000. This budget allows for off-campus housing and car maintenance.

FINANCIAL AID: The majority of students qualify for financial aid, most of which is awarded on the basis of need. Most aid is in the form of loans. Each year, several scholarships based on merit or other special criteria are offered.

UNIVERSITY OF KENTUCKY

STUDENT BODY

Type	Public
*Enrollment	388
*% male/female	62/38
*% underrepresented minorities	6
# applied (total/out)	1,363/903
†% interviewed (total/out)	56/5
†% accepted (total/out)	48/17
†% enrolled (total/out)	64/50
Average age	23

ADMISSIONS

Average GPA and MCAT Scores

Overall GPA	3.54	Science GPA	3.46
MCAT Bio	10.00	MCAT Phys	9.37
MCAT Verbal	9.49	MCAT Essay	P

Score Release Policy

Withholding score does not affect the applicant.

Application Information

Regular application	11/1
Regular notification	After interview until filled
Early application	6/1–8/1
Early notification	10/1
Transfers accepted?	Yes
Admissions may be deferred?	Yes
AMCAS application accepted?	Yes
Interview required?	Yes
Application fee	$30

COSTS AND AID

Tuition & Fees

Tuition (in/out)	$10,284/$25,674
Cost of books	$2,200
Fees	$393

Financial Aid

% students receiving aid	76
Average grant	$7,178
Average loan	$17,915
Average debt	NR

† Figures are percentages of the KY pool, not overall

*Figures based on total enrollment

LOMA LINDA UNIVERSITY
SCHOOL OF MEDICINE

Loma Linda, CA 92350
Admission: 909-824-4467 • Fax: 909-824-4146

Loma Linda University is a Seventh-Day Adventist institution, situated sixty miles East of Los Angeles in the San Bernardino area. In addition to the School of Medicine, Loma Linda features Schools of Allied Health Professions, Dentistry, Nursing, Public Health, and Graduate education. Loma Linda is unusual among United States medical schools in that it incorporates Christian principles into instruction, and seeks primarily to educate Christian Physicians. The School's emphasis on medical ethics is considered a strength. Southern California offers pleasant year-round weather and a diverse patient population.

Academics

Joint degree programs are offered to qualified students. Along with the M.D., students may earn the M.S. or Ph.D. degree in fields such as Anatomy, Biochemistry, Genetics, Immunology, Microbiology, Neuroscience, Molecular Biology, Pharmacology, and Physiology. Examinations and other methods of evaluation are given percentile scores, but the courses are graded Pass or Fail. Passing the USMLE Step 1 is a requirement for promotion to year three.

BASIC SCIENCES: Although Loma Linda's curriculum covers the basic science topics typical of most medical schools, its religious affiliation adds another dimension. In addition to learning about human biology, the nature of disease, and the appropriate treatment for disease, first- and second-year students participate in a course called Whole Person Formation, which emphasizes Biblical, ethical, and relational aspects of the practice of medicine. Patient contact occurs during the first year, in Physical Diagnosis and Interviewing. Other first-year courses are Biochemistry/Molecular Biology; Cell Structure and Function; Gross Anatomy and Embryology; Human Behavior; Information Sciences and Population-Based Medicine; Medical Applications of the Basic Sciences; and Neuroscience. Second-year courses are Human Behavior; Microbiology; Pathology; Physiology; Pathophysiology and Applied Physical Diagnosis; and Pharmacology. First- and second-year instruction takes place in facilities located on the Loma Linda campus and close to the Medical Center, giving students access to University resources and clinical activities. Computers are available in a comprehensive computer lab, and are used for instruction and research.

CLINICAL TRAINING: Third-year required rotations are Orientation to Clinical Medicine/Preventive Medicine (4 weeks); Family Medicine (4 weeks); Ob/Gyn (6 weeks); Internal Medicine (12 weeks); Pediatrics (8 weeks); Psychiatry (6 weeks); and Surgery (12 weeks). Half of the fourth year is reserved entirely for basic science and clinical electives, and half of the year is split between required clerkships and selectives. Required clerkships are Subinternship Selectives (8 weeks, selected from Family Medicine, Internal Medicine, Ob/Gyn, Pediatrics, and

Surgery); Intensive Care Unit (4 weeks); Neurology (4 weeks); Ambulatory Care (4 weeks); and Electives (16–22 weeks). Training takes place primarily at Loma Linda University Medical Center (500 beds), the Jerry L. Pettis Memorial Veterans Hospital, Riverside General Hospital, and the White Memorial Medical Center in Los Angeles. Other affiliated sites are San Bernardino County General Hospital, Kaiser Foundation Hospital, and Glendale Adventist Medical Center.

Students

Most students are members of the Seventh-Day Adventist Church. About 6 percent of students are underrepresented minorities, most of whom are African American. Generally, there is a wide age range among incoming students, with the average at about 24. Class size is 189.

STUDENT LIFE: For the most part, student life revolves around the medical school and the immediate community. When in need of a change of scenery, Los Angeles and beautiful Southern California beaches are a short drive. Perhaps as a result of a shared religious background, students are cohesive. Alcohol is not a part of the social life, as it is prohibited in the Seventh-Day Adventist Church. Beyond extracurricular activities sponsored by the medical school, students are welcome to participate in University-wide events and organizations. Medical students have access to the University's athletic facilities, and are active in intramural sports. Students live both on and off campus, and virtually all students own cars.

GRADUATES: Graduates are successful in securing residencies in all specialty fields. Loma Linda Medical Center is a popular destination for post-graduate training, offering about 25 residency programs.

Admissions

REQUIREMENTS: Prerequisite course work is eight semester hours each of Biology, General Chemistry, Organic Chemistry, and Physics. Applicants should have met the English and Religion requirements of their respective undergraduate institution. The MCAT is required, and scores should be no more than three years old. For applicants who have taken the test more than once, all sets of scores are considered.

Suggestions: Courses in the Humanities and Social Sciences are recommended, and applicants are urged to take the April rather than August MCAT. For applicants who have taken time off after college, recent course work is important. Some involvement in health care delivery is valued by the Admissions Committee. Preference is given to qualified applicants who are members of the Seventh-Day Adventist Church. However, others who demonstrate a commitment to Christian principles are also considered favorably.

Process: All AMCAS applicants are sent secondary applications. Of those returning secondaries, about 10 percent are invited to interview between November and March. Interviews consist of one or two hour-long sessions with faculty, students, and/or administrators. On interview day, lunch, a campus tour, and the opportunity to meet with current students are all provided. About 40 percent of interviewed candidates are accepted on a rolling basis, while others are rejected or wait-listed. Wait-listed candidates may send updated transcripts.

Costs

In addition to tuition costs, yearly living expenses, including books and supplies, are about $11,000 for a single student. This budget allows for on- or off-campus housing and car ownership.

Financial Aid: Though there are some merit-based scholarships; most aid is awarded on the basis of financial need. Need is assessed with the FAFSA form, which should be filed as early as possible. Most students are expected to borrow $18,500 from subsidized and unsubsidized federal loan programs before receiving institutional aid. For students with the greatest need, institutional/private assistance is available in the form of grants, scholarships, employment opportunities, and low interest loans.

LOMA LINDA UNIVERSITY

STUDENT BODY

Type	Private
*Enrollment	661
*% male/female	59/41
*% underrepresented minorities	6
# applied (total/out)	3,990/2,083
% interviewed (total/out)	10/5
% accepted (total/out)	NR/NR
% enrolled (total/out)	36/33
Average age	24

ADMISSIONS

Average GPA and MCAT Scores

Overall GPA	3.66	Science GPA	NR
MCAT Bio	9.20	MCAT Phys	8.90
MCAT Verbal	9.30	MCAT Essay	NR

Score Release Policy

The Admissions Committee will suspect that student did poorly if they withhold scores, so they do not recommend doing so.

Application Information

Regular application	11/1
Regular notification	12/15
Early application	6/1–8/1
Early notification	10/1
Admissions may be deferred?	Yes
AMCAS application accepted?	Yes
Interview required?	Yes
Application fee	$55

COSTS AND AID

Tuition & Fees

Tuition	$25,081
Cost of books	NR
Fees	$1007

Financial Aid

% students receiving aid	NR
Average grant	NR
Average loan	NR
Average debt	NR

*Figures based on total enrollment

LOUISIANA STATE UNIVERSITY

SCHOOL OF MEDICINE IN NEW ORLEANS

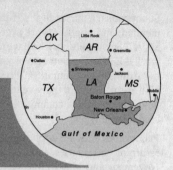

1901 Perdido Street, Box P3-4, New Orleans, LA 70112

Admission: 504-568-6262 • Fax: 504-568-7701

Email: ms-admissions@lsuhsc.edu

Internet: www.medschool.lsuhsc.edu/admissions

The Louisiana State University (LSU) Health Sciences Center has teaching, research, and health care facilities statewide. LSU includes six professional schools including the Schools of Medicine in New Orleans and Shreveport and the Schools of Dentistry, Nursing, Allied Health Professions, and Graduate Studies. The New Orleans campus is part of one of the world's largest medical complexes, spanning about 10 square blocks in the commercial area of the city. Medical students have the opportunity to learn from a large and diverse patient population.

Academics

The course of instruction leading to the M.D. extends over a four-year period. A revised first- and second-year curriculum was introduced in 1995, and changes in the third- and fourth-year clinical curriculum were implemented in 1996. An Honors Program, which involves independent research, challenges the exceptional student and is open to those who excel during their first semester of medical school. For highly qualified students interested in careers in research, a combined M.D./Ph.D. program is available. Medical students are graded with Honors, High Pass, Pass, and Fail. All students are required to pass Step 1 of the USMLE following completion of year two, and fourth-year students must pass Step 2 of the exam.

BASIC SCIENCES: Although most instruction uses a lecture format, small-group discussions and tutorials are also part of the curriculum. First year courses are Anatomy, Human Prenatal Development, Cell Biology and Micro-Anatomy, Biochemistry, Physiology, Clinical Correlation, Neuroscience, Medicine, Medical Ethics, Introduction to Clinical Medicine, Psychiatry, and Social Issues in Medicine. Electives are offered in Geriatrics, Problem Based Learning, Community Service, and Health Promotion and Wellness. Second year courses are Microbiology, Immunology and Parasitology, Pathology, Clinical Pathology, Pharmacology, and Introduction to Clinical Medicine. Basic sciences are taught in a modern building that is part of the medical center complex. Important educational resources are maintained by the LSU Division of Learning Resources, which provides audiovisual and classroom services to the downtown campus of the LSU Health Sciences Center. The medical library in New Orleans has a total of about 188,000 volumes, nearly 4,000 audiovisual titles, and approximately 2,000 periodicals. The library is fully computerized and houses individual computers that are equipped with educational software programs.

CLINICAL TRAINING: The third and fourth years are devoted primarily to clinical rotations. Lectures, conferences, and small-group discussions supplement the hands-on clinical training. Year three consists of eight and one-half days of ophthalmology course work in addition to rotations in: Medicine (12 weeks); General Surgery (8 weeks); Otolaryngology (2 weeks); Urology (2 weeks); Pediatrics (8 weeks); Family Medicine (4 weeks); Ob/Gyn (6 weeks); and Psychiatry (6 weeks). The final year consists of 36 weeks divided into nine four-week blocks, which are Ambulatory care, General Medicine, Neural Sciences, Special Topics, and an Acting Internship. The special-topics block includes Nutrition, Human Sexuality, Geriatrics, Drug and Alcohol Abuse, Office Management, and Financial Planning. The remainder of the year may include electives either in basic or clinical sciences with four weeks allowed for vacation. Most training takes place at LSU-affiliated hospitals including Charity Hospital, which has a total of 2,200 beds. Elective requirements may be fulfilled at any accredited medical school or teaching hospital in the United States or Canada. With approval, electives may also be taken at foreign institutions.

Students

All students are Louisiana residents. Approximately 15 percent of students are underrepresented minorities, most of whom are African American. The average age of entering students is about 23, and there are usually a number of students in their late 20s and 30s. Class size is 165.

STUDENT LIFE: Some medical students are active in the student government, which works closely with the faculty and the administration on a range of important issues. Others are involved in the student publication or in any number of professional clubs, honor societies, recreational groups, and community service projects. Extracurricular opportunities in New Orleans abound. The restaurants, music scene, historic and cultural sights, and annual festivals and events are world-renowned. Some students opt to live in the school's residence hall, which has its own student center. Others live off campus where housing is generally reasonably priced.

GRADUATES: The School assists and advises graduating students in obtaining suitable appointments in hospitals. LSU—New Orleans itself offers a comprehensive graduate medical-education program in more than 20 specialty fields.

Admissions

REQUIREMENTS: Louisiana residency is a requirement. Prerequisite courses are 8 semester hours each of Biology, Chemistry, Organic Chemistry, and Physics, all with associated labs. Strength in both written and spoken English is required. The MCAT is required, and scores should be from within the past three years. For applicants who have taken the exam more than once, the most recent set of scores is weighed most heavily.

SUGGESTIONS: A well-rounded undergraduate experience with course work in Humanities, Social Sciences, Math, and English is advised. Community service or medically related work or volunteer activities are valued.

PROCESS: All AMCAS applicants who are Louisiana residents are sent secondary applications. Of those returning secondaries, about 50 percent are invited to interview between October and April. The interview consists of two or three one-on-one sessions, each with a faculty member, student, or administrator. On interview day, candidates also have the opportunity to meet with students, tour the campus, and have lunch. About 60 percent of interviewed candidates are accepted on a rolling basis. Wait-listed candidates may send additional information to update their files.

Costs

Beyond tuition, the estimated yearly cost of living for a single student is about $13,000. This allows for on- or off-campus housing.

FINANCIAL AID: LSU administers a broad program of student aid, which includes awards, scholarships, and loans. Aid is given on the basis of need and/or merit or other special criteria. Generally, employment during medical school is discouraged. Each year, up to two M.D./Ph.D. students are fully funded.

LOUISIANA STATE UNIVERSITY, NEW ORLEANS

STUDENT BODY

Type	Public
*Enrollment	720
*% male/female	58/42
*% underrepresented minorities	19
# applied (total/out)	1,212/794
% interviewed	53
% accepted (total/out)	NR/NR
% enrolled (total/out)	NR/NR

ADMISSIONS

Average GPA and MCAT Scores

Overall GPA	3.60	Science GPA	3.50
MCAT Bio	9.60	MCAT Phys	9.20
MCAT Verbal	9.20	MCAT Essay	N

Score Release Policy

The school has not responded to our inquiry regarding withheld MCAT scores. Therefore, we advise caution. Contact the Admissions Office before withholding any scores.

Application Information

Regular application	11/15
Regular notification	10/15–varies
Early application	6/1–8/1
Early notification	10/1
Admissions may be deferred?	Yes
AMCAS application accepted?	Yes
Interview required?	Yes
Application fee	$50

COSTS AND AID

Tuition & Fees

Tuition (in/out)	$8,856/$11,502
Cost of books	$2,851
Fees	NR

Financial Aid

% students receiving aid	NR
Average grant	NR
Average loan	NR
Average debt	NR

*Figures based on total enrollment

LOUISIANA STATE UNIVERSITY
SCHOOL OF MEDICINE IN SHREVEPORT

PO Box 33932, Shreveport, LA 71130
Admission: 318-675-5190 • Fax: 318-675-5244
Email: shvadm@lsumc.edu • Internet: lib-sh.lsumc.edu

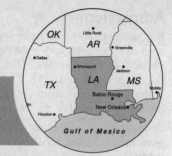

Louisiana State University in Shreveport (LSUS) is a comprehensive, urban university with a wide range of both undergraduate and graduate education programs. The School of Medicine is dedicated to providing a sound medical education to residents of Louisiana. The curriculum is designed for maximum flexibility, with opportunities for elective study during all four years. Clinical rotations include a unique, longitudinal clerkship in a student-run, primary care clinic.

Academics

The first two years are devoted to basic medical sciences with orientation to clinical applications. The second two years are devoted to clinical training and are spent primarily in hospitals and clinics. In addition to the M.D. degree, advanced studies leading to the M.D./Ph.D. are possible. The doctorate may be earned in Anatomy, Biochemistry, Microbiology, Pharmacology, and Physiology. All medical students are encouraged to take advantage of the many research opportunities available during summers and year-round. Special funds are provided for this purpose, and medical students who complete prescribed research activities are awarded diplomas with the special designation "Honors Research Participant." During summer terms, The school offers opportunities for rural, clinical electives. Medical students are evaluated with an A–F scale, with the exception of elective courses, which are Pass/Fail. Passing both steps of the USMLE is a graduation requirement.

BASIC SCIENCES: During the first year, students are in lectures, small-group seminars, labs, or other scheduled sessions for about 25 hours per week. Courses are CPR; Human Anatomy; Biometry; Ethics; Medical Neuroscience; Library Science; Family Medicine and Comprehensive Care; Radiology; Introduction to Computer-Aided Learning; Medical Genetics; Histology; Physiology and Biophysics; Psychiatry; Biochemistry and Molecular Biology; and Human Embryology. The second year is increasingly clinically oriented. Students are in class or other scheduled sessions for about 35 hours per week. Courses are Pathology; Radiology; Perspectives in Medicine; Psychiatry; Family Medicine and Comprehensive Care; Microbiology; Pharmacology; Clinical Neurology; Clinical Diagnosis; Clinical Pathology; and Clinical-Pathological Conference. A note-taking service, organized by and for students, assists with learning and retaining material. Computer-assisted instruction is a critical component of the basic-science education, and all entering students are required to own a computer.

CLINICAL TRAINING: An unusual, longitudinal clerkship called Comprehensive Care spans both the third and fourth years. In it, students work together and serve as the primary caregivers in a functioning clinic. Other third-

year required rotations are Medicine (8 weeks); Surgery (4 weeks); Surgery Subspecialties (3 weeks); Pediatrics (4 weeks); Ob/Gyn (8 weeks); Psychiatry (4 weeks); and Family Medicine (8 weeks). A minimum of 16 weeks during the fourth year are reserved for electives. Required clerkships are Medicine (6 weeks), Surgery (3 weeks), Pediatrics (3 weeks), and Neuroscience (3 weeks). Most training takes place at the LSU Hospital (650 beds), the Shreveport Veterans' Administration Hospital, and the Comprehensive Care Clinic.

Students

All students are Louisiana residents. About 5 percent of students are underrepresented minorities. There is a wide age range among entering students, including those in their late twenties or thirties. Class size is 100.

STUDENT LIFE: Outside of class, LSU offers medical students a rich campus life. The University offers more than 60 student organizations in addition to intramural sports, performing arts events, visiting speakers, and social activities. The University Center has dining facilities, a lounge, student activity rooms, and a bookstore, among other student services. Generally, it serves as a meeting place for students. The Health and Physical Education Building houses an indoor swimming pool; handball and racquetball courts; basketball; tennis, volleyball, and badminton courts; a dance studio; and fitness and weight training rooms. Shreveport is a historic Southern city with a population of more than 370,000. Museums, art galleries, parks, gardens, restaurants, bars, and shopping areas are some of its many attractions. The cities of Baton Rouge and New Orleans are easily accessible. Houston, Memphis, Little Rock, and Jackson are also within driving distance. Most medical students live off campus.

GRADUATES: An increasing proportion of graduates are entering primary care fields. The majority of graduates return to Louisiana to practice.

Admissions

REQUIREMENTS: Admission to the School of Medicine is limited to Louisiana residents. Requirements are one year each of Biology, Chemistry, Organic Chemistry, Physics, and English. All science courses must include laboratory work. The MCAT is required, and scores should be from within three years of application. For applicants who have taken the exam more than once, the most recent set of scores is generally weighed most heavily.

SUGGESTIONS: Once prerequisites are fulfilled, perspective applicants are encouraged to pursue their own interests and to develop their own special talents in gaining a broad educational background. In making admissions decisions, a candidate's motivation as well as his or her intellectual ability and preparation are assessed. Applicants must show potential of developing into mature, sensitive physicians who will inspire and deserve trust and confidence.

PROCESS: All AMCAS applicants who are Louisiana residents are sent secondary applications. Of those returning secondaries, about 30 percent are invited to interview between September and March. Interviews are given by members of the Admissions Committee, which is composed of Medical School faculty from the basic and clinical sciences as well as physicians from the community at large. The interview is used to assess personal traits and also allows candidates to see the facilities and to meet current students. Approximately 90 percent of interviewed candidates are accepted on a rolling basis. Others are rejected or wait-listed.

Costs

The estimated yearly cost of living for a single student is about $12,000. This includes all costs other than tuition and allows for off-campus housing and car maintenance. First-year students may also include the cost of a computer in their budget.

FINANCIAL AID: Various types of support are available from state, federal, and private sources for students demonstrating financial need. The School of Medicine has private funds for scholarships based on need as well as merit.

LOUISIANA STATE UNIVERSITY, SHREVEPORT

STUDENT BODY

Type	Public
*Enrollment	391
*% male/female	67/33
*% underrepresented minorities	5
# applied (total/out)	1,046/272
% interviewed	26
% accepted (total/out)	NR/NR
% enrolled (total/out)	NR/NR

ADMISSIONS

Average GPA and MCAT Scores

Overall GPA	3.50	Science GPA	3.40
MCAT Bio	8.90	MCAT Phys	8.40
MCAT Verbal	9.00	MCAT Essay	NR

Score Release Policy

The school has not responded to our inquiry regarding withheld MCAT scores. Therefore, we advise caution. Contact the Admissions Office before withholding any scores.

Application Information

Regular application	11/15
Regular notification	10/15 until filled
Early application	6/1–8/1
Early notification	10/1
Transfers accepted?	Yes
Admissions may be deferred?	Yes
AMCAS application accepted?	Yes
Interview required?	Yes
Application fee	$50

COSTS AND AID

Tuition & Fees

Tuition (in/out)	$6,551/$20,069
Cost of books	NR
Fees	$276

Financial Aid

% students receiving aid	81
Average grant	NR
Average loan	NR
Average debt	NR

*Figures based on total enrollment

University of Louisville

SCHOOL OF MEDICINE

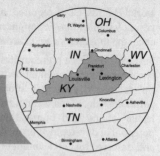

323 East Chestnut, Louisville, KY 40202

Admission: 502-852-5193

Internet: www.louisville.edu

The University of Louisville School of Medicine has a mandated statewide mission to meet the educational, research, and patient-care needs of the Commonwealth of Kentucky, within the resources available, and to cooperate with other health care teams. The educational program is designed to train physicians who are sensitive to medical ethics and who will meet the diverse health care needs of the Commonwealth of Kentucky.

Academics

Although most students complete a four-year program leading to the M.D., a few earn a combined M.D./Ph.D., which typically demands about seven years or a five-year M.D./M.B.A. Summer research scholarships allow first- and second-year students to participate in research projects alongside faculty mentors. Throughout all four years, students work closely with faculty advisers who assist with decisions related to academic and professional goals. Medical students are evaluated as Pass/Fail in both basic science and clinical courses. Passing Step 1 of the USMLE is a requirement for promotion to year three, and passing Step 2 is a requirement for graduation.

BASIC SCIENCES: The purpose of the Core Curriculum, which extends over the four-year course of study, is to provide each student with the general education and training considered essential to all physicians. It stresses understanding of concepts and general principles instead of superficial knowledge of details. It provides opportunity for correlation among the sciences so that information received in one subject can reinforce ideas and build upon concepts developed in another. The incorporation of clinical correlation into the first two years demonstrates how knowledge of the basic sciences applies directly to the solution of problems with human disease. The Core Curriculum, for the first two academic years, is divided into four quarters (one-half-semester intervals) of nine weeks each. Within these smaller subdivisions it is possible to very the balance of departmental activities to accommodate a better integrated understanding of the subject matter.

The purpose of the Preclinical Elective Program is to allow each student to extend his/her education in certain areas of scientific knowledge. The electives make it possible to construct a program of medical education that best meets the needs, abilities, and goals of the individual student. Students also are permitted to take courses as electives in divisions of the University of Louisville other than the School of Medicine, class schedule permitting. In addition to the courses listed, students with a research interest are permitted to participate in an approved research activity for credit. Elective courses constitute an integral part of the student's total program in medical school. Second-year students take two credit hours of elective courses.

CLINICAL TRAINING: Third-year required rotations are Psychiatry (6 weeks); Basic Surgery (8 weeks); Ob/Gyn (8 weeks); and Primary Care—Integrated Medicine, Pediatrics, and Family Medicine (24 weeks). Fourth-year requirements are Inpatient Medicine (4 weeks); Inpatient Surgery (4 weeks); Neurology (4 weeks); AHEC (4 weeks); Ambulatory Primary Care (4 weeks); and Ambulatory Rotation (4 weeks). The remaining 11 weeks in the fourth year are reserved for electives.

Students

In the entering class of 1999, 124 of 141 students were Kentucky residents. African Americans represented 10 percent of the class, and students older than 27 years old represented 13 percent of the class.

STUDENT LIFE: Students profit from the school's location, in the center of Louisville. Louisville is the largest city in Kentucky, offering cultural and recreational activities such as orchestra, theater, ballet, opera, numerous restaurants and bars, and shopping areas. Just outside of Louisville is the home of the Kentucky Derby. Many medical students take advantage of the university-owned Medical-Dental Dormitory and Apartment Building, which is two blocks from both the School of Medicine and the University Hospital. In this residential complex, there are apartments of all sizes as well as dorm rooms.

GRADUATES: A large proportion of practicing physicians in Kentucky are Louisville School of Medicine graduates. At Louisville itself, at least 17 post-graduate training programs are offered.

Admissions

REQUIREMENTS: Requirements are two semesters each of Biology, Chemistry, Organic Chemistry, Physics, and Calculus or other college-level Math. All science courses must include lab work. One semester of English is also required. The MCAT is required, and scores should be no more than two years old. For applicants who have retaken the exam, the most recent set of scores is considered. Thus, there is no advantage in withholding scores.

SUGGESTIONS: Approximately 90 percent of positions in each class are reserved for Kentucky residents, making out-of-state admission very competitive. Pre-medical students should develop a strong background in the Humanities, Philosophy, and the Arts. Communication and reading abilities are also important. The Committee values volunteer work, medically related experience, and evidence of strong interpersonal skills. Applicants are advised to take the April, rather than August, MCAT.

PROCESS: All Kentucky residents and highly qualified nonresidents who submit AMCAS applications are sent secondaries. Of those returning secondary applications, about one-half of Kentucky applicants are invited to interview between September and April. Ten percent of nonresidents are invited to interview. On interview day, candidates receive two 30-minute interview sessions each with a faculty member, administrator, or medical student. In addition, interviewees have a guided campus tour, lunch, and the opportunity to meet informally with current students. About 40 percent of interviewed candidates are accepted on a rolling basis. Wait-listed candidates may send information to update their files in the Spring.

Costs

The expected yearly budget for a single student is $11,846 on average. This allows for housing, transportation, and personal expenses.

FINANCIAL AID: Most financial aid is awarded on the basis of need, as determined by the FAFSA form. At least two state-sponsored scholarship programs support selected students who commit to practicing in rural areas of Kentucky. In addition, the Medical School offers privately funded scholarships awarded for superior academic performance, other merits, or special criteria. Some of these scholarships cover the full cost of tuition.

UNIVERSITY OF LOUISVILLE

STUDENT BODY

Type	Public
*Enrollment	570
*% male/female	51/49
*% underrepresented minorities	9
# applied (total/out)	1,453/1,006
% interviewed (total/out)	NR/NR
% accepted (total/out)	NR/NR
% enrolled (total/out)	NR/NR

ADMISSIONS

Average GPA and MCAT Scores

Overall GPA	3.60	Science GPA	3.5
MCAT Bio	9.20	MCAT Phys	8.60
MCAT Verbal	9.30	MCAT Essay	N–P

Score Release Policy

The Admissions Office says that students who withhold scores are at a disadvantage.

Application Information

Regular application	11/1
Regular notification	10/1–4/30
Early application	6/1–8/1
Early notification	10/1
Admissions may be deferred?	Yes
AMCAS application accepted?	Yes
Interview required?	Yes
Application fee	$25

COSTS AND AID

Tuition & Fees

Tuition (in/out)	$11,177/$28,100
Cost of books	$1,700
Fees	$286

Financial Aid

% students receiving aid	90
Average grant	NR
Average loan	NR
Average debt	NR

*Figures based on total enrollment

LOYOLA UNIVERSITY CHICAGO

STRITCH SCHOOL OF MEDICINE

2160 South First Avenue, Maywood, IL 60153
Admission: 708-216-3229
Internet www.meddean.luc.edu

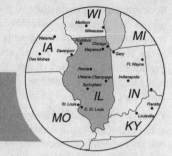

The Stritch School of Medicine is one of nine colleges within Loyola's network of educational institutions. In training future physicians, Loyola emphasizes humanism and spirituality along with academics and clinical medicine. The curriculum utilizes active learning, case-based instruction, early clinical experiences, and technological instructional aids. Through organized student communities, Loyola encourages cooperation among students and promotes positive faculty-student interaction. In their clinical rotations, students benefit from the diverse patient population of the Chicago metropolitan area.

Academics

Most students follow a four-year curriculum, leading to the M.D. A combined M.D. /Ph.D. program accepts up to three students each year. In this program, a doctorate degree may be earned in Anatomy, Biochemistry, Cell Biology, Immunology, Microbiology, Molecular Biology, Neuroscience, Pathology, Pharmacology, and Physiology. Evaluation of student performance uses Honors/High Pass/Pass/Fail. Students must pass Step 1 of the USMLE for promotion to year three, and must record a score on Step 2 in order to graduate.

BASIC SCIENCES: As a result of a comprehensive program evaluation, the School of Medicine introduced a new curriculum in 1995 that relies on small group sessions and problem-based learning as much as it does on traditional lectures and labs. Students are in class or other scheduled sessions for approximately 25 hours per week, discussing behavioral science and humanistic perspectives along with basic science concepts. First-year courses are: Cell and Molecular Biology; Structure of the Human Body; Function of the Human Body; Developmental Human Biology I; and Introduction to the Practice of Medicine I, a two-year continuum that begins with the medical interview and later covers the physical diagnosis, health promotion, medical ethics, health care finance, and legal issues in medicine. As part of the course, each student participates in special mentoring programs, spending time with a primary care physician and with a chaplain as he does his hospital rounds. Second-year courses are: Neuroscience; Mechanisms of Human Disease; Developmental Human Biology II; and Introduction to the Practice of Medicine II. Instruction takes place in the new Medical Education Building, which includes classrooms of many different sizes to accommodate different instructional modalities, labs, and other learning centers, video equipment, numerous computer clusters, lounges, study areas, and other facilities. The Medical Center Library houses about 170,000 volumes and periodicals.

CLINICAL TRAINING: Required third-year rotations are Family Medicine (6 weeks); Medicine (12 weeks); Ob/Gyn (6 weeks); Pediatrics (6 weeks); Psychiatry (6 weeks); and Surgery (12 weeks). During the fourth year, requirements are Neurology (4 weeks); Selectives in Medical Humanities (2 weeks); a subinternship (8 weeks); and 26 weeks of electives. Clinical facilities include: University Hospital and Ambulatory Center; Hines Veterans Affairs Hospital; Foster G. McGaw Hospital; Mulchy Outpatient Center; Cardinal Bernardin Cancer Center; and a Level I trauma center. Elective credits can be earned at other academic or clinical institutions. Students may arrange international clinical experiences, or take part in organized programs in the Caribbean and other locations. Often, financial assistance is available for such opportunities.

Students

At least half of students are Illinois residents. Approximately one-quarter of students took time off between college and medical school. Underrepresented minorities account for about 5 percent of the student body. Class size is 130.

STUDENT LIFE: At Loyola, not only is class cohesion strong, but interaction within the entire student body is high. In order to promote social interaction among classes, students are grouped into three equal "communities," each with representatives of all classes and each with two faculty mentors. In the Medical Education Building, communities are assigned their own lounges, kitchenettes, and study areas. Students also get to know each other through their involvement in student organizations, which provide support, recreational activities, and an opportunity to discuss professional and personal interests. During the first two years, most classes end at noon, allowing ample time for extracurricular pursuits. Many students use this time to volunteer for public clinics, homeless shelters, seniors programs, and schools. The University Ministry and other religious centers sponsor events and programs. A new Health and Fitness Center opened in 1997, featuring exercise equipment, racquetball and basketball courts, pools, tracks, classes, and a spa. Off-campus activities are plentiful, as Chicago is easily accessible from Loyola. All students live off campus, most in areas surrounding the campus.

GRADUATES: Graduates are successful in securing residency positions nationwide in both primary care and specialized fields. About 63 percent of graduates remain in the Midwest, while 23 percent go to the Western United States, 8 percent to the East, and 6 percent to the South.

Admissions

REQUIREMENTS: Prerequisites are one year each of Biology, Chemistry, Organic Chemistry, and Physics, all with associated labs. One semester of Biochemistry may be substituted for a semester of Organic Chemistry. The MCAT is required, and scores should be from within four years of anticipated entrance to medical school. For applicants who have retaken the exam, the most recent set of scores is weighed most heavily.

SUGGESTIONS: State residents are given some preference, as 50 percent of the positions in each class are reserved for them. Some recent course work is important for nontraditional applicants who have been out of school for a period of time. All students are advised to take the April MCAT so that the exam may be repeated in August if scores are not at the national average. Qualities that are sought in applicants are maturity, integrity, the ability to work with diverse populations, dedication to community service, and an awareness of the environment surrounding health care provision.

PROCESS: All applicants who meet minimum qualifications receive secondary applications. Of those returning secondaries, about 5 percent are interviewed between September and April. Interviews consist of two one-hour sessions each with a faculty member or administrator. On interview day, candidates also have lunch with current medical students and tour the campus. Among interviewed candidates, about 60 percent are accepted on a rolling basis, with notification beginning in October. Wait-listed candidates, or those in a hold category, may send additional information to update their files and indicate interest in Loyola.

Costs

Beyond tuition, the anticipated yearly cost of living for a single student is $14,000. This budget allows for off-campus housing.

FINANCIAL AID: Although most aid is awarded on the basis of need, some scholarships based on special criteria are available. The FAFSA, with parental financial disclosure, is used to determine financial need.

LOYOLA UNIVERSITY CHICAGO

STUDENT BODY

Type	Private
*Enrollment	514
*% male/female	55/45
*% underrepresented minorities	5
# applied (total/out)	8,464/6,863
% interviewed (total/out)	7/4
% accepted (total/out)	7/54
% enrolled (total/out)	43/50
Average age	23

ADMISSIONS

Average GPA and MCAT Scores

Overall GPA	3.57	Science GPA	3.50
MCAT Bio	10.00	MCAT Phys	9.70
MCAT Verbal	9.70	MCAT Essay	O

Score Release Policy

The school has not responded to our inquiry regarding withheld MCAT scores. Therefore, we advise caution. Contact the Admissions Office before withholding any scores.

Application Information

Regular application	11/15
Regular notification	10/15 until filled
Transfers accepted?	Yes
Admissions may be deferred?	Yes
AMCAS application accepted?	Yes
Interview required?	Yes
Application fee	$50

COSTS AND AID

Tuition & Fees

Tuition	$27,700
Cost of books	$2,022
Fees	$675

Financial Aid

% students receiving aid	93
Average grant	$12,300
Average loan	$38,000
Average debt	NR

*Figures based on total enrollment

MARSHALL UNIVERSITY

SCHOOL OF MEDICINE

1600 Medical Center Drive, Huntington, WV 25701-3655

Admission: 800-544-8514 • Fax: 304-691-1740

Email: warren@marshall.edu • Internet: musom.marshall.edu

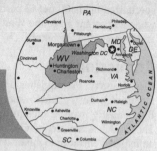

Marshall is known for its strength in rural medicine and its emphasis on ethics and the personal side of health care delivery. Clinical affiliates around the state give medical students the opportunity to learn first-hand about practicing in rural areas while they are in school. The majority of graduates enter primary care fields, ranking Marshall among the top four medical schools nationally in terms of the percentage of primary care graduates. This primary care philosophy of the school ensures that students have contact with patients beginning in the first semester and work in the community, alongside generalist physicians, throughout the four years.

Academics

The academic curriculum is influenced by the needs of rural providers, and the community's and the state's priorities and is geared toward achieving greater retention of West Virginia trained physicians in underserved communities. Although most students complete a four-year course of study leading to the M.D. degree, qualified students interested in research may concurrently pursue an M.S. or Ph.D. in Biomedical Sciences. Evaluation of student performance uses an A–F scale. Passing Step 1 of the USMLE is required for promotion to year three, and passing Step 2 is a graduation requirement.

BASIC SCIENCES: Basic science is taught primarily by using a lecture/lab format, although some time is spent in small-group discussions and clinical settings. Students are in scheduled sessions for about 30 hours per week. First-year courses are: Gross Anatomy and Embryology; Microanatomy and Ultrastructure; Neuroscience; Biochemistry; Physiology; Behavioral Medicine; Human Sexuality; Medical Cell and Molecular Biology; Medical Ethics; and Introduction to Patient Care. Second-year courses are: Pharmacology; Microbiology; Pathology; Physical Diagnosis; Introduction to Clinical Medicine; Introduction to Patient Care; Community Medicine; Psychopathology; Genetics; Medical Ethics; and Immunology. The medical education building where basic sciences are taught is self-contained, with a library and other educational resources.

CLINICAL TRAINING: Third-year students may participate in the standard curriculum or choose one of two alternative tracks that focus directly on rural, primary care medicine. In the standard curriculum, required third-year clerkships are: Medicine (8 weeks); Ob/Gyn (8 weeks); Psychiatry (8 weeks); Surgery (8 weeks); Pediatrics (8 weeks); Family Practice (8 weeks); and Transition to Primary Care (3 weeks). During the fourth year, required rotations are Medicine (4 weeks) and Surgery (4 weeks). A full 27 weeks are reserved for elective study, a portion of which must be taken in a rural area. Affiliated clinical teaching sites are numerous and include the Cabell Huntington Hospital (363 beds), St. Mary's Hospital (440 beds), and the Veterans Affairs Medical Center (100 beds).

Students

Among entering students in a recent class, 23 percent graduated from Marshall's undergraduate college. A total of 26 other undergraduate institutions were represented in the class. Seventy-one percent majored in Biology, 10 percent in Chemistry, and the remainder in other disciplines. The average age of incoming students is about 26, with an age range of 21–50. About 10 percent are minorities, mostly Asians. Class size is 48.

STUDENT LIFE: The small class size at Marshall contributes to a supportive and friendly environment. Students are active in chapters of national organizations, and in groups like the Christian Medical and Dental Society, American Medical Women's Association, and the Family Practice Interest Group. Huntington is a small city, offering the amenities and resources that students need while providing easy access to rural areas. For more recreational and cultural opportunities, the larger cities of Pittsburgh and Cincinnati are each about a four-hour drive. Medical students have access to the athletic and recreational facilities of the main University, and take part in University-wide events. On-campus housing options include University dormitories and units suitable for families. Off-campus housing is also affordable and readily available.

GRADUATES: Two-thirds of graduates enter primary care fields, which include Internal Medicine, Family Medicine, Pediatrics, and Ob/Gyn. Graduates are successful in securing residencies inside and outside of West Virginia.

Admissions

REQUIREMENTS: Prerequisites are eight semester hours each of Biology, Chemistry, Organic Chemistry, and Physics. Six semester hours each of Social Science and English are also required. An applicant's GPA is evaluated with consideration given to the academic institution and the rigor of courses taken. The MCAT is required and scores must be from within the past three years. For applicants who have retaken the exam, the latest set of scores is weighed most heavily.

Suggestions: As a state school, Marshall gives preference to West Virginia residents. A maximum of three positions in each year's class are reserved for residents of states that border West Virginia, and for candidates with strong ties to the state. The April, rather than August, MCAT is recommended. In addition to the academic record, Marshall considers personal qualities such as judgment, responsibility, altruism, integrity, and sensitivity important. Strong communication skills are valued.

Process: All AMCAS applicants receive secondary applications. Almost all West Virginia residents are interviewed, while only about 1 percent of out-of-state applicants are interviewed. Interviews take place between September and February and consist of two 30-minute sessions with members of the Admissions Committee. Acceptances are issued on a rolling basis. Wait-listed candidates may send information to update their files as the year progresses.

Costs

Beyond tuition, the expected yearly expenditures for a single student amount to about $13,500. This budget supports either on- or off-campus housing, as well as car ownership.

Financial Aid: Low tuition keeps student debt levels manageable. Most assistance is need-based, with need determined by the FAFSA and other forms. Some loans are available to students who commit to working in underserved areas in West Virginia, and a few merit-based scholarships are also offered.

MARSHALL UNIVERSITY

STUDENT BODY

Type	Public
*Enrollment	204
*% male/female	66/34
*% of all minorities	18
*% underrepresented minorities	5
# applied (total/out)	1,141/831
% interviewed (total/out)	21/1
% accepted (total/out)	7/1
% enrolled (total/out)	62/60
Average age	26

ADMISSIONS

Average GPA and MCAT Scores

Overall GPA	3.50	Science GPA	3.50
MCAT Bio	9.1	MCAT Phys	8.5
MCAT Verbal	9.0	MCAT Essay	NR

Score Release Policy

Applicants are not penalized for withholding scores from an early attempt at the MCAT.

Application Information

Regular application	6/1–11/15
Regular notification	10/15 until filled
Transfers accepted?	Yes
Admissions may be deferred?	Yes
AMCAS application accepted?	Yes
Interview required?	Yes
Application fee (in/out)	$40/$80

COSTS AND AID

Tuition & Fees

Tuition (in/out)	$8,684/$21,710
Cost of books and supplies	$3,627
Fees (in/out)	$360/$404

Financial Aid

% students receiving aid	85
Average scholarship	$6,904
Average loan	$23,723
Average debt	NR

*Figures based on total enrollment

UNIVERSITY OF MARYLAND

SCHOOL OF MEDICINE

655 West Baltimore Street, Baltimore, MD 21201

Admissions: 410-706-7478

Internet: www.som1.umaryland.edu

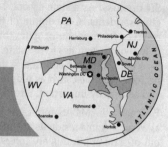

The University of Maryland School of Medicine provides a comprehensive medical education with respected programs in research and clinical medicine. The school is located in central Baltimore, only a few blocks from the revitalized Inner Harbor. The campus is also home to several other professional schools, including Schools of Nursing and Law.

Academics

Maryland changed its curriculum in 1994 to emphasize independent and small group learning, informatics, and the integration of basic and clinical science knowledge. The traditional degree program takes most students four years to complete. However, with permission of the dean, students may spend three years covering the basic sciences, and complete the degree requirements in five years. For students interested in a research career, the medical school offers a combined M.D./Ph.D. program in which the doctorate degree is offered in numerous disciplines such as Biochemistry, Biomedical Engineering, Genetics, Molecular Biology, Neuroscience, and Pharmacology. Grading is A–F. Students must pass Step 1 of the USMLE before beginning clinical training.

BASIC SCIENCES: The basic science curriculum is divided into integrated blocks by using interdisciplinary teaching with both basic and clinical science instructors. Lectures and labs rarely last longer than four hours per day; small-group and independent study are emphasized. Course work during the first year occupies 37 weeks and is organized into the following blocks: Structure and Development; Informatics; Principles of Human Development; Cell and Molecular Biology; Neuroscience; and Functional Systems. Introduction to Clinical Medicine runs concurrently throughout the year, as does Problem Based Learning. Intimate Human Behavior is also part of the first-year curriculum. The second year is particularly rigorous. Students learn pathophysiology and therapeutics by organ system, and are trained in conducting a physical diagnosis in the Introduction to Clinical Medicine course. Computers, not microscopes, are the laboratory tool of choice at Maryland. Lap tops are a required purchase, and students spend the first block of medical school in a Medical Informatics course that discusses medical applications and practical uses for the computer. The multidisciplinary laboratories seat ten students and have the latest in educational technology. The recently renovated library is among the largest medical libraries in the United States, with at least 240,000 volumes, and is fully connected to the information superhighway. The Office of Student Affairs closely monitors students and provides tutoring and other support services. In addition, a pre-matriculation summer program allows entrants to review pre-medical course work and preview first-year material.

CLINICAL TRAINING: Year three consists of seven required rotations in Family Medicine (4 weeks); Medicine (12 weeks); Surgery (12 weeks); Pediatrics (6 weeks); Psychiatry (4 weeks); Ob/Gyn (6 weeks); and Neurology/ Rehabilitation (4 weeks). The senior year includes a mandatory Ambulatory Care experience (8 weeks); a Subinternship (8 weeks); and 16 weeks of elective rotations. The majority of training takes place at University Hospital, a 747-bed tertiary care center adjacent to the Medical School. Rotations are also spent at the Baltimore VA Medical Center, Mercy Hospital, and other community hospitals. In total, 1,400 patient beds are used for teaching. One of the most popular electives is a rotation through the R. Adams Cowley Shock Trauma. Shock Trauma was the first trauma center in America and continues to be a model for the rest of the nation.

Students

The majority of students are Maryland residents, but the Medical School attracts and accepts a significant number of out-of-state applicants. In a typical class, approximately 20 of the 140 students are from out-of-state. The student body is highly diverse, with about 20 percent of students from underrepresented minority backgrounds. Increasingly, older students are making up a higher percentage of incoming classes. At least one-third of incoming classes took time off between college and medical school.

STUDENT LIFE: An extensive orientation program in rural Maryland allows entering students to get to know fellow classmates, upperclassmen, and faculty advisors. Almost half of the incoming class attends. Other organized events, such as pot-luck suppers, community activities, and meetings of student organizations all serve to bring students together. Baltimore is a lively city, with interesting neighborhoods and real character. The harbor, the commercial district (Fells Point), the Orioles baseball stadium, and other attractions are accessible to the campus. The University offers athletic facilities and housing in the form of dorms. Most students find affordable, private apartments off campus. While the surrounding area has undergone a renaissance in recent years, safety remains a concern, as in most large cities.

GRADUATES: Over half of each year's graduates enter one of the primary care fields. Graduates, however, are competitive candidates for the entire range of specialties.

Admissions

REQUIREMENTS: Maryland requires one year each of Biology, General Chemistry, Organic Chemistry, Physics, and English as prerequisite courses. A grade of C or better is mandatory in each course. While the MCAT is also required, there is no set formula for determining competitive scores. Students with a wide range of scores are accepted each year. In addition, Maryland considers the best scores for those applicants who retake the exam.

SUGGESTIONS: Maryland gives clinical experience with direct patient exposure considerable weight. Research experience and service activity are also valued.

PROCESS: Maryland uses the AMCAS application. Secondary applications are sent to all Maryland residents and almost a quarter of nonresidents. Of those who complete the secondary, approximately 33 percent are interviewed beginning in October. The interview day consists of a faculty interview, a medical student interview, and a casual lunch with students and a tour of the campus. Interviewed applicants normally receive a decision within a month after the interview. Half of those interviewed are accepted, and the other half either rejected or wait-listed.

Costs

The anticipated yearly cost of living for a single student is about $14,000. This budget allows students to live off campus. Most students own cars.

FINANCIAL AID: Financial need is based solely on the student portion of the FAFSA, and parental assets are not used when determining financial aid. In addition to need-based loans and grants, Maryland offers various merit-based scholarships.

UNIVERSITY OF MARYLAND

STUDENT BODY

Type	Public
*Enrollment	589
*% male/female	52/48
*% underrepresented minorities	20
# applied (total/out)	3,290/2,475
% interviewed (total/out)	14/6
% accepted (total/out)	8/2
% enrolled (total/out)	14/1

ADMISSIONS

Average GPA and MCAT Scores

Overall GPA	3.63	Science GPA	3.59
MCAT Bio	10.40	MCAT Phys	10.20
MCAT Verbal	9.90	MCAT Essay	NR

Score Release Policy

The Admissions Committee does not care if scores are withheld, but they add that it is not generally a good idea for students to file applications without all scores.

Application Information

Regular application	11/1
Regular notification	10/15 until filled
Early application	6/1–8/1
Early notification	10/1
Admissions may be deferred?	Yes
AMCAS application accepted?	Yes
Interview required?	Yes
Application fee	$50

COSTS AND AID

Tuition & Fees

Tuition (in/out)	$13,129/$25,145
Cost of books	NR
Fees	$1,806

Financial Aid

% students receiving aid	96
Average grant	NR
Average loan	NR
Average debt	$63,296

*Figures based on total enrollment

UNIVERSITY OF MASSACHUSETTS

MEDICAL SCHOOL

55 Lake Avenue North, Worcester, MA 01655
Admission: 508-856-2323
Email: anne.parlante@banyan.ummed.edu • Internet: www.ummed.edu

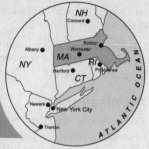

The University of Massachusetts at Worcester is one of five UMass campuses and is devoted entirely to the health sciences. The Medical School, the UMass Clinical System, the Graduate School of Biomedical Sciences and the Graduate School of Nursing comprise the medical campus. As a state-affiliated institution, the medical campus strives to meet the health care needs of Massachusetts residents. However, research at UMass addresses issues that are considered priorities at the national and global levels. The Medical School is one of 14 centers nationwide to receive the Robert Wood Johnson Generalist Physician Initiative grant, aimed at increasing the supply of primary care physicians.

Academics

The four-year program emphasizes varied educational modalities, lifelong learning, communication skills, and a generalist approach that prepares students for all medical career paths. Ethical issues are an important aspect of the education, demonstrated by the existence of an active Office of Ethics. Year-long and summer research fellowships are available, as is a joint M.D./Ph.D. program. The doctorate degree may be earned in Biomedical Sciences, Biochemistry and Molecular Biology, Cell Biology, Cellular and Molecular Physiology, Immunology and Virology, Molecular Genetics, Microbiology, Neuroscience, and Pharmacology and Molecular Toxicology. A combined M.D./M.P.H. degree program is also offered. For pre-clinical courses, grades are Honors, Near Honors, Satisfactory, Marginal, Unsatisfactory, or Incomplete, with the exception of a few courses that are taken as Credit/No Credit. During the clinical years, ratings are Outstanding, Above Expected Performance, Expected Performance, Below Expected Performance, and Failure.

BASIC SCIENCES: First-year courses are Biochemistry/Metabolism; The Gene; Human Anatomy; Cells and Tissues; Systems I; Physiology; Immunology; Mind, Brain and Behavior I; Physician, Patient and Society (PPS); and Longitudinal Preceptor Program (LPP). PPS and LPP together introduce students to medical interviewing, physician-patient relationships, physical diagnosis, medical reasoning and decision analyses, population-based medicine, ethics, epidemiology, medical informatics, and preventive medicine. Systems I covers several body/organ systems: Hematology; Cardiovascular; Respiratory; Renal and Acid/Base; Endocrine Regulation; GI/Nutrition; and Reproduction. Second-year courses focus on the biology of disease. They are General Pathology; Neoplasia; General Pharmacology; Microbiology; Mind, Brain and Behavior II; Systems II; and a continuation of PPS and LPP. In Systems II, Dermatology, Musculoskeletal/Renal, and "Pumps, Wind and Water" are among the body systems studied. Basic sciences are taught in a wing of the School's central complex. A new Learning Center houses amphitheaters, flexible classrooms, and a video conference facility. The Lamar Soutter Library holds over 239,000 volumes, subscribes to 1,500 journals, and provides access to online search and database tools. The Library Computer Area contains personal computers and workstations for computer-assisted instruction, interactive programs, and educational databases.

CLINICAL TRAINING: Third-year required rotations are Medicine (12 weeks); Surgery (12 weeks); Family and Community Medicine (6 weeks); Ob/Gyn (6 weeks); Pediatrics (6 weeks); and Psychiatry (6 weeks). Fourth-year requirements are Neurology (4 weeks), a Subinternship in Medicine (4 weeks), and 24 weeks of elective study. Clinical training takes place at the UMass hospital (388 beds), a comprehensive facility with general and specialty services. Clinical specialties include: Cancer Center; Level I Trauma Center; Kidney-Pancreas transplantation; Children's Medical Center; Center of Stone Disease; advanced laser technology; Cardiovascular Center; Breast Center; AIDS programs; burn unit; and public sector psychiatry. UMass benefits from affiliations with hospitals in and around the Worcester area: Memorial Health Care (319 beds); Saint Vincent Hospital; and Berkshire Medical Center (330 beds).

Students

All students are Massachusetts residents. The average age of incoming students is 25, and at least half of students took some time off after college. About 60 percent of students were science majors as undergraduates. Approximately 7 percent of students are underrepresented minorities. Class size is 100.

STUDENT LIFE: Recreational and athletic facilities are conveniently located in the lower level of the basic science building. Facilities include a lounge with a TV, pool and ping pong tables, study areas, and an exercise and weight room. Students are involved in organizations focused on community service, recreational interests, and professional pursuits. Worcester is a city of nearly 200,000, offering a full range of services and activities. Students live off campus, most choosing to live in the local community. Some students rely on public transportation, while others use cars.

GRADUATES: Among 1997 graduates, the most popular fields for post-graduate training were Internal Medicine (28%); Family Practice (25%); Pediatrics (15%); Emergency Medicine (7%); Ob/Gyn (4%); and Surgery (5%). A significant proportion entered residency programs in Massachusetts.

Admissions

REQUIREMENTS: Massachusetts residency is a requirement. Prerequisites are one year each of Biology, General Chemistry, Organic Chemistry, Physics, and English. All science courses should include associated labs. The MCAT is required, and scores should be from within the past two years. For applicants who have taken the exam on multiple occasions, the best scores are weighed most heavily. Thus, withholding scores is not advantageous.

SUGGESTIONS: Applications should be submitted as early as possible. In addition to requirements, course work in Computer Science; Calculus; Statistics; Sociology; and Psychology is advised. For applicants who have been out of college for a significant period of time, some recent course work is important. Medically related experiences or research may strengthen an application.

PROCESS: All in-state AMCAS applicants are sent secondary applications. Of those returning secondaries, about half are interviewed between October and March. Interviews consist of two 30-minute sessions with faculty members and/or medical students. On interview day, candidates also have a group information session and campus tour. Approximately one-third of interviewees are accepted on a rolling basis. Wait-listed candidates may send supplementary information if it serves to update their files.

Costs

Beyond tuition, the estimated yearly cost of living for a single student is about $12,000. This budget allows for off-campus housing.

FINANCIAL AID: Assistance is need-based, with need determined by the FAFSA and CCS profile. A unique program, the UMass Learning Contract, awards institutional loans and allows students to choose whether they will pay back loans or will serve in physician-shortage areas in lieu of repayment.

UNIVERSITY OF MASSACHUSETTS

STUDENT BODY

Type	Public
*Enrollment	425
*% male/female	49/51
*% underrepresented minorities	7
# applied (total/out)	814/0
% interviewed	53
% accepted (total/out)	NR/NR
% enrolled (total/out)	22/NR
Average age	25

ADMISSIONS

Average GPA and MCAT Scores

Overall GPA	NR	Science GPA	3.50
MCAT Bio	10.00	MCAT Phys	10.00
MCAT Verbal	10.00	MCAT Essay	NR

Score Release Policy

Students must submit all scores to be considered for admission.

Application Information

Regular application	11/1
Regular notification	10/15–varies
Early application	6/1–8/1
Early notification	10/1
Admissions may be deferred?	Yes
AMCAS application accepted?	Yes
Interview required?	No
Application fee	$50

COSTS AND AID

Tuition & Fees

Tuition (in/out)	$8,352/NR
Cost of books	$460
Fees	$1,835

Financial Aid

% students receiving aid	97
Average grant	NR
Average loan	NR
Average debt	$70,068

*Figures based on total enrollment

MAYO MEDICAL SCHOOL

200 First Street, SW, Rochester, MN 55905
Admission: 507-284-2316 • Fax: 507-284-2634
Internet: www.mayo.edu/education/mms/MMS_home_page.html

Mayo students have access to the resources of the nation's largest and most renowned private group practice, the Mayo Clinic. These resources are associated with the clinical and research activities at the Mayo Clinic in Rochester and at Mayo's group practices in Arizona and Florida. Other unique features of Mayo Medical School are its small class size, integrated curriculum, initiation of clinical rotations in the second year rather than the third, and emphasis on patient-centered medicine. Although Mayo offers reduced tuition to residents of states with affiliated facilities, it is a private medical school that attracts students from around the country. Mayo Medical School is in Rochester, a small city located 80 miles from Minneapolis.

Academics

Each year, 34 students begin a four-year curriculum, leading to the M.D. degree, and six students pursue a joint M.D./Ph.D. program in connection with the Mayo Graduate School. Through this program, a Ph.D. may be obtained in: Biochemistry, Biomedical Imaging, Biophysics, Immunology, Molecular Biology, Neuroscience, Pharmacology, Physiology, and Tumor Biology. Two students with D.D.S. degrees are admitted each year for training towards careers in oral and maxillofacial surgery. Courses are grouped into units, which are The Organ, The Patient, Physician and Society, The Scientific Foundation of Medical Practice, The Clinical Experience, and The Research Trimester. All students are required to write a research paper while at Mayo, and 80 percent of these works are published. Evaluation of student performance uses Honors, High Pass, Pass, Marginal Pass, and Fail. Taking the USMLE Steps 1 and 2 is a requirement for graduation.

BASIC SCIENCES: During the first five months of school, students take Molecular Biology and Genetics, Pathology and Cell Biology, Immunology, and Anatomy. The remainder of year one is organized around the following organ and physiological systems: Cutaneous System, Respiratory System, Hematopoietic System, Neuroscience, Growth and Development, Renal System, Cardiovascular System, Digestive System, Endocrine System, Allergy, and Musculoskeletal System. Patient contact begins in year one, in Introduction to the Patient and Continuity of Care. Small groups and problem-based learning enhance the lecture/lab format and account for about one-third of the 28 hours per week of scheduled class time. The second year is split between clinical and basic science education. The first block of year two includes: Microbiology and Infectious Disease, Psychopathology, and ENT, SAR/Sexual Medicine, and Bioethics. In the next block, second-year students attend lectures and seminars and rotate through several clinical departments, evaluating patients under the guidance of a preceptor. Clinical rotations are: Dermatology (3 weeks); Family Medicine (2 weeks); Musculoskeletal Medicine and Rehabilitation (3 weeks); Medicine (9 weeks); Surgery (3 weeks); Pediatrics (6 weeks); and Clinical Skills Aquisition (3 weeks). Tutoring

and a wide variety of advising services are available to students, and a formal system is in place to identify and assist students who may be experiencing academic difficulties. Scheduled classes and labs take place on the Mayo campus, while independent and computer-aided instruction is offered in the Learning Resource Center located in the Mitchell Student Center. The Mayo Medical Library houses 353,000 volumes and subscribes to 4,300 journals.

CLINICAL TRAINING: The third year is divided into three segments. The Research Trimester is a 17-week experience in which students participate in a biomedical research project and produce a related scientific paper. Two trimesters of clinical rotations are: Family Medicine (2 weeks); Internal Medicine (6 weeks); Neurology (3 weeks); Surgery (6 weeks); Pediatrics (3 weeks); Ob/Gyn (6 weeks); Radiology (3 weeks); and Psychiatry (4 weeks). Training takes place at the Mayo Clinic, Rochester Methodist, and Saint Mary's Hospitals, which together have 2,000 beds. Fourth-year requirements are six weeks of an Internal Medicine Subinternship, and three-week clerkships selected from specialties within Surgery, Pediatrics, and Internal Medicine. The remainder of year four is reserved for elective study throughout the Mayo system nationally and internationally.

Students

The student body consists of about 170 students from more than 40 states. About 15 percent of a typical class are underrepresented minorities. About one-quarter of entering students took at least a year or two off between college and medical school. Class size is 42.

STUDENT LIFE: The small class size facilitates cohesion among students. Mitchell Student Center, in addition to housing the Learning Resource Center, provides an area for relaxation and communal study. Students are involved in medically related organizations and societies, community projects, and groups organized around athletic and cultural interests. Students also play an important role in the School's administration, participating in governing committees. Rochester's population is 75,000, offering concerts, theater, museums, golf courses, and parks, among other recreational opportunities. All students live off campus.

GRADUATES: In a class of recent graduates, 39 percent entered residencies in primary care. Specialties selected by more than one student were Internal Medicine (11%); Family Medicine (8%) Ob/Gyn (11%); Dermatology (8%); Anesthesiology (8%); Diagnostic Radiology (6%), and Pediatrics (8%).

Admissions

REQUIREMENTS: Prerequisites are: Biology with lab (one year); Chemistry with lab (one year); Organic Chemistry with lab (one year); Physics (one year); and Biochemistry (one course). Consideration is given to the standing of the applicant's undergraduate institution when assessing GPA. The MCAT is required and must be no more than three years old.

SUGGESTIONS: Mayo is interested in undergraduate course work that demonstrates both aptitude in science and breadth of knowledge in social science and humanities. Strong interest in community service and leadership potential are important traits.

PROCESS: About 15 percent of AMCAS applicants are asked to submit letters of recommendation. No supplementary application is required, although some applicants will be further screened with phone interviews. About 20 percent of screened applicants are invited to interview, with interviews taking place between September and April. Applicants receive two 30–45 minute interviews with faculty, students, and/or administrators. Of interviewed applicants, about 10 percent are accepted on a rolling basis. Others are rejected or wait-listed. Additional material from wait-listed candidates is not encouraged.

Costs

The total yearly budget (excluding tuition) for a single student is about $10,000. This budget allows for car ownership.

FINANCIAL AID: Mayo's financial aid program is very generous, and is unique among medical schools. All students receive grants and/or scholarships that cover either all or half of the cost of tuition. Loans are also available to cover additional costs.

MAYO MEDICAL SCHOOL

STUDENT BODY

Type	Private
*Enrollment	167
*% male/female	45/55
*% underrepresented minorities	14
# applied (total/out)	3,322/2,990
% interviewed (total/out)	9/8
% accepted (total/out)	3/2
% enrolled (total/out)	1/.8
Average age	22

ADMISSIONS

Average GPA and MCAT Scores

Overall GPA	3.80	Science GPA	3.77
MCAT Bio	11.00	MCAT Phys	11.00
MCAT Verbal	11.00	MCAT Essay	P

Score Release Policy

Withholding scores is not recommended. The school needs to see all MCAT scores.

Application Information

Regular application	11/1
Regular notification	10/15 until filled
Early application	6/1–8/1
Early notification	10/1
Transfers accepted?	No
Admissions may be deferred?	Yes
AMCAS application accepted?	Yes
Interview required?	Yes
Application fee	$60

COSTS AND AID

Tuition & Fees

Tuition	$19,700
Cost of books and fees	$1,030

Financial Aid

% students receiving aid	100
Average grant	$16,399
Average loan	$14,678
Average debt	$60,285

*Figures based on total enrollment

MCP Hahnemann University

MCP HAHNEMANN SCHOOL OF MEDICINE

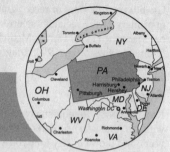

2900 Queen Lane, Philadelphia, PA 19129
Admission: 215-991-8100 • Fax: 215-843-1766
Email: admis@auhs.edu • Internet: www.mcphu.edu

MCP Hahnemann is the largest private medical school in the United States, with 250 students in each medical school class. Affiliated educational institutions include schools of nursing, public health, and health professions. The hospitals owned by Allegheny are numerous, providing excellent clinical training facilities for medical students. Medical students are from across the country, and represent diverse backgrounds. An indication of the School's interest in nontraditional students is the effort that is made to recruit students from a number of post-baccalaureate pre-medical programs. Before merging with Hahnemann, the Medical College of Pennsylvania (MCP) was the first medical school dedicated to educating women physicians. Today, MCP Hahnemann remains committed to women in medicine and to women's health issues.

Academics

Most students follow a four-year curriculum, leading to the M.D. Students gain research experience through the Summer Research Fellowship Program, which provides a stipend in exchange for full-time research in the laboratory of a participating mentor. The combined M.D./ M.H.P. program is available, as are M.D./M.S. and M.D./ Ph.D. programs, through which students may earn graduate degrees in: Bioengineering; Cardiovascular Biology; Clinical Microbiology; Interdepartmental Medical Science; Laboratory Animal Science; Medical Science Preparatory; Microbiology and Immunology; Molecular and Cell Biology; Molecular and Human Genetics; Molecular PathoBiology; Neuroscience; Pharmacology; and Physiology and Radiation Sciences. The Medical Humanities Scholars Program allows students who are particularly interested in the humanistic elements of medicine to graduate with the designation of Humanities Scholar. Several programs aimed at encouraging primary care, including a 6-year combined medical school/residency option, are offered. Medical students are evaluated with Honors/Pass/Fail, and Step 1 of the USMLE is required for promotion to year three.

BASIC SCIENCES: As an alternative to the traditional preclinical curriculum, the Program for Integrated Learning (PIL) offers a problem-based learning track to selected entering students. Students in PIL work in small groups and on their own, learning principles of basic sciences and applying them to clinical cases. Although the learning modality differs, students in both tracks cover similar topics, and are in class or other scheduled sessions for about 20 hours per week. During the first year, topics are: Biochemistry; Gross Anatomy and Embryology; Microscopic Anatomy and Cell Biology; Human and Molecular Genetics; Neuroscience and Medical Physiology; Bioethics; Nutrition; Human Sexuality; Behavioral Science; Principles of Medical Research; and Clinical Skills. Second-year topics are: Medical Microbiology; Community and Preventive Medicine; Psychopathology;

Pathology and Laboratory Medicine; Medical Pharmacology; and Introduction to Clinical Medicine, which is a continuation of the first year Clinical Skills course. The clinical continuum teaches interviewing techniques, the physical examination, and problem-solving skills that are relevant to the practice of medicine. Standardized patients and model examination rooms are some of the facilities used to enhance clinical instruction in the course. Students also spend time in the offices of primary care physicians, thereby gaining first-hand experience with patient care. All students are involved in the School's Computer-Based Learning Program, which takes advantage of extensive educational and informational software programs.

CLINICAL TRAINING: Required rotations, most of which are completed in the third year, are: Medicine (12 weeks); Surgery (12 weeks); Pediatrics (6 weeks); Ob/Gyn (6 weeks); Psychiatry (6 weeks); Neurology (4 weeks); a Subinternship (4 weeks); and Family Medicine (6 weeks). Among the clinical training sites in the Philadelphia area are: Allegheny University Hospitals Hahnemann (618 beds); Allegheny University Hospitals MCP (465 beds); Allegheny University Hospitals, City Avenue (228 beds); Allegheny University Hospitals, Elkins Park (280 beds); Allegheny University Hospitals, Mt. Sinai (235 beds); Allegheny University Hospitals, Parkview (200 beds); Allegheny University Hospitals, Rancocoas (318 beds); and St. Christopher's Hospital for Children (183 beds). In the Pittsburgh area, teaching sites include: Allegheny General Hospital (728 beds) and Allegheny University Medical Center, Forbes-Metropolitan (172 beds). There are numerous other affiliated hospitals throughout Pennsylvania and in New Jersey, in addition to community-based clinical facilities.

Students

About 17 percent of students are underrepresented minorities, and at least a quarter of students are older, having pursued other interests or careers in between college and medical school.

STUDENT LIFE: Despite the relatively large class size, students are cohesive and supportive. The School of Medicine offers a variety of clubs and activities that are both academically and nonacademically oriented. Many students are involved in community outreach activities in local public schools, health clinics, and rehabilitation centers. Students have access to a new on-site fitness center and to the local YMCA. Philadelphia is a diverse and interesting city with a large student population. For additional attractions, New York and other urban areas can be easily reached by train. There is no campus-owned housing in Philadelphia.

GRADUATES: Graduates are successful in securing residency positions. As one of 16 schools nationwide to receive an implementation grant from the Robert Wood Johnson Foundation's Generalist Physician Initiative, MCP Hahnemann is focused on training primary care physicians.

Admissions

REQUIREMENTS: Requirements are two semesters each of Biology, General Chemistry, Organic Chemistry, Physics, and English. Science courses should include associated labs. The MCAT is required, and scores should be from within the past two years. For applicants who have retaken the exam, the most recent set of scores is weighed most heavily.

SUGGESTIONS: Beyond prerequisites, recommended courses include Philosophy, Ethics, History, Psychology, and other Social Science and Humanities courses. The Admissions Committee regards an applicant's background and experience as important. Women, older students, minorities, and students from rural areas are encouraged to apply. Pennsylvania residents are given slight preference.

PROCESS: All AMCAS applicants receive secondary applications. Of those returning secondaries, about 10 percent are interviewed between September and March. The interview typically consists of two sessions, each with a faculty member or administrator. Of interviewed candidates, about one-third are accepted on a rolling basis. Wait-listed candidates may send transcripts or other material to update their files. An alternate route to admissions is through B.A./M.D. and B.S./M.D. programs organized in conjunction with Leigh and Villanova Universities. For highly qualified post-baccalaureate students at participating institutions, a provisional acceptance to the School of Medicine may be granted, contingent on successful completion of the pre-medical curriculum. Post-bacc programs at which this type of arrangement is possible are: Bryn Mawr; Bennington; Columbia; Duquesne; Goucher; University of Pennsylvania; and West Chester University.

Costs

In addition to tuition, the estimated yearly cost of living for a single student is about $11,000. While some students rely on public transportation, most own cars.

FINANCIAL AID: Financial aid, in the form of grants, loans, and work-study arrangements, is available to students with need, as determined by the FAFSA and institutional forms. Merit scholarships, offered on the basis of outstanding accomplishments, are offered each year to a number of entering students.

MCP HAHNEMANN UNIVERSITY

STUDENT BODY

Type	Private
*Enrollment	1,067
*% male/female	53/47
*% underrepresented minorities	17
#applied (total/out)	9,060/7,864
% interviewed (total/out)	11/6
% accepted (total/out)	NR/NR
% enrolled (total/out)	20/18

ADMISSIONS

Average GPA and MCAT Scores

Overall GPA	3.35	Science GPA	NR
MCAT Bio	NR	MCAT Phys	NR
MCAT Verbal	NR	MCAT Essay	NR

Score Release Policy

The school has not responded to our inquiry regarding withheld MCAT scores. Therefore, we advise caution. Contact the Admissions Office before withholding any scores.

Application Information

Regular application	12/1
Regular notification	10/15 until filled
Early application	6/1–8/1
Early notification	10/1
Admissions may be deferred?	Yes
AMCAS application accepted?	Yes
Interview required?	No
Application fee	$65

COSTS AND AID

Tuition & Fees

Tuition	$25,725
Cost of books	NR
Fees	$500

Financial Aid

% students receiving aid	NR
Average grant	NR
Average loan	NR
Average debt	NR

*Figures based on total enrollment

MEDICAL UNIVERSITY OF SOUTH CAROLINA

COLLEGE OF MEDICINE

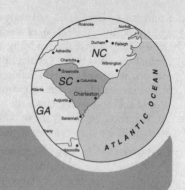

171 Ashley Avenue, Charleston, SC 29425
Admission: 803-792-3283 • Fax: 803-792-3764
Email: taylorwl1@musc.edu • Internet: www2.musc.edu

College of Medicine students at the Medical University of South Carolina (MUSC) are enriched through contact with students in five of the University colleges: Dentistry, Pharmacy, Nursing, Graduate Studies, and Health Professions. The primary goal of the College of Medicine is to train competent and caring physicians capable of succeeding in post-graduate programs in their chosen fields. The education that MUSC medicine students receive is characterized by rigorous basic science instruction, early patient interaction, and access to excellent clinical teaching facilities. Charleston is a culturally and historically rich city that also offers lovely weather and year-round outdoor activities.

Academics

Basic Sciences are taught during the first two years, through either the traditional curriculum or the parallel curriculum (PC), and are integrated with a variety of clinical experiences. All students fulfill the same clerkship requirements during the third and fourth years. Qualified students may pursue a Ph.D. degree concurrently with an M.D. as part of the Medical Scientist Training Program (M.S.T.P.). The doctorate degree is offered in a number of disciplines, including Anatomy, Biochemistry, Cell Biology, Genetics, Immunology, Microbiology, Molecular Biology, Pathology, Pharmacology, and Physiology. Evaluation is based on a 0–4 scale, with the exception of the Introduction to Clinical Medicine sequence, taken during the first two years, and clinical rotations taken during the fourth year when grades of Pass/Fail are recorded.

BASIC SCIENCES: Though most students follow a lecture-based curriculum, 18 students each year enter an alternative curriculum that covers similar topics but uses a problem-based instructional format. First-year subjects are Gross Anatomy; Biochemistry; Neuroscience; basic and Clinical Genetics; Physiology; Cell Biology/Histology; Embryology; and Introduction to Clinical Medicine. Second-year subjects are Pathology/Neuropathology; Immunology; Systemic Pathology and Laboratory Medicine; Pharmacology; Microbiology and Infectious Diseases; and Introduction to Clinical Medicine. The Clinical Medicine sequence covers a range of issues including community medicine, behavioral sciences, ethics, techniques for physical diagnosis, interviewing skills, and the computer in medicine. A student note-taking service provides documentation of lectures, allowing participating students to concentrate on the speaker and absorb information more effectively. Additionally, the school administers tutoring and study groups to reinforce basic science instruction. The University's Center for Academic Excellence provides one-on-one assistance and study skills and test-taking anxiety seminars. Month-long reviews for the USMLE Step 1 are offered to second-year students prior to the exam. The Health Affairs Library houses over 200,000 volumes and about 3,000 periodicals.

CLINICAL TRAINING: Required third-year clerkships are two months each of Medicine, Surgery, Pediatrics, Psychiatry, and Ob/Gyn in addition to one month each of Family Medicine and Neurology. During the fourth year, one month each of Surgery, Medicine, and a clinical externship are required in addition to four months of electives. Training takes place at Medical University Hospital (510 beds); Albert Florins Storm Memorial Eye Institute; Hollins Cancer Center; Veterans Affairs Hospital (431 beds); Charleston Memorial Hospital (175 beds); Children's Hospital (150 beds); and the Psychiatric Institute (50 beds).

Students

Over 90 percent of students are South Carolina residents. About 15–20 percent are underrepresented minorities, most of whom are African American. The average age of incoming students is typically around 25, and usually at least 10 percent of entering classes are over 30 years old. Class size is 135.

STUDENT LIFE: During orientation, incoming students are assigned to groups composed of first- and second-year students and a faculty member. The groups serve as informational resources for both academic and nonacademic matters. Also during the first week of school, the Activities Fair is held and introduces various student activities, groups, and events. Organizations that are popular with medical students include chapters of national medical fraternities, professionally oriented interest groups, and groups focused on health care related community service. Intramural sports are also popular. The Harper Student Center (HSC) houses student service offices, a student lounge, and a comprehensive fitness center with indoor and outdoor tracks, rooftop tennis courts, and a swimming pool, among other features. HSC is also a gathering site for students, offering happy hours and other social events. Beyond the campus, Charleston is a city known for its beauty and charm. Students enjoy the nearby beaches and other outdoor attractions. All students live off campus.

GRADUATES: Graduates are successful in securing residencies in all medical fields, with a significant number entering Family Medicine. MUSC itself offers over 20 post-graduate training programs. More than 95 percent pass USMLE Step 2.

Admissions

REQUIREMENTS: No prerequisites are specified. An applicant's GPA is evaluated with consideration given to the undergraduate institution attended and the difficulty of the course load. The MCAT is required, and scores must be from within the past five years. For applicants who have taken the exam on multiple occasions, the best set of scores is used.

SUGGESTIONS: South Carolina residents are given strong preference. The MCAT requirement suggests that applicants should have a basic science background. However, breadth of course work, including courses in the Humanities and Social Sciences, is also valued. Since the best set of MCAT scores is used, withholding scores has no advantage. Extracurricular activities, specifically those that are medically, community-service, or research related are important. During the interview, non cognitive traits such as emotional stability, integrity, honesty, and enthusiasm are evaluated.

PROCESS: All South Carolina residents, in addition to minority and highly-qualified out-of-state applicants, are asked to submit secondary applications. Of those returning secondaries, about 65 percent of state residents, and 5 percent of out-of-state residents are interviewed if they are academically qualified. Interviews are conducted from September through March, and consist of three sessions each with a faculty member or MUSC alumni. About one-third of interviewees are accepted on a rolling basis. Others are rejected or wait-listed.

Costs

The anticipated yearly cost of living and academic charges for a single in-state student is about $15,000 (about $28,000 for out-of-state students). This budget allows for shared housing and car ownership.

FINANCIAL AID: The School participates in federal and state need-based student loan programs. In addition, a wide range of private scholarships are available, some based solely on merit. Grants and loans may be awarded to students who commit to practicing in underserved areas in the state.

MEDICAL UNIVERSITY OF SOUTH CAROLINA

STUDENT BODY

Type	Public
*Enrollment	586
*% male/female	59/41
*% underrepresented minorities	15
# applied (total/out)	2,293/1,754
% interviewed (total/out)	20/4
% accepted (total/out)	NR/NR
% enrolled (total/out)	28/9
Average age	25

ADMISSIONS

Average GPA and MCAT Scores

Overall GPA	3.00	Science GPA	NR
MCAT Bio	8.00	MCAT Phys	8.00
MCAT Verbal	8.00	MCAT Essay	NR

Score Release Policy

The school has not responded to our inquiry regarding withheld MCAT scores. Therefore, we advise caution. Contact the Admissions Office before withholding any scores.

Application Information

Regular application	12/1
Regular notification	10/15–3/15
Early application	6/1–8/1
Early notification	10/1
Transfers accepted?	No
Admissions may be deferred?	Yes
AMCAS application accepted?	Yes
Interview required?	Yes
Application fee	$55

COSTS AND AID

Tuition & Fees

Tuition (in/out)	$8,280/$23,604
Cost of books	$2,068
Fees	$0

Financial Aid

% students receiving aid	79
Average grant	$3,274
Average loan	$18,862
Average debt	$54,337

*Figures based on total enrollment

MEHARRY MEDICAL COLLEGE

SCHOOL OF MEDICINE

1005 D.B. Todd Boulevard, Nashville, TN 37208
Admission: 615-327-6223 • Fax: 615-327-6228
Internet: www.mmc.edu

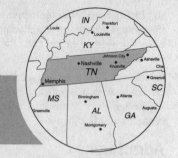

Meharry is the largest historically black institution exclusively dedicated to educating health care professionals. In addition to its program leading to the M.D. degree, Meharry offers graduate training programs in Public Health, Dentistry, Biomedical Science, and Allied Health Professions. Meharry is committed to promoting excellence in primary care and preventive medicine, with a particular emphasis on addressing the needs of underserved communities. The School of Medicine is nationally recognized for its research in areas such as Sickle Cell Anemia, hypertension, HIV/AIDS, environmental health, teen pregnancy, cancer, kidney failure, and aging.

Academics

Meharry benefits from its proximity to Fisk University and Tennessee State University. The three schools share certain facilities and together provide an active academic community. Most medical students at Meharry complete their studies in four years, although some extend their first year over a longer period of time and complete medical training in five years. Others participate in the Medical Scholars Program, which leads to the M.S. degree along with the M.D. A combined M.D./Ph.D. program is offered in Biochemistry, Biomedical Science, Microbiology, Pharmacology, and Physiology. Grades are A, B, C, and F. All medical students must pass Step 1 of the USMLE in order to be promoted to year three, and Step 2 in order to graduate.

BASIC SCIENCES: First-year courses are Anatomy, Biochemistry, Physiology, Nutrition, and Introduction to Clinical Medicine I. Students are in class or other scheduled sessions for 20–25 hours per week. Most instruction uses a lecture format, supplemented by labs and small-group discussions. Second-year courses are Microbiology, General and Clinical Pathology, Behavioral Sciences, Genetics, Pharmacology, and Introduction to Clinical Medicine II. During the second year, students are in class for about 30 hours per week, a significant proportion of which is devoted to small-group discussions. The Teaching and Learning Resource Center is located in the Student Center, serves as a comprehensive academic support unit, and provides tutoring and board review, among other services. The Library, holding over 50,000 volumes and 1,000 journals, is located in the same complex.

CLINICAL TRAINING: Third-year required rotations are Medicine (12 weeks); Surgery (8 weeks); Pediatrics (8 weeks); Ob/Gyn (8 weeks); Family and Preventive Medicine (8 weeks); and Psychiatry (4 weeks). Fourth-year subinternships are Medicine (4 weeks); Surgery (4 weeks); Family and Preventive Medicine (4 weeks); Radiology (4 weeks); and Psychiatry (4 weeks). Twelve weeks are reserved for electives. Major teaching hospitals are Metropolitan Nashville General Hospital, Alvin C. York Veterans Administration Medical Center, and Blanchefield Army Community Hospital. Other affili-

ated health care institutions are Columbia-Centennial Hospital, Memorial Hospital, Middle Tennessee Mental Health Hospital, and numerous clinics and health centers throughout the state. All students complete an ambulatory rotation in an underserved area.

Students

About 70 percent of students are African American. Students come from around the country, with about 20 percent of students from Tennessee. Class size is 80.

STUDENT LIFE: Students are supportive and cooperative, usually opting to study together in groups. There are a large number of student organizations, including honor societies, medical fraternities, support groups such as the Meharry Wives Club, groups focused on professional interests, such as the Family Practice Club, and societies focused on a common religion or ethnicity. The Daniel T. Rolfe Student Center accommodates student activities and organizations and provides a focal point for extracurricular life. Many students are involved in community activities, such as serving as mentors for high school students. Medical students interact with other Meharry students and also with peers at nearby universities. Nashville offers restaurants, nightlife, outdoor activities, and a generally student-friendly atmosphere. On-campus housing options are residence halls and apartment complexes with both one- and two-bedroom units.

GRADUATES: The College of Medicine has graduated more than 3,000 African American physicians, almost half of the total number of African American physicians who studied and who practice in the United States. About three-quarters of graduates go on to work in medically underserved rural and inner-city areas. Some graduates enter residency programs at Meharry, which has a total of 30 post-graduate positions in Family Practice, Internal Medicine, Occupational Medicine, Preventive Medicine, and Psychiatry.

Admissions

REQUIREMENTS: Required course work is eight semesters hours each of Biology, General Chemistry, Organic Chemistry, and Physics, all with associated labs. Six semester hours of English are also required. The MCAT is required, and scores should be from within the past three years. The April, rather than August, MCAT is strongly advised. For applicants who have taken the exam on multiple occasions, all sets of scores are considered.

SUGGESTIONS: Special consideration is given to underrepresented minority students and students from disadvantaged backgrounds. Meharry is interested in applicants who are dedicated to improving health care for the underserved. In addition to academic credentials, medically related or community service activities are viewed as important.

PROCESS: All qualified AMCAS applicants are sent secondary applications. Of those returning secondaries, about 10 percent are interviewed between September and May. Interviews consist of two sessions, each with a faculty member, administrator, or current medical student. On interview day, applicants also have the opportunity to meet informally with students. About one-third of interviewed candidates are accepted on a rolling basis. Others are rejected or placed on a wait-list. Wait-listed candidates may send additional information if it serves to update their files.

Costs

Beyond tuition, the estimated yearly cost of living for a single student is $10,000. On this budget, students may live on or off campus. Most students own cars.

FINANCIAL AID: Financial aid is awarded on the basis of merit and/or need, with need determined by the FAFSA form. Assistance is from both federal and institutional aid programs. About 85 percent of students qualify for assistance.

MEHARRY MEDICAL COLLEGE

STUDENT BODY

Type	Private
*Enrollment	384
*% male/female	52/48
*% underrepresented minorities	79
# applied (total/out)	4,640/4,418
% interviewed (total/out)	7/7
% accepted (total/out)	NR/NR
% enrolled (total/out)	23/21

ADMISSIONS

Average GPA and MCAT Scores

Overall GPA	NR	Science GPA	NR
MCAT Bio	7.80	MCAT Phys	7.20
MCAT Verbal	7.70	MCAT Essay	NR

Score Release Policy

The school has not responded to our inquiry regarding withheld MCAT scores. Therefore, we advise caution. Contact the Admissions Office before withholding any scores.

Application Information

Regular application	12/15
Regular notification	10/15–varies
Early application	6/1–8/1
Early notification	10/1
Admissions may be deferred?	Yes
AMCAS application accepted?	Yes
Interview required?	Yes
Application fee	$45

COSTS AND AID

Tuition & Fees

Tuition	$20,785
Cost of books	NR
Fees	$1,812

Financial Aid

% students receiving aid	NR
Average grant	NR
Average loan	NR
Average debt	NR

*Figures based on total enrollment

MERCER UNIVERSITY

SCHOOL OF MEDICINE

Office of Admissions and Student Affairs, Macon, GA 31207

Admission: 912-752-2524 • Fax: 912-752-2547

Email: kothanek.j@gain.mercer.edu

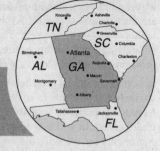

Mercer was recently recognized with an award from the American Academy of Family Physicians because well over 20 percent of its graduates enter residencies in family practice. Mercer's emphasis on primary care is in part a response to the priorities of the state and the needs of Georgians. The School of Medicine is particularly concerned with educating physicians who are interested in working with underserved populations. Instruction uses a small-group approach and emphasizes self-directed study, lifelong learning skills, and early patient contact. Mercer University is affiliated with the Baptist Church, and offers programs in Liberal Arts, Business, Engineering, Education, Pharmacy, Law, and Theology in addition to Medicine.

Academics

Each entering student is assigned to a faculty advisor who assists with the transition to medical school, with strategies for pre-clinical studies, and later with decisions involved in elective and specialty selection. Almost all students complete the M.D. curriculum in four years. Evaluation uses Satisfactory/Unsatisfactory during the first two years, and Honors/Satisfactory/Unsatisfactory during the third and fourth years. Self and Peer Evaluations are also used in some situations. Passing both steps of the USMLE is a requirement for graduation.

BASIC SCIENCES: Basic sciences are presented during the first two years as part of the Biomedical Problems Program, which uses case-based instructional techniques and computer-assisted, self-directed study. The curriculum is organized around physiological systems or "phases," which are Cells and Metabolism, Genetics and Development, Host Defense, Hematology, Neurology, Brain and Behavior, Musculoskeletal, Cardiology, Pulmonology, Gastrointestinal, Renal Endocrinology, Biology of Reproduction, and Infectious Disease. Issues related to Medical Ethics are also discussed in the context of case studies. Community Science is another important part of the first two years. Courses included in this category are Community Epidemiology; Rural Preceptorship; Managed Care and Physician Workforce; Clinical Biostatistics; and Research Design and the Medical Literature. Clinical training begins during the first year, when students learn interviewing and examination skills by working with simulated patients. Actual patient contact occurs through the Community Office Practice Program (COPP) in which students work directly with community physicians. Most basic science instruction takes place in the Medical Education Building, which, in addition to classrooms, houses the Medical Library, Mercer Health Systems (which provides clinical services), the Health Education Center, and the school's administrative offices. This physical arrangement, with basic science and clinical facilities in the same building, guarantees first- and second-year students an integrated educational experience. The library has over 90,000 volumes, 2,500 audiovisuals, and 850 current subscriptions. The Learning Resource Center offers computers, labs, and areas for clinical training using simulated patients.

CLINICAL TRAINING: Third-year required rotations are Internal Medicine (12 weeks); Surgery (8 weeks); Pediatrics (8 weeks); Ob/Gyn (6 weeks); Family Medicine (8 weeks); and Psychiatry (6 weeks). During the fourth year, students choose among fields within Surgical Subspecialities (4 weeks) and also complete clerkships in Community Science (4 weeks); Substance Abuse (2 weeks); and Critical Care (2 weeks). The remainder of the year is reserved for elective study. The primary teaching hospitals are the Medical Center of Central Georgia in Macon (518 beds) and the Memorial Medical Center in Savannah (530 beds). Other major affiliates are Floyd Medical Center in Rome, Phoebe Putney Memorial Hospital in Albany, and the Medical Center in Columbus. Training also takes place outside of major hospitals, at sites such as community hospitals, clinics, and physicians' offices throughout the state.

Students

All students are Georgia residents. About 4 percent are underrepresented minorities. The average age of incoming students is around 24, and at least 20 percent of a typical entering class took significant time off between college and medical school.

STUDENT LIFE: Medical students have access to the facilities of the greater University. These include cafeterias, athletic facilities, and recreational centers. Medical students also have their own student center, which has a snack bar and functions as a meeting place. Students may join chapters of national medical student organizations, including those that focus on the needs of women and minority medical students. Mercer offers conveniently located, campus-owned apartments to medical students on a limited basis. Affordable accommodations are also available in and around Macon. The Office of Admissions and Student Affairs helps students find suitable housing.

GRADUATES: Most graduates enter residency programs in Georgia and go on to practice in primary care fields within the state.

Admissions

REQUIREMENTS: Generally, only residents of Georgia are accepted. Required course work is one year each of Biology, Physics, Chemistry, and Organic Chemistry. The MCAT is required and scores must be no more than two years old.

SUGGESTIONS: In addition to required preparatory courses, Biochemistry is recommended. The April MCAT is strongly advised as files are not reviewed until MCAT scores are available. The Admissions Committee is interested in students who are strongly motivated to work with underserved populations and in rural areas. For applicants who have taken time off after college, some recent course work is important.

PROCESS: Secondary applications are sent to AMCAS applicants who meet minimum requirements. Typically, about 70 percent of Georgia residents who apply receive secondary applications. Of those returning secondaries, about 20 percent are invited to interview. Interviews take place between October and March, and consist of two sessions with faculty, administrators, or members of the community. About one-third of interviewees are accepted. All decisions are made before March 15, at which point a wait list is formed.

Costs

In addition to tuition, the expected yearly budget for a single student is about $18,000. This allows for on- or off-campus living and car ownership.

FINANCIAL AID: Over 90 percent of students receive financial aid in the form of grants, scholarships, and/or loans. Private and institutional assistance is awarded on the basis of need as well as for specific criteria established by donors. A significant number of students are generously funded in return for service commitments in rural areas within the state. Federal aid is based on need, as determined by the FAFSA form.

MERCER UNIVERSITY

STUDENT BODY

Type	Private
*Enrollment	221
*% male/female	63/37
*% underrepresented minorities	4
# applied (total/out)	1,311/632
% interviewed	15
% accepted (total/out)	NR/NR
% enrolled (total/out)	30/NR

ADMISSIONS

Average GPA and MCAT Scores

Overall GPA	NR	Science GPA	NR
MCAT Bio	NR	MCAT Phys	NR
MCAT Verbal	NR	MCAT Essay	NR

Score Release Policy

The school has not responded to our inquiry regarding withheld MCAT scores. Therefore, we advise caution. Contact the Admissions Office before withholding any scores.

Application Information

Regular application	11/1
Regular notification	1/24 until filled
Early application	6/1–8/1
Early notification	10/1
Admissions may be deferred?	Yes
AMCAS application accepted?	Yes
Interview required?	Yes
Application fee	$25

COSTS AND AID

Tuition & Fees

Tuition	$21,114
Cost of books	NR
Fees	$0

Financial Aid

% students receiving aid	88
Average grant	NR
Average loan	NR
Average debt	NR

*Figures based on total enrollment

UNIVERSITY OF MIAMI

SCHOOL OF MEDICINE

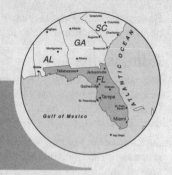

PO Box 016159, Miami, FL 33101
Admission: 305-243-3234 • Fax: 305-243-6548
Email: med.admissions@miami.edu
Internet: www.miami.edu/medical-admissions

The University of Miami School of Medicine is the oldest and largest medical school in Florida. It is now the nucleus of the nation's second busiest medical center. The Medical School campus is situated in the Civic Center area of downtown Miami, adjacent to the Jackson Memorial Hospital and other clinical affiliates. Medical students benefit from the clinical experiences that result from Miami's diverse, multicultural patient population. Though the School of Medicine is clinically oriented, it also offers varied research opportunities. Students enjoy early patient contact and an interdisciplinary approach to basic science instruction.

Academics

Most students follow a four-year curriculum, leading to the M.D. A number of students participate in a six-year B.S./M.D. program organized with Miami's undergraduate college. Up to six students each year enter a combined M.D./Ph.D. program, earning the doctorate degree in Biochemistry and Molecular Biology; Molecular, Cell, and Developmental Biology; Microbiology and Immunology; Molecular and Cellular Pharmacology; Neuroscience; or Physiology and Biophysics. Opportunities for summer research are also available to medical students. Students are graded with percentile scores during the first two years and with ratings of Honors, High Pass, Pass, and Fail during the second two years. Promotion to year three requires a passing score on the USMLE Step 1. Step 2 of the USMLE must be taken in order to graduate.

BASIC SCIENCES: Although the first two years are devoted primarily to basic sciences, students are introduced to clinical concepts and techniques from day one in the Clinical Skills course. In this two-year course, students work alongside community physician mentors, learning about the patient interview, the physical examination, and clinical diagnosis. Other first-year courses are Gross Anatomy; Genetics; Embryology; Immunology; Cell and Molecular Biology; Behavioral and Life Sciences; Physiology; Histology; Neuroanatomy; Systemic Biochemistry; Endocrine Module; and Ethics/Social Policy. Second-year courses are Microbiology, Pharmacology, Pathology, Mechanisms of Disease, Introduction to Psychiatry, and Pathology. During the first two years, students are in class or other scheduled sessions for about 24 hours per week. Lectures are the primary instructional modality, but small-group discussions are also used, and are increasingly important in the second year. Basic sciences are taught in the Rosensteil Medical Sciences Building and the Glaser Medical Research Building, which house newly renovated lecture halls, teaching laboratories, and the brand new Glaser Computer Laboratory. The Louis Calder Memorial Library has almost 200,000 volumes and 2,300 current journals and periodicals. It also offers an Electronic Class-room with computer instructional aids, and a Learning Resource Center with multimedia programs.

CLINICAL TRAINING: Required third-year clerkships are Introduction to Medicine (1 week); Radiology (1 week); Medicine (8 weeks); Surgery (8 weeks); Primary Care (8 weeks); Ob/Gyn (6 weeks); Psychiatry (6 weeks); Pediatrics (6 weeks); and Family Medicine (4 weeks). Fourth-year requirements are Geriatrics (2 weeks) and Neurology (4 weeks). The remainder of the fourth year is devoted to selectives, which must include at least eight weeks of Direct Patient Care, and electives which may be clinical or research-based. Clinical training takes place at: Jackson Memorial Hospital (1,567 beds); Veterans Affairs Medical Center (900 beds); Bascom Palmer/Anne Bates Leach Eye Hospital; Sylvester Comprehensive Cancer Center; Ryder Trauma Center; Diabetes Research Institute; and The Mailman Center for Child Development. Up to three months of the fourth year may be spent in clerkships at other institutions.

Students

A recently entering class had the following profile: age range, 18–37; women, 55 percent; underrepresented minorities, 10 percent; Florida residents, 97 percent; Science majors, 65 percent. Thirty-six colleges and universities were represented. Class size is 148.

STUDENT LIFE: Although the medical campus is separate from the main campus, medical students have access to extracurricular programs and events sponsored by the greater University. In addition, the medical campus has athletic and other recreational facilities of its own. Medical students are involved in student organizations and volunteer activities in areas such as AIDS prevention, general health education, and drug-abuse counseling. Students enjoy the good weather and multicultural environment of Miami. Medical students live off campus in various parts of Miami, and usually drive to school or take Metrorail.

GRADUATES: Graduates are successful in securing residency positions nationwide. A significant proportion enter programs at Jackson Memorial Hospital, which features at least 15 post-graduate training programs.

Admissions

REQUIREMENTS: Prerequisites are one year each of Biology, Chemistry, Organic Chemistry, Physics, Math, and English. Science courses should include associated labs. The MCAT is required and scores must be from within the past three years. For applicants who have taken the exam on multiple occasions, the best set of scores is weighed most heavily.

SUGGESTIONS: Florida residents are given preference, and only highly qualified out-of-state residents are encouraged to apply. Recommended course work includes Biochemistry, Cell and Molecular Biology, Microbiology and Immunology, Genetics, Embryology, Mammalian Physiology, and Computer Science. Students should display achievement in the humanities and social sciences as well as in the natural sciences. Beyond academic credentials, the Committee on Admissions values interpersonal skills, leadership, maturity, motivation, and compassion. Meaningful patient-contact experience is essential.

PROCESS: About 75 percent of Florida residents and 20 percent of out-of-state residents are sent secondary applications. About 300 applicants are interviewed on campus. Interviews take place on Fridays, between August and April, and consist of one session with a faculty member. About 60 percent of interviewed candidates are accepted, with notification occurring on a rolling basis. Approximately 25 positions in each entering class are reserved for participants in the University of Miami Honors Program in Medicine, a six-year B.S./M.D. program.

Costs

The anticipated yearly cost of living for a single student is about $13,000. This budget allows for off-campus housing.

FINANCIAL AID: Most financial aid is awarded on the basis of need, as determined by the FAFSA form. Assistance is in the form of loans, work-study arrangements, and grants. A few merit-based scholarships that cover part of the cost of tuition are available each year. Participants in the M.D./Ph.D. program typically receive a full-tuition scholarship in addition to a stipend for living expenses.

UNIVERSITY OF MIAMI

STUDENT BODY

Type	Private
*Enrollment	617
*% male/female	50/50
*% underrepresented minorities	11
# applied (total/out)	948/44
% interviewed (total/out)	35/15
% accepted (total/out)	60/100
% enrolled (total/out)	16/4
Average age	22

ADMISSIONS

Average GPA and MCAT Scores

Overall GPA	3.69	Science GPA	3.63
MCAT Bio	10.0	MCAT Phys	9.4
MCAT Verbal	10.0	MCAT Essay	P–Q

Score Release Policy
Scores must be released.

Application Information

Regular application	12/15
Regular notification	10/1 until filled
Early application	No
Early notification	10/1
Transfers accepted?	Yes
Admissions may be deferred?	No
AMCAS application accepted?	Yes
Interview required?	Yes
Application fee	$55

COSTS AND AID

Tuition & Fees

Tuition (in/out)	$26,440/$36,440
Cost of books	NR
Fees (in/out)	$120/$120

Financial Aid

% students receiving aid	80
Average grant	NR
Average loan	NR
Average debt	NR

*Figures based on total enrollment

MICHIGAN STATE UNIVERSITY
COLLEGE OF HUMAN MEDICINE

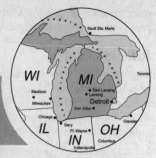

Office of Admissions, A-239 Life Sciences, East Lansing, MI 48824

Admission: 517-353-9620 • Fax: 517-432-0021

Email: M.D.Admissions@msu.edu • Internet: www.chm.msu.edu

Along with the College of Human Medicine, Michigan State University has two other medical schools, the Colleges of Osteopathic Medicine and Veterinary Medicine. The College of Human Medicine is a community-based medical school, uniquely positioned to provide students with comprehensive training in clinical settings that most closely parallel the environments in which they are likely to practice. In order to provide quality health care to Michigan's underserved populations, MSU has developed a clinical program that uses facilities located throughout the state.

Academics

The four-year curriculum is modern and highly innovative. While the first two years are spend at MSU's main campus in East Lansing, during the third and fourth years, students are assigned to one of six community-based programs for clinical training. These communities are the following: Kalamazoo, Upper Peninsula, Grand Rapids, Flint, Lansing, and Saginaw. Along with its focus on primary care, MSU is dedicated to research and offers several combined M.D./advanced degree programs including the M.S.T.P. Some of the fields in which graduate degrees may be earned are the following: Anatomy, Biochemistry, Cellular and Molecular Biology, Ecology and Evolutionary Biology, Epidemiology, Genetics, Health and Humanities, Microbiology, Neuroscience, Pathology, Pharmacology and Toxicology, and Physiology. Medical students are evaluated with Pass or Fail.

BASIC SCIENCES: In addition to mastering basic science concepts, first-year students address the doctor/patient relationship in Clinical Skills. A unique Mentor Program assigns small groups of students to a preceptor, allowing the groups to explore patient care and the complex roles of the physician. Students accompany their mentor for hospital rounds and patient visits. The course Integrative Clinical Correlations, taught by basic science faculty members and clinicians, develops problem-solving skills and allows students to apply basic science concepts to clinical case studies. Other first-year courses are the following: Anatomy, Biochemistry, Genetics, Microbiology, Neuroscience, Pathology, Pharmacology, Physiology, Histology, Human Development, and Radiology. The second year is organized around body systems and general disease categories. These are the following: Infectious Diseases; Disorders of Development and Behavior; Hematopoietic/Neoplasia; Cardiovascular; Urinary Tract; Pulmonary; Metabolic Endocrine Reproductive; Digestive; Neurological/Musculoskeletal; Major Mental Disorders; and Comprehensive, which covers topics such as AIDS and substance abuse. In the Social Context of Clinical Decisions, students take part in a series of small-group seminars dealing with the concepts of Medical Ethics; Epidemiology; Biostatistics; Critical Reasoning;

Humanities; and Social, Economic, and Organizational Issues in Medicine. The primary mode of instruction during the second year is small-group discussions/tutorials. Students are in scheduled sessions for less than 20 hours per week, allowing ample time for individual and group study. Academic facilities include the Echt Computer Lab, which offers computer-based instructional programs, the Learning Resource Center with audio/visual aids, the Clinical Center Library, and MSU's main library.

CLINICAL TRAINING: Most clerkship requirements are fulfilled during the third year and the early part of year four. Students are assigned to one of six communities during the summer of their third year. They begin with an orientation called Clinical Medicine in the Community (4 weeks) and then rotate through eight weeks of each of the following: Family Practice, Internal Medicine, Pediatrics, Surgery, Ob/Gyn, and Psychiatry. Four weeks of Advanced Medicine and Advanced Surgery are also required. Throughout the period in which students complete required clerkships, students also participate in a Core Competency Seminar, which requires 2 hours per week and provides a forum for discussion of interdisciplinary topics important to the care and health management of patients. A total of 20 weeks are reserved for elective experiences. Students may rotate to other communities in the state, to hospitals and academic centers in other states, and to clinical sites overseas. In particular, students are encouraged to spend time at the hospital at which they hope to enter post-graduate training.

Students

At least 80 percent of students are Michigan residents. Class size is 106. In a recent class, the average age of incoming students was 26, and a significant percentage of students were in their 30s.

STUDENT LIFE: First- and second-year students enjoy the activities, facilities, resources, and social life of a Big Ten university. Medical students are also involved in the greater community, volunteering at clinics and as health educators in schools. Professionally focused and special-interest organizations are numerous, as are athletic opportunities such as intramural sports. A variety of campus-owned housing options are available in Lansing. Some single students live in a graduate/professional student residence hall. Apartments of all sizes are also available, accommodating single and married students, and students with larger families. Where students spend their third and fourth years is largely determined by a lottery, though some consideration is given to special circumstances and preferences.

GRADUATES: Students typically score above the national average on the USMLE, contributing to their success in securing top-choice residency positions. Among 1997 graduates, the most prevalent fields for post-graduate training were the following: Family Practice (30%); Internal Medicine (12%); Ob/Gyn (10 %); Surgery (9%); Pediatrics (8%); Medicine-Pediatrics (7%); and Psychiatry (7%). About 50% of graduates remained in Michigan for residency programs.

Admissions

REQUIREMENTS: Prerequisites are one year each of Biology, Chemistry, Organic Chemistry, and Physics, all with associated labs. Strong skills in English and Math are required. The MCAT is required, and scores must be no more than three years old. For applicants who have retaken the exam, the most recent set of scores is used. Thus, there is no advantage in withholding scores.

SUGGESTIONS: Though Michigan residents are given preference, about 20 percent of the positions in an entering class are available to highly qualified nonresident applicants. MSU is focused on training generalist physicians and seeks applicants with an interest in primary care and community-based medicine. Important personal traits are competence, honesty, social responsibility, and compassion.

PROCESS: About one-quarter of AMCAS applicants are sent secondary applications. Of those returning secondaries, about one-third are interviewed. Interviews are conducted on Thursdays, from September through March. Interviews consist of two sessions, one with a faculty member and the other with a current medical student. On Interview Day, candidates attend informational sessions, have lunch with medical students, and tour the campus. About one-third of interviewees are accepted on a rolling basis.

Costs

The estimated yearly cost of living for a first-year, single student is about $16,000. This budget allows for on-campus housing and car maintenance.

FINANCIAL AID: Although most aid is awarded on the basis of need, some scholarships are offered to students with exceptional academic merit, leadership potential, or other special traits.

MICHIGAN STATE UNIVERSITY

STUDENT BODY

Type	Public
*Enrollment	461
*% male/female	48/52
*% underrepresented minorities	27
# applied (total/out)	3,404/2,252
% interviewed (total/out)	12/4
% accepted (total/out)	NR/NR
% enrolled (total/out)	30/17
Average age	25

ADMISSIONS

Average GPA and MCAT Scores

Overall GPA	NR	Science GPA	NR
MCAT Bio	9.10	MCAT Phys	8.60
MCAT Verbal	9.70	MCAT Essay	NR

Score Release Policy

The Admissions Committee stresses that they will see how many times a student has taken the MCAT; without the MCAT, student is not even considered.

Application Information

Regular application	11/15
Regular notification	10/15–varies
Early application	6/1–8/1
Early notification	10/1
Admissions may be deferred?	Yes
AMCAS application accepted?	Yes
Interview required?	Yes
Application fee	$55

COSTS AND AID

Tuition & Fees

Tuition (in/out)	$15,880/$33,796
Cost of books	NR
Fees	$910

Financial Aid

% students receiving aid	NR
Average grant	NR
Average loan	NR
Average debt	NR

*Figures based on total enrollment

UNIVERSITY OF MICHIGAN
MEDICAL SCHOOL

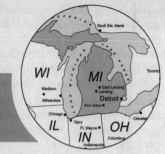

M4130 Medical Science I Building, Ann Arbor, MI 48109
Admission: 734-764-6317 • Fax: 734-763-0453
Internet: www.med.umich.edu/medschool

Although the University of Michigan is a state-supported institution, its medical school enjoys a national reputation for outstanding research, teaching, and facilities. With input from students, Michigan recently implemented a new curriculum which, among other revisions, relies more on small-group sessions for instruction. The Medical School is geared toward training physicians who are able to practice effectively in multicultural environments and who are sensitive to the needs of people from diverse backgrounds. Medical students benefit from the resources of the greater University and from the student-friendly community of Ann Arbor.

Academics

Most students follow a four-year program leading to the M.D., although a growing number opt for combined degrees. A combined M.D./Ph.D. curriculum allows students to pursue graduate studies in numerous departments, including Anatomy and Cell Biology, Biological Chemistry, Cellular and Molecular Biology, Human Genetics, Microbiology and Immunology, Neuroscience; Pharmacology, and Physiology. Some M.D./Ph.D. students are M.S.T.P. participants, while others are funded through institutional sources. For students who are interested in research, but who are not interested in earning an additional degree, summer and year-long research fellowships are available. In addition, combined programs with Public Health and Business Administration are available. Passing Step 1 of the USMLE is a requirement for promotion to year three, and passing Step 2 is a requirement for graduation.

BASIC SCIENCES: During the first year, grading is strictly Satisfactory/Fail. This promotes student cooperation and allows for variation in the level of scientific knowledge among incoming students. Throughout the first and second years, students take Introduction to the Patient, which includes interdisciplinary perspectives and the use of simulated patients, and Multidisciplinary Conferences, which provides clinical correlations for basic science concepts. Other first-year courses are Molecular and Cell Biology; Gross Anatomy; Human Genetics; Pathology; Embryology; Histology; Host Defenses; Microbiology; Pharmacology; and Physiology. Year two is organized around organ and body systems. These are Infectious Diseases; Hematology; Oncology; Cardiovascular; Respiratory; Renal; Dermatology; Gastrointestinal; Neuroscience; Endocrine; Reproduction; and Musculoskeletal. The Medical School's basic science instructional facilities include recently renovated lecture halls with audiovisual and computer equipment. A Learning Resource Center is open 24 hours per day and has over 50 computers for student use. The Taubman Medical Library is one of the largest in the United States in terms of the number of volumes, journals, and electronic resources that it

holds. The Office of Academic Enrichment provides academic counseling and organizes study groups and tutoring services.

CLINICAL TRAINING: During the second, third, and fourth years, students are evaluated with Honors, High Pass, Pass, and Fail. Third-year required rotations are Family Practice (4 weeks); Internal Medicine (12 weeks); Neurology (4 weeks); Ob/Gyn (6 weeks); Pediatrics (6 weeks); Psychiatry (4 weeks); Surgery (12 weeks). Students attend weekly conferences and discuss a range of topics including the ethical, social, and economic issues related to practicing medicine. Fourth-year requirements are Subinternship (8 weeks); Intensive Care Unit Experience (4 weeks); Advanced Basic Science Experience (4 weeks); and Electives (12–20 weeks), which are selected from more than 300 subjects. Clinical training takes place at the University Hospital (888 beds), St. Joseph Mercy Hospital (522 beds), the Veterans Affairs Hospital (486 beds), and at other affiliated institutions. With approval, students may earn elective credits at other academic or clinical sites in the United States and overseas.

Students

About 50 percent of students are Michigan residents, with the remainder of the student body coming from all regions of the country. Typically, at least 10 percent of entering students are older, having taken some time off after college. Approximately 15 percent of students are underrepresented minorities. Class size is 170.

STUDENT LIFE: Incoming medical students benefit from the support and advice of more senior medical students through a peer-counseling program called Big Sib, Little Sib. Students interact outside of the classroom through participation in organizations that focus on issues such as community service, support for minority and gay/lesbian students, and recreational and professional pursuits. The Furstenberg Student Study Center features a Well-Being Room for information and activities related to student health, computer stations, lounges, and quiet study rooms. Expansive sports and recreation centers also enrich student life on campus. Ann Arbor is an academic and cultural center, attracting scholars from around the world. To serve the University community, the area around the campus is filled with coffee shops, bookstores, restaurants, bars, and shops. In addition to commercial districts, Ann Arbor offers parks, lakes, theaters, farmers markets, and attractive residential areas. Although some limited campus-owned housing is available to medical students, most opt to live in privately owned apartment complexes that are within walking distance of the Medical Center.

GRADUATES: Medical students consistently score above the national average on both steps of the USMLE, contributing to their success in securing top residency positions. Among 1996 graduates, popular choices for specialty areas were Internal Medicine (23%); Pediatrics (12%); Surgery (11%); Family Practice (10%); Ob/Gyn (7%); and Emergency Medicine (6%).

Admission

REQUIREMENTS: Prerequisites are Chemistry (8 semester hours, to include both Organic and Inorganic); Biochemistry (3 semester hours); Biology (6 semester hours); Physics (6 semester hours); and English Composition and Literature (6 semester hours). In addition, at least 18 semester hours must be completed in areas other than the natural sciences or math.

SUGGESTIONS: In addition to the required science courses, Genetics and Cell Biology are considered useful preparation for medical school. Humanities and Social Sciences course work is also important.

PROCESS: All AMCAS applicants are sent supplementary applications. Of those returning secondaries, about 15 percent are interviewed between September and March. Interviews consist of two 30-minute sessions each with a faculty member or medical student. Candidates are also given a group informational presentation, a campus tour, and lunch with medical students. About one-third of interviewees are accepted and are notified between November and May. Others are rejected or put on a wait list. Previously, 35 high school students were admitted each year to the Inteflex Program, a combined B.S./M.D. program organized in conjunction with Michigan's undergraduate college, but admissions have been suspended for 1999.

Costs

The estimated yearly cost of living for a single student is $16,000. This budget allows for on- or off-campus housing and car maintenance.

FINANCIAL AID: Assistance in the form of scholarships and loans is granted on the basis of financial need, as demonstrated by the FAFSA and other forms. There are a few recruiting scholarships that do not require financial need. Parental financial disclosure is required for most aid.

UNIVERSITY OF MICHIGAN

STUDENT BODY

Type	Public
*Enrollment	660
*% male/female	59/41
*% underrepresented minorities	15
# applied (total/out)	5,114/4,154
% interviewed (total/out)	12/8
% accepted (total/out)	6/5
% enrolled (total/out)	NR/NR

ADMISSIONS

Average GPA and MCAT Scores

Overall GPA	3.60	Science GPA	NR
MCAT Bio	11.00	MCAT Phys	11.00
MCAT Verbal	10.00	MCAT Essay	P

Score Release Policy

The school has not responded to our inquiry regarding withheld MCAT scores. Therefore, we advise caution. Contact the Admissions Office before withholding any scores.

Application Information

Regular application	11/15
Regular notification	11/1–5/1
Early application	6/1–8/1
Early notification	10/1
Transfers accepted?	No
Admissions may be deferred?	Yes
AMCAS application accepted?	Yes
Interview required?	Yes
Application fee	$50

COSTS AND AID

Tuition & Fees

Tuition (in/out)	$17,840/$27,400
Cost of books	$791
Fees	$185

Financial Aid

% students receiving aid	NR
Average grant	NR
Average loan	NR
Average debt	NR

*Figures based on total enrollment

UNIVERSITY OF MINNESOTA, DULUTH
SCHOOL OF MEDICINE

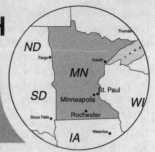

180 Med, Duluth, MN 55812
Admission: 218-726-8511 • Fax: 218-726-6235
Email: jcarls10@d.umn.edu • Internet: www.d.umn.edu/medweb

Students at the University of Minnesota School of Medicine at Duluth (UMD) spend two years at the Duluth campus, and then join medical students at the University of Minnesota, Minneapolis campus, for third- and fourth-year clinical rotations. The objective of UMD is to increase the number of well-trained physicians entering family medicine and practicing in rural areas of the state. This is accomplished by using family medicine practitioners and other primary care physicians as mentors and instructors. In addition to a full-time faculty of 45 members, part-time and voluntary clinical sciences instructors include over 250 area physicians. UMD offers several programs aimed at recruiting and training Native Americans and other underrepresented minorities for careers in medicine.

Academics

Although formal clinical rotations are not included in the two-year UMD curriculum, early patient contact and clinical correlation are important aspects of the program. Successful completion of UMD requirements guarantees transfer after year two to the Minneapolis campus. Evaluation of medical student performance uses Outstanding, Excellent, Satisfactory, Incomplete, and No Pass. Passing Step 1 of the USMLE is a requirement for promotion to the Minneapolis program.

BASIC SCIENCES: The two-year curriculum is a unique blend of basic medical and behavioral sciences and clinical "hands-on" experiences. The basic sciences, presented using an organ systems approach that begins with principles of basic science, extends to various aspects of the prevention and pathophysiology of organ system disease, and concludes with discussions of several presenting clinical symptoms and multisystems diseases. The behavioral sciences portion of the curriculum emphasizes knowledge about the psycho-social aspects of health and illness that are relevant to the clinical setting and is interwoven with the organ systems component. The clinical experience is directed by community specialists and is augmented by UMDs nationally recognized Family Practice Preceptorship program. In addition to classrooms and labs, the Learning Resource Center serves as a computer and multimedia instructional facility. It is open 24 hours per day. The Health Science Library houses 95,000 volumes, 600 current journals, and several online data bases.

CLINICAL TRAINING: In Duluth, clinical affiliates are St. Luke's Hospital and Miller-Dawn and St. Mary's Medical Centers. After successfully completing year two, students transfer to Minneapolis, where they rotate through required clerkships during their third and fourth years. These are Medicine (12 weeks); Ob/Gyn (6 weeks); Surgery (6 weeks); Pediatrics (6 weeks); Psychiatry (6 weeks); Neurology (4 weeks); Surgical Specialty (4 weeks); and Ambulatory Care (8 weeks). The remaining time is reserved for elective study. Clinical facilities include the Fairview-University Medical Center; Variety Club Heart and Research Center; Masonic Cancer Center; Veterans of Foreign Wars Cancer Research Center; Children's Rehabilitation Center; Paul F. Dwan Cardiovascular Research Center; and the Jackson/Owre/Millard/Lyon complex. Each year, through the Rural Physician Associate Program, up to 40 third-year medical students study primary health care in Minnesota communities under the supervision of local physicians. Six weeks of clinical electives may be fulfilled at nonaffiliated institutions in other parts of the country or abroad.

Students

STUDENT LIFE: Small class size, and students' shared interest in family medicine promotes a supportive and cohesive atmosphere. University recreational events, facilities, and activities are open to medical students, including the student center, the gym, intramural sports, and student organizations. Students also take advantage of the extracurricular opportunities afforded by the school's location. Activities such as cycling, running, skiing, hiking, and camping are easily accessible within or around Duluth. Duluth functions as a cultural center for Northern Minnesota, and has a symphony, a ballet, theaters, and art museums. On-campus housing is available, as are affordable off-campus housing options in the immediate area.

GRADUATES: About 95 percent of students are Minnesota residents. About 19 percent of students are underrepresented minorities, most of whom are Native American. Class size is 53. At least 70 percent of graduates enter primary care fields, and most go on to practice in rural areas.

Admissions

REQUIREMENTS: Only residents of Minnesota, selected counties in Wisconsin, and the Canadian Province of Manitoba are considered. The exception is underrepresented minority applicants who may be considered regardless of residency status. Prerequisites are one year each of Biology, General Chemistry, Physics, English, Behavioral Sciences, and Humanities/Social Sciences. One math course in Calculus or upper-level Statistics, and one Biochemistry course are also required. The MCAT is required, and scores must be no more than three years old.

SUGGESTIONS: UMD looks for applicants who demonstrate interest in entering family practice and working with underserved rural or small town communities.

PROCESS: Applicants who meet residency or minority requirements are sent secondary applications after preliminary screening of academics and MCAT scores. Of those returning secondaries, about 30 percent are invited to interview between October and April. Interviews consist of two one-hour sessions, each with a member of the Admissions Committee. Notification occurs on a rolling basis, and about 30 percent of interviewees are offered a place in the class.

Costs

Beyond tuition, the estimated yearly cost of living for a single student is $9,000. This budget allows for either on- or off-campus housing, and car ownership.

FINANCIAL AID: Currently, 96 percent of all medical students receive some form of financial assistance in the form of regional scholarships, federal loans, special loan funds, and designated prizes. Most aid is need-based, with need determined by the FAFSA form.

UNIVERSITY OF MINNESOTA, DULUTH

STUDENT BODY

Type	Public
*Enrollment	107
*% male/female	49/51
*% underrepresented minorities	12
# applied (total/out)	730/424
% interviewed (total/out)	NR/NR
% accepted (total/out)	NR/NR
Average age	NR

ADMISSIONS

Average GPA and MCAT Scores

Overall GPA	3.67	Science GPA	3.50
MCAT Bio	9.8	MCAT Phys	9.7
MCAT Verbal	9.8	MCAT Essay	NR

Score Release Policy

The school has not responded to our inquiry regarding withheld MCAT scores. Therefore, we advise caution. Contact the Admissions Office before withholding any scores.

Application Information

Regular application	11/15
Regular notification	10/15–until filled
Early application	6/1–8/1
Early notification	10/1
Transfers accepted?	No
Admissions may be deferred?	Yes
AMCAS application accepted?	Yes
Interview required?	Yes
Application fee	$50

COSTS AND AID

Tuition & Fees

Tuition (in/out)	$16,064/$29,840
Cost of books	NR
Fees	$534

Financial Aid

% students receiving aid	96
Average grant	NR
Average loan	NR
Average debt	NR

*Figures based on total enrollment

UNIVERSITY OF MINNESOTA

MEDICAL SCHOOL, MINNEAPOLIS

420 Delaware Street, SE, Minneapolis, MN 55455
Admission: 612-625-2436 • Fax: 612-626-4200
Internet: www.meded@tc.umn.edu

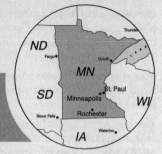

The Medical School at the University of Minnesota, in Minneapolis, benefits from resources of the greater University, excellent clinical facilities in the area, and a faculty dedicated both to teaching and research. The curriculum is unusual in that focused clinical instruction, in the form of tutorials, is integrated into basic science course work. The curriculum is also flexible, allowing students to pursue interests in areas such as research, rural medicine, or international health. Among recent graduates, 62 percent entered primary care fields.

Academics

In addition to a four-year curriculum leading to the M.D. degree, Minnesota offers joint M.D./Ph.D. programs, generally M.S.T.P.-sponsored, leading to the doctorate degree in Biochemistry, Biomedical Engineering, Biophysics, Cell Biology, Genetics, Immunology, Microbiology, Molecular Biology, Neuroscience, Pharmacology, and Physiology. Evaluation of medical student performance uses grades of Outstanding, Excellent, Satisfactory, Incomplete, and No Credit. Passing both steps of the USMLE is a graduation requirement. Faculty members serve as informal advisors to medical students throughout the four years.

BASIC SCIENCES: Basic sciences are taught as part of an interdisciplinary curriculum that also includes behavioral, social, and ethical aspects of medicine in addition to introductory clinical instruction. On average, students are in class or other scheduled sessions for 24 hours per week. First-year courses are Gross Anatomy; Human Histology; Biochemistry; Molecular and Cellular Biology; Human Nutrition; Medical Physiology; Neuroscience; Microbiology; Human Behavior; Human Sexuality; Human Genetics; Foundations of Preventive Medicine; Pathology; Pharmacology; and Clinical Medicine, the last of which focuses on history taking and the physical examination. Second-year courses are Pharmacology; Organ System Pathology; Pathophysiology; Laboratory Medicine; and Clinical Medicine. In addition, second-year students participate in four six-week tutorials in Internal Medicine, Family Practice, Pediatrics, and Neurology. First- and second-year instruction takes place in the Moos Health Tower and other buildings in the basic science complex. The Bio-Medical Library contains more than 428,000 volumes, 4,393 journals, 1,194 audiovisual programs, and 223 computer programs. The reference department has over 50 computers and has access to several online databases.

CLINICAL TRAINING: Students rotate through required clerkships during their third and fourth years: Medicine (12 weeks); Ob/Gyn (6 weeks); Surgery (6 weeks); Pediatrics (6 weeks); Psychiatry (6 weeks); Neurology (4 weeks); Surgical Specialty (4 weeks); and Ambulatory Care (8 weeks). The remaining time is reserved for elective study.

Clinical facilities include the Fairview-University Medical Center; Variety Club Heart and Research Center; Masonic Cancer Center; Veterans of Foreign Wars Cancer Research Center; Children's Rehabilitation Center; Paul F. Dwan Cardiovascular Research Center. Each year, through the Rural Physician Associate Program, up to 40 third-year medical students study primary health care in Minnesota communities under the supervision of local physicians. One-quarter of clinical electives may be fulfilled at non-affiliated institutions in other parts of the country or abroad.

Students

Of the 165 students in last year's entering class, 89 percent were Minnesota residents, and 62 percent attended college in Minnesota. About 5 percent were from underrepresented minority groups. Typically, the average age of incoming students is 24 or 25.

STUDENT LIFE: Some students work part-time as graduate research or teaching assistants while in medical school. These positions provide academic opportunities and a source of income or tuition reduction. The Medical Student Adytum (adytum is Greek for "innermost sanctuary") is a spacious, comfortable area reserved solely for medical students and their guests. Students use the facility for studying, socializing, eating, and relaxing. Medical students also have the opportunity to interact with other Health Sciences students at an alternate student center. Organizations bring students together around common interests, allow them to contribute to the community, and provide extracurricular activities. Examples of student organizations are the Marathon Training Club, which in a recent year motivated 10 percent of the student body to complete a marathon, the Student Committee on Bioethics, and the Medical Students in Community Service, which operates a health clinic. The medical school is part of the greater University, and medical students have access to its athletic and recreational facilities. Beyond the campus, the city of Minneapolis offers restaurants, shopping, cultural activities, and entertainment. Housing options include residence halls, medical fraternities, and privately owned apartments that are adjacent to the Medical Center.

GRADUATES: In the 1999 graduating class, the most popular fields for residencies were Family Practice (33%); Internal Medicine (18%); Surgery (8%); Pediatrics (7%); Emergency Medicine (5%); Ob/Gyn (4%); and Radiology (3%). Generally, at least half of graduates enter post-graduate programs in Minnesota.

Admissions

REQUIREMENTS: Prerequisites are Biology (7 semester hours); General Chemistry (8 hours); Organic Chemistry (8 hours); Physics (8 hours); English (8 hours); Math (one college level course); and Biochemistry (3 hours). In addition, at least 18 hours of Social and Behavioral Sciences and Humanities are required. This requirement is fulfilled with courses such as History, Economics, Anthropology, Psychology, Sociology, Philosophy, and Foreign Languages. The MCAT is required, and scores must be no more than three years old. For applicants who have taken the exam more than once, the highest set of scores is considered.

SUGGESTIONS: Minnesota residents are given preference. As indicated by the Social Science/Humanities requirement, breadth in undergraduate preparation is important. In addition to academic strength, applicants should demonstrate extensive volunteer/community service activity, personal integrity, high ethical standards, motivation, intellectual curiosity, enthusiasm, dedication to lifelong learning, and the ability to work well with others. Computer literacy is recommended.

PROCESS: Qualified applicants who submit AMCAS applications are sent secondaries. Of those returning secondaries, about 80 percent of Minnesota residents, and 30 percent of out-of-state applicants, are invited to interview. Interviews take place on campus from September through March and consist of one session with a faculty member. Of interviewed candidates, about 25 percent of Minnesota residents and 15 percent of out-of-state residents are offered a place in the class. Applicants are accepted on a rolling admission basis, October through April. Additional materials from wait-listed candidates are not accepted.

Costs

FINANCIAL AID: Awards are made on the basis of need, merit, a combination of the two, or, in some cases, other special criteria. Generally, financial aid packages are a combination of grants and loans. Qualified applicants from states other than Minnesota are granted a tuition waiver equal to the difference between in- and out-of-state tuition. Students from North and South Dakota are eligible for in-state tuition rates.

UNIVERSITY OF MINNESOTA

STUDENT BODY

Type	Public
*Enrollment	849
*% male/female	55/45
*% underrepresented minorities	2
# applied (total/out)	1,874/NR
% interviewed (total/out)	37/4
% accepted (total/out)	13/1
% enrolled (total/out)	68/NR
Average age	23

ADMISSIONS

Average GPA and MCAT Scores

Overall GPA	3.67	Science GPA	3.63
MCAT Bio	10.0	MCAT Phys	10.0
MCAT Verbal	10.0	MCAT Essay	N

Score Release Policy

An application will not be processed until MCAT scores are received. No application will be considered without scores.

Application Information

Regular application	11/15
Regular notification	11/1
Early application	6/1–8/1
Early notification	10/1
Admissions may be deferred?	Yes
AMCAS application accepted?	Yes
Interview required?	Yes
Application fee	$50

COSTS AND AID

Tuition & Fees

Tuition (in/out)	NR/NR
Cost of books	NR
Fees	NR

Financial Aid

% students receiving aid	90+
Average grant	NR
Average loan	NR
Average debt	NR

*Figures based on total enrollment

UNIVERSITY OF MISSISSIPPI

SCHOOL OF MEDICINE

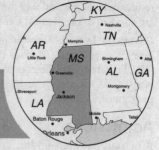

2500 North State Street, Jackson, MS 39216
Admission: 601-984-5010 • Fax: 601-984-5008
Internet: www.umsmed.edu

The School of Medicine along with Schools of Nursing, Health-Related Professions, Dentistry, and Graduate Programs in the medical and clinical health sciences are the academic components of the University of Mississippi Medical Center, which also serves as an important health care provider to Mississippi residents. The School of Medicine not only trains physicians who go on to practice in Mississippi, but also offers continuing education programs to physicians already practicing in the state. Research into biomedical developments and improvements in health care delivery systems are additional objectives of the School of Medicine. Jackson is a medium-sized, student-friendly city with a diverse patient population.

Academics

While most medical students follow a four-year curriculum leading to the M.D., some take advantage of other schools within the Medical Center and pursue joint-degree programs such as the combined M.D./Ph.D. curriculum, which leads to the doctorate, in Anatomy, Biochemistry, Microbiology, Neuroscience, Pathology, and Pharmacology. Medical students receive percentile scores and a class rank and may be awarded honors at the time of graduation. To be eligible for promotion, a student must achieve at least a 70 in each course, have a weighted average of 75 or higher, and attend 80 percent of the lectures and classes. Passing the USMLE Step 1 is a requirement for promotion to year three, and passing Step 2 is a requirement for graduation.

BASIC SCIENCES: The basic sciences are integrated with social science courses and are taught through a combination of lectures, small groups, labs, and hands-on clinical experiences. Students are in class or other scheduled activity for about 22 hours per week. First-year courses are Gross Anatomy; Histology; Neurobiology; Biochemistry; Medical Physiology; Behavioral Science and Psychiatry; and Cardiopulmonary Resuscitation. Second-year courses are Medial Microbiology; General and Systemic Pathology; Pharmacology; Biostatistics; Preventive Medicine and Public Health; Medical Genetics; Clinical Psychiatry; and Introduction to Clinical Medicine (ICM). In the ICM course students learn history-taking, examination, and diagnosis skills through classroom presentations and small-group sessions. The ICM experience helps prepare students for the clinical phase of the curriculum. Basic-science instruction facilities are central to the campus and include the Holmes Learning Resources center, which houses the Rowland Medical Library. The library is impressive, with more than 160,000 volumes and 2,500 periodicals.

CLINICAL TRAINING: Required third-year rotations are Family Medicine (6 weeks); Medicine/Neurology (12 weeks); Ob/Gyn (6 weeks); Psychiatry (6 weeks); Pediatrics (6 weeks); and Surgery (12 weeks). The fourth year is organized into 8 month-long blocks of Selectives. Students choose specialty areas from within Internal Medicine, Ob/Gyn, Pediatrics, and Surgery. In addition, 3 blocks of Selectives in an ambulatory setting and 2 blocks in inpatient settings are required. Throughout the fourth year, students participate in a Senior Seminar, which provides a forum for interdisciplinary instruction and discussion of issues relevant to modern medical practice. Clinical training takes place at the University Hospital (593 beds); Blair E. Batson Hospital for Children; the community-based University Hospital Durant; the Veterans Administration Hospital; McBryde Rehabilitation Center for the Blind; and Jackson Medical Mall with clinic, and State Health Department offices.

Students

In recent years all students have been Mississippi residents. Approximately 10 percent of students are underrepresented minorities, most of whom are African Americans. The average age of incoming students is generally around 24. Class size is 100.

STUDENT LIFE: Medical students use the resources and facilities of the University in addition to those of the greater community. As the state capital of Mississippi, Jackson offers numerous cultural and recreational attractions. Beyond clinical-care provision, the Medical School contributes directly to the community through activities such as the Base-Pair Mentorship Program, which pairs Medical School researchers and high school students and encourages them to jointly pursue academic projects. On-campus housing options include residence halls and an apartment complex with one-, two-, and three-bedroom units.

GRADUATES: Graduates are successful in securing positions in a range of specialty areas. At the University Hospital in Jackson there are more then 20 residency programs into which a number of graduates enter each year.

Admissions

REQUIREMENTS: Due to high competition in the admissions process, state residency is virtually a requirement. Required science courses are 8 semester hours each of

Biology, Chemistry, Organic Chemistry, and Physics, all with associated labs. Three semester hours of college-level Algebra and three of college-level Trigonometry, or 3 semester hours of Calculus, satisfies the Math requirement. Six semester hours of English is an additional prerequisite. The MCAT is required, and scores must be from after 1991.

SUGGESTIONS: The April, rather than August, MCAT is advised. Beyond requirements, some advanced science course work in areas such as Biochemistry, Anatomy, Embryology, Genetics, Physical Chemistry, Histology, or Advanced Physics is recommended. Other suggested courses are Advanced English, Sociology, Psychology, Philosophy, History, Geography, Foreign Language, Computer Science, and Fine Arts. Math and Science courses designed for nonscience majors are not counted toward minimum requirements.

PROCESS: All Mississippi residents who submit AMCAS applications are sent secondaries. About half of those returning secondary applications are interviewed between August and March. Candidates have three interview sessions, each with a faculty member or administrator. In addition, a tour of the campus and the opportunity to have lunch with current medical students is provided. Among interviewees, about half are accepted with notification occurring throughout the application cycle. Wait-listed candidates may send additional information to update their files.

Costs

The estimated yearly cost of living for a single student is $10,000. This does not include tuition, but allows for all other expenses.

FINANCIAL AID: Most assistance is awarded on the basis of need, but a few merit scholarships are offered. For students who are interested in practicing in underserved areas of Mississippi, the state offers a Medical Education Scholarship/Loan Program.

UNIVERSITY OF MISSISSIPPI

STUDENT BODY

Type	Public
*Enrollment	390
*% male/female	69/31
*% underrepresented minorities	10
# applied (total/out)	597/264
% interviewed	33/0
% accepted (total/out)	NR/NR
% enrolled (total/out)	48/NR
Average age	24

ADMISSIONS

Average GPA and MCAT Scores

Overall GPA	3.62	Science GPA	NR
MCAT Bio	9.00	MCAT Phys	9.00
MCAT Verbal	9.00	MCAT Essay	NR

Score Release Policy

The Admissions Committee says that it makes no difference if scores are withheld.

Application Information

Regular application	11/1
Regular notification	10/15 until filled
Early application	6/1–8/1
Early notification	10/1
Transfers accepted?	Yes
Admissions may be deferred?	Yes
AMCAS application accepted?	Yes
Interview required?	Yes
Application fee	$0

COSTS AND AID

Tuition & Fees

Tuition (in/out)	$6,837/$13,198
Cost of books	$1,850
Fees	$120

Financial Aid

% students receiving aid	80
Average grant	$6,600
Average loan	$13,000
Average debt	$46,500

*Figures based on total enrollment

University of Missouri, Columbia

SCHOOL OF MEDICINE

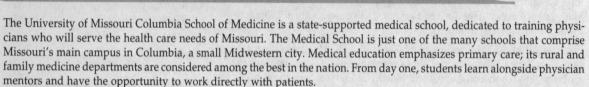

One Hospital Drive, Columbia, MO 65212
Admission: 573-882-8047 • Fax: 573-884-4808
Email: nolkej@health.missouri.edu
Internet: www.muhealth.org/~medicine

The University of Missouri Columbia School of Medicine is a state-supported medical school, dedicated to training physicians who will serve the health care needs of Missouri. The Medical School is just one of the many schools that comprise Missouri's main campus in Columbia, a small Midwestern city. Medical education emphasizes primary care; its rural and family medicine departments are considered among the best in the nation. From day one, students learn alongside physician mentors and have the opportunity to work directly with patients.

Academics

Although most students complete the M.D. curriculum in four years, some follow an extended program, leading to the M.S. or Ph.D. along with the M.D. Doctoral programs are available in diverse areas.

BASIC SCIENCES: Missouri is one of the leaders in the movement towards problem-based learning. Students learn in small groups and, with less than 20 hours per week in scheduled sessions, have ample time for self-study or individualized projects. The first two years are organized into eight 10-week blocks, each of which consists of eight weeks of instruction followed by one week of evaluation and one week of vacation. Each block is divided into two general instructional components, Problem-Based Learning and Introduction to Patient Care. Block one is devoted to the Structure of the Human Body, covering Biochemistry, Anatomy, Histology, Embryology, and Molecular Biology. Blocks two, three, and four each focus on a set of body/organ systems, which include the following: Cardiovascular, Respiratory, Renal, Gastrointestinal, Metabolism, Endocrine, Neuroscience, Liver, and Heme-Lymph. Year two is comprised of blocks 5–8, which concentrate on Pathophysiology and Clinical Management. One of the main objectives of the second year is to prepare students for clinical rotations. Grading for the first year is Satisfactory/Unsatisfactory and for the second year is Honors/Satisfactory/Unsatisfactory. The medical library and computer facilities are comprehensive and serve as educational resources for faculty, students, and the medical community.

CLINICAL TRAINING: Year three is divided into six 8-week blocks of required clerkships, which are the following: Child Health, Family Medicine, Internal Medicine, Ob/Gyn, Psychiatry/Neurology, and Surgery. A separate rural track offers up to six months of clinical experience in a rural community during the third year in lieu of some of the required rotations. Year four consists of twelve weeks of general electives and three 4-week advanced clinical selectives—one must be in a core medical specialty, and another must be in a core surgical specialty. Finally,

fourth-year students must complete 8 weeks of advanced basic science selectives. The majority of clinical training is conducted at University Hospital and Clinics, a 288-bed tertiary care facility that draws patients from throughout central Missouri. Other training sites include Children's Hospital, Ellis Fischel Cancer Center, and the Missouri Rehabilitation Center. In total, clinical training sites encompass over 1,000 patient beds. Grading for both of the clinical years is Honors/Letters of Commendation/Satisfactory/Unsatisfactory. Students must pass Step 1 of the USMLE to be promoted to year four and Step 2 in order to graduate.

Students

The University of Missouri–Columbia is a state school, and virtually all of the 96 entering students are Missouri residents. A large percentage attended the various public undergraduate colleges and universities throughout the state. Among students in the 1999 entering class, 78 percent were science majors as undergraduates. Approximately 4 percent of medical students are underrepresented minorities. The average age of incoming students is usually 23.

STUDENT LIFE: The School of Medicine is located in the heart of the University of Missouri's main campus, allowing students to take advantage of its recreational, athletic, and entertainment facilities. The new curriculum gives students flexibility within their schedules, allowing them to explore both their academic and non-academic interests. Student organizations are active, particularly the local chapter of the American Student Medical Association, which coordinates academic, social, and cultural events and sponsors community-service projects, such as Students Teaching AIDS to Students (STATS). Columbia is located within a few hours of both Kansas City and St. Louis. Most medical students live in privately owned apartments, generally a short distance from campus.

GRADUATES: About half of the graduates enter residencies in one of the primary care fields. A limited number of students seeking primary care careers are selected for a program that integrates the senior year of medical school with residency training in Family Medicine, Internal Medicine, Pediatrics, or Psychiatry.

Admissions

REQUIREMENTS: The School of Medicine requires one year each of the following courses, all of which must be taken with associated labs: Biology, General Chemistry, Organic Chemistry, and General Physics. In addition to the traditional pre-medical courses, one semester of math and two semesters of English composition are also prerequisites. The MCAT is required; scores must be from after 1993. If a student has taken the MCAT more than once, the highest total set of MCAT scores is considered.

SUGGESTIONS: Course work in biology and chemistry beyond requirements is strongly recommended. In addition, applicants are encouraged to study humanities and social sciences while in college. The Admissions Committee looks for applicants with a clear interest in primary care and rural medicine.

PROCESS: All Missouri residents who submit an AMCAS application receive a secondary, which should be submitted as soon as possible. Almost 50 percent of the Missouri-resident applicants are invited to interview between October and April. Students are interviewed one-on-one by two members of the Admissions Committee. A current medical student gives a short tour of the facilities and answers questions. About a month after interviewing, applicants may be notified of the Committee's decision. Approximately 40 percent of interviewed candidates are accepted. Wait-listed candidates are not encouraged to send supplementary information.

Costs

The estimated yearly cost of living for a single student is about $13,000. This budget allows for off-campus housing and car maintenance.

FINANCIAL AID: The majority of aid is awarded on the basis of financial need. Most students finance their education through loans, but a number of need-based scholarships and grants are also available. Each year, four entering students receive full-tuition scholarships that are not based on need.

UNIVERSITY OF MISSOURI, COLUMBIA

STUDENT BODY

Type	Public
*Enrollment	383
*% male/female	56/44
*% underrepresented minorities	4
# applied (total/out)	920/451
% interviewed (total/out)	29/4
% accepted (total/out)	13/1
% enrolled (total/out)	70/30
Average age	24

ADMISSIONS

Average GPA and MCAT Scores

Overall GPA	3.74	Science GPA	3.68
MCAT Bio	10.13	MCAT Phys	9.81
MCAT Verbal	9.61	MCAT Essay	O

Score Release Policy

It is not viewed negatively if an applicant chooses to withhold scores.

Application Information

Regular application	11/1
Regular notification	3/15
Early application	8/1
Early notification	10/1
Transfers accepted?	Yes
Admissions may be deferred?	Yes
AMCAS application accepted?	Yes
Interview required?	Yes
Application fee	$50

COSTS AND AID

Tuition & Fees

Tuition (in/out)	$14,719/$28,907
Cost of books	$1,005
Fees	NR

Financial Aid

% students receiving aid	96
Average grant	$3,000
Average loan	$21,000
Average debt	$80,300

*Figures based on total enrollment

University of Missouri, Kansas City

SCHOOL OF MEDICINE

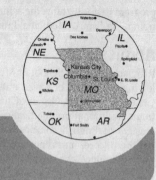

2411 Holmes, Kansas City, MO 64108
Admission: 816-235-1870 • Fax: 816-235-5277
Internet: www.med.umkc.edu

The School of Medicine at the University of Missouri, Kansas City (UMKC), does not offer a traditional four-year medical education. Instead, the School of Medicine along with the College of Arts and Sciences and School of Biological Sciences at UMKC offer a unique, combined B.A./M.D. program that allows students to save both time and money. Students enter the program directly from high school and earn their bachelor's degree and M.D. in a six-year period. Even during the baccalaureate portion of their studies, students enjoy patient contact and hands-on experience in health care settings. The primary mission of the program is to train physicians to meet the health care needs of Missouri and the nation.

Academics

Rather than distinguishing pre-medical course work, pre-clinical medical course work, and clinical instruction, the curriculum integrates liberal arts, didactic medical sciences, and clinical training. Grading is letter grade, Honors/Credit/No Credit, and narrative, and students must pass both steps of the USMLE in order to graduate.

BASIC SCIENCES: During the first two years, students focus most of their efforts on working toward a baccalaureate degree through Arts and Science course work. Seventy-five percent of classroom hours are devoted to liberal arts studies and 25 percent to introductory medical course work. Year one (35 weeks) consists of undergraduate level courses in General Chemistry, Biology, Sociology, Psychology, and Introduction to Medicine. The Introduction to Medicine course gives special attention to the effects of illness on the patient, family, and community. Students become acclimated to the hospital environment and are introduced to the medical vocabulary and to basic clinical skills such as patient interviews and simple data gathering. The second year (44 weeks) includes Organic Chemistry, Human Biochemistry, Life Cycles, Medical Physiology, Biostatistics, and ongoing introductory clinical experiences. In years three and four (both 48 weeks) students take course in Anatomy, Microbiology, Pathology, and Pharmacology and participate in clinical rotations, including a weekly continuing care clinic and family medicine preceptorship. Throughout the first four years, additional liberal arts courses are included in the curriculum that are considered part of the B.A. To assist with clinical training, a physician-scholar (or docent) instructs and advises groups of 11 or 12 students. The docent acts as a mentor, guide, and preceptor throughout the entire six years.

CLINICAL TRAINING: Students enter fifth- and sixth-year clerkships having already had significant clinical exposure. They continue their weekly continuing care clinic experience. Year five (48 weeks) is comprised of rotations

in Community Medicine/Family Practice (1 month), Psychiatry (1 month), Ob/Gyn (2 months), Pediatrics (2 months), Surgery (2 months), and Internal Medicine (2 months). One month is reserved for electives. The sixth year (48 weeks) gives students ample opportunity to explore their specific areas of interest with 6 months of elective rotations. Required rotations include Internal Medicine (2 months) and Emergency Medicine (1 month). During the fifth or sixth year, students also take 1 month of liberal arts courses. Most training takes place at Truman Medical Center, one of the clinical facilities associated with UMKC.

Students

At least 85 percent of students are Missouri residents. Others come from high schools in neighboring states and other regions of the country. Underrepresented minorities account for about 6 percent of the student body. As a result of the structure of the program, students within a class are all roughly the same age.

STUDENT LIFE: For the most part, classes run year round. Although the atmosphere is intense, students are committed and supportive of one another particularly because of the junior-senior partnership program. Students enjoy the resources of both the undergraduate campus and Kansas City. All students live on campus during the first year, but most choose to live off campus for the remainder of their studies.

GRADUATES: Graduates are successful in securing residency positions in all fields. Approximately 25 percent enter programs affiliated with UMKC.

Admissions

REQUIREMENTS: Applicants for admission at the freshman level must take the American College Test (ACT) or the SAT (out-of-state applicants only). Applicants should have completed four years of high school English, four years of Math, three years of Science including one year each of Biology and Chemistry, three years of Social Studies, one year of Foreign Language, and one year in the Fine Arts. In addition, one year of Physics and one semester of Computer Science are highly recommended by the Medical School. If Advanced Placement (AP) courses are available, these are recommended as well. A limited number of positions may be available at the year-three level owing to attrition. Applicants to year three must be Missouri residents and must have completed the standard pre-medical requirements of one year each of Biology, Chemistry, Organic Chemistry as well as other requirements. The MCAT is required of these applicants, and scores must be from within the past three years.

Suggestions: For applicants to the B.A./M.D. program and for those applying after college, some medically related experience is considered useful. High school students are encouraged to volunteer or work in a hospital or other health care environment.

Process: UMKC is not a part of AMCAS. Applications may be obtained from the address above and are due by November 15. Interviews take place between December and mid-March and consist of two sessions, each of which is one-on-one. In addition to the interview, students and their parents attend group orientation sessions that cover a range of topics including financial aid. Applicants tour the campus and have the opportunity to meet with current students. All candidates are notified of the Admissions Committee's decision on April 1. Some are accepted from a wait list later in the spring.

Costs

For the first two years, the total annual anticipated budget including tuition is about $36,000 for in-state students and $55,000 for out-of-state students. During years three through six, the annual cost is about $45,000 for in-state students and $60,000 for out-of-state students depending somewhat on lifestyle choices. Most students own cars, particularly in the later years of the program. One benefit of the UMKC curriculum is that there are considerable savings in completing both the bachelor's degree and the M.D. in six rather than eight years.

Financial Aid: Most financial aid is awarded on the basis of need, as determined by federal and institutional formulas. Each year, a number of merit-based scholarships are awarded to Missouri residents.

UNIVERSITY OF MISSOURI, KANSAS CITY

STUDENT BODY

Type	Public
*Enrollment	625
*% male/female	42/58
*% underrepresented minorities	7
# applied (total/out)	644/314
% interviewed (total/out)	44/25
% accepted (total/out)	NR/NR
% enrolled (total/out)	42/21
Average age	18

ADMISSIONS

Average GPA and MCAT Scores

Overall GPA	NR	Science GPA	NR
MCAT Bio	NR	MCAT Phys	NR
MCAT Verbal	NR	MCAT Essay	NR

Score Release Policy

The school has not responded to our inquiry regarding withheld MCAT scores. Therefore, we advise caution. Contact the Admissions Office before withholding any scores.

Application Information

Regular application	11/15
Regular notification	4/1–varies
Transfers accepted?	No
Admissions may be deferred?	No
AMCAS application accepted?	No
Interview required?	Yes
Application fee (in/out)	$25/$50

COSTS AND AID

Tuition & Fees

Tuition (in/out)	$20,059/$40,642
Cost of books	$650
Fees	NR

Financial Aid

% students receiving aid	NR
Average grant	NR
Average loan	NR
Average debt	NR

*Figures based on total enrollment for six-year program

MOREHOUSE SCHOOL OF MEDICINE

720 Westview Drive, SW, Atlanta, GA 30310
Admission: 404-752-1650 • Fax: 404-752-1512
Internet: www.msm.edu

Morehouse trains clinical and academic physicians to provide and improve health care for the medically underserved. Morehouse School of Medicine is a predominantly African American institution that enjoys a national reputation. At the same time, the School of Medicine is an integral part of its immediate community, providing clinical and other services to the local population. The original mission—to recruit, educate, and graduate students from minority and underrepresented backgrounds—is as important today as it was in 1975, when the school was founded. In response to national and local health care needs and priorities, the curriculum at Morehouse emphasizes primary care.

Academics

Most students follow a four-year curriculum leading to the M.D., although some pursue joint degree programs of M.D./M.P.H or M.D./Ph.D. To be considered for these programs, applications must be submitted to the appropriate graduate department at the time of application to medical school. Medical students are evaluated on an A–F scale. Passing the USMLE Step 1 is a requirement for promotion to year three, and passing Step 2 is a requirement for graduation.

BASIC SCIENCES: Instruction uses a lecture/lab format, and students are in class or laboratories for about 30 hours per week. First-year courses are Human Morphology, Medical Biochemistry, Neurobiology, Medical Physiology, Biostatistics and Epidemiology, Human Behavior, Human Values in Medicine, Community Health, and a weekly preceptorship with a community physician. Community Health Promotion is an examination of preventive medicine, while Human Values in Medicine addresses the behavioral, socioeconomic, and ethical aspects of medicine. Second-year courses are Introduction to Primary Care, Pathophysiology, Human Values in Medicine, Psychopathology, Microbiology and Immunology, Pathology, Pharmacology, and Nutrition. During the second year, students learn patient interview and examination techniques. Instruction takes place in the Basic Medical Sciences Building, which contains classrooms, laboratories, and administrative offices, and in the adjacent Medical Education Building. In 1996, a new Multidisciplinary Research Center opened.

CLINICAL TRAINING: Third- and fourth-year required clerkships are Internal Medicine (2 months); Pediatrics (2 months); Ob/Gyn (2 months); Psychiatry (7 weeks); Radiology (1 week); Surgery (2 months); Family Medicine (1 month); Ambulatory Medicine (1 month); Maternal Child Health (1 month); and Rural Primary Care (1 month). Five months are reserved for electives. Third-year rotations take place primarily at Grady Memorial Hospital (1,000 beds), a full-service facility for indigent patients that, for training purposes, is shared with Emory University. Other clinical sites include the Tuskegee Veterans Hospital (900 beds); Georgia Regional Hospital,

Ridgeview Institute; West Fulton Community Mental Health Center; Brawner Psychiatric Institute and HCA West Paces Ferry Hospital; and Southwest Hospital and Medical Center. A portion of elective credit may be earned at accredited medical schools other than Morehouse, and at a wide range of clinical institutions.

Students

Approximately 95 percent of students are African American. About 70 percent of students are from Georgia, while others are from a wide geographic area. Class size is 35.

STUDENT LIFE: Community service is an important part of student life, and virtually all students are involved in some sort of volunteer activity while in medical school. Students are cohesive both in and out of the classroom. A demonstration of cooperation between students is the large percentage of students who are in study groups. Students participate in local chapters of national medical school organizations and in student groups focused on professional interests. Atlanta is the cultural, financial and industrial hub of the Southeastern United States, and offers a wide range of activities and attractions including arts, sports, recreation, dining, and entertainment. The city is accessible by public transportation. Although there is no school-owned housing, students are able to locate affordable housing off campus.

GRADUATES: Graduates are successful in securing residencies in prestigious programs nationwide. Approximately 75 percent of graduates enter primary care fields, one of the highest percentages among medical schools. Most go on to work with underserved populations, either in inner cities or in rural areas.

Admissions

REQUIREMENTS: Required courses are Biology (one year); General Chemistry (one year); Organic Chemistry (one year); Physics (one year); college-level Math (one year), and English (one year). All science courses must include associated labs. Grades are assessed with consideration given to academic improvement, balance and depth of academic program, difficulty of courses taken, and overall achievement. The MCAT is required, and scores must be from within the past two years. Applicants who have taken the exam on multiple occasions are not penalized, but the most recent set of scores is weighed most heavily.

SUGGESTIONS: Of the 40 spots in a class, at least 20 are reserved for Georgia residents. Thus, competition for out-of-state residents can be intense. For all applicants, the April, rather than August, MCAT is advised. Beyond academic achievement, the committee is interested in extracurricular activities, research projects and experiences, and evidence of pursuing interests and talents in depth. Compassion, honesty, motivation, and perseverance are qualities that are considered important to the practice of medicine.

PROCESS: About 80 percent of AMCAS applicants are sent secondary applications. Of those returning secondaries, about 8 percent are invited to interview between October and March. Of Georgia residents, about 25 percent are invited to interview. Interviews generally consist of one 30-minute session with a faculty member. On interview day, candidates receive a campus tour, group orientation sessions, lunch, and the opportunity to meet with current medical students. About 10–20 percent of interviewees are accepted, with notification beginning in December. Wait-listed candidates may send supplementary material to update or strengthen their files.

Costs

Beyond tuition, the estimated yearly cost of living for a single student is about $20,000. This budget allows for off-campus housing and use of public transportation.

FINANCIAL AID: About 95 percent of students qualify for financial aid. Most assistance is need-based, with need established by the FAFSA and other forms. Parental disclosure is required for institutional assistance. Each year, a few full-tuition scholarships awarded solely on merit are available.

MOREHOUSE SCHOOL OF MEDICINE

STUDENT BODY

Type	Private
*Enrollment	148
*% male/female	40/60
*% underrepresented minorities	95
# applied (total/out)	2,586/NR
% interviewed (total/out)	9/NR
% accepted (total/out)	3.5/NR
% enrolled (total/out)	2/NR
Average age	NR

ADMISSIONS

Average GPA and MCAT Scores

Overall GPA	NR	Science GPA	NR
MCAT Bio	NR	MCAT Phys	NR
MCAT Verbal	NR	MCAT Essay	NR

Score Release Policy

The school has not responded to our inquiry regarding withheld MCAT scores. Therefore, we advise caution. Contact the Admissions Office before withholding any scores.

Application Information

Regular application	12/1
Regular notification	12/20 until filled
Early application	6/1–8/1
Early notification	10/1
Transfers accepted?	Yes
Admissions may be deferred?	Yes
AMCAS application accepted?	Yes
Interview required?	Yes
Application fee	$45

COSTS AND AID

Tuition & Fees

Tuition	$18,200
Cost of books	NR
Fees	$2,454

Financial Aid

% students receiving aid	95
Average grant	$10,273
Average loan	$22,350
Average debt	$95,251

*Figures based on total enrollment

MOUNT SINAI SCHOOL OF MEDICINE

One Gustave L. Levy Place, Box 1002, New York, NY 10029-6574
Admission: 212-241-6696 • Fax: 212-828-4135
Internet: www.mssm.edu

Mount Sinai School of Medicine's goal is not only to prepare individuals to become superb physicians, but also to help them to reach their maximum potential as caring, well-rounded people. Innovation has been a hallmark of the School since it was founded in 1963. New approaches to teaching have helped students to become effective, compassionate physicians. The curriculum has recently been revised to meet the challenges of modern medicine. The faculty/student ratio is among the most favorable in the country, and faculty members serve as instructors, advisors, role models, and mentors. New York City is an unbeatable location for clinical training and extracurricular pursuits.

Academics

Mount Sinai's approach to medical education emphasizes cooperative rather than competitive learning to prepare students for the lifelong learning that is essential for the modern medical career. Group study, small classes and, for the past 30 years, a Pass/Fail grading system for the first- and second-year students contribute to this emphasis. The majority of the students' time in the first two (pre-clinical) years is focused on the core biomedical knowledge and the basic skills of the doctor-patient relationship. Through direct patient contact during the third and fourth (clinical) years in inpatient and ambulatory settings, students develop the skills necessary for the practice of medicine. Joint degree programs, such as the M.S./M.D., are possible in conjunction with New York University. Seven students each year pursue an MSTP-sponsored Ph.D. degree along with the M.D. in conjunction with the Mount Sinai Graduate School of Biological Sciences. The Ph.D. may be earned in Biochemistry, Biomathematical Sciences, Cell Biology and Anatomy, Genetics, Immunobiology, Microbiology, Molecular Biology, Neuroscience, Pharmacology, and Physiology/Biophysics. Evaluation of student performance uses Pass/Fail for the pre-clinical courses and Honor/Pass/Fail for clinical training. Students must pass Step 1 of the USMLE for promotion to year three, and Step 2 in order to graduate.

BASIC SCIENCES: Basic sciences are taught through a combination of lectures, small-group discussions, labs, and clinical correlates. Lecture time is kept to two hours per day and students typically have three mornings or afternoons per week study time. Beginning in the first month of the first year, students apply the knowledge gained in the classroom to patient care in Introduction to Clinical Medicine. Throughout both years the emphasis is on case-based learning. Integrated with every course are numerous means for providing clinical relevance for the basic science being studied. Topics—such as ethics, pharmacology, and nutrition—that overlap many areas are incorporated into the curriculum of all four years through Courses Without Walls. First-year courses are Student Well Being, First Aid, Lifecycle, Embryology, Molecules and Cells, Histology and Physiology, and Pathogenesis and Host Defense Mechanisms. The year ends with an integrative core that focuses on translational topics, allowing students to work with faculty from the bench to the bedside on a selected and structured topic. Extensive study of Mechanisms of Disease and Therapy is the major focus of the second year. This sequence of courses addresses each of the major pathophysiology topics essential to the practice of medicine. Organs and systems covered include respiratory, cardiovascular, renal/genitourinary, breast, skin, gynecologic, hematologic, endocrine, and musculoskelatal. A section on Brain and Behavior encompasses both psychopathology and neurology and at the end of the year the focus shifts to epidemiology and biostatistics.

CLINICAL TRAINING: The curriculum in the third year is composed of four 12-week modules of clinical clerkships. The modules are Pediatrics, Obstetrics, Nursery, and Gynecology; Medicine and Geriatrics; Surgery, Pediatrics and Psychiatry; and Neurology, Anesthesia and Family Practice. Four weeks of electives are also offered in the third year. As in the first two years, an integrated case-based curriculum enriches the learning opportunities throughout the year. The fourth year begins with a four-week preparation period for Step 2 of the USMLE followed by an emergency rotation and a subinternship in medicine. A clinical Translational Fellowship combines the clinical practice of medicine with the relevant basic science. A four-week required Post-March Integrated Selective addresses issues essential for students to explore before going on to residency. A significant portion of clinical training takes place at The Mount Sinai Hospital, which includes the 625-bed Guggenheim Pavilion and a Primary Care Building with an expansive ambulatory care program. Affiliated teaching facilities include, but are not limited to, Bronx Veterans Affairs Medical Center (Queens, 561 beds), Elmhurst Hospital Center (Queens, 561 beds), Englewood Hospital and Medical Center (New Jersey, 520 beds), North General Hospital (Central and East Harlem), and Queens Hospital Center (408 beds).

Students

The class entering in 1999 came from 53 different undergraduate institutions and pursued 36 undergraduate majors. Underrepresented minorities accounted for 14 percent of the students. The average age of incoming students was 22.

STUDENT LIFE: Beginning with the Student Well-Being course, which is offered in August to incoming students, and the Big Sib program, which pairs first- and second-year students, Mount Sinai Mount Sinai provides a healthy environment and encourages the development of life-long healthy habits. Cultural diversity is respected and supported, both in and out of the classroom. Students are active in a wide range of school-related organizations, particularly those focused on community service activities, and New York City is a rich source of extracurricular life. The Recreation Office provides discounted tickets to theater, movies, sporting events, and concerts. The Aron Residence Hall offers over 600 furnished suites for single students. It is conveniently located, and features a fitness center, among other amenities. School-owned housing for students with families is also available.

GRADUATES: Among graduates of the 2000 class, 27 percent entered Internal Medicine, 13 percent entered Pediatrics, 15 percent entered Surgical Specialties, and 9 percent entered Ob/Gyn. The remainder entered a broad range of other post-graduate programs.

Admissions

REQUIREMENTS: Prerequisites are one year each of General Chemistry, Organic Chemistry, Biology, college-level Math, English, and Physics. The MCAT is required, and scores from 1997 onward are acceptable.

SUGGESTIONS: Students who have taken significant time off after college should have some recent course work. No particular extracurricular activities are specified, although successful applicants usually have some community service, research, or medically-related experience.

PROCESS: All AMCAS applicants receive secondary applications. Of those returning secondaries, about 16 percent are interviewed. Interviews are conducted from September through March, and consist of two half-hour sessions, either with two faculty members or a faculty member and a medical student. Some candidates are notified of the committee's decision shortly after the interview, while others may not hear until later in the year. About 30 percent of interviewees are ultimately accepted. Waitlisted candidates may send supplementary material to update their files. Early acceptance programs admit a limited number of sophomores from selected colleges and universities, with admission contingent upon completing undergraduate requirements.

Costs

The estimated yearly cost of living for a single student is about $12,400. On this budget, students can live comfortably in campus housing. Most students do not own cars.

FINANCIAL AID: With a few exceptions, financial aid is need-based, with need determined by the FAFSA and the Needs Access Diskette. Full parental disclosure is required for most forms of aid. State scholarships and loans are available to underrepresented minority students and to students who commit to working in physician-shortage areas.

MOUNT SINAI SCHOOL OF MEDICINE

STUDENT BODY

Type	Private
*Enrollment	451
*% male/female	51/49
*% underrepresented minorities	4
# applied (total/out)	5,206/3,856
% interviewed (total/out)	16/NR
% accepted (total/out)	5.5/NR
% enrolled (total/out)	37/NR
Average age	22

ADMISSIONS

Average GPA and MCAT Scores

Overall GPA	3.64	Science GPA	3.59
MCAT Bio	10.8	MCAT Phys	10.7
MCAT Verbal	10.3	MCAT Essay	P

Score Release Policy

The school has not responded to our inquiry regarding withheld MCAT scores. Therefore, we advise caution. Contact the Admissions Office before withholding any scores.

Application Information

Regular application	11/1
Regular notification	11/15–varies
Early application	8/1
Early notification	10/1
Transfers accepted?	No
Admissions may be deferred?	Yes
AMCAS application accepted?	Yes
Interview required?	Yes
Application fee	$100

COSTS AND AID

Tuition & Fees

Tuition	$23,750
Cost of books	$1,220
Fees	$2,275

Financial Aid

% students receiving aid	80
Average grant	$10,830
Average loan	$16,500
Average debt	$83,295

*Figures based on total enrollment

UNIVERSITY OF NEBRASKA

COLLEGE OF MEDICINE

600 South 42nd Street, Omaha, NE 68198
Admission: 402-559-2259 • Fax: 402-559-4148
Internet: www.unmc.edu/UNCOM/index.html

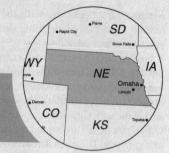

As a state-supported institution, the University of Nebraska College of Medicine is committed to improving the health of Nebraska's population through patient care, preventive medicine, and outreach efforts. In response to the needs of the state and of the nation as a whole, the College of Medicine puts considerable resources into training community-oriented physicians who are likely to enter primary care fields. In addition to the College of Medicine, the University of Nebraska Medical Center (UNMC) features Colleges of Pharmacy, Dentistry, Nursing, and Allied Health Professions. Clinical training takes place at 29 clinics and health care centers that comprise the newly formed Nebraska Health System, a merger of UNMC and Clarkson Regional Health Services.

Academics

Most medical students complete the M.D. curriculum in four years, although some may take an additional year for research projects or other activities. A combined M.D./Ph.D. program is offered to qualified students, leading to the doctorate degree in a number of fields, including Cell Biology and Anatomy, Biochemistry and Molecular Biology, Physiology and Biophysics, Pathology and Microbiology, and Pharmacology. For medical students interested in discrete research projects, summer research stipends are available on a competitive basis. Students entering in 1998 will be evaluated with letter grades, and all students whose grades place them in the upper 40 percent of the class are eligible to write an honors thesis. Passing the USMLE Step 1 is a requirement for promotion to year three, and all students must record a score on Step 2 in order to graduate.

BASIC SCIENCES: Throughout the first two years, basic sciences are integrated with introductory clinical instruction and topics are organized into blocks, referred to as Cores. Students are in class for about 32 hours per week, most of which is spent in lectures, small groups, or labs. During the first year, these are Structure and Development of the Human Body; Cellular Processes; Neuroscience; and Function of the Human Body. Throughout the first and second years, Integrated Clinical Experience (ICE) covers the history and physical examination, interviewing skills, behavioral sciences, ethics, preventive medicine, health care policy, and health care services research. Through ICE, students have the opportunity to work alongside primary care physicians in a longitudinal clinical experience and a summer preceptorship. Also spanning both years is Problem-Based Learning, in which students work in small groups and apply basic science concepts to clinical case studies. Second year Cores are Introduction to Disease Processes; Cardiology/Pulmonary/Endocrinology/Ear, Nose, and Throat; Neurology, Ophthalmology and Psychiatry; Hematology/Oncology/Musculoskeletal; Dermatology and Infectious Disease; and Genitourinary/Gastroenterology. Instruction takes place in the Eppley

Institute and in Wittson Hall, which also houses administrative offices, laboratories, and audiovisual resources. The Leon S. McGoogan Library of Medicine holds over 200,000 volumes and 2,100 current journals. Multimedia materials for computer-assisted and self-instruction are available, as are online informational systems.

CLINICAL TRAINING: Required third-year clerkships are: Internal Medicine (12 weeks); Ob/Gyn (6 weeks); Pediatrics (8 weeks); Surgery (10 weeks); Psychiatry (6 weeks); Community Preceptorship (8 weeks); Basic Science Selective (4 weeks); and a mini-clerkship in an area of choice (2 weeks). During the fourth year, a basic science selective in addition to 28 weeks of electives are required. Clinical facilities at UNMC are Nebraska Health System (650 beds); University Medical Associates, which operates over 60 primary care and subspecialty clinics throughout the greater Omaha metropolitan area; Meyer Rehabilitation Institute; Omaha Veterans Affairs Medical Center; Children's Hospital; Immanuel Hospital; and Methodist Hospital.

Students

Most students in each class are Nebraska residents. In the 1997 entering class, approximately 10 percent of students were older than 25. About 4 percent of current students are underrepresented minorities. Class size is 118.

STUDENT LIFE: Medical students are active in student organizations ranging from the Student Alliance for Global Health, to the Family Practice Club, to a group focused on alternative medicine. The local chapter of the American Medical Student Association is particularly active, organizing volunteer projects, film series, and opportunities for enhanced clinical exposure. Omaha is a city of 320,000, offering a symphony, theaters, art museums, shopping, restaurants, and parks, among other attractions. Students live off campus in the surrounding communities, where, for an urban area, housing is relatively inexpensive.

GRADUATES: Students are successful at securing residencies in both primary care and specialty areas. A significant percentage of graduates enter post-graduate programs at

UNMC, which oversees 18 residency programs. In recent years, at least 60 percent of graduates have gone on to practice in the state of Nebraska. Among students who graduated between 1981 and 1990, 130 joined the faculty at UNMC.

Admissions

REQUIREMENTS: Prerequisites are Biology (8 semester hours); General Chemistry (8 hours); Organic Chemistry (8 hours); Physics (8 hours); Humanities and/or Social Sciences (12 hours); English Composition (3 hours); and Calculus or Statistics (3 credits). All science courses must include associated labs. The MCAT is required, and scores must be from 1997 or later.

SUGGESTIONS: State residents are given preference, but other highly qualified candidates are considered, particularly if they have ties to Nebraska and are interested in practicing in underserved communities in the state. Beyond required courses, the following are recommended: Genetics, Molecular Biology, Biochemistry, Immunology and Microbiology, Communications, Ethics, and Personnel Management.

PROCESS: All Nebraska residents who apply through AMCAS, and about 5 percent of out-of-state applicants, are asked to submit supplementary materials and are interviewed. Interviews are conducted between October and March, and consist of two 30-minute sessions with a faculty member. On interview day, there is also a group information session and a campus tour. Typically, about 50 percent of Nebraska residents are accepted, with notification beginning in November. Wait-listed candidates may send additional information to update their files.

Costs

The estimated yearly cost of living for a single student is $15,000. This budget supports off-campus housing.

FINANCIAL AID: Most assistance is granted on the basis of financial need, as determined by the FAFSA form. Institutional loans and grants supplement Federal aid programs. A few merit-based scholarships are awarded each year to entering students. Joint M.D./Ph.D. students are fully funded through the Medical Scholars program.

UNIVERSITY OF NEBRASKA

STUDENT BODY

Type	Public
*Enrollment	470
*% male/female	55/45
*% underrepresented minorities	3.4
# applied (total/out)	857/577
% interviewed (total/out)	38/7
% accepted (total/out)	NR/NR
% enrolled (total/out)	29/11
Average age	22

ADMISSIONS

Average GPA and MCAT Scores

Overall GPA	3.70	Science GPA	3.71
MCAT Bio	9.40	MCAT Phys	9.40
MCAT Verbal	9.30	MCAT Essay	NR

Score Release Policy

The Admissions Committee will consider individual cases, but it is generally viewed unfavorably if scores are withheld.

Application Information

Regular application	11/1
Regular notification	11/1 until filled
Early application	6/1–8/1
Early notification	10/1
Admissions may be deferred?	No
AMCAS application accepted?	Yes
Interview required?	Yes
Application fee	$25

COSTS AND AID

Tuition & Fees

Tuition (in/out)	$11,922/$23,501
Cost of books	$700
Fees	$1,208

Financial Aid

% students receiving aid	80
Average grant	NR
Average loan	NR
Average debt	$60,000

*Figures based on total enrollment

UNIVERSITY OF NEVADA

SCHOOL OF MEDICINE

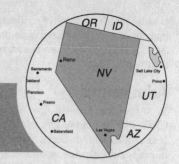

Mail Stop 357, Reno, NV 89557
Admission: 775-784-6063 • Fax: 775-784-6194
Email: asa@unr.edu • Internet: www.unr.edu/unr/med.html

With a class size of about 52, the University of Nevada School of Medicine is able to provide individual attention to its medical students. Although primarily focused on fulfilling the medical demands of the state, graduates of the University of Nevada are competitive for residencies nationwide. Students study basic sciences in Reno but rotate to Las Vegas and to rural sites for clinical training.

Academics

The first two years provide a foundation in basic clinical sciences, significant preclinical training, and clerkships that take place statewide in community clinics as well as hospital settings. The School of Medicine applicants or current medical students may apply to jointly pursue a M.D./Ph.D. program in several areas including biomedical engineering and cell and molecular biology, pharmacology, and physiology. For students interested in research without undertaking a Ph.D., projects can be arranged with faculty members.

BASIC SCIENCES: The first two years at Nevada focus on the basic sciences , but also give considerable attention to community health and social issues. Additional scientific material is presented through lectures, labs, and small group formats at the Reno campus. Students apply scientific principles to clinical challenges through problem-solving courses using case study methods. This approach promotes the development of problem-solving skills in medical students. Concurrent with basic and behavioral science courses, students learn fundamental skills in doctor-patient relationship and physical exams through weekly sessions that are supervised by physicians and senior medical students. In this way, students learn not only from full-time faculty but also from knowledgeable and experienced clinical faculty physicians throughout the state. First-year course work includes Human Biochemistry, Human Anatomy, Embryology, Histology, Neuroanatomy, Human Behavior, Medical Cell Biology, Neurosciences, Systems Physiology, Clinical Problem Solving, Nutrition, and Introduction to Patient Care. Year two courses include Human Genetics, Medical Mircobiology, Medical Pharmacology, Pathology, Laboratory Medicine, Psychiatric Medicine, Medical Ethics, Community Medicine, Introduction to Patient Care II, and Clinical Problem Solving II. Most courses are graded on a letter grade from A through F, and students must receive at least a C to be promoted. Students are evaluated on both cognitive and noncognitive factors. Two major medical libraries serve the medical students: the Savitt Medical Library on the Reno campus, containing more than 40,000 volumes, and the University Medical Center Library in Las Vegas, both of which maintain computer labs that feature an assort-

ment of general and curriculum-based software. Additional learning resource labs are available in Las Vegas in the ambulatory care centers. Students have electronic access to all of Nevada's university and community college collections through terminals located throughout the teaching sites in the state. Students are issued computer accounts for email and Internet access. In addition, the USMLE Step 1 is required passage for promotion to year three.

CLINICAL TRAINING: Training takes place at affiliated hospitals, clinics, and ambulatory care centers throughout the state. Most students have required rotations including The Practice of Medicine, which is a 24-week integrated clerkship experience that includes Family Medicine (6 weeks), Internal Medicine (12 weeks) and Pediatrics (6 weeks). The Practice of Medicine also includes a core curriculum that runs throughout the state via distance education facilities. Medical students also complete required specialty rotations of Ob/Gyn (6 weeks), Psychiatry (6 weeks), and Surgery (12 weeks). There is an increased emphasis in all of the rotations to blend ambulatory and hospital-based practice to give the students a balanced educational experience. During the fourth year, students rotate through 32 weeks of elective clerkships and 4 weeks of a required rural clerkship. Elective study can take place in Reno, Las Vegas, rural Nevada, other states, or abroad. Although the obvious emphasis and strength of the program is primary care and rural medicine, hospitals in Reno and Las Vegas treat urban and often international populations. Evaluation of clinical performance is Honors/Pass/Fail. In addition, special awards and honors are granted to students who have made unique and outstanding achievements in clinical areas. Passing the USMLE Step 2 is required for graduation.

Students

Eighty-five percent of students majored in a science-related discipline in college. About 5 percent are underrepresented minorities, most of whom are Mexican or Native American. Almost all students are Nevada residents, although many attended college in other states. About one-quarter of each class took some time off between college and medical school.

Student Life: Small class size promotes cohesion among students. A designated lounge on campus gives medical students a place to relax and interact. Athletic facilities are available: Students in the Reno area use the Lombardi Recreational Facility and, in Las Vegas, the McDermott Physical Education Facility. Student organizations include AMWA & OSR medical specialty interest groups, the Significant Others Group for partners of medical students, and the University of Nevada Student Outreach Clinic, through which medical students, with supervision, volunteer to treat patients from underserved areas. Most students have cars, and on-campus parking is free for students with registered vehicles. Beyond campus, Lake Tahoe is just an hour from Reno and offers outstanding outdoor activities all year. Virtually all medical students live off campus, where housing is affordable and comfortable.

Graduates: The majority of graduates enter residency programs outside the state. Almost all graduates ultimately become practicing clinical physicians.

Admissions

Requirements: Required course work includes Biology (12 Semester hours); Chemistry (8 hours); Organic Chemistry (8 hours); Physics (8 hours); and Behavioral Science (6 hours). The Biology and Behavioral Science requirements specify that at least 3 semester hours be upper-division credit. GPA is used, along with MCAT scores, to screen for interview invitations. The most recent MCAT scores are used, and the exam must have been taken within the past 3 years.

Suggestions: Only applicants from Nevada, from neighboring states, from Wyoming, Alaska, Montana and Idaho, and those who have close ties to Nevada are considered for admission. Nevada residents are given preference. Community-focused work and health care experience are considered important.

Process: Interviews are held from September through January. The interview is composed of two 50-minute sessions, which may be with faculty, or medical students. Of interviewed candidates, about 25 percent of Nevada residents are offered a place in the class, and about 10 percent of out-of-state applicants are accepted. The first acceptances are sent in January. Wait-listed candidates are ranked, and those in the top third are likely to be admitted.

Costs

Estimated yearly expenses for room, board, transportation, and personal needs is $15,000. This budget presumes off-campus housing and car ownership. Books and supplies are an additional $5,000.

Financial Aid: All students seeking assistance should apply for federal student aid. The University of Nevada School of Medicine Scholarships are awarded on the basis of several criteria, including academic achievement, interest in primary and/or rural health care, and financial need. Students who commit to practicing in underserved areas in Nevada have access to additional grants and low-interest loans. A limited number of scholarships are available for underrepresented minorities.

UNIVERSITY OF NEVADA

STUDENT BODY

Type	Public
*Enrollment	208
*% male/female	60/40
*% underrepresented minorities	5
# applied (total/out)	210/NR
% interviewed (total/out)	75/NR
% accepted (total/out)	NR/NR
% enrolled (total/out)	NR/NR

ADMISSIONS

Average GPA and MCAT Scores

Overall GPA	3.70	Science GPA	3.60
MCAT Bio	9.30	MCAT Phys	8.80
MCAT Verbal	9.30	MCAT Essay	NR

Score Release Policy

The school has not responded to our inquiry regarding withheld MCAT scores. Therefore, we advise caution. Contact the Admissions Office before withholding any scores.

Application Information

Regular application	11/1
Regular notification	1/15–varies
Early application	6/1–8/1
Early notification	10/1
Admissions may be deferred?	Yes
AMCAS application accepted?	Yes
Interview required?	Yes
Application fee	$45

COSTS AND AID

Tuition & Fees

Tuition	(in/out)	$8,189/$23,720
Cost of books		NR
Fees		$2,124

Financial Aid

% students receiving aid	80
Average grant	NR
Average loan	NR
Average debt	NR

*Figures based on total enrollment

UNIVERSITY OF NEW MEXICO

SCHOOL OF MEDICINE

Basic Medical Sciences Building, Room 107, Albuquerque, NM 87131
Admission: 505-272-4766 • Fax: 505-272-8239

The School of Medicine at the University of New Mexico is renowned for its innovative approach to education. UNM was among the leaders in replacing long lectures and memorization with small groups, problem-based instruction, and an emphasis on lifelong learning. The school continues to evaluate and refine its curriculum with consideration given to adult learning patterns and trends in health care. At UNM, clinical rotations begin during the second year. Students have access to a diverse patient population from Albuquerque, a relatively urban area, and from the more remote areas of the state.

Academics

The four-year curriculum is organized into three phases, all of which involve at least some basic science instruction and clinical training. In addition, all students conduct research projects under the guidance of a faculty mentor. The complete project consists of research, presentation, and a written paper. Applicants interested in pursuing a combined M.D./Ph.D. may apply to the graduate committee at the School of Medicine in addition to completing medical school admissions requirements. Medical students are evaluated as Outstanding, Good, Satisfactory, Marginal, and Unsatisfactory. The USMLE Step 1 must be passed prior to graduation, and Step 2 must be taken in order to graduate.

BASIC SCIENCES: The first year and a half (Phase I) is organized into discrete segments, most of which focus on an organ system. First-year subjects are Foundations, Musculoskeletal, GI/Nutrition/Metabolism, Renal/Endocrine, Neuroscience, and Cardiovascular/Pulmonary. During the summer following year one, students take part in a three-month Practical Immersion Experience that involves hands-on clinical work in either a rural or urban setting. Phase I continues in the first semester of year two with Molecular Genetics, Human Sex and Reproduction, Infectious Disease, and Neoplasma. A range of learning methodologies are used, including lectures, labs, discussions, tutorials, and seminars. Concurrent to basic science instruction are weekly clinical experiences in both inpatient and ambulatory settings. Here, students learn interviewing and examination techniques, and are able to improve communication and personal interaction skills. Much of Phase I and II take place in the Basic Medical Sciences Building. The nearby Health Sciences Center Library supports educational, research, and clinical activities. It houses 150,000 volumes in addition to audiovisuals, online search services, and computer software.

CLINICAL TRAINING: Phase II begins midway through year two with a three-week pharmacology block and orientation to the hospital. Clinical rotations are accompanied by ongoing small-group sessions focused on problem solving and integratinginformation. Students rotate through required clerkships throughout the spring and summer of the second year and the fall and winter of the third year.

Requirementsare Internal Medicine (8 weeks); Surgery (8 weeks); Neurology/Psychiatry (8 weeks); Family Medicine Ambulatory (8 weeks); Pediatrics Ambulatory/Inpatient (8 weeks); and Ob/Gyn Ambulatory/Inpatient (8 weeks). Phase III begins in the spring of year three and is comprised entirely of selectives and electives. A month-long, community-based preceptorship, in which students work alongside a primary care physician who serves as a mentor, is also required. Clinical training takes place at the University Hospital (370 beds) and at several affiliated sites, namely Regional Federal Medical Center (429 beds); UNM Cancer Center; UNM Mental Health Center; UNM Children's Psychiatric Hospital (73 beds); and the Carrie Tingley Hospital for children.

Students

About 25 percent of students are underrepresented minorities, most of whom are Mexican Americans. At least 90 percent of students are New Mexico residents, and about half of each class graduated from UNM's undergraduate college. In a recent class, the average age of entering students was 25, and around a third of students took time off after college. Class size is 73.

STUDENT LIFE: The medical school is located on the North campus of UNM, allowing students access to the resources and facilities of the University. The city also provides an outlet for students who need a break from studying. The greater Albuquerque metropolitan area is home to nearly a third of the state's population and offers numerous cultural and recreational opportunities. Although no on-campus housing is available, off-campus options are convenient and comfortable.

GRADUATES: About 35 percent of graduates enter residencies at UNM, which offers programs in 12 different departments. The majority of graduates enter primary care fields.

Admissions

REQUIREMENTS: Prerequisites are General Biology (8 semester hours); General Chemistry (8 semester hours); Organic Chemistry (8 semester hours); Physics (6 semester hours); and Biochemistry (3 semester hours). Competency in English and the MCAT are additional requirements.

SUGGESTIONS: Knowledge of Spanish or a Native American language is an advantage. Coursework in the Humanities and Social Sciences is important. The April, rather than August, MCAT is advised. Students are selected on the basis of academic achievement, motivation for the study of medicine, problem-solving ability, self-appraisal, ability to relate to people, maturity, breadth of interest and achievements, professional goals, and the likelihood of serving the health care needs of the state following post-graduate training.

PROCESS: All New Mexico AMCAS applicants receive secondary applications and are invited to interview. Qualified WICHE and other out-of-state applicants who apply for early decision are also sent secondary materials and invited to interview. Interviews are conducted from June through March and consist of two sessions with members of the Admissions Committee, who are either full-time faculty members or community physicians. On interview day, lunch and a tour of the facilities are provided. Of interviewed candidates, about 20–25 percent are accepted. Wait-listed candidates are ranked and notified of their position on the list.

Costs

Beyond tuition, the estimated yearly cost of living for a single student is about $17,000. This budget includes books and health insurance costs, and allows for off-campus housing and car ownership.

FINANCIAL AID: Most assistance is awarded on the basis of need, as established by the federal government's Free Application for Federal Student Aid. Before becoming eligible for grants, students must borrow $7,000 per year as part of a unit loan. In addition to Federal programs, the New Mexico Physician Loan-for-Service program targets students who commit to working in underserved areas within the state.

UNIVERSITY OF NEW MEXICO

STUDENT BODY

Type	Public
*Enrollment	304
*% male/female	46/54
*% underrepresented minorities	37.5
# applied (total/out)	1,129/810
% interviewed (total/out)	28/1
% accepted (total/out)	8/6
% enrolled (total/out)	6/1
Average age	26

ADMISSIONS

Average GPA and MCAT Scores

Overall GPA	3.47	Science GPA	NR
MCAT Bio	9.37	MCAT Phys	9.06
MCAT Verbal	9.48	MCAT Essay	NR

Score Release Policy

The school has not responded to our inquiry regarding withheld MCAT scores. Therefore, we advise caution. Contact the Admissions Office before withholding any scores.

Application Information

Regular application	6/1–11/15
Regular notification	3/15–varies
Early application	6/1–8/1
Early notification	10/1
Transfers accepted?	Yes
Admissions may be deferred?	Yes
AMCAS application accepted?	Yes
Interview required?	Yes
Application fee	$50

COSTS AND AID

Tuition & Fees

Tuition (in/out)	$6,446/$18,572
Cost of books	$1,310
Fees	$32

Financial Aid

% students receiving aid	90
Average grant	$2,800
Average loan	$16,300
Average debt	$56,500

*Figures based on total enrollment

NEW YORK MEDICAL COLLEGE

Administration Building, Valhalla, NY 10595
Admission: 914-594-4507 • Fax: 914-594-4976
Internet: www.nymc.edu

New York Medical College is located in Westchester County, an attractive suburb one-half hour north of New York City. This large private university has three schools—a School of Medicine that confers the M.D. degree and two graduate schools, the Graduate School of Basic Medical Sciences and the Graduate School of Health Sciences, which offer M.S., M.P.H., and Ph.D. degrees in 37 advanced degree programs. The university's network of 22 affiliated hospitals includes large urban medical centers, small suburban hospitals, and high-tech regional tertiary care facilities. This extensive network affords excellent clinical training. The medical school is a national leader in educating primary care physicians; it was one of only 16 schools awarded major funding from The Robert Wood Johnson Foundation to support its primary care initiatives. As a health sciences university in the Catholic tradition, the School emphasizes service to underserved populations and recognition of the worth and dignity of each person.

Academics

Students have an opportunity to earn joint degrees, combining the M.D. with an M.P.H., which is in great demand in today's managed care environment, or a Ph.D. in the basic medical sciences. Grading is Honors/High Pass/Pass/Fail. Passing Step 1 of the USMLE is a graduation requirement. In recent years, the pass rate has been 100 percent.

BASIC SCIENCES: The curriculum of the first two years, although focused on the basic sciences, maintains a consistent clinical orientation. The program has been revised to bring clinical relevance and small-group teaching into all courses. The first two years focus on developing a thorough understanding of the sciences basic to clinical medicine. The core of the first-year curriculum—Anatomy, Histology, Biochemistry, Physiology, Neural Science, and Behavioral Science—is supplemented by clinical case correlations and courses in Epidemiology and Biostatistics. The redesigned second-year curriculum, with its strong focus on Pathology/Pathophysiology, emphasizes small-group discussion, problem-based learning, and self-study, with only 25 percent of class time spent in large lectures. Clinical Skills Training, Pharmacology, and Medical Microbiology prepare students for the clerkship experience of the next two years.

CLINICAL TRAINING: While immersed in the basic science curriculum, all first-year students have ongoing, direct patient contact, working in the office of a primary care physician. This one-on-one placement gives students clinical exposure and a personal mentor relationship. This preceptorship experience can be continued throughout the second year to fulfill the clinical skills requirement.

Third-year clinical clerkships are the following: Medicine (12 weeks); Surgery (8 weeks); Pediatrics (8 weeks); Ob/Gyn (6 weeks); Psychiatry (6 weeks); Neurology (4 weeks); Family Medicine Clerkship (4 weeks); and Community and Preventive Medicine (2 weeks). The school's great location and large hospital network afford clinical-training opportunities in demographically and clinically diverse settings. About one-half of the third-year class moves into New York City for their clinical years; many live in College-owned housing in Manhattan.

Fourth-year requirements are the following: Medicine or Pediatrics Subinternship (4 weeks); Ambulatory Surgical Subspecialties (4 weeks); Geriatrics or Chronic Care Pediatrics (4 weeks); and Anesthesiology/Rehabilitation Medicine (4 weeks). The 18 weeks of electives can be taken anywhere. About 15–20 students take international electives each year.

For students with a strong interest in internal medicine, New York Medical College offers a six-year combined M.D./Internal Medicine program. Students are selected for this competitive program during their third year. Those lucky enough to be accepted, do their fourth year of medical school simultaneously with first-year residency. They not only earn a resident's salary during that year, but also have fourth-year tuition loans entirely forgiven if they practice in primary care for three years.

Students

The school's student body is generally representative of the demographic diversity of the country. First-year class size is 190 students; 47 percent of the current class is female. In the current first-year class, one-third of the students took no time off between undergraduate and medical school. About half come from public colleges and universities.

STUDENT LIFE: Most first- and second-year students live on campus in attractive garden apartments; many third- and fourth-year students live in the 95th Street residence in New York City.

The campus environment encourages a sense of community. Students participate in dozens of clubs and groups focused on professional, cultural, social, and athletic interests. These include The Arrhythmias, an *a cappella* singing group; two chamber music groups; and the Sign Language Club. There are numerous organized opportunities for tutoring and mentoring area high school students. The student newspaper; *NYMC News*, is among the first to be written and published entirely by medical students.

GRADUATES: The School of Medicine encourages students to aim high in applying for residency matches. While a growing number of students are choosing to match in primary care disciplines, there are equally impressive matches in highly competitive specialty programs. Matches for the current year can be viewed on the school's website.

Some 9,500 alumni are supported by alumni association chapters in major cities. Alumni can track University announcements of upcoming events on the Web, and they keep current on their classmates' activities via the University magazine, *Chironian*.

Admissions

REQUIREMENTS: All applicants must have taken the MCAT within the last three years and must have completed or have in progress the following prerequisites: two semesters of Biology; Chemistry; Organic Chemistry and Physics. Each of these must have been completed with lab work. Two semesters of English are also required. The most recent MCAT scores are given greatest weight. While most students have majored in the sciences, the school encourages those with strong humanities backgrounds and the necessary science requirements to apply.

SUGGESTIONS: In addition to looking carefully at academic accomplishments, the Admissions Committee is very interested in each applicant's motivation for medicine, as well as his or her interpersonal skills and personal qualities, such as maturity, integrity, and humor. The committee wants to know what an applicant has actually done—be it medically related service, community service, or research. Since interviews here are blind, or closed-file, those invited for an interview should come prepared to talk about their most meaningful experiences.

PROCESS: All AMCAS applicants receive a secondary application. Of those returning secondaries, about 20 percent are invited to interview between October and April. Interviews consist of one or two 30-minute sessions with members of the Admissions Committee. The second interviewer is often a fourth-year student. One-third of those interviewed are accepted and are generally notified within 8 weeks of the interview date. Wait-listed candidates may submit supplemental materials. The wait list is not ranked; wait-listed applicant files are reviewed fully in June and July.

Costs

Cost of living for a student living on campus is about $13,000 per year; off campus about $16,000. Tuition is $29,150 in 1999.

FINANCIAL AID: Financial aid is need-based; with need determined by the FAFSA and other applications. Most assistance is in the form of loans. Some financial awards are available for students entering primary care specialties. In addition, the top 30 students in each class are awarded scholarships and low-interest loans. As mentioned above, participants in the six-year program enjoy reduced costs.

NEW YORK MEDICAL COLLEGE

STUDENT BODY

Type	Private
*Enrollment	789
*% male/female	54/46
*% underrepresented minorities	6
# applied (total/out)	10,985/8,832
% interviewed (total/out)	12/10
% accepted (total/out)	5/5
% enrolled (total/out)	32/33
Average age	23

ADMISSIONS

Average GPA and MCAT Scores

Overall GPA	3.50	Science GPA	3.40
MCAT Bio	10.60	MCAT Phys	10.40
MCAT Verbal	9.60	MCAT Essay	NR

Score Release Policy

There is no policy regarding withheld MCAT scores.

Application Information

Regular application	12/1
Regular notification	Rolling
Early application	8/1
Early notification	10/1
Transfers accepted?	Yes
Admissions may be deferred?	Yes
AMCAS application accepted?	Yes
Interview required?	Yes
Application fee	$100

COSTS AND AID

Tuition & Fees

Tuition	$29,150
Cost of books	$1,464
Fees	$1,952

Financial Aid

% students receiving aid	90
Average grant	$15,000
Average loan	$40,000
Average debt	$140,000

*Figures based on total enrollment

NEW YORK UNIVERSITY

SCHOOL OF MEDICINE

PO Box 1924, New York, NY 10016
Admission: 212-263-5290 • Fax: 212-263-0720
Internet: www.med.nyu.edu

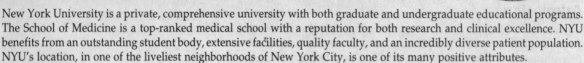

New York University is a private, comprehensive university with both graduate and undergraduate educational programs. The School of Medicine is a top-ranked medical school with a reputation for both research and clinical excellence. NYU benefits from an outstanding student body, extensive facilities, quality faculty, and an incredibly diverse patient population. NYU's location, in one of the liveliest neighborhoods of New York City, is one of its many positive attributes.

Academics

The goal of the curriculum is to train physician-scholars who will approach the profession of medicine with intellectual rigor and who also understand the humanistic and ethical aspects of the field. Selected students may pursue a curriculum leading to both the M.D. and Ph.D. degrees in a minimum of six years. The doctorate degree may be earned in a basic medical science field or in a social science discipline. An honors program permits students who are following the standard four-year M.D. curriculum to supplement formal classwork with summer research or ongoing projects and to receive credit for doing so. Grading during the preclinical years is Pass/Fail. Letter grades are given during the clinical clerkship.

BASIC SCIENCES: In the fall of 1997, the School of Medicine implemented a new basic science curriculum organized into interdisciplinary modules. Year one has three modules. The first module is comprised of Molecular Biology/ Genetics and Biochemistry; Anatomy; and Embryology. Module Two includes Cellular Biology; Physiology; Histology; and Immunology. Module Three is Organ Physiology; Histology of Tissues/Organs; Microbiology; Immunology; and Parasitology. Throughout the first year, students take Behavioral Science/Introduction to Clinical Medicine, which addresses the interrelationship among patients, their families, environments, their particular illness, and their care. The first year also includes a new course, The Skills and Science of Doctoring. This includes a preceptorship in the office of a practicing physician and serves to integrate basic science concepts with clinical applications. First-semester, second-year courses are the following: Neuroscience, General Pathology, and Psychopathology. In second semester, Pathophysiology; Systemic Pathology; Pharmacology and Biostatistics/ Epidemiology are integrated in a Human Organ System module. During the first two years, class time is divided between lectures and small-group discussions. Laboratory work and computer-assisted instruction enhance learning. In total, first- and second-year students are in class or other scheduled sessions for about 20 hours per week. There is a newly established Division of Academic Computing, which has resulted in increased integration of bioinformatics into the curriculum. Each of the courses

has a Web page, and students can access all course materials, including lecture slides, through the Web. Instruction takes place in the Medical Science Building and adjacent facilities, which provide laboratory space, lecture halls, rooms for small-group discussions, and conference rooms. The Frederick L. Ehrman Medical Library occupies three stories in the Medical Science Building and has areas that are open to students 24 hours a day. Its collection includes over 160,000 volumes and 2,000 current serial titles.

CLINICAL TRAINING: Required clerkships must be completed during year three and the first part of year four. These are the following: Medicine (10 weeks); Pediatrics (8 weeks); Surgery (10 weeks); Ob/Gyn (6 weeks); Psychiatry (6 weeks); Neurology (4 weeks); and Ambulatory Care Medicine (4 weeks). During the fourth year, all students take six weeks of advanced medicine. The remainder of the year is reserved for elective study, which typically involves a research project. Clinical training takes place at Bellevue Hospital Center and New York University Medical Center Complex and at affiliated institutions. In total, the complex has a capacity of 5,400 beds. A portion of electives may be taken at other hospitals in the United States or abroad.

Students

Approximately 50 percent of students are New York residents. Others come from all regions of the country. About 7 percent of students are underrepresented minorities, most of whom are African American. Though the majority of students are in their early 20s, each class has several nontraditional students who pursued careers or other activities between college and medical school. Class size is 160.

STUDENT LIFE: In terms of extracurricular life, medical students at NYU have the best of all worlds. Because most students live in University-owned housing, they interact outside of class and are able to enjoy a real student community. The neighborhood around NYU is filled with restaurants, cafes, bars, shops, galleries, and other attractions. New York is a cultural, artistic, commercial, and entertainment center with virtually unlimited recreational opportunities. The entire city is accessible by public transportation. The School of Medicine operates housing facilities for students, assuring that all NYU medical students can afford convenient and comfortable housing. Both residence halls and apartments are available.

GRADUATES: Of 1999 graduates, the most prevalent fields for post-graduate training were the following: Categorical Internal Medicine (37%); General Surgery (10%); Ob/Gyn (9%); Pediatrics or Medicine/Pediatrics (8%); Psychiatry (8%); Radiology (8%); and Dermatology (4%). Many graduates enter residency programs at top institutions nationwide.

Admissions

REQUIREMENTS: Prerequisites are six semester hours each of General Chemistry, Organic Chemistry, Physics, Biology, and English. All science courses must include laboratory work. The MCAT is required, and scores should be from the post-1997 version of the test. For applicants who have retaken the exam, the best set of scores is considered.

SUGGESTIONS: Biochemistry is strongly recommended. Other recommended courses are Calculus, Quantitative and Physical Chemistry, Genetics, Embryology, and Spanish, particularly if the applicant intends on practicing in the New York area. Experience in a health care setting is considered valuable.

PROCESS: NYU does not participate in AMCAS. Rather, applications should be requested from the Office of Admissions and must be submitted between August 7 and November 17. About 20 percent of applicants are invited to interview between November and February. Interviews consist of one session with a faculty member or administrator. On interview day, applicants also tour the campus and have lunch with medical students. About 25 percent of interviewed candidates are accepted, with notification occurring about one month after the interview. Others are rejected or put on hold and either accepted or wait-listed later in the year. Wait-listed candidates may send information to update their files.

Costs

The estimated yearly cost of living for a single student is about $11,000. This budget assumes on campus housing and use of public transportation.

FINANCIAL AID: All financial aid is awarded on the basis of financial need, as determined by the FAFSA and institutional forms. Generally, students are expected to borrow $18,500 in Federal Stafford Loans before qualifying for other sources of assistance. Parental financial disclosure is required.

NEW YORK UNIVERSITY

STUDENT BODY

Type	Private
*Enrollment	692
*% male/female	55/45
*% underrepresented minorities	7
# applied (total/out)	3,471/NR
% interviewed (total/out)	25/NR
% accepted (total/out)	8/NR
% enrolled (total/out)	NR/NR

ADMISSIONS

Average GPA and MCAT Scores

Overall GPA	3.60	Science GPA	3.60
MCAT Bio	13.00	MCAT Phys	13.00
MCAT Verbal	11.00	MCAT Essay	Q

Score Release Policy

Committee only evaluates the score they have. Doesn't matter if student withholds score. They usually don't even notice that factor during evaluation.

Application Information

Regular application	11/17
Regular notification	12/20 until filled
Transfers accepted?	Yes
Admissions may be deferred?	Yes
AMCAS application accepted?	No
Interview required?	Yes
Application fee	$75

COSTS AND AID

Tuition & Fees

Tuition	$29,984
Cost of books	$800
Fees	$4,450

Financial Aid

% students receiving aid	80
Average grant	$3,000
Average loan	$15,000
Average debt	$75,000

*Figures based on total enrollment

University of North Carolina at Chapel Hill

SCHOOL OF MEDICINE

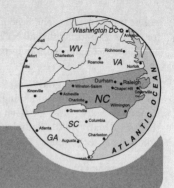

CB#7000 130 MacNider Hall, Chapel Hill, NC 27599-7000
Admission: 919-962-8331
Email: admissions@med.unc.edu • Internet: www.med.unc.edu

The University of North Carolina School of Medicine prepares students for the broad range of professional activities open to physicians. Graduates of the UNC School of Medicine become practitioners in the community, formulate health policy at the highest state and national levels, and make seminal contributions in research, both at the bench and in the clinic. The range and quality of departments and centers within the School of Medicine and our close association with other schools, such as the School of Public Health and mission-oriented Centers (e.g., Lineberger Cancer Center, Neuroscience Center) provide students with unusually rich educational opportunities.

Academics

The core curriculum gives students the required comprehensive education before they embark on the next stage of their careers. In addition, many students pursue focused research training in the clinic or at the bench. Research stipends are available through training grants or individual research grants. Students with a particular interest in research may apply for the MSTP-supported M.D./Ph.D. program at UNC. Other students take the opportunity to combine an advanced degree in Public Health, Law, or Business with their medical studies.

Courses in the first two years are graded on an Honors, Pass, Fail basis. Students are required to pass the USMLE Step 1 examination before promotion to the third year and to pass Step 2 before graduation.

BASIC SCIENCES: The first two years are devoted primarily to studying the scientific basis of clinical practice, with emphasis on demonstrating clinical implications and correlation. Clinical instruction begins early in the first year with the two-year course, Medical Practice and the Community (MPAC), in which students have the opportunity to develop the clinical skills (e.g., history-taking, physical examination) and problem-solving abilities needed for the clinical years. MPAC also serves as a forum for discussion of a wide range of crosscutting topics, such as substance abuse, domestic violence, and computing in medicine. Other first-year courses are Biochemistry, Cell Biology, Gross Anatomy, Histology, Immunology, Introduction to Pathology, Medical Embryology, Medical Physiology, Medicine and Society, Microbiology, and Neurobiology. Many of the courses in the second year are organized around the pathophysiology of particular organ systems, such as Cardiovascular, Endocrine, Gastrointestinal, Hematology/Oncology, Neurology and Special Senses, Reproductive Biology, Respiratory, Skin, Musculoskeletal, and Urinary. Closely integrated with the study of particular organ systems are courses in Pathology, Genetics, Humanities and Social Sciences, and Psychiatry.

Throughout the first and second years, students participate in small-group discussions, lectures, labs, clinical practice sessions, and real clinical experiences. The needs of the curriculum are well served by continuous training in information technology coupled with the requirement that each student have a laptop computer. The Health Sciences Library serves the Schools of Dentistry, Medicine, Nursing, Pharmacy, and Public Health and the UNC Hospitals. The library has approximately 300,000 volumes, 4,000 serial titles, and 9,000 audiovisual and microcomputer software programs.

CLINICAL TRAINING: Students rotate through six major clinical disciplines during their third year. These are Medicine (12 weeks), Ob/Gyn (6 weeks), Pediatrics (8 weeks), Family Medicine (6 weeks), Psychiatry (6 weeks), and Surgery (8 weeks). An additional requirement is Life Support Skills (1 week). The purpose of the fourth-year program is to offer a flexible educational experience that can be tailored to the career goals and intellectual interests of each student. Requirements are an Ambulatory Care Selective (4 weeks), an Acting Internship (4 weeks), a Neuroscience Selective (4 weeks), and a Critical Care/Surgery Selective. A total of 28 weeks of electives are required, some of which may be completed at other universities or clinical settings, either in the United States or overseas.

Students

Approximately 90 percent of students are North Carolina residents. The School of Medicine is committed to admitting students who are representative of the diversity of the population of North Carolina. About one-third of entering students have pursued other interests or careers before applying to medical school.

STUDENT LIFE: The School of Medicine is responsive to students' needs and provides a range of support services. Faculty advisors are assigned to entering students and serve as mentors and academic counselors throughout all four years. The School of Medicine has 26 student organizations, including the student body government, student chapters of national medical professional organizations, community-service groups, and special interest groups. Students are particularly active in outreach efforts such as Habitat for Humanity, the Domestic Violence Coalition, and Physicians for Social Responsibility. During the academic year, scheduled events bring faculty, students, families, and the community together. The university offers single-room accommodations for some graduate students in a building near the Medical Center. Other students live off campus in surrounding neighborhoods.

GRADUATES: Among 1999 graduates, 53 percent entered primary care fields, and 32 percent chose post-graduate training programs within North Carolina. Eighty-four percent of the class of 1999 matched with one of their top three choices for residency training.

Admissions

REQUIREMENTS: Prerequisites are eight semester hours of Biology, at least four hours of which must be accompanied by a lab. Students are strongly encouraged to have taken at least one course in molecular and cell biology. Eight semester hours of General Chemistry, Organic Chemistry, and Physics, all with lab, are also required in addition to six semester hours of English. The MCAT is required.

SUGGESTIONS: Preference is given to residents of North Carolina. Thus, successful applicants who are not residents of North Carolina typically have outstanding qualifications.

PROCESS: Approximately 50 percent of AMCAS applicants who are North Carolina residents, and fewer than 10 percent of nonresidents, are sent secondary applications and are invited to interview. Interviews take place between August and March and consist of two sessions with faculty members. On interview day, candidates also meet currently enrolled medical students and tour the campus.

Costs

The estimated first-year cost of living for a single student is about $19,000. This figure covers all expenses other than tuition. Because many components of the curriculum are computer-based, all first-year medical students are required to have their own computer. This expense is included in the first-year budget.

FINANCIAL AID: Financial aid includes school-funded scholarships, school emergency loans, and federally subsidized loans. In part because of extremely low in-state tuition, the school has been able to meet the cost of education for all students.

UNIVERSITY OF NORTH CAROLINA AT CHAPEL HILL

STUDENT BODY

Type	Public
*Enrollment	624
*% male/female	51/49
*% underrepresented minorities	17
# applied (total/out)	5,859/5,153
% interviewed (total/out)	9/5
% accepted (total/out)	NR/NR
% enrolled (total/out)	NR/NR

ADMISSIONS

Average GPA and MCAT Scores

Overall GPA	NR	Science GPA	NR
MCAT Bio	9.30	MCAT Phys	9.10
MCAT Verbal	9.80	MCAT Essay	NR

Score Release Policy

The school has not responded to our inquiry regarding withheld MCAT scores. Therefore, we advise caution. Contact the Admissions Office before withholding any scores.

Application Information

Regular application	11/15
Regular notification	10/15 until filled
Early application	6/1–8/1
Early notification	10/1
Admissions may be deferred?	Yes
AMCAS application accepted?	Yes
Interview required?	Yes
Application fee	$55

COSTS AND AID

Tuition & Fees

Tuition (in/out)	$2,502/$26,500
Cost of books	NR
Fees	$791

Financial Aid

% students receiving aid	NR
Average grant	NR
Average loan	NR
Average debt	NR

*Figures based on total enrollment

UNIVERSITY OF NORTH DAKOTA
SCHOOL OF MEDICINE AND HEALTH SCIENCES

501 North Columbia Road, Box 9037, Grand Forks, ND 58202

Admission: 701-777-4221 • Fax: 701-777-4942

Email: jdheit@medicine.nodak.edu • Internet: www.med.und.nodak.edu

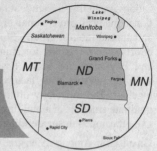

The University of North Dakota is the largest college or university in the Dakotas, Montana, Wyoming, and Western Minnesota. One of the key objectives of its School of Medicine is training primary care physicians to meet the health care demands of the North Dakota population. The State Office of Rural Health is part of the University, providing information and services related to promoting rural health care. The 1998–1999 academic year initiates the school's new "patient-centered learning" (PCL), characterized by early patient contact and small-group instruction. The School of Medicine administers a minority program, Indians Into Medicine (INMED), which offers instruction to Native Americans from around the country who are interested in health care professions and introduces them to the University of North Dakota and the Indian Health Service.

Academics

Pre-clinical instruction takes place at the University of North Dakota campus in Grand Forks, and clinical training takes place throughout the state. After students have been admitted to the M.D. program, they may apply to pursue a joint M.D./Ph.D. program in Anatomy, Biochemistry, Cell Biology, Immunology, Microbiology, Molecular Biology, Pathology, and Pharmacology. Evaluation of students is with ratings of Satisfactory or Unsatisfactory. Both steps of the USMLE must be passed in order to graduate.

BASIC SCIENCES: The basic sciences are taught through a combination of lectures, labs, and small-group sessions. The new curriculum puts significant emphasis on active student participation and early clinical experience. Social science courses that address topics such as statistics, human behavioral patterns, and social issues that are relevant in North Dakota and other rural areas are integrated into the basic science and clinical curriculum throughout the first and second years. The first-year courses are organized into blocks, namely: Functional Biology of Cells and Tissues; Biology of Organ Systems I; Biology of Organ Systems II; and Biology of the Nervous System. These blocks are offered in the morning. The afternoons are reserved for self-study, or Introduction to Patient Care (IPC), which is the clinical component and is also organized into blocks, such as IPC Block I-Interviewing and Professionalism. The same format continues into the second year. Second-year students have the opportunity to take electives, and are required to complete their first clinical rotation, Introduction to Inpatient and Ambulatory Practice of Medicine (3 weeks). Most instruction takes place in the Medical Sciences North buildings, which house administrative offices, classrooms, labs, and the library. The Harley E. French Library of the Health Sciences has over 80,000 books, periodicals, and audiovisual programs. It is fully automated, and offers computers for informational and research purposes. The proximity of basic science instructional facilities to the clinical and research facilities of the North Dakota Medical Center

promote an integrated learning experience during the first two years.

CLINICAL TRAINING: Third-year, required clerkships are Medicine (8 weeks); Surgery (8 weeks); Pediatrics (8 weeks); Ob/Gyn (8 weeks); Psychiatry (8 weeks); Family Medicine (8 weeks); and Clinical Epidemiology, which is taken throughout the year. During the third and fourth years, students train at regional sites in Bismarck, Fargo, Minot, and Grand Forks. Each site has a campus, is affiliated with from 10 to 22 hospitals, and provides health care services to anywhere from nine to 18 counties. The fourth year is reserved for electives. Fourth-year students train at sites throughout the state, including community hospitals, clinics that are part of the Indian Health Service, and physicians' offices. The University of North Dakota's Center for Rural Health focuses on policy analysis and research on rural health care delivery at the state, regional, and national level.

Students

Most students are North Dakota residents, though five to six in each class may be from other Western states. Up to seven students in each class are Native American, admitted as part of INMED. In total, underrepresented minorities account for about 17 percent of the student body. About 30 percent of an entering class is composed of older students who took time off between college and medical school. Class size is 57.

STUDENT LIFE: Grand Forks is a community of 50,000 people, located in the Red River Valley on the border between North Dakota and Minnesota. The city is affordable and safe, and offers the services that students need. Students have access to the facilities of the greater University, and are encouraged to participate in student organizations, including the local chapters of national medical student organizations. On-campus housing is available, although many students opt to live off campus. Since clinical training takes place around the state, students will experience a variety of living situations throughout their four years.

GRADUATES: Most graduates enter residency programs in primary care fields, and a significant number go on to practice in North Dakota. Post-graduate training programs are offered at all the regional training sites.

Admissions

REQUIREMENTS: State residency is a requirement, with the exception of applicants certified by the Western Interstate Commission for Higher Education (WICHE) and Native Americans who may be admitted through the INMED program. Minnesota residents are also given some consideration. Prerequisite course work is General Chemistry (8 semester hours); Organic/Biochemistry (8 hours); Biology (8 hours); Physics (8 hours); Psychology/Sociology (3 hours); Language Arts (6 hours) and College Algebra (3 hours). A minimum GPA of 3.0 is expected. The MCAT is required, and scores must be no more than three years old. For applicants who have retaken the test, the most recent set of scores is considered.

SUGGESTIONS: Preference is given to students who are broadly educated in the Sciences and Humanities. For students who have been out of college for a period of time, some recent course work is suggested. Computer literacy is also advised. The April, rather than August, MCAT is recommended.

PROCESS: North Dakota does not participate in AMCAS. Applications should be requested from the address listed above. About 40 percent of applicants are invited to interview in December or January. The committee consists of faculty, administrators, community members, practicing physicians, and medical students. After interviewing, candidates are notified of the committee's decision within 4–6 weeks. About 40 percent of interviewees are accepted. Wait-listed candidates are not encouraged to send supplementary information.

Costs

The anticipated yearly cost of living for a single student is about $11,000. This does not include tuition. On such a budget, a student may live off campus and maintain a car.

FINANCIAL AID: Each year, several full-tuition, merit-based scholarships are offered. Other assistance is need- and/or merit-based, in the form of loans, scholarships, and grants.

UNIVERSITY OF NORTH DAKOTA

STUDENT BODY

Type	Public
*Enrollment	230
*% male/female	55/45
*% underrepresented minorities	17
# applied (total/out)	306/152
% interviewed (total/out)	50/16
% accepted (total/out)	19/10
% enrolled (total/out)	87/13
Average age	25

ADMISSIONS

Average GPA and MCAT Scores

Overall GPA	3.63	Science GPA	NR
MCAT Bio	9.4	MCAT Phys	9.1
MCAT Verbal	9.0	MCAT Essay	O

Score Release Policy
The school has not responded to our inquiry regarding withheld MCAT scores. Therefore, we advise caution. Contact the Admissions Office before withholding any scores.

Application Information

Regular application	11/1
Regular notification	12/15 until filled
†Transfers accepted?	No
Admissions may be deferred?	Yes
AMCAS application accepted?	No
Interview required?	Yes
Application fee	$35

COSTS AND AID

Tuition & Fees

Tuition (in/out)	$10,995/$29,249
Cost of books	$2,250
Fees	$793

Financial Aid

% students receiving aid	98
Average grant	$1,000
Average loan	$25,000
Average debt	NR

† Some very limited consideration under extenuating circumstances. (Must be a ND resident.)

*Figures based on total enrollment

NORTHEASTERN OHIO UNIVERSITIES
COLLEGE OF MEDICINE

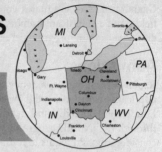

PO Box 95, Rootstown, OH 44272-0095
Admission: 330-325-6270 • Fax: 800-686-2511
Email: admission@neoucom.edu • Internet: www.neoucom.edu

Northeastern Ohio Universities College of Medicine (NEOUCOM) is a state-supported institution that capitalizes on the strengths, assets, and facilities of three major public universities—the University of Akron, Kent State University, and Youngstown State University. Most students enter NEOUCOM through a combined B.S./M.D. program organized with one of these three universities. NEOUCOM and its clinical affiliates provide health-related services to 17 counties in Northeastern Ohio. Although NEOUCOM is focused on primary care and preparing physicians to practice medicine at the community level, it is also involved in biomedical and behavioral science research.

Academics

While most students participate in the 6- or 7-year B.S./M.D. program, about 15–25 students each year enter the four-year M.D. program. A combined M.D./Ph.D. program is offered in collaboration with either Kent State or the University of Akron, leading to the doctorate degree in biomedical engineering or a number of medically related science fields. A Summer Fellowship Program provides a stipend to selected medical students who undertake research or clinical education projects related to community health. Medical students are evaluated with marks of Honors, Satisfactory, Conditional-Unsatisfactory, or Unsatisfactory for most courses. Passing the USMLE Step 1 is a requirement for promotion to year three, and passing Step 2 is a requirement for graduation.

BASIC SCIENCES: Basic sciences are taught primarily in a lecture/lab format, although some courses also utilize small-group discussions and tutorials. On average, students are in class or other scheduled sessions for 32 hours per week. First-year courses are Human Anatomy/Embryology, Microscopic Anatomy, Neurobiology, Biochemistry and Molecular Pathology, Physiology, Behavioral Science, Microbiology and Infection/Immunology, General Pathology, Medical Genetics, and Problem-based Learning. Second-year courses are Introduction to Clinical Medicine (ICM), Systemic Pathology, Pharmacology, Principles of Medical Sciences, and Radiology. The ICM course focuses on clinical problems, fundamental doctor-patient communication skills, the physical examination, and clinical evaluation. NEOUCOM's approach to instruction in this transitional year allows for extensive clinical exposure and patient contact. As part of ICM, students spend three days per week in family practice centers. Students benefit from academic support and counseling services offered by the Office of Student Services. The Oliver Ocasek Regional Medical Information Center, on the Rootstown campus, houses more than 91,000 books and journals in addition to computerized information systems. The Center is electronically linked to libraries in the teaching hospitals and consortium universities.

CLINICAL TRAINING: Third-year required rotations are Internal Medicine (10 weeks); Surgery (10 weeks); General Pediatrics (8 weeks); Ob/Gyn (8 weeks); Psychiatry (6 weeks); and Family Medicine (6 weeks). During the fourth year, additional requirements are Primary care Preceptorship (4 weeks); Medical Humanities (4 weeks); Community Medicine Clerkship (4 weeks); and 20 weeks of electives. Training takes place at affiliated hospitals: Lodi Community Hospital; Wadsworth-Rittman Hospital; Akron General Medical Center; Barberton Citizens Hospital; Children's Hospital Medical Center; Edwin Shaw Hospital; Summa Health System; Robinson Memorial Hospital; Hillside Rehabilitation Hospital; Trumbull Memorial Hospital; St. Elizabeth Health Center; Western Reserve Care System; Salem Community Hospital; Aultman Hospital; Massillon Psychiatric Center; and Columbia Mercy Medical Center. In addition, students train at community-based centers that are part of the Area Health Education Center Program.

Students

Approximately 95 percent of students are Ohio residents. About 105 students in each class are admitted through the B.S./M.D. program, and up to 25 are admitted through the traditional route. Although most entering students are in their early twenties, there are a few older or nontraditional students in each class. Underrepresented minorities account for about 4 percent of the student body.

STUDENT LIFE: Rootstown is a small town located about fifteen miles east of Akron. On the Medical School campus are recreation and exercise centers, student lounges, a picnic area, and tennis, basketball, and volleyball courts. Student groups include chapters of national medical student organizations, groups focused on professional interests, student-to- student support groups, and a recreation club. On-campus housing, including residence halls and apartments, is available on all three campuses.

GRADUATES: NEOUCOM graduates usually score well above the national average on the USMLE. Of the 1,350 graduates currently in residency or practice, 55 percent have remained in Ohio. About half of graduates enter primary care fields.

Admissions

REQUIREMENTS: Prerequisites are one year each of Organic Chemistry and Physics, although success on the MCAT probably requires preparation in Biology and General Chemistry as well. The MCAT is required, and scores must be no more than two years old. For applicants who have retaken the exam, the most recent set of scores is considered. Thus, there is no advantage to withholding scores.

SUGGESTIONS: Ohio residents are given strong preference in the admissions process, and slight preference is given to graduates of consortium schools. Highly qualified applicants are encouraged to apply to the early decision program. Beyond requirements, recommended course work includes Biochemistry, Calculus, Community Health, Embryology, General Biology, General Chemistry, Humanities, Microbiology, Molecular Biology, Physiology, Psychology, Sociology, and Statistics. For applicants who have taken time off after college, some recent course work is advised.

PROCESS: High school students interested in the combined B.S./M.D. program apply in the fall of the senior year to NEUOCOM, and complete a condensed undergraduate experience at Kent State, University of Akron, or Youngstown State before arriving at the Rootstown campus. As a result of attrition from this program, a limited number of seats are available for college graduates interested in the four-year M.D. program. These applicants must apply through AMCAS. About 30 percent of AMCAS applicants are sent secondary applications. Of those returning secondaries, about 40 percent are interviewed between November and March. On interview day, candidates receive one interview with a panel of members of the Admissions Committee, a tour of the campus, lunch with current students, and a group informational session. Of interviewed candidates, about 10 percent are accepted on a rolling basis. Wait-listed candidates may update their files with transcripts.

Costs

The estimated yearly cost of living for a single medical student is $11,000. This budget allows for on- or off-campus housing. Most students own a car. B.S./M.S. students save money by completing both degrees in six rather than eight years.

FINANCIAL AID: Financial assistance is available through loan, grant, and scholarship programs. While most aid is awarded on the basis of need, NEUOCOM offers some merit scholarships. In exchange for a service commitment, students interested in practicing in medically underserved areas of Ohio may be eligible for state tuition remission programs.

NORTHEASTERN OHIO UNIVERSITIES

STUDENT BODY

Type	Public
*Enrollment	422
*% male/female	56/44
*% underrepresented minorities	4
# applied (total/out)	1,104/325
% interviewed (total/out)	10/2
% accepted (total/out)	NR/NR
% enrolled (total/out)	NR/NR
Average age	22

ADMISSIONS

Average GPA and MCAT Scores

Overall GPA	3.60	Science GPA	3.46
MCAT Bio	9.30	MCAT Phys	8.90
MCAT Verbal	9.20	MCAT Essay	NR

Score Release Policy

The school has not responded to our inquiry regarding withheld MCAT scores. Therefore, we advise caution. Contact the Admissions Office before withholding any scores.

Application Information

Regular application	11/1
Regular notification	10/15 until filled
Early application	6/1–8/1
Early notification	10/1
Transfers accepted?	Yes
Admissions may be deferred?	No
AMCAS application accepted?	Yes
Interview required?	Yes
Application fee	$30

COSTS AND AID

Tuition & Fees

Tuition (in/out)	$11,244/$22,488
Cost of books	$1,000
Fees	$564

Financial Aid

% students receiving aid	80
Average grant	$1,000
Average loan	$15,000
Average debt	$67,300

*Figures based on total enrollment

NORTHWESTERN UNIVERSITY
MEDICAL SCHOOL

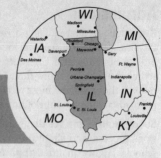

303 East Chicago Avenue, Room 1-606, Chicago, IL 60611
Admission: 312-503-8206 • Email: med-admissions@northwestern.edu
Internet: www.nums.northwestern.edu

Northwestern University Medical School is located in the heart of Chicago, steps away from the Magnificent Mile and Lake Michigan. Northwestern has adopted a basic science curriculum that emphasizes independent and problem-based learning and is designed to produce responsible physicians with a broad understanding of medicine. Northwestern is a private university that attracts students from all regions of the country.

Academics

The medical curriculum retains the best aspects of traditional medical education and incorporates innovative, interactive methods designed for the independent adult learner. Students may benefit from clinical exposure that begins on day one. Although most students complete studies in four years, some enter joint-degree programs such as the M.D./M.P.H. and M.D./M.M. (Master of Management from the Kellogg Graduate School of Management) offered in conjunction with other graduate and professional schools at Northwestern. Qualified students interested in careers in medical research can pursue a Ph.D. along with the M.D. in the Medical Scientist Training Program. A Medical Student Research Program facilitates the arrangement of post–first-year summer research experiences. Students are also encouraged to seek extended, year-long research opportunities.

BASIC SCIENCES: The first- and second-year curriculum is composed of four major courses, each presented in a series of discreet, topically focused units. Each course and nearly every unit is interdisciplinary and draws faculty from a number of departments. Two courses are in the basic medical sciences. Each involves approximately 10 hours of lecture per week for the entire academic year, complemented by problem-based learning sessions, laboratories, and small-group discussions and tutorials. Structure-Function, the first-year course, begins with a review of cell and molecular biology, genetics, and signal transduction, then addresses gross and microscopic anatomy, biochemistry, and physiology in a consecutive sequence of organ systems. The Scientific Basis of Medicine in the second year begins with an overview of immunology, microbiology, and infectious diseases and then details the pathology, pathophysiology, and pharmacology specific to each organ system. The Medical Decision-Making course occupies three short blocks of time: the initial week of the first year, one week later in the first year, and the final portion of the second year. This innovative course allows students to develop the knowledge and skills in information management, epidemiology and biostatistics, and clinical problem solving essential to the contemporary practice of medicine. The Patient, Physician, and Society course is devoted to the development of clinical

skills and professional perspectives, and provides each student the opportunity to develop mentoring relationships with a variety of faculty preceptors. The class is divided into four "colleges," each led by an experienced clinician. Colleges meet two afternoons per week throughout the first two years. One afternoon offers learning experiences centered around clinical skills development and the provision of an integrated biopsychosocial perspective on illness and patient care. The other afternoon's course sequence addresses medical ethics and humanities, public health, and health policy. Activities in both afternoon tracks incorporate health promotion and disease prevention as a guiding principle of the practice of medicine.

CLINICAL TRAINING: The third year consists of 49 weeks of required clerkships. Students gain experience in: Medicine (12 weeks), Surgery (6 weeks), surgical specialties (6 weeks), Pediatrics (6 weeks), Ob/Gyn (6 weeks), Psychiatry (4 weeks), Neurology (4 weeks), and Primary Care (4 weeks). A one-week Introduction to Clinical Clerkships provides orientation to the clerkship teaching format. During the fourth year, students complete a six-week acting internship in Medicine, Pediatrics, or Surgery and a two-week clerkship in Physical Medicine and Rehabilitation. The remainder of the fourth year is elective. The majority of clinical rotations are taught at Northwestern Memorial Hospital, one of the major tertiary care facilities in Chicago. Other affiliated health care centers include Catholic Health Partners, the Rehabilitation Institute of Chicago, VA Chicago Healthcare System—Lakeside Division, Evanston Northwestern Healthcare, and Children's Memorial Hospital.

Students

Northwestern draws students from all regions of the country. Students enrolled in the Northwestern University Honors Program in Medical Education constitute approximately on-fourth of the class. These students enter medical school after completion of three years of undergraduate education at Northwestern. About 8 percent of students are underrepresented minorities. Though the Honors Program lowers the mean age of entering students, there is a wide age range, and in each class there is a contingent of students in their late 20s, 30s, and older. Class size is 170.

STUDENT LIFE: Northwestern students spend less time in class than students at many other schools and more time in outside preparation and group and independent learning. Students are also encouraged to pursue supplemental academic interests, community service endeavors, and other activities. The school's location, in one of the most vibrant cities in the country, is an important asset. A good public transportation system makes Chicago's museums, shopping areas, parks, restaurants, clubs, theaters, and other attractions easily accessible. About half the medical students live in on-campus housing facilities, located within walking distance of the school and Northwestern Memorial Hospital; others live in a variety of neighborhoods throughout the city.

GRADUATES: Northwestern graduates are accepted to competitive residencies throughout the nation. Today there are more than 12,000 medical school alumni living in the United States and around the world. Northwestern alumni are particularly well represented in academic medicine.

Admissions

REQUIREMENTS: Minimum requirements are one year each of Chemistry, Organic Chemistry, Physics, and Biology, all with associated labs. The MCAT is required, and scores should be from within the past three years. Clinical experience is also required.

SUGGESTIONS: Research experience is recommended. A well-rounded undergraduate background is important, and applicants who have majored in nonscience areas are appreciated.

PROCESS: Approximately 70 percent of AMCAS applicants are sent a supplementary application. Of those returning secondaries, about 10 percent are offered interviews between October and March. The interview day begins with a group interview that demonstrates interpersonal skills among other qualities. The group interview is among three applicants and a three-person team chosen from faculty, current students, and administrators. It is followed by a short individual interview, tour, lunch, and financial aid session. Notification of committee decision usually occurs within a few weeks of the interview. Applicants are either accepted, declined, or placed on the alternate list. About 50 percent of the interviewed candidates are ultimately accepted. Alternate candidates may send additional material that serves both to update their files and to express interest in attending Northwestern. An alternate route to admission is the Northwestern University Honors Program in Medical Education. This combined B.A./M.D. program targets highly qualified high-school students.

Costs

In addition to tuition, the anticipated first-year expenditure for a single student is about $13,000. This allows for on-campus housing and use of public transportation. Tuition is charged for twelve quarters. Up to an additional two quarters of clinical or research electives may be added for no additional tuition.

FINANCIAL AID: Financial need is determined from the income and assets of a student and those of his or her parents. The majority of aid comes in the form of loans and in-school subsidies. A number of need-based scholarships are available for entering students. In addition, at the time of graduation, those students whose need-based borrowing has been greatest over their four-year medical education share a sizeable pool of scholarships to bring the indebtedness of each to as low a common level as possible.

NORTHWESTERN UNIVERSITY

STUDENT BODY

Type	Private
*Enrollment	686
*% male/female	56/44
*% underrepresented minorities	8
# applied (total/out)	7,803/6,835
% interviewed (total/out)	8/7
% accepted (total/out)	3/3
% enrolled (total/out)	35/54
Average age	23

ADMISSIONS

Average GPA and MCAT Scores

Overall GPA	3.7	Science GPA	3.6
MCAT Bio	11.2	MCAT Phys	11.4
MCAT Verbal	10.2	MCAT Essay	P

Score Release Policy

Interview decisions will not be made without MCAT scores.

Application Information

Regular application	10/15
Regular notification	12/17
Transfers accepted?	Yes
Admissions may be deferred?	Yes
AMCAS application accepted?	Yes
Interview required?	Yes
Application fee	$65

COSTS AND AID

Tuition & Fees

Tuition	$30,417
Cost of books	$2,199
Fees	$1,311

Financial Aid

% students receiving aid	70
Average grant	NR
Average loan	NR
Average debt	NR

*Figures based on total enrollment

OHIO STATE UNIVERSITY
COLLEGE OF MEDICINE AND PUBLIC HEALTH

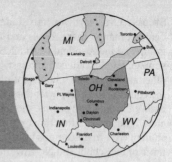

270A Meiling Hall, Columbus, OH 43210-1238
Admission: 614-292-7137 • Fax: 614-292-1544
Email: admiss-med@osu.edu • Internet: www.med.ohio-state.edu

The Ohio State University is the major comprehensive academic institution in the State of Ohio. As Ohio's land-grant institution, it serves the entire state through its central campus in Columbus, four regional campuses, educational telecommunications programs, Agriculture and Technical Institute, cooperative extension service, and health care programs. Its fundamental mission—teaching, research, and public service—is designed to enhance the quality of human life through the development of the individual capacity for enlightened understanding, thought, and action. In addition to the College of Medicine and Public Health, the Medical Center complex includes Colleges of Optometry, Dentistry, Pharmacy, and Nursing. The complex also includes a School of Allied Medical Professions, School of Public Health, and School of Biomedical Science consisting of six departments: Anatomy and Medical Education, Molecular Virology, Immunology and Medical Genetics, Neuroscience, Physiology and Cell Biology, Pharmacology, and Molecular and Cellular Biochemistry, and numerous other hospitals and health science facilities. The College of Medicine and Public Health consists of 15 clinical departments, including Anesthesiology, Emergency Medicine, Family Medicine, Internal Medicine, Neurology, Obstetrics and Gynecology, Ophthalmology, Orthopedics, Otolaryngology, Pathology, Pediatrics, Physical Medicine and Rehabilitation, Psychiatry, Radiology, and Surgery. The Health Sciences Library is one of the 14 campus libraries. It contains approximately 220,00 books, receives 2,300 journals, and is fully computerized.

Academics

All students begin with a 12-week course in Human Anatomy. This includes cadaver dissection, cross-sectional anatomy, multimedia for self-directed learning, imaging technology, and clinical correlation's. Students also initiate their study of the Medical Humanities and Behavioral Sciences during this period. After the conclusion of the first 12-week academic experience, students enter one of three pre-clinical pathways: Lecture Discussion, Problem-Based Learning, or Independent Study. A program emphasizing a Family Medicine enrichment experience is also available. Passage of Step 1 of the USMLE is required for progression to year three. A hallmark of Ohio State's M.D. curriculum is the opportunity for students to select experiences that fit with their individual learning styles and long-term career goals. The curriculum provides a variety of analytical and managerial skills specifically designed to be applicable in the health services setting.

BASIC SCIENCES: Joint-degree programs include three options. The Medical Scientist Program (MSP), a 7-year combined M.D./Ph.D. degree for highly qualified and motivated students who have excellent academic backgrounds, motivation for a career in academic medicine, and a commitment to or demonstrated aptitude for a research career. The Master of Public Health (M.P.H.), a combined 5-year program allows students to simultaneously earn the M.D. and M.P.H. degrees, with instruction in Epidemiology/Biometrics, Environmental Health Sciences, Health Services Management/Policy, and Health Promotion. The Master of Health Administration (M.H.A.) is a joint 5-year program that allows students to simultaneously earn the M.D. and M.H.A. degrees.

CLINICAL TRAINING: Clinical rotations begin with the Introduction to Clinical Medicine (ICM). The goal of this clerkship is to enable students to better use their major and elective experiences to become excellent physicians. The third-year curriculum is delivered in clinical blocks— Ambulatory and Adult Emphasis (Block I); Surgery and Ob/Gyn (Block II); Child and Adolescent Medicine (Block III); and Neurology and Psychology (Block IV). Curriculum in the fourth year includes five 4-week experiences called the Differentiation of Care Selectives (DOCS). DOC 1 is the Undifferentiated Patient; DOC 2 is the Differentiated Ambulatory Patient; DOC 3 is the Chronic Care Patient; DOC 4 is the Acute Medical Care Patient, and DOC 5 is the Acute Surgical Care Patient. Other fourth-year requirements include the Dean's Colloquium, other elective opportunities, and vacation allowances. Training occurs in 24 affiliated hospitals, including the University Hospital, The Cleveland Clinic, and The Arthur G. James/ Richard J. Solove Cancer Hospital and Research Institute. Passage of Step 2 of the USMLE is required for graduation.

Students

The class profile for 1999 reflects a class size of 210 entering students, with 81 percent from Ohio, 40 percent women, and 7 percent underrepresented minority students. The average GPA was 3.59 with an MCAT average above 10.

STUDENT LIFE: There are currently 37 medical student organizations. Medical students have access to all of the resources and facilities of the University. Campus and city bus transportation is free with the presentation of student ID. Computerized housing opportunities are available free of charge through the Off-Campus Student Services. University graduate residence halls and family housing are also available.

Graduates: PGY-1 Match Results for 2000 reflect 60 percent of the graduating class plan to enter primary care residencies, and 47 percent matched with Ohio residency programs.

Admissions

Requirements: One year of Biology with labs, Chemistry, Organic Chemistry with labs, and Physics are required. Also recommended are courses in Biochemistry and Molecular Genetics.

Application through AMCAS and MCAT test with scores that are no more than 3 years old are required.

Suggestions: The Admissions Committee evaluates candidates according to competitive standards. Applicants are judged on the basis of academic performance as well as personal qualities such as integrity, leadership, and interpersonal skills. Clinically related experiences, as well as research positions, are encouraged.

Process: Applications are reviewed upon receipt from AMCAS. Competitive applicants are sent secondary applications. Approximately 680 applicants are interviewed between September and April. On interview day, applicants tour the Medical Center and have lunch with current medical students.

Costs

Ohio resident tuition for 1999 was $12,414. Estimated off-campus living expenses with a roommate are $916 per month (rent, utilities, telephone, groceries, laundry, clothing, transportation, insurance, with approximately $100 for miscellaneous expenses).

Financial Aid: Although most assistance is based on need, some merit scholarships are also awarded each year. Need is determined through the FAFSA. Parental financial disclosure is required for most grants and scholarships. Students have a variety of opportunities to explore their research interests through Roessler Scholarships, pathology fellowships, internal medicine fellowships, student research assistantships, as well as the student research honorary organization, the Landacre Society.

OHIO STATE UNIVERSITY

STUDENT BODY

Type	Public
*Enrollment	852
*% male/female	62/38
*% underrepresented minorities	7
# applied (total/out)	3,308/2,104
% interviewed (total/out)	21/11
% accepted (total/out)	12/6
% enrolled (total/out)	5/2
Average age	21

ADMISSIONS

Average GPA and MCAT Scores

Overall GPA	3.60	Science GPA	3.54
MCAT Bio	10.40	MCAT Phys	10.40
MCAT Verbal	9.76	MCAT Essay	P

Score Release Policy

Applications with MCAT scores that have been withheld or scores three years of prior to intended date of entry are closed.

Application Information

Regular application	11/1
Regular notification	10/15 until filled
Early application	6/1–8/1
Early notification	10/1
Transfers accepted?	Yes
Admissions may be deferred?	Yes
AMCAS application accepted?	Yes
Interview required?	Yes
Application fee	$30

COSTS AND AID

Tuition & Fees

Tuition (in/out)	$12,414/$34,380
Cost of books	$1,200
Fees	$357

Financial Aid

% students receiving aid	80
Average grant	$2,000
Average loan	$17,000
Average debt	$63,000

*Figures based on total enrollment

MEDICAL COLLEGE OF OHIO

3045 Arlington Avenue, Toledo, OH 43614
Admission: 419-383-4229 • Fax: 419-383-4005
Internet: www.mco.edu

The Medical College of Ohio (MCO) encompasses Schools of Medicine, Allied Health, Nursing, and Graduate Studies. The student body is cohesive and supportive, and the School of Medicine emphasizes positive interaction between faculty and students. Both faculty and students contribute to the greater community and benefit from the friendly environment of Toledo and the surrounding areas. Primary care is emphasized.

Academics

Although most students follow a four-year program, some educationally disadvantaged students enter the Flexible Curriculum Program, which permits extension of the M.D. curriculum over a five-year period. Joint-degree programs offered in conjunction with affiliated schools are available, including the M.D./M.S. and M.D./Ph.D. through which a doctorate degree may be earned in the following areas: Anatomy, Biochemistry, Microbiology, Neuroscience, Pathology, Pharmacology, Physiology, and numerous other fields. Medical students are evaluated with ratings of Honors, High Pass, Pass, and Fail. Passing Step 1 of the USMLE is a requirement for promotion to year three. In order to graduate, a score on Step 2 must be recorded.

BASIC SCIENCES: The first two years are devoted to an integrated approach to the basic sciences, behavioral sciences, primary care preceptorships, introductory clinical experiences, and problem-based learning (PBL) for all students. First-year courses are the following: Cellular and Molecular Biology; Human Structure and Development; Neuroscience and Behavioral Science; Integrated Pathophysiology I (PBL); and Physician, Patient, and Society I. During the first year, students are in class for about 30 hours per week, most of which is either lecture or lab periods. Second-year courses are Introduction to Primary Care; Immunity and Infection; Organ Systems; Integrated Pathophysiology II (PBL); and Physician, Patient, and Society II. Physician, Patient, and Society includes Introduction to Primary Care; Introduction to Clinical Medicine; and a series of courses that address topics in medical ethics, managed care, medical decision-making, nutrition, geriatrics, and substance abuse disorders. The ICM course covers practical skills such as taking patient histories and conducting physical examinations. It also serves as a forum for correlating basic science principles with clinical case studies and for discussing ethical issues related to practicing medicine. Second-year students are in class for about 20 hours per week. Basic science instruction takes place in the Health Sciences Teaching and Laboratory Building and the Health Education Building. The Mulford Library holds 125,000 volumes and 1,800 journals and, along with the Computer Learning Resource Center, provides educational and informational resources to students.

CLINICAL TRAINING: Third-year required clerkships are the following: Medicine (12 weeks); Surgery (12 weeks); Pediatrics (6 weeks); Psychiatry (6 weeks); Family Medicine (6 weeks); and Ob/Gyn (6 weeks). During the fourth year, one Basic Science Selective (4 weeks) and one Neurology clerkship (4 weeks) are required. The remaining 28 weeks are reserved for elective study. Three teaching hospitals operate on campus, the Medical College of Ohio Hospital (258 beds), Coghlin Rehabilitation Hospital (36 beds), and Lenore W. and Marvin S. Kobacker Center (25 beds, a children's psychiatric hospital). Other associated hospitals include St. Vincent Mercy Medical Center; The Toledo Hospital/Children's Medical Center of Northwest Ohio; Flower Hospital; and Northwestern Psychiatric Hospital. Through the Area Health Education Center clerkships, MCO students also have the opportunity to train in rural and inner-city communities.

Students

At least 80 percent of students are Ohio residents although many attended undergraduate institutions outside of the state. Underrepresented minorities, mostly African Americans, account for approximately 10 percent of the student body. Among entrants, there are significant numbers of older individuals, some of whom are in their late thirties and early forties. Typically, about 80 percent of medical students were science majors in college.

STUDENT LIFE: In addition to providing academic resources, the Office of Student Affairs supports students in and outside of the classroom, organizing events such as an annual orientation for incoming students. There are countless student associations, ranging from one that administers a community care clinic, to a student-to-student support group, to organizations focused on personal, recreational, religious, cultural, and professional interests. MCO is situated on 475 acres of land, with ponds, streams, trees, and open areas. The campus offers extensive athletic and recreational facilities. Major attractions in Toledo are easily reached on public transportation and include riverside restaurants and bars, museums, parks with golf courses and other facilities, a zoo, theaters, and shopping areas. Further distraction is found in Detroit, Cincinnati, Pittsburgh, Cleveland, and Chicago all of which are in driving distance of MCO. Students live off campus, usually in the surrounding residential neighborhood.

Graduates: About 40 percent of graduates go on to practice in Ohio. In recent years, about 60 percent of graduates have entered primary care fields.

Admissions

Requirements: Prerequisites are one year each of Biology, General Chemistry, Organic Chemistry, Physics, Math, and English. All science courses must include labs. The MCAT is required. For applicants who have retaken the exam, the best set of scores is weighted most heavily. Thus, withholding scores is not advantageous.

Suggestions: As a state-supported institution, MCO gives preference to Ohio residents. Additional preparation in Biology is recommended as are courses in the Humanities and Social Sciences. For students who have been out of school for a significant period of time, some recent course work is advised. Community service and medically related experience involving patient contact are both considered valuable.

Process: About 75 percent of AMCAS applicants are sent secondary applications. Of those returning secondaries, about 25 percent of Ohio residents and 10 percent of nonresidents are invited to interview. Interviews take place between October and April and consist of two hour-long sessions each with a faculty member, medical student, or school administrator. Also on interview day, candidates tour the campus, hear group informational sessions, and have the opportunity to meet informally with current students. About one-third of interviewees are accepted, with notification occurring throughout the year. Wait-listed candidates may send additional information, such as transcripts and test scores, to update their files.

Costs

The estimated yearly cost of living for a single student is about $13,000. This budget allows for off-campus housing and car maintenance.

Financial Aid: Most financial assistance is awarded on the basis of need, as determined by federal and other forms. A few merit-based scholarships are offered each year.

MEDICAL COLLEGE OF OHIO

STUDENT BODY

Type	Public
*Enrollment	565
*% male/female	70/30
*% underrepresented minorities	10
# applied (total/out)	3,698/2,472
% interviewed (total/out)	NR/NR
% accepted (total/out)	NR/NR
% enrolled (total/out)	NR/NR
Average age	23

ADMISSIONS

Average GPA and MCAT Scores

Overall GPA	3.55	Science GPA	3.48
MCAT Bio	9.48	MCAT Phys	9.34
MCAT Verbal	9.42	MCAT Essay	NR

Score Release Policy

The school has not responded to our inquiry regarding withheld MCAT scores. Therefore, we advise caution. Contact the Admissions Office before withholding any scores.

Application Information

Regular application	11/1
Regular notification	10/15 until filled
Early application	6/1–8/1
Early notification	10/1
Transfers accepted?	Yes
Admissions may be deferred?	Yes
AMCAS application accepted?	Yes
Interview required?	Yes
Application fee	$30

COSTS AND AID

Tuition & Fees

Tuition (in/out)	$10,512/$22,966
Cost of books	$741
Fees	$2,054

Financial Aid

% students receiving aid	90
Average grant	$6,000
Average loan	$18,500
Average debt	NR

*Figures based on total enrollment

UNIVERSITY OF OKLAHOMA

COLLEGE OF MEDICINE

PO Box 26901, Oklahoma City, OK 73190
Admission: 405-271-2331 • Fax: 405-271-3032
Email: Dotty-Shaw@ouhsc.edu • Internet: www.ouhsc.edu

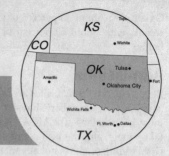

The College of Medicine, six other colleges including a College of Public Health, four hospitals, two research institutes, and the state's Public Health Department comprise the University of Oklahoma Health Science Center (OUHSC), which is geared toward meeting the health care needs of the state's population. The system features two geographic sites—one in Oklahoma City, one in Tulsa. The College of Medicine also benefits from a large network of affiliated clinical providers and research institutes. OUHSC emphasizes patient care, and its curriculum involves student-patient interaction starting with the first week of classes. Oklahoma City, with a population of more than one million, has extensive resources and attractions.

Academics

All students spend their first two years on the Oklahoma City campus. On completion of year two, about 25 percent of the class enter clinical rotations at sites affiliated with the University of Oklahoma's Tulsa campus. Tulsa is particularly well-equipped for primary care and community-based medical instruction. Qualified students may pursue the joint M.D./Ph.D. degree from any graduate department. OUHSC also offers a joint M.D./Master's in Public Health and Health Administration. Medical students are evaluated on an A–F scale. They must pass Step 1 of the USMLE in order to be promoted to year three, and graduates must take, but not necessarily pass, Step 2 to earn their diploma.

BASIC SCIENCES: Basic sciences are taught through lectures, labs, computer-assisted instruction, and small group discussions. During the first two years, students are in class or other scheduled sessions for 20–25 hours per week, allowing ample time for self-directed study. First-year courses are Gross Anatomy, Embryology, Microanatomy, Medical Molecular Genetics, Biochemistry/Molecular Biology, Physiology, Neuroscience, Human Behavior I, Medical Statistics, and Principles of Clinical Medicine I. Second-year courses are Microbiology and Immunology, Principles of Clinical Medicine II, Human Behavior II, Pharmacology, Introduction to Human Illness, and Professional Ethics and Professionalism. Basic sciences are taught in the Basic Sciences Education Building, which, in addition to classrooms and labs, houses a study area. The Robert Bird Library contains more than 212,000 books, journals, and audiovisuals and has two special collections—the Indian Health Collection and the Rare Book Collection. Students can access a number of online catalogs and databases from the library.

CLINICAL TRAINING: Third-year rotations are Medicine (8 weeks); Surgery (8 weeks); Ob/Gyn (6 weeks); Psychiatry (6 weeks); Pediatrics (6 weeks); Family Medicine (4 weeks); Specialty Elective (4 weeks); and Neuroscience (2 weeks). Fourth-year clerkships are: Otorhinolaryngology (2 weeks); Dermatology (2 weeks); Ophthalmology (1 week); Adult Ambulatory Medicine (4 weeks); and a Rural Preceptorship (4 weeks). Clinical affiliates and training sites are OUHSC; Oklahoma Medical Center; Department of Veterans Affairs Medical Center; Oklahoma Medical Research Foundation; Oklahoma City Clinic; Oklahoma Allergy Clinic; Columbia/Presbyterian Hospital; Dean A. McGee Eye Institute; Oklahoma Blood Institute; State Medical Examiner's Office; Department of Mental Health; and Oklahoma State Department of Health. At the Tulsa campus, clinical facilities contain more than 2,000 patient beds. There are also family medicine training sites in Enid and Bartlesville, and additional rural training sites are currently being developed. The Oklahoma Telemedicine Network is among the largest medical communications systems in the world, successfully bringing information and expertise to rural physicians, clinics, and hospitals.

Students

At least 85 percent of students must be Oklahoma residents, but generally only 5 or 10 students are from out of state. There is a wide age range among incoming students, and students older than 35 are not unusual. About 26 percent of students are underrepresented minorities, most of whom are Native Americans. Class size is 150.

STUDENT LIFE: Students are cohesive, both inside and outside of the classroom. A student-run note service is one example of cooperation among students. The OUHSC Student Center facilitates both social and academic interaction. It features an exercise room, study areas, computers, a food service court and common rooms. For a fee, medical students also have access to the recreational center at the nearby Norman campus. Medical students are active in student organizations that offer support and focus on recreational pursuits, professional goals, or community service. Students are eligible for intercollegiate athletic tickets and other University-wide events. Though OUHSC has no campus housing; off-campus housing is affordable and comfortable. University-owned housing for married and single students is available on the Norman campus. Downtown Oklahoma City is 1 mile from the OUHSC campus and offers a range of activities and attractions.

GRADUATES: Typically, about half of graduates enter residencies in Oklahoma. Others are successful in securing positions nationwide. There are about ten OUHSC-affiliated post-graduate programs in Tulsa, and nearly 20 in Oklahoma City.

Admissions

REQUIREMENTS: Prerequisites are General Zoology/Biology with lab (1 semester); Embryology, Genetics, Anatomy, Cellular Biology, or Histology (1 semester); Inorganic Chemistry (1 year); Organic Chemistry (1 year); General Physics (1 year); English (3 semesters), and three semesters of any combination of Sociology; Psychology, Anthropology; Humanities; Philosophy; or Foreign Language. The MCAT is required, and scores must be from after 1991. For applicants who have retaken the exam, the most recent set of scores is considered. Basic computer skills are required.

SUGGESTIONS: Strong preference is given to Oklahoma residents, making competition intense for out-of-state residents. Applicants are encouraged to take additional courses in Social Sciences, Humanities, Fine Arts, Computer Sciences, and English. In addition to academic achievement, a candidate's personality, maturity, and character are evaluated. Admissions decisions are made with recognition of the importance of social and cultural diversity.

PROCESS: All AMCAS applicants receive secondary applications. Of those returning secondaries, about 20 percent are interviewed. Interviews are conducted between November and January, and consist of one session with a panel of three members of the Admissions Committee. On interview day, applicants tour the campus and have the opportunity to meet informally with current students. Of interviewed candidates, about 80 percent (not including wait-listed candidates) are accepted on a rolling basis. Wait-listed candidates may send updated transcripts.

Costs

The anticipated yearly cost of living for a single student is about $12,000. This budget allows for off-campus living and maintenance of a car.

FINANCIAL AID: In addition to Federal loan programs, Oklahoma offers a number of state and institutional financial aid opportunities. Among these are the Regents' Scholarships Fee Waiver program, which provides assistance to underrepresented minority students, and the Rural Medical Education Loan and Scholarship fund, which assists students who commit to practicing in rural, underserved communities.

UNIVERSITY OF OKLAHOMA

STUDENT BODY

Type	Public
*Enrollment	587
*% male/female	59/41
*% underrepresented minorities	26
# applied (total/out)	912/553
% interviewed (total/out)	19/2
% accepted (total/out)	NR/NR
% enrolled (total/out)	53/30

ADMISSIONS

Average GPA and MCAT Scores

Overall GPA	3.59	Science GPA	NR
MCAT Bio	9.00	MCAT Phys	8.80
MCAT Verbal	9.60	MCAT Essay	NR

Score Release Policy

The most recent score is considered for admissions. The applicant must reveal the most recent score, but it is OK not to release earlier scores.

Application Information

Regular application	10/15
Regular notification	12/1 until filled
Early application	8/1
Admissions may be deferred?	No
AMCAS application accepted?	Yes
Interview required?	Yes
Application fee	$50

COSTS AND AID

Tuition & Fees

Tuition (in/out)	$9,552/$23,606
Cost of books	NR
Fees	$636

Financial Aid

% students receiving aid	94
Average grant	NR
Average loan	NR
Average debt	NR

*Figures based on total enrollment

OREGON HEALTH SCIENCES UNIVERSITY
SCHOOL OF MEDICINE

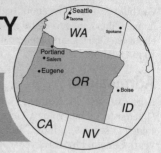

3181 SW Sam Jackson Park Road, Portland, OR 97201
Admission: 503-494-2998 • Fax: 503-494-3400
Internet: www.ohsu.edu/som-Dean/admit.html

Oregon Health Sciences University (OHSU) plays a critical role in health care delivery to Oregon's population and to people throughout the Pacific Northwest. OHSU includes the Schools of Dentistry, Medicine, and Nursing. The School of Medicine is unusually progressive, demonstrated both by its curriculum, which is entirely modern, and its extracurricular offerings, which include an active Multicultural Affairs Office and student-run interest groups. As a state-affiliated institution, OHSU is interested in training physicians who will help meet the demand for health care in Oregon, particularly in underserved, rural areas. Both the admissions policies and the curriculum, which includes preceptorships in the community and a rural health clerkship, support this goal.

Academics

Although most students complete a four-year M.D. curriculum, others follow alternative courses of study, including joint-degree programs. The five-year M.D./M.P.H. Degree Program is offered by the School of Medicine's Department of Public Health and Preventive Medicine in conjunction with appropriate departments at Oregon State University and Portland State University. Generally, students indicate their interest in this program when they apply to the School of Medicine. First-year medical students may pursue an Epidemiological and Biostatistical track, which also serves as preparation for careers in public health. The joint-degree program is the M.D./Ph.D. in the following fields: Biochemistry and Molecular Biology, Cell Biology and Anatomy, Molecular and Medical Genetics, Medical Psychology, Molecular Microbiology and Immunology, Pharmacology and Physiology, and Neuroscience. Grades are Honors, Near Honors, Satisfactory, Marginal, and Fail. Taking both steps of the USMLE is a requirement for graduation.

BASIC SCIENCES: Students spend two hours per day in lecture. An additional two hours each day are used for small-group sessions and/or laboratory activities. One afternoon each week is devoted to Principles of Clinical Medicine in which students work one-on-one with physicians and an additional afternoon studying issues related to public health, behavioral sciences, history taking and learning physical diagnosis skills. First-year courses are Anatomy, Embryology and Imaging; Cell Structure and Function; Systems Process and Homeostasis; Biological Basis of Disease; and Principles of Clinical Medicine, which continues into the second year. The second year is organized around organ systems and physiological concepts, which include Blood, Circulation, Neuroscience and Behavior, Metabolism, and Human Development and Life Cycle. The first two years are spent largely in the Basic Sciences and Education buildings, which have facilities for lectures, discussions, computer learning, and laboratories. The library contains over 150,000 volumes and 2,500 periodicals.

CLINICAL TRAINING: Required third-year rotations are Transition to Clerkship (1 week); Medicine (12 weeks); Primary Care (6 weeks); Ob/Gyn (6 weeks); Child Health (6 weeks); Psychiatry (6 weeks); Family Medicine (6 weeks); and Surgery (6 weeks). During the fourth year, students fulfill advanced clerkship requirements in Medicine, Surgery, Child Health, and Neurology (4 weeks each) in addition to Selectives and Electives. The fourth year culminates in Transition to Physician, a week-long experience. Clinical training takes place at the University Hospital and Clinics and at affiliated institutions, which include Doernbecher Children's Hospital and Portland's Veterans Affairs Medical Center. The School of Medicine's research touches all realms of modern medical sciences. Some investigate the causes and treatments of learning disorders, addiction, heart disease, stroke, cancer, infertility, movement disorders, and emotional disorders. Others work at the molecular and cellular levels to unravel the most basic aspects of human health.

Students

About 6 percent of students at OHSU are from underrepresented minority backgrounds. The average age of incoming students is around 25. Class size is 96.

STUDENT LIFE: Portland is an ideal location for students, offering the comforts of a medium-sized city and proximity to spectacular outdoor destinations. Close to campus are parks and other places to run, walk, or bike ride. A bit further are mountains for hiking and skiing. For an urban area, Portland is relatively affordable and safe. On-campus activities are also popular with medical students. The newly renovated Fitness and Sports Center includes a full weight room, racquetball and squash courts, aerobics classes, swimming pools, and a spa. The Office of Multicultural Affairs supports students of ethnic and international backgrounds with supplemental counseling services, recreational activities, workshops, and classes. Numerous clubs and organizations bring students together around professional or extracurricular interests.

Although student housing is available on a limited basis in the Residence Hall, most opt to live off campus.

GRADUATES: Graduates are successful in securing residency positions at prestigious institutions all over the country. However, most enter programs in the Western United States. Over half enter primary care residencies.

Admissions

REQUIREMENTS: Required courses are Chemistry/Organic Chemistry (2 years); Biology (1year); Physics (1 year); college-level Math (1 semester); English (1 year); Humanities (1 year); and Social Science (1 year). GPAs from all four-year undergraduate institutions are evaluated equally, although factors such as the breadth of education, rigor of major, GPA trends, course load, and extracurricular activities are considered. The MCAT is required and scores must be from within three years of the year of matriculation.

SUGGESTIONS: Preference is given to residents of Oregon and certified WICHE states. Applicants with exceptional qualifications, applicants from underrepresented ethnic/racial groups, and applicants to the M.D./Ph.D. and M.D./M.P.H. programs are considered even if they are not residents of preferred states. For students applying to the M.D./Ph.D. program, advanced course work in Chemistry and Biology and courses in Psychology and Statistics are recommended in addition to requirements for M.D./M.P.H. For all applicants, some medically related experience is important.

PROCESS: About half of AMCAS applicants receive secondaries, and about 40 percent of candidates in this group are interviewed. Interviews consist of two 30-minute sessions with members of the faculty or Admissions Committee. Interviewees are invited to lunch with medical students, and are given a tour of the campus. Approximately 20 percent of interviewees are accepted on a rolling basis. Wait-listed candidates are ranked and have a fairly good chance of being accepted later in the spring.

Costs

In addition to tuition, the yearly expenditure for a single student is estimated at $8,000. This budget covers basic living and personal expenses, in addition to the cost of books and materials. It allows for either on- or off-campus living and car ownership.

FINANCIAL AID: In almost all cases, assistance is awarded on the basis of financial need, as determined by federal and institutional forms. A few scholarships may be available.

OREGON HEALTH SCIENCES UNIVERSITY

STUDENT BODY

Type	Public
*Enrollment	420
*% male/female	55/45
*% underrepresented minorities	6
# applied (total/out)	2,474/2,156
% interviewed (total/out)	17/9
% accepted (total/out)	7/4
% enrolled (total/out)	59/37
Average age	24

ADMISSIONS

Average GPA and MCAT Scores

Overall GPA	3.60	Science GPA	3.6
MCAT Bio	10.00	MCAT Phys	10.00
MCAT Verbal	9.00	MCAT Essay	NR

Score Release Policy

The school has not responded to our inquiry regarding withheld MCAT scores. Therefore, we advise caution. Contact the Admissions Office before withholding any scores.

Application Information

Regular application	10/15
Regular notification	11/1 until filled
Transfers accepted?	No
Admissions may be deferred?	No
AMCAS application accepted?	Yes
Interview required?	Yes
Application fee	$60

COSTS AND AID

Tuition & Fees

Tuition (in/out)	$14,400/$30,351
Cost of books	$3,000
Fees	$1,844

Financial Aid

% students receiving aid	90
Average grant	$1,000
Average loan	$10,000
Average debt	$60,000

*Figures based on total enrollment

PENNSYLVANIA STATE UNIVERSITY
COLLEGE OF MEDICINE

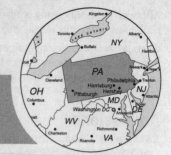

500 University Drive, Hershey, PA 17033
Admission: 717-531-8755 • Fax: 717-531-6225
Email: hmcsaff@psu.edu • Internet: www.hmc.psu.edu

Penn State College of Medicine, located in Hershey, Pennsylvania, is a relatively new addition to the Pennsylvania State University system. Although the College of Medicine receives some state funding, it was founded with the support of the Milton S. Hershey Foundation and is technically considered a private institution. The Medical Center includes Schools of Medicine, Nursing, Basic Science Graduate Studies, and health care–related professions, and also functions as an important health care provider to the population of Central Pennsylvania. Penn State is nationally recognized for its interdisciplinary approach to teaching, its emphasis on primary care, and its medically related research contributions.

Academics

Penn State was one of the first medical schools in the country to institute departments of Humanities and Behavioral Science and to incorporate these perspectives into the basic science and clinical education programs. The College of Medicine was also among the first to develop a separate Family and Community Medicine department. A combined M.D./Ph.D. program is offered, allowing students to earn the doctorate degree in Biochemistry, Biomedical Engineering, Cell Biology, Genetics, Immunology, Microbiology, Molecular Biology, Pharmacology, and Physiology. There are also numerous opportunities to pursue discrete research projects as electives or during summers. Grading designations are Honors, High Pass, Pass, and Fail. Students must pass USMLE Step 1 after the pre-clinical years, and Step 2 in order to graduate.

BASIC SCIENCES: During the first and second years, students are in class or other scheduled sessions for approximately 23 hours per week. This schedule gives students the opportunity for independent and collaborative study. Clinical problems are used as a means of applying and correlating the basic science information that is presented in lectures or discussions. Labs and computer-assisted learning are also important parts of the curriculum. First-year courses are Structural Basis of Medical Practice; Cellular and Molecular Basis of Medical Practice; Biological Basis of Disease; and Physicians, Patients and Society, which touches on the psychological, social, ethical, legal, and humanistic aspects of medicine. Second-year courses are Pharmacology; Microbiology; Immunology; Psychiatry; Pathology; Introduction to Medicine III and IV; Physical Diagnosis; and Issues in Medical Practice. Instruction takes place in the Medical Sciences Building, which houses classrooms and laboratories. The Harrell Library is open 24 hours a day, and holds approximately 125,000 volumes and 2,000 periodicals in addition to modern computer and audiovisual resources.

CLINICAL TRAINING: Third-year required clerkships are Internal Medicine (8 weeks); Surgery (8 weeks); Pediatrics (6 weeks); Ob/Gyn (6 weeks); Psychiatry (4 weeks); Family and Community Medicine (4 weeks); selectives (8 weeks); and Primary Care (4 weeks). The fourth year is devoted to electives and selectives, which are chosen from clinical or research departments. An overseas elective program allows a number of fourth-year students to fulfill elective requirements at clinical sites in Asia, Africa, and Latin America. Generally, clinical training takes place at the University Hospital (463 beds), Children's Hospital, the Rehabilitation Center, and at other hospitals and clinics affiliated through an organized health network called Alliance Health. Additional facilities on campus are a Sports Medicine Center, the General Clinical Research Center, an Animal Research Center, and a Trauma Center.

Students

About 40 percent of students are Pennsylvania residents. Over 25 percent of students are underrepresented minorities, a tribute to the school's commitment to recruiting a diverse student body. The average age of incoming students is 23, with a wide age range. Class size is 110.

STUDENT LIFE: Educational facilities, clinical teaching sites, campus housing and recreational centers are within walking distance of one another. The College of Medicine is an attractive campus, occupying 550 acres. Hershey provides a comfortable, student-friendly community that is relatively safe. As a tourist destination, Hershey offers a variety of dining and entertainment possibilities. Medical students are involved in organizations such as honor societies, professional interest groups, local chapters of national organizations, and groups focused on community service or recreational pursuits. When in need of urban distractions, the state capital, Harrisburg, is 12 miles away, and both Philadelphia and Pittsburgh are easily accessible. On-campus housing options include one-, two-, and three-bedroom apartments.

GRADUATES: Graduates are successful at securing residencies nationwide. Penn State emphasizes primary care and encourages students to consider post-graduate training programs in primary care fields.

Admissions

REQUIREMENTS: Prerequisites are one year each of Biology, Physics, Chemistry, Organic Chemistry, and college-level Math. All science courses should have associated labs. One semester each of Social Sciences and Humanities is also required. The MCAT is required, and scores must be no more than two years old. For applicants who have taken the exam on multiple occasions, all sets of scores are considered.

SUGGESTIONS: Beyond requirements, course work in Calculus, Psychology, Statistics, Sociology, Genetics, and Anthropology are recommended. The April, rather than August, MCAT is strongly advised. Health care related experience is valued, as are interpersonal and communication skills. State residency is not a consideration in the application process.

PROCESS: All AMCAS applicants are sent secondary applications. About 10 percent of those returning secondaries are interviewed between September and March. Interviews consist of two or three sessions each with a faculty member. On interview day, candidates also tour the campus and have lunch with current medical students. About one-third of interviewees are accepted on a rolling basis. Another group is wait-listed. Wait-listed candidates are not encouraged to send supplementary material.

Costs

The estimated yearly budget for a single student is about $10,000. This does not include tuition, but allows for either on- or off-campus housing and car ownership. Tuition is less for Pennsylvania residents.

FINANCIAL AID: Most assistance is need based, with need determined by the FAFSA and other forms. Aid is in the form of grants and loans. A few scholarships based on special criteria or academic achievement are available each year.

PENNSYLVANIA STATE UNIVERSITY

STUDENT BODY

Type	Public
*Enrollment	423
*% male/female	56/44
*% underrepresented minorities	28
# applied (total/out)	6,615/5,509
% interviewed (total/out)	9/6
% accepted (total/out)	6/59
% enrolled (total/out)	31/28
Average age	23

ADMISSIONS

Average GPA and MCAT Scores

Overall GPA	3.58	Science GPA	3.65
MCAT Bio	10.10	MCAT Phys	9.55
MCAT Verbal	9.16	MCAT Essay	NR

Score Release Policy

The school has not responded to our inquiry regarding withheld MCAT scores. Therefore, we advise caution. Contact the Admissions Office before withholding any scores.

Application Information

Regular application	11/15
Regular notification	10/1 until filled
Early application	6/1–8/1
Early notification	10/1
Transfers accepted?	Yes
Admissions may be deferred?	Yes
AMCAS application accepted?	Yes
Interview required?	Yes
Application fee	$40

COSTS AND AID

Tuition & Fees

Tuition (in/out)	$16,824/$24,550
Cost of books	$1,306
Fees	$0

Financial Aid

% students receiving aid	89
Average grant	$13,580
Average loan	$25,035
Average debt	$98,061

*Figures based on total enrollment

UNIVERSITY OF PENNSYLVANIA

SCHOOL OF MEDICINE

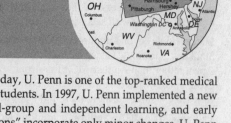

Edward J. Stemmler Hall, Suite 100, Philadelphia, PA 19104

Admission: 215-898-8001 • Fax: 215-573-6645

Internet: www.med.upenn.edu

The University of Pennsylvania founded the nation's first medical school. Today, U. Penn is one of the top-ranked medical schools, known for its clinical facilities, research, and the high caliber of its students. In 1997, U. Penn implemented a new curriculum that emphasizes lifelong learning skills, problem-solving, small-group and independent learning, and early patient contact. Unlike a number of medical schools whose acclaimed "revisions" incorporate only minor changes, U. Penn has adopted an entirely modern approach that responds to the complex demands of today's health care environment. Medical students benefit from the academic and nonacademic resources of the greater U. Penn campus and community.

Academics

The four-year curriculum is organized into five modules, some of which overlap. Patient contact begins on day one, and clinical rotations begin midway through the second year. Research and scholarly projects are encouraged, and may be pursued in a wide range of areas including biomedical science, clinical medicine, behavioral science, and public-health related fields. For qualified students, combined M.D./Ph.D. and M.D./Master's degree programs are available. Among other disciplines, graduate degrees may be earned in Cell and Molecular Biology, Neuroscience, Chemical/Structural Biology and Biophysics, Immunology, Pharmacological Sciences, Psychology, Bioengineering, Epidemiology, Health Care Systems, Public Policy and Management, History and Sociology of Science, and Philosophy. Another option is a joint M.D./M.B.A. in conjunction with the Wharton School of Business. Grading is Pass/Fail during module one and Honors/High Pass/Pass/Fail during the remaining modules.

BASIC SCIENCES: Basic sciences are taught primarily through an integrated organ/disease system model, correlated with clinical examples and hands-on experiences. Module one occupies the first semester and is devoted to Core Principles. Courses are Developmental and Molecular Biology; Cellular Physiology, Metabolism, and Pharmacological Processes; Human Body Structure and Function; Host Defenses; and Pharmacological Responses. Module two spans the second semester of the first year and the first semester of the second year. It is entitled Integrative Systems and Disease, and is organized around body or organ systems. These are Cardiology/Pulmonary; Skin/Connective tissue/Musculoskeletal/Hematology/Oncology; Gastrointestinal and Nutrition; Brain and Behavior; and Endocrinology and Reproduction. Throughout the entire first year and a half, students are introduced to clinical medicine in Module Three, The Technology, Art, and Practice of Medicine. In addition to providing training in basic clinical techniques, Module Three addresses ethics, technological issues, population-based medicine, public health, and humanistic perspectives. Classroom instruction is enhanced by various academic resources, including multimedia, video, and computerized instructional programs. The Biomedical Science Library houses over 100,000 volumes and receives more than 2,000 periodicals.

CLINICAL TRAINING: Students rotate through required clerkships during Module Four, which covers the second semester of year two and the first semester of year three. These are Internal Medicine (9 weeks); Family Medicine (3 weeks); Ob/Gyn (6 weeks); Pediatrics (6 weeks); Surgery/Anesthesia (9 weeks); Emergency Medicine (3 weeks); and Psychiatry/Substance Abuse (6 weeks); Neurology (3 weeks); and Clinical Specialists (3 weeks). Module Five begins in the second semester of year three and continues until graduation at the end of year four. It includes a subinternship, advanced electives, and a required three-month scholarly or research experience. A large portion of clinical training takes place at the Hospital of the University of Pennsylvania, also the site of research institutions and labs. Other training sites are Children's Hospital of Philadelphia; Veterans Affairs of Philadelphia Hospitals; Phoenixville Hospital; Penn Medicine at Radnor; Chestnut Hill Health Care; Chester County Hospital; Friends Hospital; Holy Redeemer Health System; and the Presbyterian-University of Pennsylvania Medical Center.

Students

The student body at U. Penn is nationally represented. About 16 percent of students are underrepresented minorities, and about 20 percent of students took significant time off after college. Class size is 150.

STUDENT LIFE: Pass/Fail grading in the first semester contributes to the high degree of cooperation among students. U. Penn, a comprehensive private university, offers a wide range of extracurricular activities on and around campus, and students are involved both in school and community organizations. Medical students have access to all recreational facilities, including athletic centers. Philadelphia is an important urban center, and is also the home of a very large number of universities. The student community is vast, and the city serves the student community well. Other metropolitan areas such as New York,

Baltimore, and Washington, D.C., are easily accessible by train, and mountains and beaches are a short drive. The Graduate Towers and High Rise North is a University-owned graduate student apartment complex available to medical students. However, most students choose to live off campus.

GRADUATES: During a recent three-year period, the most prevalent residency programs selected were Medicine (22% of graduates); Surgical Specialties (17%); General Surgery (8%); Pediatrics (14%); Family Practice (4%); Ob/Gyn (5%); Orthopedics (3%); Radiology (4%); Emergency Medicine (5%); and Psychiatry (3%).

Admissions

REQUIREMENTS: No prerequisites are specified, although the MCAT is required, suggesting a comprehensive science preparation. U. Penn recommends that applicants submit MCAT scores from the spring, but no later than the summer, of the calendar year prior to entrance.

SUGGESTIONS: Recommended undergraduate preparation includes courses in Biology, Chemistry, Organic Chemistry, Physics, Math, History, Philosophy, Ethics, Anthropology, Political Science, and Economics. For applicants who have taken time off after college, some recent course work is advised. Experience in hospitals, clinics, or community service projects is important.

PROCESS: All AMCAS applicants receive secondary applications. Of those returning secondaries, about 20 percent are interviewed between October and February. Interviews consist of two sessions, one with a student and one with a faculty member. On interview day, candidates tour the campus, attend group informational sessions, and have the opportunity to meet informally with students. Of interviewed candidates, about 10–20 percent are accepted. Wait-listed candidates may send additional information to update their files.

Costs

In addition to tuition, the estimated yearly cost of living for a single student is $13,500. This budget allows for on- or off-campus housing. Many students rely on public transportation.

FINANCIAL AID: Most aid is need-based, with financial need determined by the FAFSA and Penn institutional forms. The Twenty-First Century Gamble Scholars Program awards six four-year, full-tuition scholarships annually to entering students who demonstrate outstanding achievement in academic, intellectual, community-service, or other realms. M.D./Ph.D. students are generally fully funded, either through the M.S.T.P. or institutional programs.

UNIVERSITY OF PENNSYLVANIA

STUDENT BODY

Type	Private
*Enrollment	710
*% male/female	57/43
*% underrepresented minorities	15
# applied (total/out)	6,617/5,843
% interviewed (total/out)	12/14
% accepted (total/out)	NR/NR
% enrolled (total/out)	15/14
Average age	23

ADMISSIONS

Average GPA and MCAT Scores

Overall GPA	3.78	Science GPA	3.77
MCAT Bio	11.7	MCAT Phys	11.8
MCAT Verbal	10.7	MCAT Essay	Q

Score Release Policy

The Admissions Committee is inclined to look unfavorably on withheld scores, both because it raises questions about how bad the score is and because it delays the application process.

Application Information

Regular application	11/1
Regular notification	3/1 until filled
Transfers accepted?	No
Admissions may be deferred?	Yes
AMCAS application accepted?	Yes
Interview required?	Yes
Application fee	$65

COSTS AND AID

Tuition & Fees

Tuition	$30,830
Cost of books	$835
Fees	$1,680

Financial Aid

% students receiving aid	80
Average grant	NR
Average loan	NR
Average debt	$96,000

*Figures based on total enrollment

UNIVERSITY OF PITTSBURGH

SCHOOL OF MEDICINE

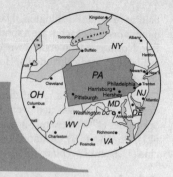

518 Scaife Hall, Pittsburgh, PA 15261

Admission: 412-648-9891 • Fax: 412-648-8768

Email: admissions@fsl.dean-med.pitt.edu

Internet: www.dean-med.pitt.edu

The University of Pittsburgh is one of a handful of medical schools to have fully and successfully implemented an integrated, organ-based curriculum organized around physiological systems rather than traditional academic divisions. Although considered a premier research institution, the School of Medicine regards patient care as the most important element of a medical education. Pittsburgh recognizes the individuality of students and is responsive to their needs and career goals. It is a state-affiliated school that, nonetheless, admits significant numbers of out-of-state residents. The city of Pittsburgh provides a diverse, urban patient population and is a dynamic, yet affordable, place to live.

Academics

The four-year curriculum encourages personal interaction among students, between faculty and students, and between patients and students. Students can obtain joint master's degrees in Medical Ethics and Public Health with nearby Carnegie-Mellon University. The M.S.T.P.-funded M.D./Ph.D. is offered in conjunction with Carnegie-Mellon Uniersity.

BASIC SCIENCES: During the first two years, students take classes that are grouped into blocks. Year one has four blocks: the Patient-Doctor Block, which covers ethical, behavioral, and sociological issues related to medicine; the Basic Science Block, which covers the biological elements of medicine; the Organ Systems Block, which includes Host Defenses and the Musculoskeletal System; and the Introduction to Patient Care Block, which encompasses Physical Diagnosis. The Blocks are synchronized so that single topics are approached in an interdisciplinary way. The blocks in year two are Patient-Doctor Relationship, Patient Care, and Organ Systems, which includes the following systems: Homeostasis; Digestion; Endocrine; Dermatology; Reproductive; and Neuroscience. As in year one, the blocks are planned to complement each other. The final segment of year two integrates all the organ systems and, while doing so, reviews important points of the previous two years. Lectures, small-group sessions, conferences, labs, and tutorials are the instructional methods used during the first two years, and students are in a structured learning environment for about 28 hours per week. Problem-based learning is used with most instructional methods. With the exception of clinical work, instruction is given in Scaife Hall, a renovated building with classrooms, labs, and a library, which has 220,000 volumes and subscribes to the major online medical informational services. Grades during the first two years are Honors/Pass/Fail. The USMLE Steps 1 and 2 are required for graduation.

CLINICAL TRAINING: Patient contact begins in year one during the Patient Care Block. Third-year rotations begin in July immediately following year two. These are Ambulatory Subspecialties (6 weeks—includes Dermatology, Neurosurgery, Ophthalmology, Orthopedics, Otolaryngology, Pediatric Surgery, Plastic Surgery, and Urology); Family Medicine (4 weeks); Ob/Gyn (6 weeks); Pediatrics (8 weeks); Psychiatry (6 weeks); Surgery (6 weeks); and Elective (4 weeks). The fourth year is made up solely of Selectives and Electives. Clinical training takes place at the University Health Center, which is composed of five major hospitals: the Presbyterian University Hospital, Montefiore Hospital, the Eye and Ear Institute, the Western Psychiatric Institute, and the University of Pittsburgh Cancer Institute. The passing rate for students at the University of Pittsburgh on both parts of the USMLE is higher than that for medical schools nationally, and for the past two years 100 percent of all students passed both Step 1 and 2.

Students

About 9 percent of students are underrepresented minorities, most of whom are African Americans. Approximately half of the students in each class are Pennsylvania residents. There is a large age range within the student body, and many students took some time off before entering medical school. Class size is 148.

STUDENT LIFE: The structure of the curriculum promotes student interaction and collegiality. In addition, medical students get to know each other through involvement in organizations and extracurricular activities. Some of the many student groups on campus are Pitt Women in Medicine, the Christian Medical Society, and the History of Medicine Society. Medical students have access to all facilities of the University of Pittsburgh, including athletic facilities. Pittsburgh is an accessible and exciting city, and, although on-campus housing is available, most medical students choose to live off campus.

GRADUATES: Graduates are successful in gaining admittance to some of most prestigious residency programs in the country. In 1999, 78 percent of the graduating class obtained one of their top three choices in the National

Residency Matching Program. About 50 percent of graduates enter primary care fields.

Admissions

REQUIREMENTS: Requirements are one year each of Biology, Physics, Chemistry, and Organic Chemistry, all with associated labs, and English. In assessing grades, consideration is given to the undergraduate institution attended and the course load taken. The MCAT is required and must be no more than three years old.

SUGGESTIONS: Competence in math is valued as is evidence of success in Social Science and Humanities courses. The University of Pittsburgh looks for interpersonal skills and commitment to community service in applicants. For applicants who graduated college several years ago, some recent course work is advised.

PROCESS: Secondary applications are sent selectively to AMCAS applicants. About 20 percent of Pennsylvania residents, and 10 percent of out-of-state residents, are interviewed. Interviews are conducted from September through April and consist of two sessions, one with a faculty member and one with a medical student. Notification occurs towards the end of February. Wait-listed candidates may send additional information to strengthen their applications and to indicate interest in the school.

Costs

Beyond the tuition, fees, and book costs, the estimated expenses for a single student are $1,100 per month. This budget allows for off-campus housing and modest car maintenance.

FINANCIAL AID: Virtually all financial aid is awarded on the basis of demonstrated financial need. However a few merit-based scholarships are awarded each year to incoming freshman. Students seeking need-based aid must first utilize their eligibility for the annual maximum Federal Stafford Student Loan. Need-based institutional scholarships and loans, for which full parental resources are considered, are awarded to 25–30 percent of the student body each year.

UNIVERSITY OF PITTSBURGH

STUDENT BODY

Type	Private
*Enrollment	595
*% male/female	52/48
*% underrepresented minorities	9
# applied (total/out)	4,176/3,340
% interviewed (total/out)	16/13
% accepted (total/out)	10/8
% enrolled (total/out)	33/48

ADMISSIONS

Average GPA and MCAT Scores

Overall GPA	3.67	Science GPA	3.66
MCAT Bio	10.8	MCAT Phys	10.5
MCAT Verbal	10.2	MCAT Essay	NR

Score Release Policy

The Admission Committee has no preference about students withholding scores.

Application Information

Regular application	12/1
Regular notification	End of February
Early application	6/1–8/1
Early notification	10/1
Transfers accepted?	Yes
Admissions may be deferred?	Yes
AMCAS application accepted?	Yes
Interview required?	Yes
Application fee	$60

COSTS AND AID

Tuition & Fees

Tuition (in/out)	$21,985/$26,999
Cost of books	$2,000
Fees	$500

Financial Aid

% students receiving aid	77
Average grant	$6,800
Average loan	NR
Average debt	$88,011

*Figures based on total enrollment

UNIVERSITY OF ROCHESTER
SCHOOL OF MEDICINE AND DENTISTRY

Medical Center Box 601A, Rochester, NY 14642
Admission: 716-275-4539 • Fax: 716-756-5479
Email: mdadmish@urmc.rochester.edu
Internet: www.urmc.rochester.edu/smd

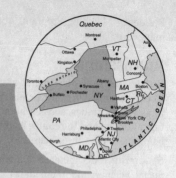

The School of Medicine and Dentistry, the School of Nursing, Strong Memorial Hospital, and the Eastman Dental Center comprise the University of Rochester Medical Center. Long recognized for excellence and innovation in medical education, Rochester continues its leading role with a comprehensive curriculum revision that began with the entering class of 1999. The "Double Helix Curriculum" captures the integrated strands of basic and clinical medicine as they are woven throughout the four-year curriculum. Each element of the curriculum strengthens Rochester's biopsychosocial tradition by fostering knowledge, skills, attitudes, and behaviors of the physician/scientist/humanist, by combining cutting-edge evidence-based medical science with the relationship-centered art that is medicine's distinctive trademark.

Academics

Special emphasis is placed on skills acquisition and use, with a commitment to lifelong learning. Sensitivity to the world of the patient is encompassed in the biopsychosocial integration of the curriculum and the learning experience, with mechanisms in place for continuous curricular improvement through the collaboration of students and faculty. By ensuring adequate and early electivity for students to enhance their special interests, along with rigorous training and assessment of all of the competencies demanded by modern medical practice, the curriculum generates a knowledge base characterized by depth, breadth, rigor, and flexibility. Students interested in careers in medical science may participate in the fully funded Medical Scientist Training Program (M.D./Ph.D.), or joint-degree programs including the M.P.H./M.D. and M.B.A./M.D. program in Health Care Management in conjunction with the William E. Simon Graduate School of Business Administration. Vacation and full-year fellowships facilitate student research or international medicine experiences. Evaluation of student performance uses Satisfactory/Fail, except in the required clerkships, where Honors/High Pass/Pass/Fail grades are used. Passing the USMLE is not required for promotion to the third year.

BASIC SCIENCES: An introductory module at the beginning of year one prepares students in the acquisition, management, and presentation of medical information. Students learn how to meet the challenges of active and independent learning by becoming competent in data management, information technology, and critical evaluation of the medical literature. Every course is interdisciplinary; basic sciences are integrated with one another and basic and clinical sciences are woven together as the strands of the Double Helix Curriculum throughout the four years. Clinical skills training from day one leads not to shadowing or preceptor experiences in clinics, but to real clinical work as part of the health care team while still in the first year. Not just "paper cases," but students' actual clinical cases drive the learning of science through the school-wide use of multidisciplinary problem-based learning (PBL) cases. Three two-hour PBL tutorials per week and an average of no more than 10 hours of lecture per week, with adequate time for self-study, and the use of labs, conferences, seminars, and computer-assisted learning—all these things characterize the classroom setting of the curriculum. Electives are available during all four years, including electives in Medical Humanities, International Medicine, and community outreach programs. The Edward G. Miner Library holds over 225,000 volumes and a modern, computer-based learning resource center.

CLINICAL TRAINING: Beginning in year one, students complete their introduction to clinical medicine in the fall and then participate in an Ambulatory Clerkship Experience beginning in the spring. This experience, unlike any other in the country, includes all the ambulatory components of Family Medicine, Pediatrics, Internal Medicine, Women's Health, Psychiatry, and Ambulatory Surgery, and is completed by the end of the second year. Inpatient clerkships are completed by December of the fourth year and focus on acute illness experiences in adult medicine, women's and children's health, mind/brain/behavior, and urgent/emergent care. Strong Memorial Hospital (700 beds) is the principal site for clinical teaching, along with a newly completed Ambulatory Care Center and five affiliated hospitals (2,000 beds) covering acute and chronic care.

Students

Students come from all regions of the country. About 13 percent are underrepresented minorities. The average age of incoming students is 24; one-third have majored in areas outside the sciences, and 100 students are accepted each year.

STUDENT LIFE: Most medical students have active lives outside of the classroom. Many participate in community outreach programs, international medicine electives, and student organizations and events. Students have access to resources of the University campus and athletic facilities in the medical center. Located on the southern shore of Lake Ontario, in the Finger Lakes wine-producing region of upstate New York, Rochester is a progressive, metropolitan community of more than one million people. Rochester has a rich cultural life, is an affordable and friendly city, and is a haven for boaters and other outdoor enthusiasts.

GRADUATES: Among the 2000 graduates, the most popular residencies were Internal Medicine (32%), Pediatrics (22%), Surgery (9%), Emergency Medicine (6%), Ob/Gyn (3%), and Psychiatry (3%). About 12 percent stayed in the Rochester area, while an additional 20 percent remained in New York State. The remainder went to 20 other states.

Admissions

REQUIREMENTS: Prerequisite science courses are one year of Biology, Physics, General Chemistry, and Organic Chemistry, all associated with labs. One semester of Biochemistry may be substituted for one semester of Organic. One year of English or expository writing is also required. Rochester belongs to AMCAS, and the MCAT exam is required; scores should be from the past three years. The best set of scores is considered.

SUGGESTIONS: In addition to required science courses, 12–16 credit hours in the Humanities and/or Social Sciences are required. Experiences in research, clinical settings, and the community are strongly recommended. Rochester looks for evidence of leadership, excellent interpersonal skills, a love of learning, appreciation of diversity, and outstanding scholarship.

PROCESS: Rochester is an AMCAS school. About 10 percent of applicants are interviewed between September and February. Interviews consist of two sessions with faculty, and applicants have a tour, lunch with current students, and a financial aid presentation. About 35 percent of the interviewed applicants are offered acceptance, with notification beginning in November and continuing through May. About 15 positions in each class are reserved for students from several programs, such as the Rochester Early Medical Scholar program and the Bryn Mawr post-baccalaureate program.

Costs

The standard student budget, beyond tuition, is about $15,000. This budget supports a single student living on or off campus and owning a car.

FINANCIAL AID: Assistance is need-based. Financial need is determined by the FAFSA and the Needs Access Diskette, and parental disclosure is required if applying for scholarships.

UNIVERSITY OF ROCHESTER

STUDENT BODY

Type	Private
*Enrollment	400
*% male/female	52/48
*% underrepresented minorities	13
# applied (total/out)	5,842/4,715
% interviewed (total/out)	12/18
% accepted (total/out)	6/5
% enrolled (total/out)	35/29
Average age	24

ADMISSIONS

Average GPA and MCAT Scores

Overall GPA	3.61	Science GPA	3.55
MCAT Bio	11.0	MCAT Phys	10.9
MCAT Verbal	10.5	MCAT Essay	NR

Score Release Policy

The school has not responded to our inquiry regarding withheld MCAT scores. Therefore, we advise caution. Contact the Admissions Office before withholding any scores.

Application Information

Regular application	10/15
Regular notification	11/1 until filled
Transfers accepted?	Yes
Admissions may be deferred?	Yes
AMCAS application accepted?	Yes
Interview required?	Yes
Application fee	$75

COSTS AND AID

Tuition & Fees

Tuition	$28,000
Cost of books	$1,300
Fees	$1,760

Financial Aid

% students receiving aid	85
Average grant	$10,185
Average loan	$26,608
Average debt	$96,000

*Figures based on total enrollment

RUSH MEDICAL COLLEGE OF RUSH UNIVERSITY

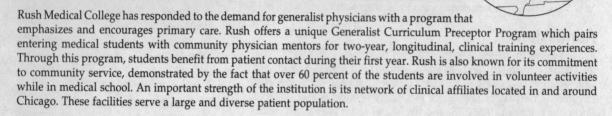

600 South Paulina Street, Chicago, IL 60612
Admission: 312-942-6913 • Fax: 312-942-2333

Rush Medical College has responded to the demand for generalist physicians with a program that emphasizes and encourages primary care. Rush offers a unique Generalist Curriculum Preceptor Program which pairs entering medical students with community physician mentors for two-year, longitudinal, clinical training experiences. Through this program, students benefit from patient contact during their first year. Rush is also known for its commitment to community service, demonstrated by the fact that over 60 percent of the students are involved in volunteer activities while in medical school. An important strength of the institution is its network of clinical affiliates located in and around Chicago. These facilities serve a large and diverse patient population.

Academics

Students follow a four-year curriculum, except those pursuing a Ph.D. along with the M.D. degree. Joint M.D./Ph.D. programs are offered in many disciplines, including Anatomy, Biochemistry, Immunology, Microbiology, Neuroscience, Pharmacology, and Physiology. Medical students are evaluated with Honors/Pass/Fail, and passing the USMLE Step 1 is a requirement for promotion to year three. Entering students are assigned a faculty member as an academic advisor to assist with education and career development.

BASIC SCIENCES: Students learn basic sciences through the Traditional Curriculum, which relies on lectures and labs for instruction, or the Alternate Curriculum, which is entirely case-based and emphasizes self-directed learning and problem-solving skills. About 24 students enter the Alternate Curriculum each year. All students participate in the Generalist Curriculum, which involves one-on-one mentorships with physician preceptors. Topics covered in the first year are Anatomy; Behavioral Science; Biochemistry; Ethics and Law in Medicine; Histology; Neurobiology; Physiology; General Pathology; Health and the Public; Primary Care Preceptorship; Physical Diagnosis; and Interviewing and Communication. Second-year subjects are Psychopathlogy; Clinical Pathophysiology; Pathology; Pharmacology; Preventive Medicine; Immunology; Microbiology; Primary Care Preceptorship; Physical Diagnosis; and Interviewing and Communication. To enhance classroom instruction, the McCormick Learning Resource Center offers audiovisual and computer-based learning aids. Academic Computer Resources operates a personal computer laboratory and a computer-assisted instruction laboratory that is available 24 hours a day. The Tutoring Program provides additional instruction and study tips from faculty, classmates, or upperclass students.

CLINICAL TRAINING: All students fulfill the same clerkship requirements during the third and fourth years. Third-year rotations are Internal Medicine (12 weeks); Surgery (12 weeks); Ob/Gyn (8 weeks); Pediatrics (8 weeks); Psy-

chiatry (6 weeks); Family Practice (6 weeks); and Neurology (4 weeks). Fourth-year students participate in an advanced, primary care subinternship, choosing from Family Medicine, Internal Medicine, or Pediatrics (4 weeks). At least 18 weeks are reserved for electives. Most clinical training takes place at Rush-Presbyterian-St. Luke's Hospital (903 beds), a not-for-profit hospital with over 30 specialty areas. Other affiliated institutions, in urban, suburban, and rural locations, are Illinois Masonic Medical Center; Rush North Shore Medical Center; Rush-Prudential Health Plans; Cook County Hospital; Hinsdale Hospital; LaGrange Memorial Hospital; MacNeal Memorial Hospital; and Westlake Hospital.

Students

Approximately 85 percent of students are Illinois residents. About 10 percent of students are underrepresented minorities, and about 30 percent are older or "nontraditional," having taken time off between college and medical school. Class size is 120.

STUDENT LIFE: Student life, both on and off campus, is varied and exciting. Campus facilities are designed to encourage student interaction. For example, student lounges provide space for socializing, relaxing between classes, or special events. The Academic Facility is open to Rush students 24 hours a day, and is a good spot for group or individual study. Student organizations are numerous, ranging from the Rush Golf Club, to the Multicultural Affairs Coalition, to chapters of national medically oriented organizations. The Rush Community Service Initiative Program (RCSIP) is a student-run umbrella organization for many projects and activities, all of which allow students to contribute to the community. RCSIP activities include free clinics, health education programs, and big sibling relationships with children who have HIV. Students have access to athletic and recreational facilities at Rush and at the University of Illinois, including indoor tennis courts, swimming pools, a bowling alley, and pool tables. Chicago is an ideal city for students, as it is relatively affordable and can be accessed with public transportation. Convenient and comfortable housing options are available both on and off campus.

GRADUATES: Rush has met its stated goal that at least 50 percent of graduates will enter primary care fields. Graduates are successful in securing residencies all over the country. Rush graduates practice in 50 states and in a number of foreign countries.

Admissions

REQUIREMENTS: Prerequisites are eight semester hours each of Biology, General Chemistry, Organic Chemistry, and Physics. The MCAT is required and scores must be from within the past four years. For applicants who have retaken the exam, recent scores are most heavily weighed.

SUGGESTIONS: Preference is given to residents of Illinois, although up to 20–30 out-of-state applicants are accepted each year. Beyond requirements, Rush suggests undergraduate courses in Math, Social Sciences, and English. The committee looks for social and intellectual maturity, personal integrity, motivation, and concern in applicants. Applicants are encouraged to take the MCAT in April of the year of application.

PROCESS: All AMCAS applicants receive secondary applications. About 500 applicants, or 10 percent of the applicant pool, are interviewed between September and March. Interviews consist of two sessions with faculty members, in addition to a tour of the campus and the opportunity to meet with current students. Of interviewed candidates, about half are accepted on a rolling basis. Wait-listed candidates may submit supplementary material to update their files.

Costs

The estimated yearly cost of living for a single student is about $13,000, not including tuition. This allows for either on- or off-campus housing.

FINANCIAL AID: Financial need is determined by the FAFSA and the CCS needs analysis form. Students with financial need are first required to borrow a specified amount, called the Unit Loan, from federal sources before becoming eligible for institutional grants and loans. Residents of Illinois who commit to practicing primary care in underserved areas in the state may be eligible for additional financial assistance.

RUSH MEDICAL COLLEGE OF RUSH UNIVERSITY

STUDENT BODY

Type	Private
*Enrollment	494
*% male/female	56/44
*% underrepresented minorities	10
# applied (total/out)	5,069/3,365
% interviewed (total/out)	9/2
% accepted (total/out)	NR/NR
% enrolled (total/out)	24/16

ADMISSIONS

Average GPA and MCAT Scores

Overall GPA	NR	Science GPA	NR
MCAT Bio	9.10	MCAT Phys	9.40
MCAT Verbal	9.60	MCAT Essay	NR

Score Release Policy

The school has not responded to our inquiry regarding withheld MCAT scores. Therefore, we advise caution. Contact the Admissions Office before withholding any scores.

Application Information

Regular application	11/15
Regular notification	10/15 until filled
Early application	6/1–8/1
Early notification	10/1
Admissions may be deferred?	Yes
AMCAS application accepted?	Yes
Interview required?	Yes
Application fee	$50

COSTS AND AID

Tuition & Fees

Tuition	$25,824
Cost of books	NR
Fees	$1,332

Financial Aid

% students receiving aid	80
Average grant	NR
Average loan	NR
Average debt	NR

*Figures based on total enrollment

SAINT LOUIS UNIVERSITY
SCHOOL OF MEDICINE

1402 South Grand Boulevard, St. Louis, MO 63104
Admission: 314-577-8205 • Fax: 314-577-8214
Email: mcpeters@slu.edu • Internet: www.slu.edu/colleges/med

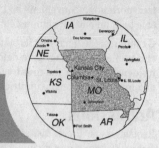

St. Louis University (SLU) is a private, Jesuit institution located in the heart of downtown St. Louis. The School of Medicine is part of the Health Sciences campus that includes the St. Louis University Hospital, a large urban medical center. In addition to teaching basic science and clinical skills, SLU ensures that students understand the humanistic side of medicine. The Center for Health Care Ethics offers programs that support this ideal.

Academics

The medical curriculum is continually evolving to respond to the rapid changes in the health care field and to reflect national trends in medical education. Current students enjoy a program of study that uses problem-based learning and emphasizes small-group and independent study. SLU offers several options for students interested in research. Qualified students may enter an M.D./Ph.D. program, allowing them to complete both degrees within 6–7 years. The doctorate is offered in Anatomy, Biochemistry, Cell Biology, Genetics, Immunology, Microbiology, Molecular Biology, Neuroscience, Pathology, Pharmacology, and Physiology. Students interested in summer or elective research experiences may graduate in four years, earning an M.D. with distinction in research. Medical students are evaluated with Honors, Pass, or Fail throughout all four years. Passing the USMLE Step 1 is a requirement for promotion to year three, and passing Step 2 is a requirement for graduation.

BASIC SCIENCES: The first and second years each consist of 36 weeks of instruction, which includes laboratories, demonstrations, discussion groups, didactic lecture sessions, and preceptorships at clinical sites. Students are in class or other scheduled sessions for about 20 hours per week, providing ample time for self-directed learning. First-year courses are Introduction to Human Anatomy; Cell Biology; Metabolism; Microbes and Host Responses; Molecular Biology and Genetics; Principles of Pharmacology; Health Information Resources; and Patient, Physician, and Society, which covers topics such as bioethics, community medicine, medical communication, and the physical diagnosis. Second-year courses are Introduction to Clinical Psychiatry; Introduction to Medicine; Microbiology; Neuroscience; Pathology; Pharmacology; Preventive and Social Medicine; and Patient, Physician, and Society, which includes both clinical and sociological/psychological topics. An important resource for students is the Learning Resources Center, which houses both the Health Sciences Center Library and the Clinical Skills Center, where both diagnostic and treatment skills are taught.

CLINICAL TRAINING: The third year consists of core clerkships in most basic medical fields. These are Internal Medicine (12 weeks); Surgery (8 weeks); Ob/Gyn (6 weeks); Pediatrics (8 weeks); Family Medicine (4 weeks); Psychiatry (6 weeks); and Neurology (4 weeks). The fourth year is flexible, allowing students to pursue elective opportunities in both clinical and research areas. A minimum of 36 weeks of instruction must be completed. Required rotations are in Intramural Floor Service (4 weeks) and Surgery Subspecialty Selective (4 weeks). Most training is conducted at the St. Louis University Hospital, a 365-bed tertiary care facility. It is also a Level I trauma center. Other affiliated institutions include the Cardinal Glennon Children's Hospital, the Anheuser-Busch Eye Institute, and the St. Louis Veterans Affairs Medical Center. A portion of electives may be taken at other academic and clinical institutions.

Students

Although students come from all regions of the country, a large number are from the Saint Louis area. About 10 percent of students are underrepresented minorities and about 10 percent are nontraditional, having pursued other careers or interests between college and medical school.

STUDENT LIFE: SLU students can pursue their health-related interests by taking part in research forums or by participating in the School's many organizations. The campus ministry is particularly strong. Those who need a break from academic and career pursuits can take advantage of the resources of the main campus, including the award-winning Simon Recreational Center or the well-subscribed intramural sports program. St. Louis also offers a wide variety of extracurricular activities. Tower Grove Park and the Missouri Botanical Gardens are a few blocks from the Medical School. Nearby Forest Park, one of the nation's largest metropolitan parks, is the home of the St. Louis Zoo, the Art Museum, and the Science Center. St. Louis also has its own opera, theater, and ballet, in addition to professional baseball and hockey teams. Although the school has some housing facilities, most medical students choose to live off campus, where housing is affordable and comfortable.

GRADUATES: The majority of graduates enter primary care residencies. Students are competitive applicants for specialty fields as well.

Admissions

REQUIREMENTS: Requirements are one year each of Chemistry, Biology, Organic Chemistry, and Physics. In addition, 6 semester hours of English and 12 hours of Humanities or Behavioral Science are expected. The MCAT is required, and scores must be from the new version of the test. For applicants who have taken the exam more than once, the best set of scores is considered. Thus, there is no advantage to withholding scores.

SUGGESTIONS: Students should apply early in the application cycle as interviews and acceptances are given on a rolling basis. Both hospital and research experience is highly valuable. Activities that demonstrate a commitment to serving others is also useful.

PROCESS: All AMCAS applicants receive secondary applications. Of the approximately 4,200 students who return secondaries, about 21 percent are interviewed on a rolling basis. Interviews are one hour in length and are conducted by a faculty member. The remainder of the interview day includes a tour of the campus, group informational sessions, and lunch with current students. Applicants are notified of committee decisions within a few weeks of the interview and are either accepted, rejected, or put into a hold category. Approximately 35 percent of the interviewed group is accepted. For wait-listed applicants, additional grades or new MCAT scores are useful supplementary information

Costs

Tuition and living expenses at St. Louis University amounts to approximately $40,000 per year. St. Louis is a relatively inexpensive city, and living comfortably off campus on such a budget is possible. Most students have cars.

FINANCIAL AID: Financial need is determined from both the student's and parents' income and assets. Most assistance is in the form of loans.

SAINT LOUIS UNIVERSITY

STUDENT BODY

Type	Private
*Enrollment	605
*% male/female	58/42
*% underrepresented minorities	10
# applied (total/out)	6,206/5,797
% interviewed (total/out)	15/14
% accepted (total/out)	5/24
% enrolled (total/out)	49/18

ADMISSIONS

Average GPA and MCAT Scores

Overall GPA	3.65	Science GPA	3.68
MCAT Bio	10.8	MCAT Phys	10.6
MCAT Verbal	9.9	MCAT Essay	P

Score Release Policy

The school has not responded to our inquiry regarding withheld MCAT scores. Therefore, we advise caution. Contact the Admissions Office before withholding any scores.

Application Information

Regular application	12/15
Regular notification	10/15 until filled
Early application	6/1–8/1
Early notification	10/1
Transfers accepted?	Yes
Admissions may be deferred?	Yes
AMCAS application accepted?	Yes
Interview required?	Yes
Application fee	$100

COSTS AND AID

Tuition & Fees

Tuition	$31,430
Cost of books	$1,500
Fees	$1,275

Financial Aid

% students receiving aid	89
Average grant	$7,000
Average loan	$32,000
Average debt	NR

*Figures based on total enrollment

University of South Alabama

COLLEGE OF MEDICINE

University of Admissions, 2015 MSB, Mobile, AL 36688
Admission: 334-460-7176 • Fax: 334-460-6278

The University of South Alabama College of Medicine has two priorities, training physicians to meet the needs of the state and conducting research that addresses medical concerns at the state and national levels. The allocation of state resources to specific departments in the Medical School reflects the medical demands of the state. The School of Medicine fulfills its mandate, demonstrated by the fact that half of the graduates enter residencies in Alabama, and almost 70 percent choose primary care fields. To meet specified goals, the University of South Alabama offers excellent clinical and research facilities, small class size, and a dedicated faculty. The University is a state-supported institution located in Mobile, a historic Southern city. The School of Medicine benefits from the resources and the cultural/social life of the greater University, which occupies a 1,200- acre campus and serves a large student population. The University Medical Center has operated since 1831 and has provided medical education for more than a century.

Academics

The curriculum is semi-traditional, and uses a lecture format for most of the pre-clinical instruction. Although some early clinical exposure is offered, during the first two years, the program focuses on ensuring a solid understanding of the basic sciences. Combining medical and doctorate studies is possible if pursuing a Ph.D. degree in a medically related discipline. About one-quarter of the class enters the School of Medicine via a combined undergraduate-medical school program that is open to both Alabama and out-of-state high school seniors.

BASIC SCIENCES: The school operates on a quarter system. During the first year, lecture courses are Gross Anatomy, Histology, Developmental Anatomy, Physiology, Neuroanatomy, and Biochemistry. Generally, students are in lecture for about 25 hours per week. The course Medical Ethics is taught by using both lecture and small-group format. Medical Practice and Society and Physical Diagnosis use lectures and a case-based approach. During the second year, traditional lecture/lab courses include Microbiology, Pharmacology, Pathology, and Genetics. Introduction to Behavioral Sciences and a course covering principles of Public Health are also part of the curriculum. In addition, students take part in weekly sessions in clinical settings, as part of an introductory course in Clinical Medicine. Basic sciences are taught in the Medical Sciences Building, which contains administrative offices, classrooms, and laboratories. The Biomedical Library houses 65,000 volumes and offers computer and online services. Grading is A–F for most courses, and promotions are based not only on grades but also on faculty evaluation of students' ethical and personal maturity. Medical students are involved in the Schools' administrative affairs through an elected student governing body, which also participates in issues relating to the greater University. The schedule for the first two years is relatively firm, and students are encouraged to focus on their studies, rather than pursue employment or other activities during this period. The USMLE Step 1 is required following the basic-science portion of study.

CLINICAL TRAINING: Year three is composed entirely of required clerkships: Medicine (12 weeks); Surgery (8 weeks); Ob/Gyn (8 weeks); Psychiatry (6 weeks); Pediatrics (8 weeks); and Family Practice (6 weeks). The fourth year is also 48 weeks but is composed of elective rather than required rotations. Students must select a one-month rotation from each broad field: Neuroscience; Surgical Subspecialties; Ambulatory Care; Primary Care; and in-house elective. Students train at University-affiliated hospitals that together constitute the largest medical complex along the Gulf Coast and that contain a total of 880 beds. All levels of trauma care and surgery are available, and patients come not only from around the state but from neighboring states as well. In downtown Mobile, the Children's and Women's Hospital offers clinical rotations in pediatric services and neonatal care. The hospital system serves managed care clients, among others, ensuring a client base. Cancer Research and Treatment, Organic Transplant, Aeromedical Transport, and Preventative Care are a few of the noteworthy services available through the University network. Students receive grades of A–F for clinical performance during required rotations and Honors/Pass/Fail during elective rotations. The USMLE Step 2 is required for graduation. Few students take part in rotations at out-of-state institutions or overseas.

Students

At least 90 percent of medical students must be Alabama residents. Reflecting the state's demographics, about 9 percent are underrepresented minorities, most of whom are African American. Each year, about 15 students enter who have taken time off after college. The student body is diverse in terms of undergraduate majors, and class size is relatively small, at 65–70 students.

STUDENT LIFE: Students take advantage of the University campus with its recreational facilities and activities. Students also use nearby municipal recreational facilities, which include a golf course. The School of Medicine provides opportunities for students to participate in medically related projects and events, such as volunteer activities and special seminars. University housing consists of more than 700 two- and three-bedroom houses, appropriate for married students, in an area adjacent to the campus. Furnished dormitories provide living accommodations that are within walking distance of the Medical School. In addition to the typical medical student associations, the Military Medical Students Society operates a chapter on campus.

GRADUATES: Of the graduating class of 1997, 66 percent chose primary care specialties; 18 percent went into Internal Medicine; 35 percent into Family Medicine; 11 percent into Pediatrics; and 2 percent chose Medicine/Pediatrics. Ob/Gyn, Pathology, and Surgery were also popular choices.

Admissions

REQUIREMENTS: Requirements are one year each of General Chemistry, Organic Chemistry, Biology, and Physics, all with associated labs; and one year each of Math, Humanities, and English. In total, 90 semester hours of undergraduate course work are required. The quality of the undergraduate institution is considered in evaluating GPA. Generally, courses taken abroad are not counted. The MCAT is required and should be no more than three years old. The most recent score is considered, and there is no preference for the April or August MCAT.

SUGGESTIONS: Preferably, the Math requirement should be fulfilled with Calculus. Nontraditional students who have taken time off after college are advised to demonstrate recent course work, particularly in the sciences. The goal of the Admissions Committee is to select candidates who have the potential to address the wide spectrum of needs faced by the medical profession, suggesting that diverse backgrounds are valued in addition to medically related experience. Because spots are few, out-of-state candidates should be competitive on a national level.

PROCESS: All Alabama residents receive a secondary application, which is sent upon receipt of the AMCAS application. About one-quarter of out-of-state residents receive a secondary. The secondary application is due on November 15, but the School of Medicine advises applicants to submit it as soon as possible. Fifty percent of Alabama residents, and about 10 percent of out-of-state residents, are interviewed. Interviews are held on campus from September through March. Students receive three half-hour interviews, which may vary in format. The interview day provides applicants and faculty an opportunity to become acquainted and is considered a two-way process. Of those interviewed, about 30 percent are accepted and 20 percent are placed on a ranked wait list. Candidates are accepted on a weekly basis, beginning in December.

Costs

Cost of living is determined for the individual student and is approximately $9,000 per year, not including tuition. Most medical students live on campus and most own cars.

FINANCIAL AID: Information pertaining to the student and his or her family income is considered in designing need-based loan packages, which consist of both grants and loans. The State of Alabama offers merit-based scholarships of up to $5,000 per year to exceptional students. In addition, students who commit to practice in rural Alabama have access to very low-interest, state-sponsored loans. Many private scholarships directed at Alabama residents are also available.

UNIVERSITY OF SOUTH ALABAMA

STUDENT BODY

Type	Public
*Enrollment	256
*% male/female	62/38
*% underrepresented minorities	9
# applied (total/out)	1,128/654
% interviewed (total/out)	20/1
% accepted (total/out)	NR/NR
% enrolled (total/out)	27/58
Average age	24

ADMISSIONS

Average GPA and MCAT Scores

Overall GPA	3.65	Science GPA	NR
MCAT Bio	10.00	MCAT Phys	10.00
MCAT Verbal	10.00	MCAT Essay	NR

Score Release Policy

The school has not responded to our inquiry regarding withheld MCAT scores. Therefore, we advise caution. Contact the Admissions Office before withholding any scores.

Application Information

Regular application	11/15
Regular notification	11/15 until filled
Early application	6/1–8/1
Early notification	10/1
Transfers accepted?	Yes
Admissions may be deferred?	Yes
AMCAS application accepted?	Yes
Interview required?	Yes
Application fee	$50

COSTS AND AID

Tuition & Fees

Tuition (in/out)	$7,000/$14,000
Cost of books	NR
Fees	$1,975

Financial Aid

% students receiving aid	NR
Average grant	$3,000
Average loan	$18,500
Average debt	$52,000

*Figures based on total enrollment

University of South Carolina
SCHOOL OF MEDICINE

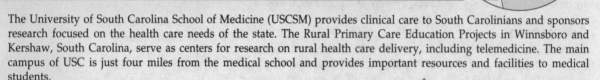

Columbia, SC 29208
Admission: 803-733-3325 • Fax: 803-733-3328
Internet: www.med.sc.edu

The University of South Carolina School of Medicine (USCSM) provides clinical care to South Carolinians and sponsors research focused on the health care needs of the state. The Rural Primary Care Education Projects in Winnsboro and Kershaw, South Carolina, serve as centers for research on rural health care delivery, including telemedicine. The main campus of USC is just four miles from the medical school and provides important resources and facilities to medical students.

Academics

In addition to the M.D., the School of Medicine offers the M.S. and Ph.D. degrees in Biomedical Science with specialization in Anatomy, Cell Biology, Experimental Pathology, Microbiology and Immunology, Pharmacology, and Physiology. For qualified students, a combined M.D./Ph.D. program is possible. A combined M.D./M.P.H. program, offered in conjunction with the School of Public Health at USC, is available. Also offered is the M.S. in Genetics Counseling, Biomedical Science with specialization in Nurse Anesthesia, and Rehabilitation Counseling. The M.D. curriculum stresses psychological and social perspectives along with biological principles. Elective opportunities are available throughout all four years to assist students in pursuing individual interests and career goals. Medical students are evaluated with an A–F scale. Passing Step 1 of the USMLE is a requirement for promotion to year three, and passing Step 2 is a graduation requirement.

BASIC SCIENCES: Throughout the first two years, clinical case studies are correlated with basic-science material. The two-year Introduction to Clinical Practice course emphasizes active, independent, and cooperative learning and uses a small-group format. Other first-year courses are Gross Anatomy, Microscopic Anatomy, Biochemistry, Neuroanatomy, and Physiology. Second-year courses are Microbiology, Pathology/Pathophysiology, and Pharmacology. An important resource is the USCSM Library, which has a collection of more than 90,0000 volumes. Medical students also use the USC Thomas Cooper Library, which has more than 2.5 million bound volumes.

CLINICAL TRAINING: Clerkship experiences in the third year include eight week rotations in Medicine, Surgery, Ob/Gyn, Psychiatry, Family Medicine, and Pediatrics. During the fourth year, required clerkships are four weeks each in Neurology and Surgery and eight weeks in Medicine. A four-week, multidisciplinary rotation concludes undergraduate clinical training and prepares students for the transition to residency and clinical practice. The remainder of the year is reserved for electives and selectives, many of which may be completed at locations around the state, at other medical schools, with federal and state agencies, and through an international elective program.

While the majority of students complete core clinical training at the five affiliated hospitals in Columbia, about 12 students in each class train at the Greenville Hospital System in Greenville, South Carolina. In the Columbia area, teaching hospitals include Palmetto Richland Memorial Hospital (649 beds); Dorn Veterans Hospital (447 beds); and the William S. Hall Psychiatric Institute (270 beds).

Students

Approximately 98 percent of students are South Carolina residents. About 9 percent of students are underrepresented minorities, most of whom are African American. Typically, about 25 percent of students in each entering class are nontraditional, having taken time off or pursued other careers or interests after college.

STUDENT LIFE: Because the School of Medicine is an important component of a comprehensive research university, medical students have many opportunities for interaction with students in other disciplines and can take advantage of the numerous student organizations, intramural sporting events, and social opportunities of the main University. Medical student organizations include chapters of the AMSA and the American Medical Women's Association, in addition to professionally focused groups such as the Internal Medicine, Family Practice, Emergency Medicine, and Pediatrics Clubs and the Psychiatry/Behavioral Science Society. Medical students have initiated a number of community service activities, including participation in the Columbia Free Medical Clinic, tutoring and social events at area children's homes, and the Health Education Leadership Program for primary school students. The School of Medicine has its own fitness center, but medical students also have access to all athletic facilities of the main campus. Columbia is a city with a population of almost 500,000, providing a wide variety of recreational and cultural activities. Both the ocean and the Great Smoky Mountains are within a few hours drive. On-campus housing is available for married couples, although most students live off campus in the area adjacent to the USC campus.

GRADUATES: Two-thirds of USCSM graduates go on to practice in primary care fields, making the School of Medicine a leader among U.S. medical schools in the percentage of graduates entering primary care. A large number enter residency programs in South Carolina or return to the state after completion of post-graduate training.

Admissions

REQUIREMENTS: Prerequisites are 8 semester hours each of General Biology or Zoology, Inorganic Chemistry, Organic Chemistry, and General Physics, all with associated labs. In addition, 6 semester hours of college-level Math and English are required. The MCAT is required, and scores must be no more than two years old. For applicants who have taken the exam more than once, the most recent set of scores is weighed most heavily.

SUGGESTIONS: A maximum of 6–8 positions in each class are open to residents of states other than South Carolina. Thus, nonresident applicants should be highly qualified. USCSM looks for applicants who are interested in primary care and who are likely to serve within the state.

PROCESS: All competitive AMCAS applicants who are South Carolina residents are sent secondary applications. About 40 percent of nonresident AMCAS applicants are sent secondaries. Of those returning secondaries, about 25 percent are interviewed between August and April. Interviews consist of two sessions, each with a member of the Admissions Committee. Candidates also have lunch with medical students and attend informational presentations. Notification of the Committee's decision occurs on a rolling basis, beginning in October. Approximately one third of interviewed candidates are accepted. Others are rejected or put on hold and possibly accepted later in the year.

Costs

The estimated yearly budget including tuition for a single student is about $26,053 per year. This budget allows for either on- or off-campus housing and car maintenance.

FINANCIAL AID: Federal loans and institutional grants are available to students with demonstrated financial need. Each year, several scholarships are awarded on the basis of academic merit or other special criteria.

UNIVERSITY OF SOUTH CAROLINA

STUDENT BODY

Type	Public
*Enrollment	295
*% male/female	60/40
*% underrepresented minorities	18
# applied (total/out)	1,304/869
% interviewed (total/out)	25/5
% accepted (total/out)	9/.6
% enrolled	76

ADMISSIONS

Average GPA and MCAT Scores

Overall GPA	NR	Science GPA	NR
MCAT Bio	NR	MCAT Phys	NR
MCAT Verbal	NR	MCAT Essay	NR

Score Release Policy

The school requires that all scores be released.

Application Information

Regular application	12/1
Regular notification	10/15 until filled
Early application	6/1–8/1
Early notification	10/1
Transfers accepted?	Yes
Admissions may be deferred?	Yes
AMCAS application accepted?	Yes
Interview required?	Yes
Application fee	$45

COSTS AND AID

Tuition & Fees

Tuition (in/out)	$9,000/$26,078
Cost of books	NR
Fees	NR

Financial Aid

% students receiving aid	89
Average grant	$5,068
Average loan	$18,616
Average debt	$67,877

*Figures based on total enrollment

UNIVERSITY OF SOUTH DAKOTA

SCHOOL OF MEDICINE

414 East Clark Street, Vermillion, SD 57069

Admission: 605-677-6886 • Fax: 605-677-5109

Internet: www.usd.edu/med/

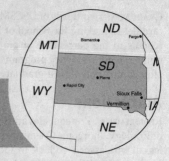

The University of South Dakota (USD) is a comprehensive university, with undergraduate, graduate, and professional programs, including Schools of Law and Business, in addition to the School of Medicine. The School of Medicine (USDSM) is focused on providing a high-quality, broad-based medical education with an emphasis on family practice for South Dakota residents. In recognition of the need for primary care physicians in rural areas within the state, USDSM emphasizes ambulatory and community-based health care. Medical students study basic sciences in Vermillion, a town of about 10,000, but have access to clinical training facilities throughout the state.

Academics

Most students complete the M.D. curriculum in four years. However, some students pursue joint degrees, such as the M.D./Ph.D. Graduate degrees may be earned in Anatomy, Biochemistry, Microbiology, Physiology, and Pharmacology. Medical students have the opportunity to undertake clinical or basic science research projects, arranged through the Summer Research Program. This program teams qualified students with physician/faculty mentors, and offers fellowship support. USD Medical students are evaluated with letter and numerical grades. Passing the USMLE Steps 1 and 2 is a requirement for graduation.

BASIC SCIENCES: The basic sciences are taught largely through lectures, labs, and small-group discussion, with an emphasis on clinical correlation. Students are in class or other scheduled sessions for about 30 hours per week. First-year courses are Biochemistry, Gross Anatomy and Embryology, Histology, Neuroanatomy, Physiology, and Introduction to Clinical Medicine (ICM). The ICM course is an interdisciplinary sequence that continues into the second year. During the first year, the course is entitled Introduction to the Patient: Personal and Professional Issues. The focus is on integrating biological, social, and psychological models and introducing the patient in all stages of the life cycle. Students also learn doctor/patient communication skills. Second-year courses are Behavioral Science, ICM, Laboratory Medicine, Microbiology, and Pharmacology. During year two, ICM focuses on the clinical skills necessary to provide basic patient care, such as the physical examination. Students also take part in a four-week preceptorship with a family practitioner from a rural community within the state. Basic sciences are taught in the Lee Memorial Medical Science Building on USDSM's main campus in Vermillion. The Lomman Health Sciences Library houses 96,000 volumes and 800 journals in addition to extensive computer resources.

CLINICAL TRAINING: During the third and fourth years, students rotate through hospitals and clinics in Sioux Falls, Rapid City, or Yankton. Standard third-year clerkships are Ob/Gyn (9 weeks); Medicine (10 weeks); Surgery (10 weeks); Pediatrics (8 weeks); Psychiatry (8 weeks); Neurology (1 week); Family Medicine (4 weeks); Radiology (2 hours per week); and a Longitudinal Ambulatory Clinic (4 hours per week for 50 weeks). Alternatively, third-year students may enter a unique, primary care curriculum in Yankton. The Yankton Model Program is a year-long, ambulatory-based, problem-oriented curriculum that emphasizes community involvement and self-directed learning. Students follow patients throughout the year, and present their findings to small groups of students and faculty. Students are exposed to the specialties of Family Medicine, Internal Medicine, Pediatrics, Ob/Gyn, Surgery, and Psychiatry. Fourth-year required clerkships for all students are Family Medicine (4 weeks); Emergency Room (4 weeks); and Surgical Specialties (7 weeks). An additional 21 weeks are reserved for electives. As a community-based medical school, the clinical facilities utilized by USD for teaching are neither owned nor operated by the School of Medicine. Rather, the school maintains strong affiliations with a range of health care providers throughout the state, including Rapid City Regional Hospital; Sioux Valley Health System and McKennen Hospital both in Sioux Falls; Sacred Heart Hospital in Yankton; several Veterans Hospitals (Sioux Falls, Fort Meade, Hot Springs); Ellsworth Air Force Base; and Yankton Medical Clinic.

Students

All admitted students are either South Dakota residents or have significant personal ties to South Dakota. About 4 percent of students are underrepresented minorities, most of whom are Native Americans. The average age of incoming students is about 23, and typically approximately one-quarter of entering students take some time off between college and medical school. Class size is 50.

STUDENT LIFE: The small class size encourages cohesion and interaction among students, as well as between faculty and students. First- and second-year students have access to the recreational and athletic facilities of the University. USD has over 127 student organizations, and the School of Medicine maintains chapters of national medical student organizations. Third- and fourth-year students have varied lifestyles, depending upon where their clinical training takes place. On-campus residence halls and apartments are available in Vermillion.

GRADUATES: Graduates are successful in securing residencies nationwide, with 70 to 80 percent matching to their first choice. At least 60 percent of graduates enter primary care fields.

Admissions

REQUIREMENTS: Prerequisites are one year each of Biology, Chemistry, Organic Chemistry, Physics, and college-level Math. The MCAT is required, and scores must be no more than three years old. For applicants who have retaken the exam, the most recent set of scores is compared to previous scores.

SUGGESTIONS: Residents of South Dakota, nonresidents with strong personal ties to the state (for example, they graduated from high school in South Dakota, or their parents live in-state,) and applicants of Native American descent who can demonstrate enrollment in federally recognized tribes in South Dakota or in border states are invited to submit secondary applications. Beyond academic credentials, exposure to the medical profession, volunteer activities, and interest in practicing primary care medicine and working with underserved communities are all valued.

PROCESS: All qualified AMCAS applicants who meet residency criteria are sent secondary applications. Of those returning secondaries, all are invited to interview with the admissions committee between October and March. Interviews consist of two one-hour-long sessions, each with a faculty member who is also part of the admissions committee. Of interviewed candidates, about 30 percent are accepted, with notification beginning in December. Wait-listed candidates are not encouraged to send additional information.

Costs

Beyond tuition, the estimated yearly cost of living for a single student is $14,580. This budget allows for on- or off-campus housing and travel expenses.

FINANCIAL AID: Although there are some merit-based scholarships, most aid is awarded on the basis of need, as determined by the FAFSA form.

UNIVERSITY OF SOUTH DAKOTA

STUDENT BODY

Type	Public
*Enrollment	208
*% male/female	54/46
*% underrepresented minorities	4
# applied (total/out)	643/519
% interviewed (total/out)	23/5
% accepted (total/out)	10/1
% enrolled (total/out)	81/1
Average age	23

ADMISSIONS

Average GPA and MCAT Scores

Overall GPA	3.65	Science GPA	3.61
MCAT Bio	9.10	MCAT Phys	8.70
MCAT Verbal	9.10	MCAT Essay	NR

Score Release Policy

The Admissions Office emphasizes that MCAT scores must be submitted.

Application Information

Regular application	11/15
Regular notification	12/15 until filled
Transfers accepted?	Yes
Admissions may be deferred?	Yes
AMCAS application accepted?	Yes
Interview required?	Yes
Application fee	$15

COSTS AND AID

Tuition & Fees

Tuition (in/out)	$10,408/$25,103
Cost of books	$2,500
Fees	$2,282

Financial Aid

% students receiving aid	94
Average grant	$2,324
Average loan	$28,500
Average debt	$91,206

*Figures based on total enrollment

University of South Florida

COLLEGE OF MEDICINE

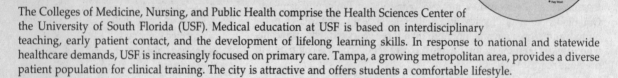

12901 Bruce B. Downs Boulevard, Tampa, FL 33612
Admission: 813-974-2229 • Fax: 813-974-4990

The Colleges of Medicine, Nursing, and Public Health comprise the Health Sciences Center of the University of South Florida (USF). Medical education at USF is based on interdisciplinary teaching, early patient contact, and the development of lifelong learning skills. In response to national and statewide healthcare demands, USF is increasingly focused on primary care. Tampa, a growing metropolitan area, provides a diverse patient population for clinical training. The city is attractive and offers students a comfortable lifestyle.

Academics

The four-year curriculum is designed to permit the student to learn the fundamental principles of medicine, to acquire skills of critical judgment based on evidence and experience, and to develop an ability to use principles and skills wisely in solving problems of health and disease. Medical students interested in careers in research may pursue a combined M.D./Ph.D. program, earning the doctorate in a number of biomedical fields. For students interested in public and community health issues, a combined M.D./M.P.H. program is offered in conjunction with the College of Public Health. Medical students are evaluated with Honors, Pass with Commendation, Pass, and Fail. Passing Step 1 of the USMLE is a requirement for promotion to year three, and passing Step 2 is a graduation requirement.

BASIC SCIENCES: First-year students focus mainly on basic sciences and are instructed in a variety of ways including lectures, labs, small-group conferences, and interdisciplinary methods. Computers are also an important educational resource. In addition to science courses, first-year students investigate ethical and behavioral aspects of medicine in the courses Behavioral Medicine and Medical Ethics. In the second semester, they begin to learn patient-interaction skills through a Physical Diagnosis course that extends into the second year. Other first-year courses are Gross Anatomy; Biochemistry; Microscopic Anatomy; Human Embryology; Molecular Biology and Human Genetics; Medical Neuroscience; and Physiology. The second year is a continuation of basic sciences with increased emphasis on clinical correlation. The remainder of Physical Diagnosis and Introduction to Clinical Medicine further develop patient examination and evaluation skills and prepare students for the clinical phase of the curriculum. Other second-year courses are Medical Microbiology and Immunology, Pathology and Laboratory Medicine, Clinical Correlation, and Pharmacology. Students are in class or other scheduled sessions for about 25 hours per week. In between the first and second year, there are opportunities for involvement in research.

CLINICAL TRAINING: Third-year required clinical rotations are eight weeks each of the following: Internal Medicine, Surgery, Pediatrics, Psychiatry, Ob/Gyn, and Family Medicine. The fourth year is devoted primarily to electives, a portion of which may be taken at other academic or clinical institutions at locations around the state, country, or overseas. Most clinical training takes place at Tampa General Hospital (1000 beds); H. Lee Moffitt Cancer Center and Research Institute (162 beds); James A. Haley Veterans Hospital (577 beds); the USF Psychiatry Center; USF Medical Clinic; All Children's Hospital (168 beds); USF Eye Institute; University Diagnostic Institute; Shriners Hospital for Crippled Children; Bayfront Medical Center (518 beds); and Bay Pines Veterans Medical Center (520 beds). A number of community-based clinics are also used as clinical training facilities.

Students

All students are Florida residents. About 7 percent of students are underrepresented minorities. Although most students enter shortly after college graduation, there is a wide age range in each class. Class size is 96.

STUDENT LIFE: Students are cooperative, often studying together and interacting outside of the academic setting. The Medical School sponsors student events and organizations, and has a strong emphasis on involvement in school and community activities. The Medical School is located on the main USF campus, giving students access to the amenities of a large university. Tampa has many cultural and recreational opportunities and is generally a popular city among students. Most students live off campus, where housing is relatively affordable and comfortable.

GRADUATES: Graduates are successful in securing residency positions in all specialty areas. At USF, post-graduate training programs are offered in more than 10 fields.

Admissions

REQUIREMENTS: Science requirements include one year each of basic introductory courses and laboratories in Biological Science, General Chemistry, Organic Chemistry, and Physics. One year of both English and Mathematics is also required. The MCAT is required, and scores should be from within the past three years. For applicants who have taken the exam more than once, the best set of scores is weighed most heavily. Thus, there is no advantage in withholding scores.

SUGGESTIONS: State residency is a requirement. Courses that are recommended, but not required, include Physical or Biological Chemistry, Biochemistry, Embryology, Cell Biology, Comparative Anatomy, Genetics, Statistics, Logic, and Rhetoric. Knowledge of calculus, computer science and statistics is useful. Consideration is given to a student's participation in honors courses, independent study, and scientific research. All applicants are advised to apply as early as possible because the application process is rolling.

PROCESS: All AMCAS applicants who are residents of Florida, and who meet minimum standards, are sent secondary applications. About 15 percent of those who return secondaries are invited to interview between September and April. Interviews are one-on-one with a faculty member. On interview day, candidates have the opportunity to tour the campus and to meet informally with current medical students. About 50 percent of interviewees are accepted, with notification occurring on a rolling basis. Others are rejected or wait-listed. Wait-listed candidates may send additional information to update their files.

Costs

The estimated yearly cost of living for a single student is about $15,000. This figure allows for off-campus housing. Most students own cars.

FINANCIAL AID: All assistance is provided on the basis of demonstrated financial need. Need is determined by a standardized analysis of both students' and parents' income and assets. Aid is in the form of loans and grants.

UNIVERSITY OF SOUTH FLORIDA

STUDENT BODY

Type	Public
*Enrollment	391
*% male/female	65/35
*% underrepresented minorities	7
# applied (total/out)	1,750/409
% interviewed (total/out)	22/0
% accepted (total/out)	NR/NR
% enrolled (total/out)	25/NR
Average age	23

ADMISSIONS

Average GPA and MCAT Scores

Overall GPA	3.70	Science GPA	3.70
MCAT Bio	10.30	MCAT Phys	10.10
MCAT Verbal	9.70	MCAT Essay	NR

Score Release Policy

National Board of Medical Examiners (USMLE Steps 1 & 2 may be reflected by the student only)

Application Information

Regular application	12/1
Regular notification	10/15 until filled
Early application	6/1–8/1
Early notification	10/1
Transfers accepted?	Yes
Admissions may be deferred?	Yes
AMCAS application accepted?	Yes
Interview required?	Yes
Application fee	$20

COSTS AND AID

Tuition & Fees

Tuition and fees (in/out)	$10,457/$28,108
Cost of books	$1,844

Financial Aid

% students receiving aid	82
Average grant	$5,000
Average loan	$18,500
Average debt	$65,000

*Figures based on total enrollment

UNIVERSITY OF SOUTHERN CALIFORNIA
SCHOOL OF MEDICINE

1975 Zonal Avenue (KAM 100-C), Los Angeles, CA 90033

Admission: 213-342-2552

Email: medadmit@hsc.usc.edu

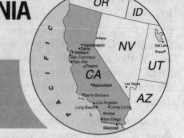

The University of Southern California (USC) School of Medicine is a private medical school located on the USC Health Sciences Campus in northeast Los Angeles, seven miles from the undergraduate campus. The school's primary clinical teaching facility, Los Angeles County and USC Medical Center, is one of the busiest teaching hospitals in the nation, with a large, diverse patient population representative of Los Angeles itself. USC also boasts extensive research facilities and specialty hospitals.

Academics

While the majority of students earn their M.D. in four years, USC offers a variety of joint-degree programs. The M.D./Ph.D. program is administered by the USC Graduate School and the School of Medicine, allowing students to earn the doctorate in Anatomy, Biochemistry, Biomedical Engineering, Biophysics, Cell Biology, Genetics, Immunology, Microbiology, Molecular Biology, Neuroscience, Pathology, Pharmacology, and Physiology. For those interested in more discrete research projects, the Research Scholar Program allows students to spend one year involved in research at USC or another approved institution. Students also have the option of entering a combined M.D./M.P.H. program.

BASIC SCIENCES: Lectures, labs, and periodic small-group discussions are the instructional modalities used during the first two years. Currently, the faculty and students are working together to design a revised curriculum which may depend more on small-group sessions and problem-based learning. The first year (38 weeks) begins with an introductory review course entitled Human Biology, which is followed by a sequence of courses based on organ systems. They are Cardiovascular, Endocrine/Reproduction, Gastrointestinal/Liver, Renal/Respiratory/Skin, Neuroscience, and Blood. Students benefit from patient contact from the very beginning in Introduction to Clinical Medicine. The second year (37 weeks) is also organized around body/organ systems and is dedicated to studying the mechanisms of disease. Key coursewait list ology, Microbiology, and Pharmacology. USC's library is comprehensive and has an ample supply of computers. Computers with course material, online resources, and other study aids are also available in individually assigned laboratory spaces, which serve as student study areas. Grading for the first two years is Honors/Satisfactory/Unsatisfactory. Students must pass Step 1 of the USMLE in order to be promoted to year three.

CLINICAL TRAINING: The clinical years are the hallmark of USC's education. The majority of teaching takes place in L.A. County and USC Medical Center. It is among the major public hospitals for Los Angeles and receives pa-

tients with every imaginable illness and injury. Students are allowed extensive patient contact. The curriculum of required courses and electives is continuous over the third and fourth years and is individually designed. Required clerkships are Internal Medicine (2 of 6 weeks each); Family Medicine (6 weeks); Pediatrics (6 weeks); Ob/Gyn (6 weeks); General Surgery (6 weeks); Psychiatry (6 weeks); Neurology (4 weeks); Specialized Surgery (2–3 weeks); and a Basic or Clinical Sciences Clerkship (4 weeks). An additional 12 weeks of selectives are required. Students may take up to 16 weeks of electives at approved institutions throughout the nation. In addition to LAC and USC Medical Center, clinical facilities include Children's Hospital Los Angeles, USC University Hospital, and USC/Norris Comprehensive Cancer Center. Grading during the clinical years is Honors/Near Honors/Satisfactory/Unsatisfactory. In order to graduate, students must record a score on the USMLE Step 2.

Students

Of the 150 students in each class, almost 80 percent are California residents. About 16 percent of students are underrepresented minorities. The average age of incoming students is about 24, with a wide age range including significant numbers of students in their thirties.

STUDENT LIFE: The Medical School campus is not situated in an ideal residential area, and the majority of students commute to school from surrounding communities. Nonetheless, USC has a cohesive and cooperative student body. Many first-year students attend a camping retreat prior to the beginning of classes, during which they are introduced to each other and to returning students. During the academic year, students typically study in groups, and spend time together outside of school. The School of Medicine offers a wide range of extracurricular activities, including volunteer programs, intramural sports, and student clubs and organizations. USC's main campus is easily accessible by car, and medical students regularly use its extensive recreational facilities. University-sponsored activities, such as intercollegiate sporting events, films, and parties, are also popular with medical students.

GRADUATES: Graduates are successful in securing positions nationwide, in both specialty and primary care fields. Most enter residency programs in California.

Admissions

REQUIREMENTS: Prerequisites are two semesters each, with associated labs, in Biology, General Chemistry, Organic Chemistry, and Physics. In addition, applicants must have completed a course in Basic Molecular Biology and an additional 30 semester hours in a combination of Social Sciences, Humanities, and English Composition. The MCAT is required, and scores must be from within the previous two years.

SUGGESTIONS: The Admissions Committee looks very favorably upon hospital or other medical experience that involves patient care and demonstrates a commitment to service. Research experience is also helpful. USC strongly recommends additional course work in Statistics and higher mathematics.

PROCESS: All AMCAS applicants are asked to submit a supplemental application. Of those students who return supplemental applications, approximately 800 are invited for interviews. The interview day consists of a tour, lunch with medical students, and one or two hour-long interviews with faculty and/or medical students. Initial acceptances are sent at the beginning of January, but most students are placed in a hold category, with the majority of acceptances offered in May. About 40 percent of interviewed candidates are accepted. Wait-listed candidates may send additional information to update or strengthen their files.

Costs

In addition to tuition, living expenses and fees are estimated at $13,000 to $14,000. This allows for off-campus living and car ownership.

FINANCIAL AID: Around 75 percent of the student body receives some form of financial aid. Both the student's and parents' need is considered when determining financial need. A variety of loans and scholarships are awarded. Although most are based on financial need, some merit-based scholarships may be available.

UNIVERSITY OF SOUTHERN CALIFORNIA

STUDENT BODY

Type	Private
*Enrollment	637
*% male/female	58/43
*% underrepresented minorities	16
# applied (total/out)	6,174/2,488
% interviewed (total/out)	11/NR
% accepted (total/out)	NR/NR
% enrolled (total/out)	21/NR
Average age	24

ADMISSIONS

Average GPA and MCAT Scores

Overall GPA	3.56	Science GPA	NR
MCAT Bio	10.60	MCAT Phys	10.60
MCAT Verbal	10.00	MCAT Essay	NR

Score Release Policy

The school has not responded to our inquiry regarding withheld MCAT scores. Therefore, we advise caution. Contact the Admissions Office before withholding any scores.

Application Information

Regular application	11/1
Regular notification	1/1 until filled
Early application	6/1–8/1
Early notification	10/1
Transfers accepted?	Yes
Admissions may be deferred?	Yes
AMCAS application accepted?	Yes
Interview required?	Yes
Application fee	$70

COSTS AND AID

Tuition & Fees

Tuition	$30,468
Cost of books	$2,200
Fees	$1,096

Financial Aid

% students receiving aid	75
Average grant	$10,000
Average loan	$29,800
Average debt	$93,000

*Figures based on total enrollment

SOUTHERN ILLINOIS UNIVERSITY

SCHOOL OF MEDICINE

PO Box 19624, Springfield, IL 62794-9624
Admission: 217-524-6013 • Fax: 217-785-5538
Email: egraham@siumed.edu • Internet: www.siumed.edu

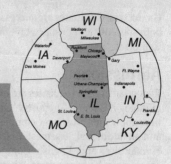

Southern Illinois University School of Medicine is committed to educating future physicians who will help meet the health care needs of Central and Southern Illinois. SIU is renowned for its effective use of simulated patients in clinical instruction and its inclusion of Medical Humanities in the curriculum. In order to take full advantage of available resources, first-year courses are taught at the Carbondale campus, while the remaining three years are spent in Springfield and at clinical affiliates in the region.

Academics

SIU offers a case-based, small group–oriented curriculum with an abundance of patient contact and early clinical exposure. In cooperation with the SIU School of Law, a joint M.D./J.D. degree program is also offered. Medical students are evaluated on Pass/Fail and with honors system. The USMLE Step 1 must be passed as a graduation requirement.

BASIC SCIENCES: The instructional format emphasizes small-group instruction, self-directed study, and a case-based approach, but also incorporates lectures and an organ system organizational scheme. Topics covered in the first year are cardiovascular, respiratory, renal, endocrine, reproductive, gastrointestinal, and sensorimotor systems and behavior. In Carbondale, basic science instruction takes place in Lindegren Hall. Early clinical experiences are offered at Memorial Hospital in Carbondale (151 beds), the Carbondale Clinic, offices of local physicians, and at the VA Hospital (171 beds). In Springfield, the Medical Instructional Facility contains lecture halls, classrooms, labs, and a teaching museum. A four-year doctoring curriculum (physicians conduct and attitude, clinical skills development, and medical humanities issues) begins immediately. Both simulated and real patients are used. Topics covered in the second year include circulation, infection and host diseases, neoplasia, population health and preventitive medicine, neuromuscular, and medicine behavior. Computer-assisted instruction is used as a learning aid, and computers are available in the Student Computer Lab and at other sites. The Morris Library at Carbondale houses more than 100,000 volumes, while the Medical Instruction Facility in Springfield contains 113,000 volumes.

CLINICAL TRAINING: Third-year required multidisciplinary rotations are Internal Medicine and Surgery (22 weeks); Family and Community Medicine, Primary Care, Psychiatry, and Neurology (12 weeks); Obstetrics, Gynecology, and Pediatrics (12 weeks). At the conclusion of the third year, students must pass an examination that evaluates their skills in assessing and managing patient problems. During the fourth year, students complete one additional required clerkship (Anesthesiology, 2 weeks). Thirty-one weeks are reserved for elective studies. Clinical training sites include Memorial Medical Center (580 beds), St. John's Hospital and Pavilion (715 beds), and the clinics and offices of faculty and community physicians. Electives may be taken off campus, and SIU has an institutional agreement with overseas universities—including locations in Germany and the Netherlands—that facilitate training overseas.

Students

At least 95 percent of students are Illinois residents. The average age of incoming students is 23. Underrepresented minorities account for about 8 percent of the student body. Class size is 72.

STUDENT LIFE: On-campus recreational facilities at Carbondale include a complete fitness room, swimming pools, racquetball courts, and a student center. Taking part in intramural sports and attending intercollegiate sporting events are popular extracurricular activities for medical students. St. Louis, with the amenities of a large city, is a two-hour drive. The surrounding area features a state park and the Shawnee National Forest, where students can hike, bike, camp, canoe, or enjoy the beach. In Springfield, medical students enjoy discounts to health clubs such as the YMCA. Lake Springfield offers fishing, swimming, boating, and sailing. Parks, golf courses, and cultural and historical sites are other local attractions. All students live off campus in both Carbondale and Springfield.

GRADUATES: Among the 2000 graduating class, the most prevalent fields for post-graduate training were Family Practice (25%), Pediatric Medicine (21%), and Ob/Gyn (10%). Students generally score around the national mean on the USMLE, making them well-positioned for securing residency positions.

Admissions

REQUIREMENTS: In order to do well on the MCAT, students should have taken at least one year each of Biology, Chemistry, Organic Chemistry, Physics, English, and Math, the last of which should have included some Statistics. The

MCAT is required and scores must be no more than two years old. For applicants who have taken the exam on multiple occasions, the most recent set of scores is considered.

SUGGESTIONS: As a state school, preference is given to applicants from Central and Southern Illinois who are interested in practicing in the region. Applicants are expected to have a good foundation in the natural sciences, social sciences, and humanities in addition to sound English skills. The Admissions Committee looks beyond scholastic achievement for evidence of responsibility, integrity, compassion, motivation, interest in medicine, community service, and sound interpersonal skills. The Medical Education Preparatory Program (MEDPREP) is a nondegree post-baccalaureate program that assists disadvantaged students with meeting the requirements for the SIU School of Medicine.

PROCESS: About one-fifth of AMCAS applicants are interviewed, the vast majority of them Illinois state residents. Interviews are conducted between August and April, and consist of two sessions with individual faculty and/or administrators. About 33 percent of interviewed candidates are accepted on a batch basis. Others are rejected or wait-listed. Wait-listed candidates may send supplemental material to update their files.

Costs

Beyond tuition, the estimated yearly cost of living for a single student is $10,804. This budget supports off-campus housing.

FINANCIAL AID: Most aid is need-based, with financial need determined by the FAFSA form. Parental disclosure is required for some forms of assistance.

SOUTHERN ILLINOIS UNIVERSITY

STUDENT BODY

Type	Public
*Enrollment	291
*% male/female	59/41
*% underrepresented minorities	7
# applied (total/out)	1,271/350
% interviewed (total/out)	19/1
% accepted (total/out)	9/1
% enrolled (total/out)	57/0
Average age	23

ADMISSIONS

Average GPA and MCAT Scores

Overall GPA	3.51	Science GPA	3.43
MCAT Bio	9.5	MCAT Phys	8.5
MCAT Verbal	9.0	MCAT Essay	O

Score Release Policy

The school has not responded to our inquiry regarding withheld MCAT scores. Therefore, we advise caution. Contact the Admissions Office before withholding any scores.

Application Information

Regular application	11/15
Regular notification	10/15–varies
Transfers accepted?	Yes
Admissions may be deferred?	Yes
AMCAS application accepted?	Yes
Interview required?	Yes
Application fee	$50

COSTS AND AID

Tuition & Fees

Tuition (in/out)	$15,134/$36,402
Cost of books	$1,554
Fees	$1,144

Financial Aid

% students receiving aid	89
Average grant	$9,022
Average loan	$7,083
Average debt	$71,649

*Figures based on total enrollment

STANFORD UNIVERSITY
SCHOOL OF MEDICINE

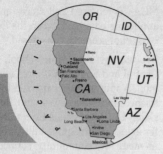

251 Campus Drive, MSOB X309, Stanford, CA 94305-5404
Admission: 650-723-6861 Fax: 650-725-7855
Internet: www.med.stanford.edu

Stanford boasts some of the best-reputed graduate departments in the nation. The Medical School is no exception and benefits from its position within the University. Students are encouraged to pursue research in their areas of interest, in either the sciences or interdisciplinary fields. In fact, the opportunities for research are so enticing that most students spread out the four-year curriculum into five, freeing up time and allowing them to take advantage of the tremendous resources of the University. This flexibility, combined with the charms of Northern California, the ease of suburban life, and the premier clinical teaching facilities, available makes Stanford a popular choice.

Academics

Generally, about 60 percent of Stanford students receive their M.D. in five rather than four years, which allows for individual research and elective study. In addition to the M.D., departmental joint degrees include an M.D./Ph.D. in Biochemistry, Developmental Biology, Genetics, Microbiology and Immunology, Molecular and Cellular Physiology, Molecular Pharmacology, and Structural Biology. Interdepartmental joint degrees are also possible, and include an M.S. in Biomechanical Engineering and Health Services Research, an M.S. and Ph.D. in Epidemiology and Medical Information Sciences, and a Ph.D. in Biophysics, Cancer Biology, Immunology, and Neuroscience. There are about six to eight M.S.T.P. slots available. In addition to formal degree programs, students may take electives in nonmedical departments. Through the Medical Student Scholars Program and other programs, students enjoy a range of research opportunities, most of which are remunerated.

BASIC SCIENCES: Stanford operates on a quarter system, and pre-clinical studies are organized into 6 quarters. During this period of rigorous science course work, students are gradually introduced to clinical care and have clinical training opportunities throughout. Classes demand 20–35 hours per week, with considerable variation from quarter to quarter. During the fall (first) quarter of the first year, students typically take Human Anatomy and Development, which includes an introduction to the Physical Examination, Structure of Cells and Tissues, and Introduction to Psychiatry, which involves patient interviews. Winter (second) quarter offers Biochemistry, Biostatistics and Epidemiology, Neurobiology, Health Systems/Policy, Clinical Psychiatry, and Physicians and Patients, a course exploring interdisciplinary topics and continuing medical interviews. During the spring (third) quarter, Molecular Biology, Genetics, Cardiovascular Physiology, Pathology, and Host Parasites and Defense are taken. The second-year fall (fourth) quarter introduces students to Infectious Basis of Disease, Physiology, Pharmacology, and more Pathology. In addition, preparation for Clinical Medicine begins. The fifth quarter

innnonresidentgy, Endocrine Physiology, Pathophysiology, and more Pharmacology and Pathology. Students make the transition into their clinical studies during this quarter and the second year (sixth quarter) with Clinical Problem Solving, presented in a case-based, small-group format and a Preceptor Program including general and psychiatric patient care. The Lane Medical Library, which is soon to benefit from substantial remodeling and enlargment, currently houses 3,000 journal titles, 350,000 volumes, and online data management services. Computer, audiovisual and other learning aids are accessible to students at the Fleischmann Learning and Resource Center. Videotapes of most pre-clinical courses are available, and appear to substitute for student-organized note services. Grading is strictly Pass/Fail, and mid-quarter exams are optional. A week-long reading period prior to final exams allows students uninterrupted study time. Step 1 of the USMLE must be passed no later than one year prior to graduation, and Step 2 must be passed in order to graduate.

CLINICAL TRAINING: Patient contact begins in the fall quarter of the first year, and there are opportunities for clinical experiences during the first two years. Third- and fourth-year clerkships take place at the major affiliated teaching hospitals, which include Stanford Hospital (479 beds), the Lucile Salter Packard Children's Hospital (162 beds), Santa Clara Valley Medical Center (644 beds), three VA Hospitals, Kaiser Permanente (336 beds), and Columbia San Jose Medical Center (529 beds). These facilities serve both rural and urban populations with diverse needs. Students complete 15 months of clinical clerkships, including nine months of required core clerkships in Medicine, Surgery, Pediatrics, Ob/Gyn, Psychiatry, and Family Medicine. Three months are spent training in areas related to required clerkships through "selectives," in which students choose from Basics In Clinical Care, Ambulatory Care, and Subinternship. The final three months are designated as elective clerkships.

Students

Stanford students are often characterized as being less cut throat than those attending other top-ranked schools, perhaps because the flexible curriculum encourages students to focus beyond the classroom. Special effort is made to recruit students from underrepresented minority backgrounds, and student organizations support these and other student groups. With 86 students per class, Stanford is relatively small.

Student Life: The campus and the surrounding area offer excellent sports and other outdoor activities. San Francisco is an hour away and is accessible by train. Numerous on-campus housing options exist, including family housing, apartments, dormitories, and co-ops. However, high rent in the vicinity of Stanford makes student housing competitive.

Graduates: Stanford itself offers excellent residency programs, and many graduates opt for post-graduate training at Stanford. Perhaps as a result of the teaching and research experience students gain while in school, many go on into academic medicine. Increasingly, graduates are entering primary care fields.

Admissions

Requirements: Biology with lab (1 year); Chemistry/Organic Chemistry with labs (2 years); and Physics with lab (1 year). The quality of an undergraduate institution is considered in evaluating the academic record. The MCAT must be no more than three years old. The most recent set of scores is used.

Suggestions: Biochemistry, Calculus, and Behavioral Sciences are recommended, as is knowledge of a second language. No preference is given to California residents or to Stanford undergraduates. Successful applicants generally have significant medical, health-related, research, or community service experience.

Process: Secondary applications are long, requiring many short responses. They are sent out on a rolling basis, with information due between 2–4 weeks. Interviews involve two semi-structured, 60-minute sessions, one with a faculty member and one with a medical student. Of interviewed candidates, about one-third are accepted, one-third rejected, and one-third put on a wait list, with responses given within 6 weeks of the interview. During the past few years, from 0–15 applicants were eventually accepted off of the wait list.

Costs

The average cost of living per quarter is estimated at $4,488, reflecting high rent. This presumes on-campus living or shared accommodations off campus, although individual needs are considered in determining a student's budget. Most students own cars.

Financial Aid: Financial aid is need-based. Assistance is in the form of grants and loans, grants being given after students meet a minimum level of "self-help" funding through personal earnings, employment, or loans. Students who conduct research are typically remunerated. Parents' incomes are assessed and parental contribution is generally expected if feasible. For "middle income" families who qualify for financial assistance, but do not qualify for substantial grant assistance, there is a parental matching formula used in which grants are made to match parental giving up to $15,000 a year. There are no merit-based scholarships.

STANFORD UNIVERSITY

STUDENT BODY

Type	Private
*Enrollment	473
*% male/female	52/48
*% underrepresented minorities	14
# applied (total/out)	6,430/4,182
% interviewed (total/out)	9/5
% accepted (total/out)	3/2
% enrolled (total/out)	43/52
Average age	23

ADMISSIONS

Average GPA and MCAT Scores

Overall GPA	3.76	Science GPA	3.70
MCAT Bio	11.00	MCAT Phys	11.00
MCAT Verbal	10.00	MCAT Essay	NR

Score Release Policy

The school has not responded to our inquiry regarding withheld MCAT scores. Therefore, we advise caution. Contact the Admissions Office before withholding any scores.

Application Information

Regular application	11/1
Regular notification	10/15 until filled
Early application	6/1–8/1
Early notification	10/15
Transfers accepted?	No
Admissions may be deferred?	Yes
AMCAS application accepted?	Yes
Interview required?	Yes
Application fee	$65

COSTS AND AID

Tuition & Fees

Tuition	$29,706
Cost of books	$1,314
Fees	$733

Financial Aid

% students receiving aid	70
Average grant	$18,000
Average loan	$12,000
Average debt	$68,000

*Figures based on total enrollment

State University of New York
Health Science Center at Brooklyn
COLLEGE OF MEDICINE

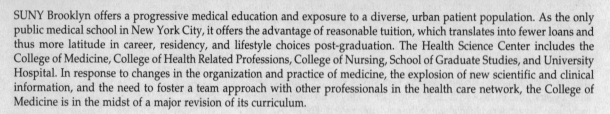

450 Clarkson Avenue-Box 60M, Brooklyn, NY 11203

Admission: 718-270-2446 • Fax: 718-270-7592

Email: admissions@netmail.hscbklyn.edu • Internet: www.hscbklyn.edu

SUNY Brooklyn offers a progressive medical education and exposure to a diverse, urban patient population. As the only public medical school in New York City, it offers the advantage of reasonable tuition, which translates into fewer loans and thus more latitude in career, residency, and lifestyle choices post-graduation. The Health Science Center includes the College of Medicine, College of Health Related Professions, College of Nursing, School of Graduate Studies, and University Hospital. In response to changes in the organization and practice of medicine, the explosion of new scientific and clinical information, and the need to foster a team approach with other professionals in the health care network, the College of Medicine is in the midst of a major revision of its curriculum.

Academics

The new curriculum emphasizes the development of clinical reasoning and problem-solving skills, it integrates basic and clinical sciences, and exposes students from the first week of the first year to patient care. In this "doctoring experience," each student spends one afternoon each week in a physician's private office or clinic; the practicing physician serves as the student's clinical mentor for the entire year. Students are also encouraged to participate in research. Opportunities are available throughout the 4 years of medical school. Those who make a significant research contribution are eligible to graduate with Distinction in Research. An M.S.T.P.-sponsored M.D./Ph.D. program is open to four students each year in one of two modern biomedical science areas, Neuroscience or Molecular and Cell Biology. Medical students are evaluated with an Honors/High Pass/Pass/Fail system. Students must pass Step 1 of the USMLE in order to be promoted to year three. Students are encouraged to take Step 2 prior to graduation, but it is not a requirement.

BASIC SCIENCES: Basic science courses have been integrated into "topics" or blocks. Each block is taught using a combination of traditional lectures, case-based, small-group sessions, laboratories, conferences, and a weekly clinical experience. First year topics are Genes to Cells, Skin and Connective Tissue, Musculoskeletal System, Blood/Hematopoiesis/ Lymphoid, Cardiovascular System, Respiratory System, Gastrointestinal System/ Intermediary Metabolism, Renal/Urinary System, Endocrine and Reproduction Systems, Head and Neck, and Neuroscience. The current second-year curriculum includes courses in Pathology, Pathophysiology, Pharmacology, Microbiology and Immunology, Preventive Medicine,

Preparation for Clinical Medicine, Psychopathology, and Nutrition. With the exception of the last two, each course runs throughout the full academic year, with each discipline presenting material related to specific organ systems. The Office of Academic Development promotes students' academic success through seminars, workshops, and individual tutoring. The Health Science Education Building holds two floors of study carrels, which serve as "home base" to students during the first two years. In the same building is the Medical Research Library, one of the largest medical school libraries in the country, and a 500 seat auditorium. A Learning Resource Center has 90 computer work stations loaded with an array of medical applications.

CLINICAL TRAINING: The current third-year clerkships (to be revised 2000–2001) are Medicine (12 weeks); Surgery (12 weeks, including 2 weeks in Anesthesia); Pediatrics (8 weeks); Ob/Gyn (6 weeks); Psychiatry (6 weeks); and Neurology (4 weeks). Fourth-year requirements are Ambulatory Care (6 weeks); a Subinternship (4 weeks), and at least 20 weeks of electives. Training takes place at a number of major affiliates, University Hospital, and Kings County Hospital. Electives can be completed at those institutions or at extramural hospitals or medical centers.

Students

This year's first-year class is 180 students from more than 60 individual colleges. About 96 percent are New York State residents. Approximately 13 percent of students are underrepresented minorities. The age range of the 1998 entering class is 20–39, with an average of 24.

STUDENT LIFE: All entering students are assigned a clinical faculty mentor who provides guidance and support throughout the first year. The focal point for recreational, social, and cultural activities on campus is the Student Center, which has lounges, a piano room, an athletic center, a swimming pool, squash courts, and a spa. Student organizations focus on professional, ethnic, service related, social, and recreational interests, and also provide support for groups of students. For example, the Daniel Hale Williams Society, named for a prominent black physician, is a voice for minority students on campus and also brings students together to participate in educational, social, and service-related goals. Brooklyn is a culturally rich, active community that provides an exciting extracurricular life for medical students. Manhattan is easily accessible on the subway. On-campus housing options are single or shared studios, or dormitory rooms. Students who live off campus often reside in the nearby neighborhood of Park Slope.

GRADUATES: SUNY Brooklyn graduates perform above the national average in terms of securing residency positions at top institutions nationwide. Alumni hold faculty positions at universities such as Harvard, Case Western, Stanford, Yale, Hopkins, Columbia, Cornell, and the University of Pennsylvania, among other prestigious institutions. Fifty-one percent of 1999 graduating students entered residency programs in primary care. More than 73 percent of graduates chose to stay within New York State.

Admissions

REQUIREMENTS: Fifteen positions in each class are reserved for students in a B.A./M.D. program organized with Brooklyn College. Five positions are reserved for early assurance applicants from Queens College and the College of Staten Island. New York residents are given strong preference for the remaining spots. Prerequisites are eight semester credits each of Biology, Chemistry, Organic Chemistry, and Physics, all with associated labs. Six semester hours of English are also required. The MCAT is required and scores must be from within three years of the date of anticipated enrollment. Component scores for each MCAT series are looked at individually.

SUGGESTIONS: In addition to required courses, one year each of college-level Math, Biochemistry, and another advanced science are recommended. Medically related experience and demonstrated commitment to social service and community outreach activities are important factors in admission.

PROCESS: All AMCAS applicants are sent secondary applications. About 20 percent of those returning secondaries are interviewed between September and April. Interviews consist of one one-hour session with a faculty member. On interview day, candidates also have a group orientation session, lunch with current students, and a campus tour. Of interviewed candidates, about 40 percent are accepted on a rolling basis. Wait-listed candidates are not encouraged to send supplementary information.

Costs

The estimated first-year budget, including tuition and fees, is $30,500.

FINANCIAL AID: Virtually all assistance is need-based, with need determined by federal formulas. Most aid is in the form of loans. State programs that award scholarships in exchange for work in underserved areas are available.

STATE UNIVERSITY OF NEW YORK HEALTH SCIENCE CENTER AT BROOKLYN

STUDENT BODY

Type	Public
*Enrollment	757
*% male/female	56/44
*% underrepresented minorities	15
# applied (total/out)	3,505/1,159
% interviewed (total/out)	16/1
% accepted (total/out)	10/1
% enrolled (total/out)	48/30
Average age	24

ADMISSIONS

Average GPA and MCAT Scores

Overall GPA	3.58	Science GPA	3.50
MCAT Bio	10.5	MCAT Phys	10.2
MCAT Verbal	9.0	MCAT Essay	NR

Score Release Policy

The school has not responded to our inquiry regarding withheld MCAT scores. Therefore, we advise caution. Contact the Admissions Office before withholding any scores.

Application Information

Regular application	12/15
Regular notification	10/15 until filled
Early application	6/1–8/1
Early notification	10/1
Admissions may be deferred?	Yes
AMCAS application accepted?	Yes
Interview required?	Yes
Application fee	$65

COSTS AND AID

Tuition & Fees

Tuition (in/out)	$10,840/$21,940
Cost of books	NR
Fees	$320

Financial Aid

% students receiving aid	80
Average grant	$2,642
Average loan	$21,000
Average debt	NR

*Figures based on total enrollment

STATE UNIVERSITY OF NEW YORK
HEALTH SCIENCE CENTER AT SYRACUSE
COLLEGE OF MEDICINE

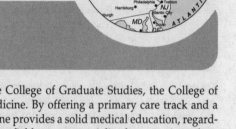

155 Elizabeth Blackwell Street, Syracuse, NY 13210

Admission: 315-464-4604 • Fax: 315-464-8867

Internet: www.hscsyr.edu

Academic institutions at the Health Science Center at Syracuse include the College of Graduate Studies, the College of Health Related Professions, the College of Nursing, and the College of Medicine. By offering a primary care track and a research track in addition to the traditional curriculum, the College of Medicine provides a solid medical education, regardless of whether a student is interested in going on to practice in a primary care field, a more specialized area, or intends to work in research or academic medicine. Syracuse provides rigorous training coupled with genuine concern for the well-being of students.

Academics

An alternative track that involves clinical training in Binghamton is geared toward students who are interested in primary care and ambulatory medicine. About one-quarter of entering students participate in this track and diverge from the rest of the group for their third and fourth years. Opportunities for research include the Academic Research Track, electives that are research-based, summer research projects and the combined M.D./Ph.D. program. The Ph.D. is offered in Anatomy, Biochemistry, Cell Biology, Immunology, Microbiology, Molecular Biology, Neuroscience, Pharmacology, and Physiology. Each year, two M.S.T.P. positions are available in addition to other funding options. A joint M.D./M.B.A. program is also possible. Medical students are evaluated with Honors/Pass/Fail, and both steps of the USMLE must be passed in order to graduate.

BASIC SCIENCES: First-year courses are Embryology, Gross Anatomy, Microscopic Anatomy, Physiology, Biochemistry, Cell and Molecular Biology, Neuroscience, Genetics, and Medicine and Society I. During the first year, students are in class or other scheduled sessions for 35 hours per week. The majority of class time is devoted to lectures and labs, supplemented with small-group discussions. Second-year courses are Medicine and Society II, Microbiology and Immunology, Nutrition, Pathology, Pharmacology, Epidemiology, Introduction to Clinical Medicine, Family Practice, and Behavioral Sciences. During the second year, students are in class for about 30 hours per week, with less emphasis on laboratory work and more time spent in small group sessions. Basic science instruction takes place in Weiskotten Hall, which is adjacent to the school's main clinical affiliates. The library houses over 171,000 volumes and features online reference services. Microcomputers and audiovisual equipment are available as learning resources.

CLINICAL TRAINING: The third and fourth years are considered as a continuum. For students at the Syracuse campus, required clerkships are Medicine (12 weeks); General Surgery (6 weeks); Pediatrics (6 weeks); Ob/Gyn (6 weeks); Neurology/Neurosurgery/Ophthalmology (6 weeks); Psychiatry (6 weeks); Radiology (3 weeks); Orthopedic Surgery/ENT/Anesthesia (4 weeks); Preventive Medicine (2 weeks); and Urology (2 weeks). Training takes place at State University Hospital (350 beds); U.S. Veteran's Administration Medical Center (379 beds); Crouse-Irving Memorial Hospital (490 beds); Community-General Hospital (350 beds); Richard H. Hutchings Psychiatric Center; and St. Joseph's Hospital and Health Center (472 beds). Students interested in a community-oriented clinical experience may opt to spend their third and fourth years in Binghamton, referred to as the Clinical Campus. Here, students establish close working relationships with community physicians and have enhanced opportunities for training in ambulatory care settings. Required clerkships are Advanced Skills (2 weeks); Ambulatory Surgery (4 weeks); General Surgery (6 weeks); Internal Medicine (12 weeks); Neuroscience (2 weeks); Psychiatry (6 weeks); Ob/Gyn (6 weeks); Pediatrics (6 weeks); and Radiology (2 weeks). Other elements of the curriculum include a longitudinal primary care clerkship (one half day per week) and a course dealing with social aspects of medicine. Typically, two required clerkships, Gerontology/Geriatric Medicine and Preventive Medicine/Community Health, are taken during the fourth year. Affiliates in Binghamton are Wilson Memorial Hospital (350 beds); Binghamton General Hospital (250 beds); Our Lady of Lourdes Memorial Hospital (acute care/hospice); and Robert Packer Hospital (366 beds). In both tracks, a minimum of 24 weeks of electives are required. A portion of these may be taken in nonuniversity settings in the area, around the country, and overseas.

Students

From 90 to 95 percent of students are New York residents. About 5 percent of students are underrepresented minorities, and about 15 percent took some significant time off between college and medical school. Class size is 150.

STUDENT LIFE: SUNY Syracuse recognizes the need for nonacademic opportunities and encourages a range of student activities. The Campus Activities Building is a hub for extracurricular pursuits and student interaction. Its athletic facilities include a comprehensive gym, a swimming pool, squash courts, tennis courts, running tracks, and pool tables. Other attractions are the snack bar, lounge, bookstore, and outdoor patio. Intramural sports, and campus-sponsored events, such as movies and happy hours, provide further distractions to medical students in need of a break from studying. Student organizations include chapters of national associations in addition to a number of groups based on ethnic or religious background, professional goals, or recreational interests. Syracuse is a medium-sized city surrounded by countryside. It is a one-hour drive to Lake Ontario's beaches, and five hours to New York City. Binghamton is conveniently situated about three hours from New York City, Philadelphia, and Buffalo. Modern residence halls at the Syracuse campus provide dormitory rooms, studios, and one-bedroom apartments for single and married students. In Binghamton, students live off campus.

GRADUATES: Graduates are successful in securing residencies in all fields. Increasingly, graduates are entering primary care fields.

Admissions

REQUIREMENTS: Prerequisites are Chemistry (6–8 semester hours); Organic Chemistry (6–8 hours); Biology (6–8 hours); Physics (6–8 hours); and English (6 hours).

SUGGESTIONS: Academic work in the Humanities and Social Sciences is considered equally as important as science course work.

PROCESS: All applicants are sent secondary applications. Of those returning secondaries, about 20 percent are invited to interview between September and February. Interviews consist of two sessions each with faculty members, administrators, students or alumni. About 20 percent of interviewed candidates are accepted on a rolling basis, while others are admitted later in the year.

Costs

Beyond tuition, the yearly cost of living for a single student is $11,000-$12,000. This budget allows for on-campus, or shared off-campus housing and transportation to clinical sites.

FINANCIAL AID: The financial aid office seeks to ensure that medical school is financially possible for all students. Financial aid is need-based, with need determined by the FAFSA form. About 90 percent of students receive financial aid, most of which is in the form of loans.

STATE UNIVERSITY OF NEW YORK HEALTH SCIENCE CENTER AT SYRACUSE

STUDENT BODY

Type	Public
*Enrollment	606
*% male/female	54/46
*% underrepresented minorities	5
# applied (total/out)	2,760/NR
% interviewed (total/out)	23/2
% accepted (total/out)	13/10
% enrolled (total/out)	25/6

ADMISSIONS

Average GPA and MCAT Scores

Overall GPA	3.57	Science GPA	3.67
MCAT Bio	9.7	MCAT Phys	9.4
MCAT Verbal	8.7	MCAT Essay	NR

Score Release Policy

This school has not responded to our inquiry regarding withheld MCAT scores. Therefore, we advise caution. Contact the Admissions Office before withholding any scores.

Application Information

Regular application	11/1
Regular notification	10/15–varies
Early application	6/1–8/1
Early notification	10/1
Transfers accepted?	Yes
Admissions may be deferred?	Yes
AMCAS application accepted?	Yes
Interview required?	Yes
Application fee	$100

COSTS AND AID

Tuition & Fees

Tuition (in/out)	$10,840/$21,940
Cost of books	$1,765
Fees	$990

Financial Aid

% students receiving aid	90
Average grant	$2,487
Average loan	$19,784
Average debt	$81,835

*Figures based on total enrollment

STATE UNIVERSITY OF NEW YORK AT STONY BROOK

SCHOOL OF MEDICINE HEALTH SCIENCES CENTER

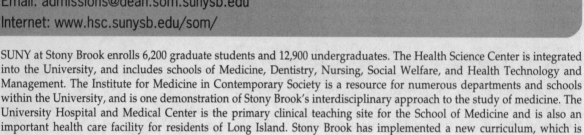

Committee on Admissions, Level 4, Room 147, Stony Brook, NY 11794

Admission: 631-444-2113 • Fax: 631-444-6032

Email: admissions@dean.som.sunysb.edu

Internet: www.hsc.sunysb.edu/som/

SUNY at Stony Brook enrolls 6,200 graduate students and 12,900 undergraduates. The Health Science Center is integrated into the University, and includes schools of Medicine, Dentistry, Nursing, Social Welfare, and Health Technology and Management. The Institute for Medicine in Contemporary Society is a resource for numerous departments and schools within the University, and is one demonstration of Stony Brook's interdisciplinary approach to the study of medicine. The University Hospital and Medical Center is the primary clinical teaching site for the School of Medicine and is also an important health care facility for residents of Long Island. Stony Brook has implemented a new curriculum, which is problem-based and organized around body systems.

Academics

Most students earn the M.D. degree in four years. Students who engage in relevant projects or course work may be eligible for the M.D. with Recognition in Research, the M.D. with Recognition in Primary Care, or the M.D. with Recognition in Humanities. A combined M.D./Ph.D. program is offered as part of the M.S.T.P. The doctorate degree may be earned in Anatomy, Biochemistry, Biomedical Engineering, Cell Biology, Genetics, Immunology, Microbiology, Molecular Biology, Neuroscience, Pathology, Pharmacology, and Physiology. Medical students are evaluated with Honors/Pass/Fail and must take both steps of the USMLE in order to graduate.

BASIC SCIENCES: Taken throughout all four years, the course Medicine in Contemporary Society addresses a range of social issues as they relate to medical training. Other first-year courses are Preventive Medicine; The Body; Cell, Genes and Molecules; Organ Systems; Neuroscience; Introduction to Human Behavior; Pathology; Nutrition; and Introduction to Clinical Medicine, which teaches fundamental clinical skills and provides early patient contact. Second-year courses are Microbiology/Infectious Diseases; Pharmacology; Introduction to Clinical Medicine II; and A Systems Approach to Medicine, which is organized around body systems. Students are in class or scheduled sessions for 20–25 hours per week. Class time is divided between lectures, labs, small group discussions, and clinical experiences, which serve to enrich learning and motivate students. The Health Sciences Center Library houses approximately 273,000 volumes and 2,750 health science–related periodicals, in addition to networked and online computer resources.

CLINICAL TRAINING: Third-year required clerkships are Medicine/Radiology (12 weeks); Surgery (8 weeks); Pediatrics (8 weeks); Ob/Gyn (6 weeks); Psychiatry (4 weeks); Family Medicine (6 weeks); Radiology (2 weeks); and Emergency Medicine (2 weeks). During the fourth year, a one-month subinternship, a one-month rotation in Neurology, one month of a didactic course, one month of Surgical Specialties, and two weeks of Psychiatry in Medicine are required. The remainder of the year is reserved for electives. Most training takes place at the University Hospital (504 beds); the Northport Veterans Affairs Medical Center (832 beds); Nassau County Medical Center (615 beds); and Winthrop-University Hospital (533 beds). As a way of learning about and relating to the community, all Health Sciences students must spend some time working with a Long Island health and welfare agency. Generally, students enjoy considerable flexibility in how and where they earn clinical elective credits.

Students

Typically, close to 100 percent of students are New York residents. About 10 percent are underrepresented minorities. There is a wide age-range among students, and at least 5–10 students in each class are in their thirties. Class size is 100.

STUDENT LIFE: Stony Brook is located on the North Shore of Long Island, just over an hour's train ride from Manhattan. Students enjoy both the comfort of their school's suburban location and its proximity to the city. The campus offers a vast sports complex, and the immediate area offers bike trails, beaches, and parks. The Stony Brook Union is the campus center for hundreds of activities, including eating, socializing, watching TV, taking art and other noncredit classes, playing billiards and table tennis, and shopping. It is also the home of student organizations, student government, and informational services. On-campus child care is available to students. University-owned housing includes residence halls and several apartment complexes with units of all sizes. Most students own cars, which are particularly important during the clinical years.

GRADUATES: Among 1999 graduates, the most prevalent fields for residencies were: Medicine (34%); Surgery (7%); Pediatrics (17%); Family Medicine (15%); Ob/Gyn (7%); and Emergency Medicine (7%). About 25 percent entered programs at University-affiliated hospitals.

Admissions

REQUIREMENTS: With the exception of M.S.T.P. applicants, New York residency is virtually a requirement. Academic prerequisites are one year each of Biology, Physics, Chemistry, Organic Chemistry, and English. Science courses must include associated labs. The MCAT is required, and scores must be no more than 5 years old. For applicants who have taken the exam more than once, the best scores are considered. Thus, there is no advantage in withholding scores.

SUGGESTIONS: Applicants who have taken significant time off after college should have some recent course work. For all applicants, some medically related experience is important, and patient contact is particularly valued.

PROCESS: All AMCAS applicants receive secondary applications. About 25 percent of those returning secondaries are interviewed between September and March. Interviews consist of one session with a member of the Admissions Committee in addition to a group orientation session, tour, and the opportunity to meet with current medical students. About 40 percent of interviewed candidates are accepted, with notification occurring on a rolling basis. An alternate admissions path is through the B.A./M.D. scholars for Medicine Program, which admits a limited number of high school students via the Honors College into an eight-year combined program. In addition, seven post-bacc programs, including Bryn Mawr, Goucher, Stony Brook, NYU, Queens, and Hunter, have admission arrangements with Stony Brook through a linkage program.

Costs

Expenses vary a great deal, depending largely on the student's housing situation. A single student can expect to spend about $17,000 per year in addition to tuition. This budget allows for either on- or off-campus shared housing and car ownership.

FINANCIAL AID: Assistance may be in the form of grants, loans, or employment opportunities. Although most financial aid is awarded solely on the basis of need, some programs are designed to encourage graduates to work in physician-shortage areas and are based on service commitments.

SUNY AT STONY BROOK

STUDENT BODY

Type	Public
*Enrollment	417
*% male/female	55/45
*% underrepresented minorities	10
# applied (total/out)	3,285/1,110
% interviewed (total/out)	22/NR
% accepted (total/out)	8/NR
% enrolled	35
Average age	24

ADMISSIONS

Average GPA and MCAT Scores

Overall GPA	3.55	Science GPA	3.6
MCAT Bio	11.00	MCAT Phys	11.00
MCAT Verbal	10.00	MCAT Essay	Q

Score Release Policy

This school has not responded to our inquiry regarding withheld MCAT scores. Therefore, we advise caution. Contact the Admissions Office before withholding any scores.

Application Information

Regular application	11/15
Regular notification	10/15 until filled
Early application	6/1–8/1
Early notification	10/1
Admissions may be deferred?	Yes
AMCAS application accepted?	Yes
Interview required?	Yes
Application fee	$75

COSTS AND AID

Tuition & Fees

Tuition (in/out)	$10,840/$21,940
Cost of books	$1,250
Fees	$250

Financial Aid

% students receiving aid	85
Average grant	$1,518
Average loan	$20,000
Average debt	$72,000

*Figures based on total enrollment

TEMPLE UNIVERSITY
SCHOOL OF MEDICINE

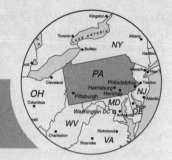

3400 N Broad Street, Philadelphia, PA 19140
Admission: 215-707-3656 • Fax: 215-707-6932
Internet: www.temple.edu/medschool

Temple stands out for its apparent emphasis on teaching. Resources are also directed toward objectives that relate to research and clinical care. The curriculum is modern, incorporating small group sessions, problem-based learning, early opportunities for elective study and patient care, and the integration of basic science and clinical training. Students participate in curriculum development and have a strong voice in school administration. Temple is an urban campus, and benefits from affiliations with clinical facilities in Philadelphia, around Pennsylvania, and in neighboring states. Admissions polices favor applicants with very strong personal qualities, creating a student body that is supportive and dedicated.

Academics

The academic program has options that appeal to all students, be they interested in research and/or intensive clinical training. Summer research projects in both basic and clinical sciences are encouraged and are often funded. Qualified students may pursue a Ph.D. concurrently with an M.D. in the following fields: Anatomy, Biochemistry, Immunology, Microbiology, Molecular Biology, Pathology, Pharmacology, and Physiology. Temple's system of student evaluation uses Honors/High Pass/Pass/Conditional/Fail. A grade of Pass or higher is required for promotion, and passing both steps of the USMLE is a graduation requirement.

BASIC SCIENCES: During the first two years, students are assigned to basic science faculty advisors who are available to discuss academic matters as well as personal issues. Students are in class for about 25 hours per week, with about half of scheduled sessions utilizing a lecture format. Other instructional methods include small-group discussions, labs, and interactive clinical training. A student-run note service operates, wherein each student takes responsibility for course notes on specified days and then shares notes with the other participants. First-year courses are Anatomy, Behavioral Science, Biochemistry, Physiology, Fundamentals of Clinical Care I, and a choice of electives. Second-year courses are Pathology, Microbiology, Fundamentals of Clinical Care II & III, Pharmacology, Pathophysiology, Behavioral Medicine, Genetics, and a wide choice of electives. The current library system includes clinical and research journals and texts; an electronic reference/information center; a microcomputer learning center; and access to online Internet informational services. Plans are in progress for a new library.

CLINICAL TRAINING: When clinical training begins, students are assigned to a clinical faculty advisor who assists with decisions about electives and post-graduate training. Third-year required rotations are Anesthesiology (1 week); Internal Medicine (12 weeks); Ob/Gyn (6 weeks); Pediatrics (6 weeks); Family Medicine (6 weeks); Psychiatry (6 weeks); Surgery (8 weeks); and Surgical

Subspecialties (3 weeks). During the fourth year, 20 weeks of electives are required, in addition to clerkships in Emergency Medicine (4 weeks) and Neuroscience (4 weeks), and a subinternship in Internal Medicine, Pediatrics, or Surgery (8 weeks). Training takes place at the Temple University Hospital (500 beds), a busy emergency room, and several specialized centers, such as a Sports Medicine Center and one of the nation's largest Heart Transplantation Programs. The new Temple University Children's Medical Center opened in January, 1998. Other affiliated hospitals include the Albert Einstein Medical Center, the Fox Chase Cancer Center, the Reading Hospital and Medical Center, Abington Memorial Hospital, St. Luke's Hospital, Mercy Hospital, Lehigh Valley Hospital, and Moss Rehabilitation Hospital.

Students

Approximately 60 percent of students are Pennsylvania residents. About 17 percent of students in a typical class are underrepresented minorities. In particular, Temple has a strong contingent of African American and Latino students. Class size is 180.

STUDENT LIFE: Temple students benefit from rich extracurricular offerings both on and off campus. Both Temple Medical School and the main Temple campus have comprehensive athletic and recreational facilities. Medical students are active in school governance, and are members of the Curriculum, Financial Affairs, and Admissions Committees. There are numerous student organizations that range from support groups for minority medical students, to community outreach organizations, to a rugby club. Philadelphia is a historically and culturally rich city. It is also a very student-friendly city, where medical students in particular abound. Most students live off campus.

GRADUATES: About half of Temple's graduates enter residency programs in Pennsylvania. Among students who graduated in 1998, the most prevalent specialty choices were Family Practice (26%); Internal Medicine (22%); Surgery (16%); Pediatrics (9%); Ob/Gyn (8%); Transitional (4%); Emergency Medicine (4%); and Orthopedics (4%).

Admissions

REQUIREMENTS: One year each of Biology, Chemistry, Organic Chemistry, and Physics are required. The MCAT is required, and scores must be no more than three years old.

SUGGESTIONS: As a "state-related" school, Temple gives some preference to Pennsylvania residents, although significant numbers of out-of-state applicants are admitted. For applicants who have been out of college for a period of time, some recent course work is important. The April, rather than August, MCAT is advised. Medically related and community service activities are valued, and the Admissions Committee is serious about selecting students who will make supportive class members and caring physicians.

PROCESS: There is no GPA or MCAT cut off, and all applications are reviewed by a member of the Admissions Committee. All AMCAS applicants receive requests for secondary application materials, and about 15 percent of those returning secondaries are invited to interview. Interviews take place between September and Mawait list onsist of one hour-long session with a faculty member or administrator. On interview day, applicants receive a campus tour and have lunch with current medical students. About one-third of interviewees are accepted, with notification occurring on a rolling basis. Wait-listed candidates are generally not encouraged to send supplementary material. Admission may also be gained through programs with post-baccalaureate, pre-medical programs at Temple, Goucher, Duquesne, Bryn Mawr, Columbia, Scripps, and the University of Pennsylvania.

Costs

The anticipated budget for a single student, not including tuition is about $14,000 per year. This allows for shared, off-campus housing, and car ownership.

FINANCIAL AID: About 80 percent of students receive financial aid, which is awarded primarily on the basis of need. Need is determined by the FAFSA form and additional institutional applications.

TEMPLE UNIVERSITY

STUDENT BODY

Type	Private
*Enrollment	739
*% male/female	62/38
*% underrepresented minorities	17
# applied (total/out)	8,278/7,060
% interviewed (total/out)	14/11
% accepted (total/out)	NR/NR
% enrolled (total/out)	16/8

ADMISSIONS

Average GPA and MCAT Scores

Overall GPA	3.40	Science GPA	3.40
MCAT Bio	10.20	MCAT Phys	10.00
MCAT Verbal	9.60	MCAT Essay	NR

Score Release Policy

We follow NBME rules concerning USMLE scores.

Application Information

Regular application	12/1
Regular notification	10/15 until filled
Early application	6/1–8/1
Early notification	10/1
Transfers accepted?	Yes
Admissions may be deferred?	Yes
AMCAS application accepted?	Yes
Interview required?	Yes
Application fee	$55

COSTS AND AID

Tuition & Fees

Tuition	$22,240
Cost of books	NR
Fees	$444

Financial Aid

% students receiving aid	80
Average grant	$3,000
Average loan	$25,000
Average debt	$105,475

*Figures based on total enrollment

University of Tennessee, Memphis

COLLEGE OF MEDICINE

790 Madison Avenue, Memphis, TN 38163
Admission: 901-448-5559 • Fax: 901-448-1740
Internet: www.utmem.edu/medicine

The University of Tennessee (UT) Memphis is one of the largest academic health science centers in the Southeastern United States. In addition to the College of Medicine, UT Memphis features Colleges of Allied Health Sciences, Dentistry, Graduate Health Sciences, Nursing, and Pharmacy. The curriculum offers many options to students, accommodating those interested in primary care and those seeking careers in medical research.

Academics

Most students follow a four-year curriculum, leading to the M.D. The Optional Expanded Academic Program allows students to expand the first two years into three. The Clinical Scholars Program provides special educational and financial assistance to entering students interested in careers in Family Medicine, General Internal Medicine, General Pediatrics, Medicine and Pediatrics (Med-Peds), or Ob/Gyn. Students are encouraged to pursue research, either during the summer following year one or as ongoing projects. For students interested in intensive research, an M.D./Ph.D. program is available. Medical students generally receive percentage scores on exams and are evaluated with an A–F scale. Examinations in some courses are administered by computer. Passing both steps of the USMLE is a requirement for graduation.

BASIC SCIENCES: The basic sciences are taught during the first two years primarily through lectures and lab work. Students are in class or other scheduled sessions for about 23 hours per week. First-year science courses are the following: Biochemistry; Fundamentals of Cellular and Molecular Biology; Medical Genetics; Gross Anatomy; Histology; Neuroanatomy; and Physiology. Other first-year courses are Behavioral Sciences and Preventive Medicine, both of which involve small-group discussions. Throughout the first and second years, students take Introduction to Clinical Skills, which correlates basic science concepts with actual medical cases and teaches students introductory clinical techniques. Students also participate in a longitudinal, community-based clinical program. Second-year courses are Microbiology, Neuroscience, Nutrition, Pathology, Pathophysiology, and Pharmacology. Most of the first two years is spent in the Cecil C. Humphreys General Education Building that houses classrooms, labs, and a computer center. A three-year longitudinal community program will begin in 1999 and incorporate content of five current courses: Behavorial Science, Preventive Medicine, Nutrition, and ICS and Longitudinal Community-based Clinical Program. An important educational resource is the Plane Tree Center with multimedia software technologies for learning Anatomy, Embryology, Histology, EKG readings, and lung and heart sounds. Plane Tree also provides health-oriented books, audiovisuals, and Internet connections.

The Health Sciences Library is used by students both for research purposes and for studying. It is fully computerized, subscribes to approximately 1,550 current periodicals, and contains a total volume count of over 170,000.

CLINICAL TRAINING: Third-year required clerkships are two months each of the following: Family Medicine, Medicine, Ob/Gyn, Pediatrics, Psychiatry, and Surgery. The fourth year is composed of five one-month clerkships and three months of electives that provide students the opportunity to select the clinical or basic science experiences to best meet their particular career goals. Electives allow for increased responsibility in patient care as well as the opportunity to pursue areas of individual interest. Fourth-year required clerkships are Ambulatory Care Medicine, Neurology, and a Senior Clerkship in Medicine and Surgical Subspecialties. As part of a Selective requirement, one month of either Family Medicine, Medicine, Pediatrics, Ob/Gyn, Psychiatry, or Surgery is also required. All students must spend a minimum of 10 months of clerkship and elective time on the Memphis campus. This requirement allows a maximum of 10 months (excluding option months) to be spent at Knoxville, Chattanooga, and/or Nashville. Two of the 10 months away from the Memphis campus may be taken at another institution, either in the United States or overseas.

Students

At least 90 percent of students are Tennessee residents. Others are usually from the eight states contiguous to Tennessee. These are Mississippi, Arkansas, Missouri, Kentucky, Virginia, North Carolina, Georgia, and Alabama. The average age of incoming students is typically about 24 with a wide age range among students. Underrepresented minorities account for about 12 percent of students. Class size is 165.

STUDENT LIFE: Medical students are cohesive and supportive of one another. As part of the Big Sib program, incoming medical students are assigned to senior students as mentors. Typically, the Big Sibs will pass along their class notes to the new students to use as a guide during basic science lectures. Medical students are part of a larger community that includes students of all professional schools and programs. The Student Alumni Center (SAC) is the focal point of campus life, providing meeting areas, a restaurant, lounges, a television room, shopping areas, and other services. More than 35 campus-wide organizations are open to medical students. Students enjoy a fitness center that houses a multipurpose gym, a swimming pool, spa, racketball courts, and a weight room. An outdoor complex has playing fields, volleyball courts, tennis courts, golf-practice facilities, and a track. Intramural sports are popular, as is the Outdoor Adventures Program, which leads canoeing, hiking, rafting, and camping trips. Memphis is a festive city, renowned for its music scene. Other attractions include riverside areas, parks, restaurants, a lively arts community, and quiet residential neighborhoods. UT Memphis offers both residence halls and apartment-style facilities for single students. The University assists married students with finding housing in the city.

GRADUATES: Among 1999 graduates, the most popular fields for residencies were the following: Internal Medicine (31%); Pediatrics (10%); Family Practice (21%); Ob/Gyn (21%); Surgery (12%); Radiology (6%); Medicine/Pediatrics (8%). A significant proportion of graduates remains in Tennessee for post-graduate training.

Admissions

REQUIREMENTS: Prerequisite course work is 8 semester hours each of: Biology, General Chemistry, Organic Chemistry, and General Physics, all taken with associated labs. In addition, six hours of English is required. The MCAT is required and scores must be no more than 5 years old. For applicants who have taken the exam more than once, all sets of scores are considered.

SUGGESTIONS: Residents of Tennessee are given preference. Children of UT alumni are also considered, regardless of their state of residence. As a state-supported institution, no more than 10 percent of students may be nonresidents. Thus, nonresident applicants should be highly qualified. Students are encouraged to take courses in the humanities, fine arts, and social sciences. Demonstration of analytic ability and independent thinking is important.

PROCESS: All AMCAS applicants who are considered competitive are sent supplemental applications. Of those returning supplementals, approximately 400 applicants are invited to interview between October and March. The interview gives insights into the applicant's character and how well he or she has formulated plans for the study of medicine. Interviews consist of two sessions, each with a faculty member or current medical student. On interview day, applicants have lunch, attend group informational sessions, sit in on classes, and tour the campus. Of interviewed candidates, about 60 percent are accepted on a rolling basis. Others are either rejected or placed on a wait list.

Costs

The estimated yearly living expenses for a single student is $10,770 if living in a residence hall, and $11,670 if living in an apartment.

FINANCIAL AID: The College of Medicine has substantial scholarship awards available to highly qualified medical students, including grants that involve service commitments in designated underserved areas in Tennessee. Approximately 84 percent of students receive some form of assistance, most of which is in the form of loans.

UNIVERSITY OF TENNESSEE, MEMPHIS

STUDENT BODY

Type	Public
*Enrollment	686
*% male/female	61/39
*% underrepresented minorities	15
# applied (total/out)	1,700/1,054
% interviewed (total/out)	22/6
% accepted (total/out)	14/4
% enrolled (total/out)	67/47
Average age	24

Score Release Policy

The school has not responded to our inquiry regarding withheld MCAT scores. Therefore, we advise caution. Contact the Admissions Office before withholding any scores.

ADMISSIONS

Average GPA and MCAT Scores

Overall GPA	3.60	Science GPA	3.50
MCAT Bio	9.40	MCAT Phys	9.00
MCAT Verbal	9.40	MCAT Essay	0

Application Information

Regular application	11/15
Regular notification	10/15–4/1
Transfers accepted?	Yes
Admissions may be deferred?	Yes
AMCAS application accepted?	Yes
Interview required?	Yes
Application fee	$50

COSTS AND AID

Tuition & Fees

Tuition (in/out)	$9,718/$19,248
Cost of books	$1,800
Fees	$212

Financial Aid

% students receiving aid	84
Average grant	$13,647
Average loan	$16,929
Average debt	$63,000

*Figures based on total enrollment

THE TEXAS A&M UNIVERSITY SYSTEM HEALTH SCIENCE CENTER
COLLEGE OF MEDICINE

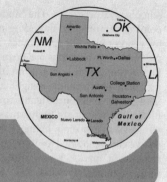

159 Joe Reynolds Medical Building, College Station, TX 77843-1114

Admission: 409-845-7743 • Fax: 409-845-5533

Email: med-stu-aff@tamu.edu • Internet: hsc.tamu.edu

Although the College of Medicine is relatively small, with 64 students per class, it is affiliated with Texas A&M University, which enrolls 43,000 students. The College of Medicine is able to provide personal attention to its students, who also profit from the resources of the larger University. Texas A&M is a public university and is among the top ten universities in the nation in terms of research expenditures. Students spend their first two years at the main campus in College Station.

Academics

Students may pursue a joint M.D./Ph.D. in conjunction with graduate departments of the University in the following fields: Anatomy, Biochemistry, Biomedical Engineering Biophysics, Cell Biology, Genetics, Immunology, Microbiology, Molecular Biology, Neuroscience, Pathology, Pharmacology, and Physiology. Clinical instruction is integrated into the basic science curriculum, as are sessions that emphasize the social and ethical aspects of medicine.

BASIC SCIENCES: The first year is organized into semesters. Year one, fall semester consists of the following: Gross Anatomy (lecture/lab); Biochemistry and Genetics (lecture); Humanities in Medicine (small-group); and Introduction to Patients (small-group), which discusses clinical care. In the spring, students take Microanatomy (lecture/lab); Neuroscience (all methods of instruction); Physiology (lecture/small-group); and Physical Diagnosis (small-group). Throughout the year, students participate in an innovative course that encourages community involvement, Leadership in Medicine (small-group). Working with Patients, which introduces the patient interview, spans part of each semester. During year one, students are in class for about 27 hours per week. Year two is organized into trimesters. Throughout year two, students take Pathology (lecture/lab); Pediatrics (lecture); Ob/Gyn (lecture); and the Primary Care Preceptorship (clinical). Humanities (small-group) is taken during the first trimester. For the duration of the first two trimesters, Microbiology (lecture/lab) and Pharmacology (lecture/small-group) are studied. Clinical Medicine and Psychiatry (lecture) are taken during the final trimester. Students are in class for about 29 hours per week during year two. Tutoring is available to all students, and is conducted by professors and qualified students. Study facilities include the Learning Resources Unit, which contains instructional videos and computer programs, as well as 1,200 basic science text and reference books; the Medical Sciences Library, which houses over 100,000 books and numerous computer databases; and Evans Library, which has over 2 million books. Evaluation of performance during years one and two uses an A–F scale. Passing the USMLE Step 1 is required for promotion to year three. The passing rate for Texas A&M Medical Students exceeds the national average.

CLINICAL TRAINING: Patient contact begins in year one, in Working with Patients and continues through year two, in the preceptorship for Primary Care program. Early informal patient contact is possible for those who engage in certain community service or volunteer activities. Year three begins with a week-long orientation, followed by required rotations: Ob/Gyn (6 weeks); Pediatrics (6 weeks); Family Medicine (12 weeks); and Surgery (12 weeks). Year four consists of electives plus four required clerkships: Neurology (4 weeks); Alcohol and Drug Dependence (2 weeks); acting internship in a 10 case, 10 care specialty (4 weeks); and Becoming a Clinician (3 weeks). Training takes place at several sites including Scott & White Hospital, based in Temple with 17 affiliated rural clinics; Central Texas Medical Centers (a consortium of hospitals totaling 2,271 beds); Teague Veterans' Center (serves veterans in a 35-county service area); the Darnall Army Community Hospital (serves the largest armored installation in the United States); and Driscoll Children Hospital (serves the children of Corpus Christi and South Texas). Libraries are available for third- and fourth-year students at the Teague Veterans' Center and the Scott & White Hospital. During year three, students are evaluated by using an A–F scale. During year four, most rotations are evaluated with Pass/Fail. Passing the USMLE Step 2 is required for graduation.

Students

The vast majority of students are from Texas. About 10 percent of students are underrepresented minorities, most of whom are of Mexican American descent. About 90 percent of the student body were science majors of some type as undergraduates.

STUDENT LIFE: Each medical school class selects and sponsors human service organizations, at which students volunteer. This, along with social activities sponsored by the School and the University, unifies the class and gives students extracurricular activities to pursue together. The University's recreational facilities are outstanding, offering every possible athletic activity. Students live off campus, generally in apartments.

GRADUATES: Of those who graduated between 1991 and 1995, the following residencies were the most popular: Family Practice (21% of graduates); Internal Medicine (13%); Surgery (12%); Ob/Gyn (9%); Pediatrics (9%); Psychiatry (7%); Anesthesiology (7%) and Radiology (6%). Half of the graduates enter residency training programs at University-affiliated hospitals or elsewhere in the state.

Admissions

REQUIREMENTS: The College of Medicine considers for enrollment individuals who have completed at least 90 credit hours of undergraduate course work. By state mandate, enrollment of out-of-state residents may not exceed 10 percent. Each year 64 entering students are enrolled. The following courses are required with at least a grade of "C": General Biology with Lab (8 hours), Additional Biological Sciences (3 hours), General Chemistry with Lab (8 hours), Organic Chemistry with Lab (8 hours), General Physics with Lab (8 hours), English (6 hours), and Calculus (3 hours). The MCAT is required and must have been taken no earlier than five years before the expected date of enrollment. The most recent set of test scores is considered in the evaluation process. Applicants should not withhold previous test scores.

SUGGESTIONS: Although the MCAT is offered twice each year, in April and August, we strongly encourage applicants to take the MCAT in April. Official scores must be released directly to the Texas Medical and Dental Schools Application Service in Austin, Texas. Involvement in community service and health-related work that involves patient and physician contact are helpful. For applicants who have been out of school for several years, some recent course work is recommended.

PROCESS: Approximately 30 percent of Texas applicants are interviewed, and 20 percent of those interviewed are offered a place in the class. About 5 percent of out-of-state residents are interviewed, and only a few are accepted each year. Interview sessions typically are scheduled from August to December. Each applicant is given two 30-minute interviews. Tender of acceptance is made on January 15. The College of Medicine participates in the Texas Medical Schools Matching Program employed by the Texas Medical and Dental Schools Application Service. A ranked wait list is established in February. The Texas Medical and Dental Schools Application Service (TMDSAS) processes all applications. Application materials may be obtained after May 1 online at http://dpweb1.dp.utexas.edu/mdac/.

Costs

The expected yearly cost of living ranges from $8,200 to $9,700 depending mostly on housing choices. This budget does not necessarily allow for car ownership.

FINANCIAL AID: Ninety percent of students receive some form of financial aid. Federal loans and state loans and grants are the primary sources of aid. Parental disclosure is required for some financial aid. There are no merit scholarships.

TEXAS A&M UNIVERSITY HEALTH SCIENCE CENTER

STUDENT BODY

Type	Public
*Enrollment	256
*% male/female	52/48
*% underrepresented minorities	39
# applied (total/out)	1,419/102
% interviewed (total/out)	31/5
% accepted (total/out)	NR/1.6
% enrolled (total/out)	33/3

ADMISSIONS

Average GPA and MCAT Scores

Overall GPA	3.70	Science GPA	NR
MCAT Bio	10.30	MCAT Phys	9.60
MCAT Verbal	9.30	MCAT Essay	NR

Score Release Policy

The most recent score is considered, but progress is also taken into great consideration.

Application Information

Regular application	11/1
Regular notification	11/15 until filled
Transfer accepted?	Yes
Admissions may be deferred?	Yes
AMCAS application accepted?	No
Interview required?	Yes
Application fee	$45

COSTS AND AID

Tuition & Fees

Tuition (in/out)	$6,650/$19,650
Cost of books	$1,600
Fees	$1,042

Financial Aid

% students receiving aid	92
Average grant	$1,750
Average loan	$16,000
Average debt	$65,921

*Figures based on total enrollment

University of Texas Southwestern Medical Center at Dallas

SOUTHWESTERN MEDICAL SCHOOL

5323 Harry Hines Boulevard, Dallas, TX 75390-9162
Admission: 214-648-5617 • Fax: 214-648-3289
Internet: www.swmed.edu/medapp

The University of Texas Southwestern Medical School's mission emphasizes the importance of training primary care physicians, educating doctors who will practice in medically underserved areas of Texas, and preparing physician-scientists for careers in academic medicine and research. Through its outstanding resources, facilities, and faculty, UT Southwestern offers strong and extensive clinical training, beginning in the pre-clinical years, as well as opportunities for medical students to pursue their research interests through funded summer positions or a well-established Medical Scientist Training Program leading to the combined M.D./Ph.D.

Academics

The vast majority of students follow a four-year path leading to the M.D. degree. A small number of students each year enter a joint M.D./Ph.D. program in conjunction with the Southwestern Graduate School of Biomedical Sciences. For the most part, students are evaluated using an A–F scale in which a C is required to pass. Fourth-year courses are taken Pass/Fail.

BASIC SCIENCES: During the first two years, a variety of teaching/learning formats are used, including lectures, small-group, problem-based learning, computerized curriculum, and standardized patient interviews. First-year courses include Biology of Cells and Tissues; Human Anatomy and Embryology; Integrative Human Biology; Medical Biochemistry; Human Behavior; and Endocrinology and Human Reproduction. In addition, Clinical Ethics in Medicine exposes first-year students to the ethical, behavioral, and clinical perspectives of medicine in a problem-based learning format. During the 10-week period between the first and second years, numerous clinical and research opportunities are available for students who wish to participate. Clinical exposure continues in the second year through Clinical Medicine: Principles and Practice when students learn about the physical examination and experience direct, one-on-one, patient contact. Second-year courses also include Immunology and Medical Microbiology; Anatomic and Clinical Pathology; Medical Pharmacology; and Psychopathology. On average, students are in scheduled sessions for 25–30 hours per week. The campus where pre-clinical instruction takes place is also part of a large medical complex that includes several hospitals, research centers, and the medical school library, which holds more than 229,000 volumes and currently subscribes to almost 2,000 journals. Passing the USMLE Step 1 is required in order to progress to the fourth year.

CLINICAL TRAINING: Building upon the clinical experiences in the first two years, the third and fourth years offer intense clinical experiences involving medical students in direct patient care. Third-year required clinical rotations are Surgery (8 weeks); Pediatrics (8 weeks); Obstetrics and Gynecology (6 weeks); Internal Medicine (12 weeks); Psychiatry (6 weeks); and Family Practice (4 weeks). The fourth year is organized into 4-week periods filled with electives, selectives, and a few remaining required rotations. Requirements include Neurology (4 weeks); Internal Medicine (4 weeks of a subinternship and 4 weeks of ambulatory care); and Women's Health Care (4 weeks). Four 4-week periods remain, two of which are for selectives and two of which are reserved for electives. Clinical training takes place at University sites and affiliated institutions, including Parkland Memorial Hospital; the James Aston Ambulatory Care Center; Zale Lipshy University Hospital; Children's Medical Center; Dallas Veterans Affairs Medical Center; Southwestern Institute of Forensic Sciences; Baylor University Medical Center; Presbyterian Hospital of Dallas; Methodist Hospitals of Dallas; St. Paul Medical Center; Texas Scottish Rite Hospital for Children; and John Peter Smith Hospital in Fort Worth. Students may fulfill many of their senior rotations at academic or medical institutions in other parts of the state, the country, or the world.

Students

At least 90 percent of the student body are Texas residents. Underrepresented minorities account for about 10 percent of the population. The average age of incoming students is usually 24; the range of ages is typically 20 to 45. Incoming class size at UT Southwestern is 200 students.

STUDENT LIFE: The Skillern Student Union has exercise and recreational facilities and offers students a convenient place to relax and socialize. Dynamic campus activity programming includes intramural sports, special-interest organizations, recreational and cultural events, and parties. Students also join groups based on professional and academic interests or participate in community service projects. Dallas is an exciting city with a diverse population and many kinds of cultural, recreational, and entertainment activities. All students live off campus, and most students own cars.

GRADUATES: Graduates are successful in securing residencies at prestigious institutions all over the country. The majority of graduates go on to become practicing physicians, typically with a large percentage choosing primary care specialties. Some go into academic medicine or research.

Admissions

REQUIREMENTS: Prerequisite courses include one semester of Calculus, two semesters of English, two semesters of Physics (with lab), four semesters of Biology (two of which should be with lab and one of which may be Biochemistry), and four semesters of Chemistry (with lab), which should be equally divided between Organic and Inorganic Chemistry. The MCAT is required, and scores must be no more than five years old. For applicants who have retaken the exam, the best set of scores is used.

SUGGESTIONS: Admission for out-of-state applicants is highly competitive, as Texas law requires that no more than 10 percent of each class be nonresidents. In addition to academic credentials (GPA, MCAT score, relative rigor of the undergraduate curriculum, letters of recommendation), the Admissions Committee considers extracurricular activities, socioeconomic background, any time spent in outside employment, personal integrity and compassion for others, the ability to communicate in English, motivation for a career in medicine, and other personal qualities and individual factors such as leadership, insightful self-appraisal, determination, social/family support, and maturity/coping capabilities. Applicants are also evaluated for the demonstration of significant interest and experiences that parallel the mission of UT Southwestern.

PROCESS: UT Southwestern does not participate in the AMCAS system. A common application is available for the University of Texas System medical schools (Southwestern at Dallas, Galveston, Houston, and San Antonio), Texas A&M University College of Medicine, and Texas Tech University School of Medicine. An online application is available at http://dpweb1.dp.utexas.edu/mdac/homepage.htm.

Applications must be submitted between May 1 and October 15. About one-quarter of the applicants are invited to interview, with interviews taking place between September and December. Interviews consist of two sessions with individual faculty members. About 40 percent of interviewed candidates are accepted, with notification beginning on January 15.

Costs

The anticipated yearly student expenses range from $20,000 to $24,000. This budget allows for tuition, fees, books and supplies, off-campus housing, transportation, and personal expenses (for in-state studenwait list sonal computer is required of all incoming students and may be included in financial aid packages.

FINANCIAL AID: No student should allow the pressures of financial constraint to cause a postponement of educational plans without first consulting with the Office of Student Financial Aid. The office can provide the student with necessary applications, forms, and advice concerning the rules and regulations of available federal, state, and institutional financial aid programs.

UNIVERSITY OF TEXAS SOUTHWESTERN MEDICAL CENTER AT DALLAS

STUDENT BODY

Type	Public
*Enrollment	807
*% male/female	65/35
*% underrepresented minorities	13
# applied (total/out)	2,591/473
% interviewed (total/out)	26/19
% accepted (total/out)	15/12
% enrolled (total/out)	52/53
Average age	24

ADMISSIONS

Average GPA and MCAT Scores

Overall GPA	3.76	Science GPA	3.74
MCAT Bio	11.20	MCAT Phys	11.20
MCAT Verbal	10.10	MCAT Essay	0

Score Release Policy

UTSMC does not have a policy on score release for the MCAT. The school cautions students that delays due to score review prior to release have rendered student applications incomplete past the point of consideration for the incoming class.

Application Information

Regular application	10/15
Regular notification	1/15 until filled
Transfers accepted?	Yes
Admissions may be deferred?	Yes
AMCAS application accepted?	No
Interview required?	Yes
Application fee (in/out)	$55/$90

COSTS AND AID

Tuition & Fees

Tuition (in/out)	$6,920/$20,020
Cost of books	$1,685
Fees	$846

Financial Aid

% students receiving aid	85
Average grant	$3,400
Average loan	$14,700
Average debt	$60,600

*Figures based on total enrollment

TEXAS TECH UNIVERSITY HEALTH SCIENCES CENTER
SCHOOL OF MEDICINE

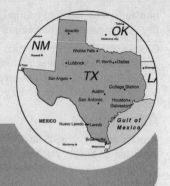

3601 4th Street, Office of Admissions–2B116, Lubbock, TX 79430
Admission: 806-743-2297 • Fax: 806-743-2725
Internet: www.ttuhsc.edu

Established in 1969, the School of Medicine is part of the Texas Tech University Health Sciences Center, which also includes Schools Of Nursing, Allied Health, and Pharmacy. The Health Sciences Center is a sister institution of Texas Tech University, which has an enrollment of 24,000 students. To extend services to a large region in West Texas—much of which is medically underserved—the School of Medicine has campuses in Amarillo, El Paso, Lubbock, and Odessa. Students spend the first two years in Lubbock but receive clinical training in Lubbock, El Paso, or Amarillo. The Midland–Odessa campus has residency training only.

Academics

Most students complete a four-year curriculum designed to prepare physicians with a broad base of medical knowledge and sound analytic and problem-solving skills. It is organized in two stages—basic science and clinical training. Some students devote an additional year to research and earn the M.D. degree in five years. Others are involved in summer research projects. Qualified students interested in Biomedical research or academic medicine can earn a Ph.D. along with the M.D. degree. To address the needs of a rapidly changing health care system, students can participate in an M.D./M.B.A. joint-degree program in which both degrees are earned in four years. Medical students are graded on a numerical system and must maintain a weighted average of 75 for promotion and graduation.

BASIC SCIENCES: First-year courses are Gross Anatomy; Histology; Biochemistry; Physician in Society; Neuroscience; Physiology; and Concepts in Community and Ambulatory Care, which serves as an introduction to clinical medicine and uses physician community mentors. First-year students also have the opportunity to take an elective. Second-year courses are Microbiology; Pharmacology; Pathology; Integrated Approach to Patient Care; Introduction to Medicine; and Introduction to Psychiatry. During the first and second years, instruction primarily uses a lecture/lab format. However, some concepts are addressed in small-group sessions. Students are in classes or other scheduled sessions for about 27 hours per week. All instruction takes place in medical education buildings on the Lubbock campus.

CLINICAL TRAINING: Third-year required rotations are Internal Medicine (12 weeks); Surgery (12 weeks); Pediatrics (6 weeks); Family Medicine (6 weeks); Ob/Gyn (6 weeks); and Psychiatry (6 weeks). Fourth-year requirements are Neurology (4 weeks); Selectives (8 weeks); a Subinternship (4 weeks); and 16 weeks of electives. After successful completion of years one and two, approxi-

mately 35 students go on to Amarillo for clinical training, 35 stay in Lubbock, and 50 go to El Paso. Amarillo, El Paso, and Lubbock all serve both urban and rural populations. Multiple clinical affiliations of each site provide a wealth of training opportunities for students. El Paso serves an urban border population of more than 700,000 and provides a unique multicultural educational opportunity. Training sites include Thomason Hospital and other community and military facilities. In Lubbock, students benefit from recreational and cultural opportunities available on the Texas Tech University campus of the main University. The primary teaching hospital is University Covanant Health–Lakeside. Other affiliated hospitals include Mary of the Plains Hospital, Charter Plains Hospital, and the Veterans Administration Outpatient Clinics. Amarillo provides exposure to medicine primarily from a private hospital perspective. Teaching hospitals include Northwest Texas Health Care System, Baptist-St. Anthony Health Care System, and Veterans Administration Hospital. In total, Texas Tech affiliates provide almost 3,000 teaching beds.

Students

The 1998 entering class had the following characteristics: 100 percent Texas residents; 23 percent underrepresented minorities; 75 percent science majors. Typically, about 20 percent of students in an entering class are a bit older, having taken time off after college. Class size is 120.

STUDENT LIFE: During their first two years, students benefit from the resources of the Health Science Center and from being adjacent to Texas Tech University, a major undergraduate institution. Medical students are supportive of one another, as demonstrated by a student-initiated, peer-tutoring program. First- and second-year students are often involved in community service projects, which provide early clinical exposure. Student life during the third and fourth years varies according to location.

GRADUATES: Approximately 21 percent of graduates enter Texas Tech residency programs, which operate on all four campuses. Others are successful in obtaining positions throughout Texas and at institutions in other regions of the country. Eighty-one percent of 1998 graduates matched with one of their top three residency choices.

Admissions

REQUIREMENTS: Requirements are Biology (12 semester hours); Biology lab (2 semester hours); General Chemistry with lab (8 semester hours); Organic Chemistry with lab (8 semester hours); Physics with lab (8 semester hours); English (6 semester hours), and Calculus (3 semester hours). All prerequisite courses require a grade of C or better. The MCAT is required, and should be taken within the past five years. For applicants who have taken the exam more than once, the most recent set of scores is weighed most heavily, but all scores must be reported. Texas residents and residents of neighboring counties in New Mexico and Oklahoma, which comprise the service areas of the school, are given preference in admission. Only nonresident applicants with GPAs of 3.60 or higher, and MCAT scores of 29 or higher will be considered for admission.

SUGGESTIONS: The April, rather than August, MCAT is advised. In addition to high intellectual ability and a record of strong academic achievement, the committee looks for qualities and traits, such as compassion, motivation, communication skills, maturity, and personal integrity.

PROCESS: Texas Tech does not participate in AMCAS. Texas Tech participates with five other state-supported medical schools in the Texas Medical and Dental Application Service (TMDAS). A single application is sent to the TMDAS for processing and then is forwarded to any or all of the participating schools as requested by the applicant. A secondary application is also required by Texas Tech. Both applications will be available via the internet. In addition, application forms may be requested from: Texas Medical and Dental Application Service, 702 Colorado Street, Suite 6400, Austin, TX 78701. About 38 percent of applicants are interviewed between September and January. Interviews consist of two sessions, each with an admissions committee/faculty member. On interview day, applicants tour the campus, attend group information sessions, meet current students, and have the opportunity to attend classes. Notification begins on October 15 and continues until the class is filled.

Costs

In addition to tuition and fees, the estimated yearly cost of living for a single student is $12,000. This budget allows for off-campus housing and car maintenance.

FINANCIAL AID: Financial aid is available to students who demonstrate need. More than 90 percent of the student body receives some type of financial assistance. Employment, other than during the summer, is discouraged. Scholarships are awarded to students who demonstrate financial need and/or academic qualifications.

TEXAS TECH UNIVERSITY HEALTH SCIENCES CENTER

STUDENT BODY

Type	Public
*Enrollment	489
*% male/female	72/28
*% underrepresented minorities	22
# applied (total/out)	1,558/30
% interviewed (total/out)	26/13
% accepted (total/out)	23/4
% enrolled (total/out)	33/3
Average age	23

ADMISSIONS

Averawait list MCAT Scores

Overall GPA	3.57	Science GPA	3.5
MCAT Bio	9.83	MCAT Phys	9.63
MCAT Verbal	9.58	MCAT Essay	NR

Score Release Policy
Scores are not released without express written consent of students.

Application Information

Regular application	10/15
Regular notification	1/15
Early application	8/1
Early notification	10/1
Transfers accepted?	Yes
Admissions may be deferred?	Yes
AMCAS application accepted?	No
Interview required?	Yes
Secondary Application fee	$40

COSTS AND AID

Tuition & Fees

Tuition (in/out)	$6,550/$19,650
Cost of books	$1,012
Fees	$1,557

Financial Aid

% students receiving aid	90
Average grant	$2,898
Average loan	$23,785
Average debt	$85,000

*Figures based on total enrollment

UNIVERSITY OF TEXAS—GALVESTON

MEDICAL BRANCH AT GALVESTON

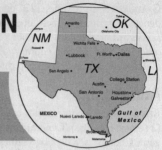

G-210 Ashbel Smith Building, Galveston, TX 77555
Admission: 409-772-3517 • Fax: 409-772-5753
Email: pwylie@utmb.edu • Internet: www.utmb.edu

The University of Texas Medical Branch at Galveston (UTMB) has grown to encompass 73 major buildings, seven hospitals, more than 100 outpatient clinics, four academic institutions, a major medical library, and numerous research facilities. It is the nation's ninth-largest health care complex and is committed to education, patient care, and research. As one of only 14 medical schools in the nation to receive a Generalist Physician Initiative Grant from the Robert Wood Johnson Foundation, UTMB puts considerable emphasis on primary care. For example, a Multidisciplinary Ambulatory Clerkship teaches third-year students the range of skills needed to practice effectively as a modern-day, generalist physician.

Academics

In addition to the standard four-year M.D. curriculum, UTMB offers a combined M.D./Ph.D. program for students interested in training for a career in biomedical research. Generally, about five students enter this program each year and receive full funding for the duration of their studies. Summer and year-long research projects are also open to medical students. As an alternative to the primarily lecture-based basic-science curriculum, 24 incoming students each year enter an Interactive Learning Track, which relies on small-group instruction.

BASIC SCIENCES: First-year courses are the following: Gross Anatomy and Developmental Anatomy; Microanatomy; Biochemistry, Cells and Genes; Physiology and Biophysics; Neuroscience; Medical Ethics; Community Continuity Experience; and Introduction to Patient Evaluation. Second-year courses are Endocrinology; Microbiology; Pharmacology and Toxicology; Pathology; Introduction to Patient Evaluation; Immunology; Introduction to Clinical Medicine; and Community Continuity Experience. During the first and second years, students are in class or other scheduled sessions for about 30 hours per week. In addition to teaching basic-science principles, the pre-clinical curriculum involves practical problem-solving experiences and case studies that demonstrate the interrelationship between the basic and clinical sciences. The Community Continuity Experience gives first- and second-year students the opportunity to work with primary care physicians, interact with patients, and apply and expand knowledge and skills gained in the classroom. Educational support services include academic counseling, peer-tutorials, study skills workshops, and stress management workshops. An Educational Support Center provides medical students with computer-assisted educational support. For research purposes, and as a place to study, students use the Moody Medical Library, which is the oldest medical library in Texas and one of the largest medical research centers in the Southwest. Collections include nearly 250,000 volumes in addition to computerized informational services.

CLINICAL TRAINING: Third-year required clerkships are Internal Medicine (8 weeks); Surgery (8 weeks); Pediatrics (4 weeks); Ob/Gyn (6 weeks); Psychiatry (6 weeks); Family Medicine (6 weeks); and a Multidisciplinary Ambulatory Clerkship (12 weeks). Lectures in Anesthesiology, Medical Jurisprudence, Ophthalmology, and Otolaryngology are also part of the third-year curriculum. Fourth-year required clerkships are Neurology (4 weeks); Surgery (4 weeks); Emergency Medicine (4 weeks); Radiology (2 weeks); Dermatology (2 weeks); and an Acting Internship Selective (4 weeks). At least 20 weeks are reserved for elective study. Clinical training takes place primarily at UTMB hospitals and clinics. Some electives may be taken at other institutions.

Students

At least 90 percent of students are Texas residents. Typically, about 10 percent of entering students are a bit older, having taken significant time off after college. Approximately 15 percent of students are underrepresented minorities. Class size is 200.

STUDENT LIFE: Students benefit from the resources and facilities of a large, modernized campus. The Lee Hage Jamail Student Center serves as a meeting place for medical students. It has a cafeteria, meeting rooms, study areas, and recreational facilities. Coed medical fraternities located close to campus offer housing, meals, and social opportunities to medical students. The UTMB Alumni Fields House features a variety of indoor and outdoor facilities, including tennis courts, baseball diamonds, volleyball courts, an outdoor basketball court, racquetball courts, fitness centers, spa facilities, an outdoor track, and an Olympic size pool. UTMB has more than 50 student organizations that range from support groups for minority students, to community service oriented groups, to professional organizations. The University operates both dormitories and apartments for single students.

GRADUATES: Graduates are successful in securing residencies at top institutions nationwide.

Admissions

REQUIREMENTS: A grade of at least a C must be earned in all of the prerequisite courses. These are: English (one year); Biology (two years); Math (one semester of college-level); Physics (one year); Chemistry (one year); and Organic Chemistry (one year). All science courses must include laboratory work. The MCAT is required, and scores should be from within the past year. For applicants who have taken the exam on multiple occasions, the most recent set of scores is considered.

SUGGESTIONS: As a state-supported institution, UTMB gives preference to Texas residents. Applicants are encouraged to take the spring MCAT because late receipt of scores from the fall cycle may delay application processing. Medical experience, volunteer activities, and research are all helpful.

PROCESS: The University of Texas does not participate in the AMCAS system. Applications may be obtained from:

> The University of Texas System
> Medical/Dental Application Center, Suite 6400
> 702 Colorado Street
> Austin, TX 78701
> Phone: 512-499-4785

Applications must be submitted between May 15 and October 15. About 1,000 applicants are invited to interview during November and December. Candidates receive two interviews, each with a faculty member. On interview day, there are also orientation sessions, a campus tour, and several opportunities to meet informally with current medical students. About 20 percent of interviewed candidates are accepted. Others are rejected or placed on a wait list and possibly accepted later in the year.

Costs

The estimated yearly cost of living for a single student is about $15,000. This allows for on- or off-campus housing.

FINANCIAL AID: Most financial aid is in the form of loans and is granted on the basis of financial need. Some scholarships are available that involve service commitments, and others are offered on the basis of merit or other special criteria.

UNIVERSITY OF TEXAS—GALVESTON

STUDENT BODY

Type	Public
*Enrollment	821
*% male/female	59/41
*% underrepresented minorities	15
# applied (total/out)	2,772/485
% interviewed (total/out)	48/1
% accepted (total/out)	NR/NR
% enrolled (total/out)	17/5

ADMISSIONS

Average GPA and MCAT Scores

Overall GPA	3.57	Science GPA	NR
MCAT Bio	NR	MCAT Phys	NR
MCAT Verbal	NR	MCAT Essay	NR

Score Release Policy

Not viewed negatively if student does not reveal scores. Committee only deals with the last MCAT.

Application Information

Regular application	10/15
Regular notification	1/15 until filled
Admissions may be deferred?	Yes
AMCAS application accepted?	No
Interview required?	Yes
Application fee (in/out)	$45/$80

COSTS AND AID

Tuition & Fees

Tuition (in/out)	$6,550/$19,650
Cost of books	NR
Fees	$465

Financial Aid

% students receiving aid	NR
Average grant	NR
Average loan	NR
Average debt	NR

*Figures based on total enrollment

UNIVERSITY OF TEXAS—HOUSTON

MEDICAL SCHOOL

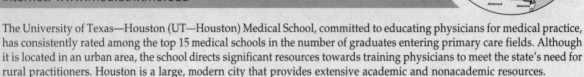

PO Box 20708, Houston, TX 77225
Admission: 713-500-5116 • Fax: 713-500-0604
Internet: www.med.uth.tmc.edu

The University of Texas—Houston (UT—Houston) Medical School, committed to educating physicians for medical practice, has consistently rated among the top 15 medical schools in the number of graduates entering primary care fields. Although it is located in an urban area, the school directs significant resources towards training physicians to meet the state's need for rural practitioners. Houston is a large, modern city that provides extensive academic and nonacademic resources.

Academics

Although most medical students complete studies in four years, some follow an Alternate Pathway curriculum, which extends first-year courses over a two-year period and which leads to the M.D. degree in five years. Others follow a six-year program leading to both the M.D. and the Ph.D. degrees, while others earn a Master's in Public Health along with the M.D. in five years. Summer research opportunities are available, most of which are paid. Medical students are evaluated with Honors, High Pass, Pass, Marginal Performance, and Fail. All students must take the USMLE Steps 1 and 2.

BASIC SCIENCES: First-year courses are Biochemistry, Gross Anatomy, Developmental Anatomy, Histology, Immunology, Introduction to Clinical Medicine (ICM), Microbiology, Neuroscience, and Physiology. The ICM course introduces students to interviewing, history-taking, and physical-examination skills. Instructional methods used during the first year include lectures, small-group sessions, tutorials, and labs. A new, problem-based learning curriculum links basic and clinical sciences and allows second-year students to begin addressing complex medical problems. Problem-based learning is an important part of the second-year curriculum, serving to integrate the various courses and provide clinical skills. Second-year courses are Behavioral Science, Genetics, Fundamentals of Clinical Medicine, Pathology, Pharmacology, Physical Diagnosis, and Reproductive Biology. During the first two years, students are in class or other scheduled sessions for about 22 hours per week. The Learning Resource Center has textbooks, audiovisuals, anatomical models, audiotapes and videotapes of lectures, computers, files of past exams, USMLE review materials, and other instructional aids. Networked computers with free access to computer-based services and instructional materials are also provided.

CLINICAL TRAINING: Third-year required rotations are Radiology (1 week); Medicine (12 weeks); Surgery (8 weeks); Ob/Gyn (8 weeks); Pediatrics (8 weeks); Psychiatry (8 weeks); and Family Medicine (4 weeks). During the fourth year, required rotations are Family Practice (1 month); Medicine (1 month); Neurology (1 month); and Surgery (1 month). Fourth-year students also take one month of didactic courses covering epidemiology; legal and ethical issues related to medicine; and fourth-year technical skills. Clinical training takes place primarily at the numerous hospitals, clinics, and care centers associated with the Texas Medical Center in Houston and in a city/county hospital in northeast Houston. There is flexibility in terms of where elective credits may be earned, and some students opt to study elsewhere in the country or at one of several international programs.

Students

At least 90 percent of students are Texas residents. Most students are recent college graduates, although there is typically a wide age range among incoming students. In terms of ethnic backgrounds, students represent the diverse population of the state.

STUDENT LIFE: There are numerous student organizations, focusing on areas such as public service projects, professional interests, religious and ethnic interests, athletics, and recreation. Medical students serve on important committees, such as the Admissions Committee, the Faculty-Student Relations Committee, and the Curriculum Committee. Houston is an exciting city for students, with a wide range of entertainment, recreational attractions, restaurants, shopping areas, and facilities for outdoor activities. The University offers apartments a short distance from school, and a free shuttle runs throughout the week.

GRADUATES: Of approximately 4,000 UT—Houston Medical School graduates, about 59 percent go on to practice in Texas. Among 2000 graduates, the most popular fields for residencies were Internal Medicine (11%); Pediatrics (11%); Family Practice (10%); Surgery (10%); Anesthesiology (9%); Emergency Medicine (3%); Ob/Gyn (6%); Medicine/Pediatrics (5%); Radiology (4%); Psychiatry (4%); and Ophthalmology (3%).

Admissions

REQUIREMENTS: Prerequisites are one year of English, one semester of college-level Calculus, one year of Physics with lab, two years of Biology with lab, one year of General Chemistry with lab, and one year of Organic Chemistry with lab. The MCAT is required, and scores should be from within the past 5 years. For applicants who have retaken the exam, the last three scores will be reviewed.

SUGGESTIONS: No more than 10 percent of students may be nonresidents. Thus, admission is very competitive for nonresidents. A liberal arts background is important, and as long as science requirements are fulfilled, students are encouraged to pursue a major in their area of interest while in college. Technological, vocational engineering, or business courses of study are not viewed as favorably as those providing a broad educational background. Important traits include intellectual capacity, interpersonal and communication skills, breadth and depth of pre-medical educational experience, potential for service to the State of Texas, motivation, and integrity.

PROCESS: The University of Texas does not participate in the AMCAS system. Applications may only be made online at the Texas Medical and Dental Schools Application Service website:

http://dpweb1.dp.utexas.edu/mdac

Applications must be submitted between May 1 and October 15. Additional information about the admissions process may be obtained from:

Texas Medical and Dental Schools Application Service
702 Colorado Street, Suite 6400
Austin, TX 78701
Phone: 512-499-4785

Applications must be submitted between May 15 and October 15. About 1,250 applicants are interviewed at UT—Houston between August and December. Applicants receive two one-on-one interviews, each with a faculty member. On interview day, candidates also have lunch with medical students, tour the campus, and attend group orientation sessions. About one-fifth of interviewees are accepted, with notification occurring on January 15. A few wait-listed candidates are accepted later in the spring.

Costs

The anticipated yearly cost of living for a single student is about $17,000. This budget allows for on- or off-campus living and car maintenance costs.

FINANCIAL AID: Most aid is from federal or state sources and is in the form of loans. However, some scholarships based on merit or other special criteria are also available.

UNIVERSITY OF TEXAS—HOUSTON

STUDENT BODY

Type	Public
*Enrollment	831
*% male/female	58/42
*% underrepresented minorities	18
# applied (total/out)	2,868/564
% interviewed (total/out)	41/1
% accepted (total/out)	23/3
% enrolled (total/out)	17/0
Average age	23

ADMISSIONS

Average GPA and MCAT Scores

Overall GPA	3.63	Science GPA	NR
MCAT Bio	9.7	MCAT Phys	9.2
MCAT Verbal	9.2	MCAT Essay	O

Score Release Policy
The Admissions Committee will review the last 3 scores released.

Application Information

Regular application	10/15
Regular notification	1/15 until filled
Transfers accepted?	No
Admissions may be deferred?	No
AMCAS application accepted?	No
Interview required?	Yes
Application fee (in/out)	$55/$100

COSTS AND AID

Tuition & Fees

Tuition (in/out)	$7,450/$20,550
Cost of books/supplies	$1,380
Fees	$872

Financial Aid

% students receiving aid	81
Average grant per student	$1,558
Average loan per student	$18,000
Average debt	$65,703

*Figures based on total enrollment

UNIVERSITY OF TEXAS—SAN ANTONIO

MEDICAL SCHOOL AT SAN ANTONIO

7703 Floyd Curl Drive, San Antonio, TX 78284
Admission: 210-567-2665 • Fax: 210-567-2685
Email: msprospect@uthscsa.edu • Internet: www.uthscsa.edu

The University of Texas (UT) Health Science Center at San Antonio is an important regional center for patient care, research, and education. It is comprised of the Dental School, Medical School, School of Allied Health Sciences, School of Nursing, and the Graduate School of Biomedical Sciences. UT San Antonio ranks about eighth in the nation in the proportion of graduates who enter primary care fields and also has one of the highest percentages of underrepresented minorities within the student body. The Health Science Center is dedicated to community service and delivers millions of dollars of donated care to underserved populations in the region. As a result of the School's location, medical students at San Antonio learn clinical skills through work with a diverse and interesting patient population.

Academics

Almost all medical students follow a four-year curriculum leading to the M.D. A few students enter combined M.D./Ph.D. programs after their first year of medical school. Grading for most courses uses an A–F system. All students must pass Step 1 of the USMLE for promotion to year three.

BASIC SCIENCES: Basic sciences are primarily covered during the first two years, although introductory clinical training also begins in year one. San Antonio operates on a semester system, with a break scheduled around Christmas. First-year, first-semester courses are the Clinical Integration Course, Biochemistry, Gross Anatomy and Embryology, Microscopic Anatomy, and Microbiology. Second-semester courses are Neuroscience and Physiology. Other first-year courses use a combination of lectures, labs, and small-group sessions. Students are in class or other scheduled sessions for about 21 hours per week during year one. During the second year, the curriculum is increasingly clinically oriented. First semester courses are Behavioral Sciences; Pathology; and Pharmacology. Second-semester courses are Pathology and Psychopathology. During year two, students are in class for about 19 hours per week, providing ample study time. An important resource for students, faculty, and the community is the Dolph Briscoe Library, which houses more than 200,000 books and journals.

CLINICAL TRAINING: The Clinical Integration course is an interdisciplinary program that starts with the first month of medical school and extends through the second year. Students learn basic clinical skills in the initial month of the program, spend time with community physicians, rotate with third-year students, and assume patient responsibilities to gain experience in continuity of care. The third and fourth years are devoted primarily to clinical clerkships. However, didactic instruction is also an important part of the curriculum. Topics covered are Clinical Orientation; Basic Cardiac Life Support; Emergency Medicine; Radiology; Patient Rehabilitation; Clinical Pathology; Medical Jurisprudence; Advanced

Cardiopulmonary Resuscitation; Medial Humanities; Infectious Disease; Genetics; and Epidemiology. Third-year required rotations are Ob/Gyn (6 weeks); Medicine (12 weeks); Pediatrics (6 weeks); Psychiatry (6 weeks); Surgery (12 weeks); and Family Practice (6 weeks). Fourth-year requirements are Medicine (8 weeks); Surgery (4 weeks); a choice of Pediatrics, Ob/Gyn, Psychiatry, or Family Practice (4 weeks); and other selectives (16 weeks). An additional 8 weeks are reserved for electives. The primary teaching hospital is the University Hospital, which has 547 beds. Training also takes place at the facilities of the South Texas Veterans Health Care System and at other affiliates. University-affiliated patient care covers a geographical area from San Antonio to the Rio Grande Valley and is delivered in clinics, hospitals, traveling vans, as well as in sites in schools and churches. The Health Science Center serves the entire South Texas/Border region.

Students

At least 90 percent of students are Texas residents. Underrepresented minorities account for 16 percent of the student population. Mexican-Americans are particularly well represented. The student body is slightly older than at many other medical schools. The average age of incoming students is usually about 24, and about 15 percent of students in each class are in their thirties or older.

STUDENT LIFE: Medical students enjoy a collegial environment and appreciate the diversity within the student body. Mentoring and peer-support programs help incoming students with the transition to medical school, and special programs are available to assist underrepresented minority students. Students are very active in community service programs and events. Activities range from volunteering at clinics to participating in health education programs in schools. All students live off campus. San Antonio offers affordable housing accessible to the Medical Center by public transportation.

GRADUATES: More than half of graduates enter primary care fields, and a significant number go on to practice in Texas.

Admissions

REQUIREMENTS: Required courses are one semester of Calculus, one year each of English and Physics, two years of Biology (one of which may be Biochemistry), and two years of Chemistry (which should include both Organic and Inorganic Chemistry). The MCAT is required, and scores must be from 1997 or later. For applicants who have taken the exam more then once, the best set of scores is weighed most heavily. Thus, there is no advantage in withholding scores.

SUGGESTIONS: In addition to academic requirements, personal traits and an applicant's background are considered. Some type of medically related experience or research is required.

PROCESS: The University of Texas medical schools do not participate in AMCAS. Rather, applications may be obtained from:

> The Texas Medical and Dental Application Service
> 702 Colorado, Suite 6400
> Austin, Texas 78701

Applications must be completed by October 15.

About one-third of applicants are interviewed between August and December. Interviews consist of two half-hour sessions with Admissions Committee members who may be faculty or senior students. On interview day, candidates also have lunch with students, attend group-orientation sessions, and tour the campus. The initial group of accepted candidates are notified in January. Others are notified later in the spring. An alternate pool of applicants is established and candidates are admitted as positions become available.

Costs

The estimated yearly cost of living for a single student is about $27,603. This budget allows for off-campus housing and car maintenance.

FINANCIAL AID: All students with financial need must file a FAFSA form. In addition to federal programs, institutional and private assistance is available in the form of scholarships, grants, employment opportunities, and loans. All financial aid is awarded on the basis of need.

UNIVERSITY OF TEXAS— SAN ANTONIO

STUDENT BODY

Type	Public
*Enrollment	824
*% male/female	51/49
*% underrepresented minorities	17
# applied (total/out)	2,647/399
% interviewed (total/out)	38/10
% accepted (total/out)	25/8
% enrolled (total/out)	8/8
Average age	24

ADMISSIONS

Average GPA and MCAT Scores

Overall GPA	3.43	Science GPA	NR
MCAT Bio	10.00	MCAT Phys	9.00
MCAT Verbal	9.00	MCAT Essay	NR

Score Release Policy

The school has not responded to our inquiry regarding withheld MCAT scores. Therefore, we advise caution. Contact the Admissions Office before withholding any scores.

Application Information

Regular application	10/1
Regular notification	1/15 until filled
Transfers accepted?	Yes
Admissions may be deferred?	No
AMCAS application accepted?	No
Interview required?	Yes
Application fee (in/out)	$45/$80

COSTS AND AID

Tuition & Fees

Tuition (in/out)	$6,550/$19,650
Cost of books	NR
Fees	$1,410

Financial Aid

% students receiving aid	NR
Average grant	NR
Average loan	NR
Average debt	NR

*Figures based on total enrollment

TUFTS UNIVERSITY
SCHOOL OF MEDICINE

136 Harrison Avenue, Boston, MA 02111
Admission: 617-636-6571
Internet: www.tufts.edu/med

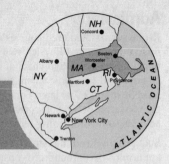

Tufts is a private medical school, featuring the standard M.D. curriculum in addition to a range of innovative combined-degree programs. Tufts has implemented a revised curriculum that reflects important developments in the health care field, such as the increase in health information technology and the growth of managed care. Weekly problem-based learning sessions are an important aspect of the curriculum, ensuring that students are able to apply their acquired knowledge and that they have the tools for lifelong learning. For clinical training, students benefit from exposure to a diverse, urban patient population. Boston is a student-centered city, offering a wide range of academic and nonacademic activities.

Academics

The majority of students follow a four-year curriculum leading to the M.D. degree. Students with an interest in public health have the opportunity to earn an M.P.H. along with their M.D. This combined M.D./M.P.H. program may be completed in four years. Other combined-degree programs include the four year M.D./M.B.A. in Health Management in partnership with Brandeis University and Northeastern University, the M.D./Ph.D. in conjunction with the Sackler School of Graduate Biomedical Sciences, and the B.S. in Engineering and combined M.S./M.D. in Engineering degree program, a collaborative effort of the Tufts College of Engineering and the Tufts University School of Medicine. The doctorate may be earned in the following fields: Anatomy, Biochemistry, Biophysics, Cell Biology, Genetics, Immunology, Microbiology, Molecular Biology, Neuroscience, Pathology, Pharmacology, and Physiology. Each year, four funded M.D./Ph.D. positions are available. A primary care preceptorship program allows students with a particular interest in primary care to experience early patient contact.

BASIC SCIENCES: In addition to required courses, first- and second-year students choose among pre-clinical selectives. These are graded as Pass/Fail and allow students to explore their interests early on in the program. A new Principles and Practice of Medicine Program (PPM) was developed to enhance the first- and second-year curriculum. PPM integrates basic science topics with interdisciplinary subjects such as Information Management, Computer Literacy, Negotiation/Team Building Skills, Health Care Economics, and Ethics. PPM also introduces important clinical techniques such as the patient interview, examination, and physical diagnosis. First-year courses are the following: Gross Anatomy; Histology; Biochemistry; Genetics; Epidemiology Biostatistics; Molecular Biology; Physiology; Cell Biology; Immunology; Hematology; Problem-Based Learning; Pre-clinical Selectives; and PPM. Second-year courses are the following: Pathology; Pathophysiology/Infectious Disease; Neuroscience; Psychopathology; Pharmacology;

Microbiology; Problem-Based Learning; Addiction Medicine; Pre-clinical Selectives; and PPM, which focuses on clinical skills and serves as an important transition to third-year clerkships. During the first and second years, instruction involves lectures, labs, and small-group sessions. As an important learning aid, Tufts Health Sciences Library developed the Health Sciences Database. It contains the full text of many syllabi, lecture slides, reserve slide collections, lecture recordings, and other multimedia and resource materials.

CLINICAL TRAINING: Third-year required clerkships are the following: Medicine (12 weeks); Surgery (12 weeks); Ob/Gyn (6 weeks); Pediatrics (6 weeks); and Psychiatry (6 weeks). About four weeks are available for elective study during the third year. Fourth-year requirements are a 4-week primary care clerkship and a 4-week Neurology elective. At least 32 weeks of electives are also required, 20 of which must be completed at Tufts facilities. Twelve weeks of electives may be taken at other academic and clinical institutions. Some students fulfill a portion of elective requirements overseas.

Students

In last year's entering class, about 28 percent of students were Massachusetts residents, and about 14 percent of students went to Tufts as undergraduates. Another 28 percent of students were California residents, and 10 percent were New York residents. Approximately 30 percent of students were at least 23 years old, and 15 percent were 25 or older. Women accounted for 41 percent of the class, and underrepresented minorities accounted for about 11 percent.

STUDENT LIFE: Medical students at Tufts are generally cohesive and supportive of one another. Some students are involved in clubs or in local chapters of national medical student organizations. Off campus, students enjoy the offerings of Boston, a city filled with students, bookstores, coffee shops, restaurants, parks, and cultural activities. Residence facilities are available on a limited basis in Posner Hall, located close to the Medical School campus.

Students who live off campus generally share apartments in neighborhoods that are convenient to the School.

GRADUATES: Graduates are successful in securing residency positions at institutions in all regions of the country. Tufts prepares graduates for careers in both primary care and specialty areas.

Admissions

REQUIREMENTS: Requirements are 8 semester credits of Biology, Chemistry, Organic Chemistry, and Physics all with associated labs. Applicants must possess the ability to speak and write English correctly. The MCAT is required, and scores should be from within the past three years. For applicants who have taken the exam on multiple occasions, the best scores are used.

SUGGESTIONS: In addition to prerequisite courses, recommended course work includes Calculus, Statistics, Computer Science, English, and Biochemistry. The selection of candidates for admissions is based not only on performance in the required pre-medical courses, but also on the applicant's entire academic record and extracurricular experiences.

PROCESS: All AMCAS applicants are sent secondary applications. Of those returning completed applications, about 12 percent are invited to interview between November and March. Interviews consist of two sessions, each with a faculty member, school administrator, or senior medical student. On interview day, applicants also attend informational sessions and a reception with current medical students. Approximately half of interviewed candidates are accepted. Notification occurs on a rolling basis and is completed by May. Wait-listed candidates are generally not encouraged to send additional information.

Costs

The estimated yearly cost of living for a single student is about $16,000. This does not include tuition or fees, but covers room, board, transportation, and other living expenses.

FINANCIAL AID: All aid is need-based, with financial need determined by the FAFSA and institutional forms. Parental financial disclosure is required for all institutional forms of aid. Funds for grants and scholarships are very limited, and most aid is in the form of loans.

TUFTS UNIVERSITY

STUDENT BODY

Type	Private
*Enrollment	689
*% male/female	59/41
*% underrepresented minorities	11
# applied (total/out)	9,338/8,336
% interviewed (total/out)	10/7
% accepted (total/out)	NR/NR
% enrolled (total/out)	20/18

ADMISSIONS

Average GPA and MCAT Scores

Overall GPA	NR	Science GPA	NR
MCAT Bio	9.80	MCAT Phys	9.60
MCAT Verbal	9.10	MCAT Essay	NR

Score Release Policy

The school has not responded to our inquiry regarding withheld MCAT scores. Therefore, we advise caution. Contact the Admissions Office before withholding any scores.

Application Information

Regular application	11/1
Regular notification	10/15 until filled
Early application	6/1–8/1
Early notification	10/1
Admissions may be deferred?	Yes
AMCAS application accepted?	Yes
Interview required?	Yes
Application fee	$95

COSTS AND AID

Tuition & Fees

Tuition	$32,865
Cost of books	NR
Fees	$460

Financial Aid

% students receiving aid	75
Average grant	NR
Average loan	NR
Average debt	NR

*Figures based on total enrollment

TULANE UNIVERSITY
SCHOOL OF MEDICINE

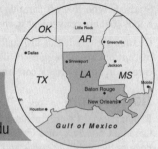

1430 Tulane Avenue, New Orleans, LA 70112

Admission: 504-588-5187 • Fax: 504-988-6735

Email: medsch@tmc.pop.tmc.tulane.edu • Internet: www.mcl.tulane.edu

Tulane is a private institution that attracts students from around the country. The School of Medicine profits from the affiliated research and educational institutions of the Medical Center, such as the renowned School of Public Health and Tropical Medicine, through which many medical students pursue a master's degree along with the M.D. The School of Medicine identifies its objectives as education, research, and patient care. By way of an innovative curriculum, these components are integrated, preparing students for a vast array of medical career paths. Tulane is situated in downtown New Orleans, a city with a great deal to offer, including world-famous jazz.

Academics

The School of Medicine is one of many schools of Tulane University. In addition to joint-degree programs with the School of Pubic Health, arrangements can be made with the Graduate School. Doctorate degrees may be earned along with the M.D. in approximately 6 years in the following fields: Anatomy, Biochemistry, Biomedical Engineering, Cell Biology, Genetics, Immunology, Microbiology, Molecular Biology, Neuroscience, Pharmacology, and Physiology. The vast majority of students earn their M.D. in four years.

BASIC SCIENCES: First-year courses are the following: Anatomy; Histology; Embryology; Neuroscience; Physiology; Biochemistry; Introduction to Clinical Computing and Communications; and Foundations in Medicine, which provides clinical experience both on campus and in community settings and introduces concepts of human behavior, preventive medicine, and ethics. Second-year courses are the following: Pharmacology, Pathology, Microbiology, Immunology, Parasitology, Genetics, and Foundations in Medicine. In addition to required courses, students participate in elective study for 3 afternoons each week beginning in the second semester of year one and continuing throughout year two. This allows students to explore their areas of interest, to take part in research, or to pursue an M.P.H. degree. Most courses have integrated a variety of teaching modalities into their structure. Thus, problem-based learning sessions, small-group and panel discussions, case-based methods, computerized instructional programs, lectures, and labs are all used throughout the first two years. On average, students are in class for 24 hours per week during their first two years. Basic science instruction takes place in the Medical School Building, central to the clinical and research facilities. Computers are used as learning aids and research tools and for communication during the basic science years, and a Computing Center serves the needs of the campus. The Rudolph Matas Library houses 130,000 volumes and receives 1,200 periodicals. The grading scale is Honors/High Pass/Pass/Conditional/Fail. This grading system is employed throughout all four years of medical school.

Students are required to record a grade on USMLE Step 1, but are not required to pass for promotion. Step 2 is not required for graduation.

CLINICAL TRAINING: Patient contact begins in year one in Foundations in Medicine. Physical Diagnosis is taught with the extensive use of standardized (surrogate) patients throughout the first two years. While clinical training is interwoven into the first two years, formal clinical training begins with the third year and consists of the following required eight-week rotations: Family/Community Medicine, Internal Medicine, Ob/Gyn, Pediatrics, Psychiatry/Neurology, and Surgery. During the fourth year, students will have a four-week internship, which focuses on the undifferentiated patient; this internship will allow students to experience ambulatory care in several settings. Also in the fourth year, students do a subinternship in ward management (4 weeks) and are allowed to have six selectives, which may include either domestic or international sites. International sites include locations in Africa, South and Central America, and Asia. Formal exchange programs exist with organizations in Sweden, Germany, and Japan. Clinical training takes place at numerous sites, including the Tulane University Hospital, Charity Hospital, and New Orleans VA Hospital. Along with the Medical School and the University Hospital, the Tulane Medical Center includes the School of Public Health and Tropical Medicine, the Tulane Hospital for Children, the University Health Service, the Primate Research Center, the U.S.-Japan Biomedical Research Laboratories, ad the Tulane/Xavier Center for Bioenvironmental Research.

Students

Students of the 1999 entering class represented 38 states, Washington, D.C., and the Virgin Islands, with 17 percent of the class from Louisiana, 14 percent from California, 8 percent from Florida, and 5 percent from Utah, New York, and Pennsylvania. Seventeen percent received undergraduate degrees from Tulane. Sixty-one percent of students were either science or engineering majors in college. The average age of incoming students was 24, with an age range from 20 to 30. About 10 percent of students are underrepresented minorities, most of whom are African American. Class size is 150.

STUDENT LIFE: Students take part in both on- and off-campus activities. The Medical Center is located in the central business district of New Orleans, within walking distance of the famous French Quarter. New Orleans has many parks and other areas suitable for fishing, biking, running, tennis, and other outdoor activities, which are possible year-round. The uptown Tulane University campus, which includes the College of Arts and Sciences, is accessible to the Medical Center by shuttle bus. At the uptown campus, a large athletic facility is available for medical student use. Organizations based on academics, specialties, religion, hobbies, ethnicity, social life, or athletics bring medical students together around shared interests and provide support. A housing facility, located adjacent to the Tulane Medical Center Hospital, makes over 250 apartments available to medical students. University-owned housing for single and married students is also available, although most opt to live off campus, where houses and apartments are affordable and attractive.

GRADUATES: Of the 1999 graduating class, the most popular residencies were Internal Medicine (22%); Surgery (8%); Pediatrics (13%); Ob/Gyn (7%); Family Practice (8%); Emergency Medicine (3%); and Otolaryngology (3%). Forty-eight percent of the class entered fields considered to be primary care. Popular states for post-graduate training were Louisiana, California, and Texas.

Admissions

REQUIREMENTS: Required subjects for admission are English (6 semester hours); Chemistry (6 hours); Organic Chemistry (6 hours); Physics (6 hours); and Biology (6 hours). All science courses must include labs. The MCAT is required and should be no more than three years old. The best set of scores is considered.

SUGGESTIONS: The April, rather than August, MCAT is strongly advised. The Admissions Committee considers the substance and level of courses taken in college, as well as the applicant's improvement in scholastic performance throughout college. There is no preference for particular majors. Activities that demonstrate strong interpersonal skills and some exposure to the medical field are valued.

PROCESS: All applicants receive secondary applications shortly after submitting AMCAS applications. Of those who return secondaries, about 20 percent are interviewed. Interviews take place from September through February and may consist of one session with a dean, one session with a member of the faculty, and one session with a medical student. Notification occurs on a rolling basis. Of those interviewed, about 30 percent are offered a place in the class. Candidates who are wait-listed may send additional information if it strengthens their files.

Costs

Beyond tuition and fees, the anticipated yearly budget for a single student is about $13,000. This allows for either on- or off-campus living.

FINANCIAL AID: Twenty-seven entering students each year receive merit-based scholarships, renewable for all four years. Most aid is need-based, and need is established by federal and institutional formulas. Tulane offers need-based scholarships and interest-free loans. The average debt of Tulane graduates in 1999 was $118,000.

TULANE UNIVERSITY

STUDENT BODY

Type	Private
*Enrollment	602
*% male/female	55/45
*% underrepresented minorities	12
# applied (total/out)	8,271/7,753
% interviewed (total/out)	908/787
% accepted (total/out)	4/1
% enrolled (total/out)	48/46
Average age	24

ADMISSIONS

Average GPA and MCAT Scores

Overall GPA	3.53	Science GPA	3.56
MCAT Bio	10.6	MCAT Phys	10.3
MCAT Verbal	10.0	MCAT Essay	P

Score Release Policy

The school has not responded to our inquiry regarding withheld MCAT scores. Therefore, we advise caution. Contact the Admissions Office before withholding any scores.

Application Information

Regular application	12/15
Regular notification	10/15 until filled
Early application	6/1–8/1
Early notification	10/1
Transfers accepted?	Yes
Admissions may be deferred?	Yes
AMCAS application accepted?	Yes
Interview required?	Yes
Application fee	$95

COSTS AND AID

Tuition & Fees

Tuition	$29,147
Cost of books & microscope	$1,000
Fees	$1,777

Financial Aid

% students receiving aid	87
Average grant	$10,000
Average loan	$29,704
Average debt	$118,000

*Figures based on total enrollment

UMDNJ, New Jersey Medical School

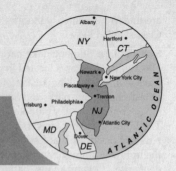

185 South Orange Avenue, Newark, NJ 07103
Admission: 973-972-4631 • Fax: 973-972-7986
Email: njmsadmiss@umdnj.edu • Internet: www.umdnj.edu/njmsweb

The New Jersey Medical School is the largest medical institution in the state. As a public entity, its priorities are providing an outstanding medical education to New Jersey residents and fulfilling its role as a major health care provider to the state's population. Several years ago, the college introduced a revised curriculum featuring greater clinical correlation during the first two years, increased emphasis on behavioral, social, and environmental aspects of medicine, and patient contact during the first year. Research is also emphasized, demonstrated by the fact that more than half of the students undertake summer research projects between the first and second years. Newark is an urban center, providing a diverse patient population and intensive clinical training. The city is a 20-minute train ride to downtown Manhattan.

Academics

Qualified students may enter a joint M.D./Ph.D. program, earning the doctorate degree in Physiology, Pharmacology, Pathology, Neuroscience, Molecular Biology, Microbiology, Immunology, Genetics, Cell Biology, Biomedical Engineering, Biochemistry, and Anatomy. Additional joint degree programs may include M.D./M.P.H., M.D./J.D., M.D./M.B.A.

BASIC SCIENCES: During the first two years, small group sessions and tutorials account for about one-third of scheduled sessions, with the remainder of class time used for lectures and labs. Students are paired with physicians in the community, working with them one afternoon each week as part of primary care preceptorships. Courses demand about 27 hours per week, in addition to individual study time. First-year courses are Biochemistry and Molecular Biology; Cell and Tissue Biology; Genetics; Gross and Developmental Anatomy; Neuroscience; Physiology; Psychiatry; Public Health; The Art of Medicine; Problem-Based Learning; and Clinical Skills, which focuses on the physical examination. During the second year, topics are coordinated among courses and are organized around organ systems. Courses are Clinical Preventive Medicine and Nutrition; Immunology; Microbiology; Pathology; Pharmacology; Introduction to Clinical Sciences; and Psychiatry and the Clinical Interview. The Medical Sciences Building, where basic sciences are taught, is connected to the University Hospital and the George F. Smith Library, the latter of which houses 70,000 volumes and over 2,000 periodicals. The proximity of clinical facilities to classrooms and labs encourages first- and second-year students' involvement in clinical activities. The Office of Student Affairs provides services ranging from personal counseling to guidance on elective and residency selection.

CLINICAL TRAINING: Required third-year clerkships are Internal Medicine (12 weeks); General Surgery (8 weeks); Pediatrics (8 weeks); Ob/Gyn (8 weeks); Psychiatry (6 weeks); and Family Medicine (6 weeks). During the fourth year, 16 weeks of electives are required in addition to Neurology (4 weeks); Emergency Medicine (4 weeks); Substance Abuse (2 weeks); Physical Medicine and Rehabilitation (2 weeks); Ophthalmology, Orthopedics, Otolaryngology, Urology (1 week each); and an acting internship in Medicine, Pediatrics, Family Medicine, Obstetrics, or Surgery (4 weeks). Most clinical training takes place at the contiguous 518-bed University Hospital, which serves the needs of the immediate community and, with its specialized care units, attracts patients from around the state. Other affiliated teaching hospitals are Hackensack University Hospital, Morristown Memorial Hospital, Veterans Affairs Health Care System–East Orange, and Kessler Institute for Rehabilitation.

Students

Generally, about 90 percent of entering students are New Jersey residents. Underrepresented minorities, most of whom are African American or Puerto Rican, account for about 13 percent of the student body. There is a large age range within each class. Class size is 170.

STUDENT LIFE: Students take advantage of the school's athletic and recreational facilities, and are involved in intramural sports and organized student events. Each entering student is assigned to a peer group of first- and second-year students. These groupswait list odically, providing support for students and assistance with academic and personal issues. Students initiate and develop service activities such as Community 2000, which conducts clinical screening and health education with local churches. Students are actively involved in community service projects through the CHARE center. NJMS was recognized in 1994 by the AAMC with the "Outstanding Community Service" award. Newark is an up-and-coming city with inexpensive ethnic restaurants, performing arts, jazz clubs, and diverse neighborhoods. New York City is an easy train ride and serves as a convenient distraction for medical students. All students live off campus, in Newark or in the surrounding suburbs, and the Office of Student Affairs actively assists students in securing housing.

GRADUATES: Each year, graduates are successful in obtaining residencies at prestigious institutions such as Massachusetts General, Columbia Presbyterian and Children's Hospital in Washington, D.C. The alumni association is very enthusiastic, and among its activities is the provision of scholarships and research stipends to medical students.

Admissions

REQUIREMENTS: Eight semester hours of Biology and Physics, 16 of Chemistry/Organic Chemistry, and six of English are required. The MCAT is required, and all sets of scores are considered. Although not a requirement, preference is given to New Jersey residents.

SUGGESTIONS: Research or experience in a health care setting is useful. Personal traits, such as compassion, dedication, and interpersonal skills, are very important.

PROCESS: In previous years, a secondary application has not been part of the admissions process. About one-quarter of applicants are invited to interview, with interviews conducted between August and April. Interviews consist of one hour-long session with a faculty member. About 30 percent of interviewees are accepted, with notification occurring on a rolling basis. Wait-listed candidates are generally not encouraged to send supplementary material. As an alternative admissions route, New Jersey residents who attend participating undergraduate institutions may apply for the Baccalaureate/M.D. Program. This program allows students to earn both degrees within a more compact time frame.

Costs

As a Northeastern city, Newark can be a relatively expensive place to live. However, the student budget reflects the costs, and the Financial Aid Office responds to them.

FINANCIAL AID: About 70 percent of students receive financial aid, which is awarded on the basis of need. A limited number of private, merit-based scholarships are available.

UMDNJ, NEW JERSEY MEDICAL SCHOOL

STUDENT BODY

Type	Public
*Enrollment	699
*% male/female	58/42
*% underrepresented minorities	18
# applied (total/out)	2,290/1,810
% interviewed (total/out)	NR/NR
% accepted (total/out)	NR/NR
% enrolled (total/out)	NR/NR

ADMISSIONS

Average GPA and MCAT Scores

Overall GPA	3.52	Science GPA	NR
MCAT Bio	10.40	MCAT Phys	10.20
MCAT Verbal	9.70	MCAT Essay	NR

Score Release Policy
The school has not responded to our inquiry regarding withheld MCAT scores. Therefore, we advise caution. Contact the Admissions Office before withholding any scores.

Application Information

Regular application	12/1
Regular notification	10/15 until filled
Early application	6/1–8/1
Early notification	10/1
Admissions may be deferred?	Yes
AMCAS application accepted?	Yes
Interview required?	Yes
Application fee	$75

COSTS AND AID

Tuition & Fees

Tuition (in/out)	$15,509/$24,270
Cost of books	NR
Fees	$900

Financial Aid

% students receiving aid	70
Average grant	NR
Average loan	NR
Average debt	NR

*Figures based on total enrollment

UMDNJ, ROBERT WOOD JOHNSON MEDICAL SCHOOL

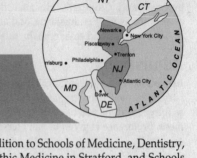

675 Hoes Lane, Piscataway, NJ 08854
Admission: 732-235-4576 • Fax: 732-235-5078
Internet: www.umdnj.edu/rwjms.html

UMDNJ encompasses the Robert Wood Johnson Medical School in Piscataway in addition to Schools of Medicine, Dentistry, Nursing, Health Related Professions, and Medicine in Newark; a School of Osteopathic Medicine in Stratford, and Schools of Biomedical Sciences in both Newark and Piscataway. The goals of the Robert Wood Johnson Medical School include educating quality physicians, contributing to important research developments, and addressing the health care needs of the people of New Jersey. The Main Medical Science Complex, where all basic science takes place, is in Piscataway. Clinical training takes place in two programs based in two principal teaching hospitals in New Brunswick and Camden. The curriculum integrates traditional and modern approaches, uses clinical staff to assist with basic science instruction, and includes problem-based learning as a way to apply basic science lessons.

Academics

Although most students complete their studies in four years, there are several possible variations on the standard program. A new flexible curriculum allows selected students to rearrange the timing of certain courses, thereby enabling them to pursue joint degrees with affiliated institutions, relevant projects, personal interests, employment, or research. Joint degree possibilities are the M.D./M.P.H, M.D./J.D., M.D./M.S., and the M.D./Ph.D. The M.D./M.S. is offered in Jurisprudence and Medical Informatics. An M.D./M.B.A. program is also available. The Ph.D. is offered in Biochemistry, Cell Biology, Biomedical Engineering, Microbiology, Molecular Biology, Pharmacology, Physiology, and Public Health. Grading uses Honors/High Pass/Pass/Low Pass/Fail, and both steps of the USMLE are required for graduation.

BASIC SCIENCES: During the first two years, clinical correlates and psychosocial perspectives enrich the basic science curriculum. First-year courses are Cell Biology and Histology, Gross and Developmental Anatomy, Neuroscience, Biological Chemistry, Environmental and Community Medicine, Medical Ethics, Introduction to the Patient, Case-Based Learning, Biochemistry of Nutrition, Medical Physiology, Medical Microbiology, and Immunology. Second-year courses are Behavioral Science and Psychiatry, Biostatistics/Epidemiology, Clinical Pathophysiology, Human Sexuality, Pathology and Laboratory Medicine, Physical Diagnosis and Clinical Decision-Making, Physical Diagnosis and Clinical Decision-Making in Psychiatry, Pharmacology, Case-Based Learning, Clinical Prevention, and Environmental Medicine. There is a vast array of electives which students may take during the preclinical curriculum, including Issues in Women's Health, Community and Child Health, Emergency Room Elective, Geriatric Issues, and Alternative and Complementary

Medicine to name a few. The Medical Science Complex includes research, clinical, and administrative facilities in addition to classrooms and modern laboratories.

CLINICAL TRAINING: Required third-year rotations are Introduction to the Clinical Experience (1 week) and eight weeks each of Family Medicine; Medicine; Ob/Gyn; Pediatrics; Psychiatry; and Surgery. During the fourth year, four weeks each of Medicine, Surgery, Neurology, and a Subinternship are required. Three weeks of Clinical Community and Professional Correlates and 16–20 weeks of electives are also required. A Student Scholars Program allows students to engage in research or teaching or to participate in off-campus activities, such as working with the Indian Health Service. Most clinical training takes place at the Robert Wood Johnson University Hospital in New Brunswick, which has areas for didactic instruction in addition to clinical facilities. Other affiliated sites are the Eric B. Chandler Health Center, a family-oriented community health center; the Cancer Institute of New Jersey; the Mental Health Center at Piscataway; the Clinical Research Center (advanced biotechnology and medicine); the Cardiovascular Institute; and 80 additional hospitals throughout the state. About one-third of each class trains at hospitals and/or clinics in the Camden area.

Students

Approximately 87 percent of the students are New Jersey residents. Almost 20 percent are underrepresented minorities, most of whom are African American. Typically, 10–20 percent of an incoming class took significant time off between college and medical school. Class size is 142.

STUDENT LIFE: Medical students have access to Rutgers University athletic facilities, which include several swimming pools and gyms, in addition to squash, racquetball, and volleyball courts. Rutgers also offers social, cultural, and recreational distractions for medical students. Chapters of the major national medical student organizations are active at UMDNJ, as are other types of groups. Some organizations volunteer services to activities such as blood drives and health-education seminars in schools, while others are focused on common interests and providing support for students. Although there is no medical student housing, the school helps students to secure accommodations in the area.

GRADUATES: Many graduates enter primary care fields, but all specialties are represented. UMDNJ has an extensive network of clinical affiliates, many of which offer post-graduate training. Medical School graduates are particularly successful in securing positions in these programs.

Admissions

REQUIREMENTS: One year each of Physics, Chemistry, Organic Chemistry, Biology, and English are required, as is one semester of college-level Math. The MCAT is required, and must be no more than four years old. For applicants who have taken the exam more than once, all scores are considered, but the most recent set is given the most weight.

SUGGESTIONS: Coursework in the Behavioral Sciences and Humanities is recommended. Medically related experiences, research, and community service are all valued by the Admissions Committee.

PROCESS: In the past, UMDNJ has not administered a supplementary application. About one-half of New Jersey resident applicants, and 5 percent or less of out-of-state residents, are interviewed on campus. Interviews are held between September and March and consist of one session with a faculty member, and possibly an additional session with a medical student. Of those interviewed, about one-third are accepted, with notification occurring on a rolling basis. Wait-listed candidates should not submit additional material unless requested. An alternate means of admissions for sophomores at Rutgers University is through a combined B. A./M.D. program.

Costs

In addition to tuition, the estimated yearly expenditure for a single student is $18,000. This includes all fees, living, and personal expenses. This budget allows for comfortable living accommodations and car ownership.

FINANCIAL AID: Most aid is need-based, with need determined primarily through the FAFSA form. Although parental disclosure is not required for all assistance, most grants and scholarships require it. Private sources of financial aid, such as a foundation affiliated with the school, offer some merit-based assistance.

UMDNJ, ROBERT WOOD JOHNSON MEDICAL SCHOOL

STUDENT BODY

Type	Public
*Enrollment	622
*% male/female	52/48
*% underrepresented minorities	20
# applied (total/out)	2,471/1,427
% interviewed (total/out)	29/10
% accepted (total/out)	15/7
% enrolled (total/out)	6/1
Average age	24

ADMISSIONS

Average GPA and MCAT Scores

Overall GPA	3.59	Science GPA	3.53
MCAT Bio	10.20	MCAT Phys	10.10
MCAT Verbal	9.10	MCAT Essay	P

Score Release Policy

Students are not disadvantaged by withholding scores.

Application Information

Regular application	12/1
Regular notification	10/15 until filled
Early application	6/1–8/1
Early notification	10/1
Transfers accepted?	Yes
Admissions may be deferred?	Yes
AMCAS application accepted?	Yes
Interview required?	Yes
Application fee	$75

COSTS AND AID

Tuition & Fees

Tuition (in/out)	$16,052/$25,119
Cost of books	$1,151
Fees	$1,372

Financial Aid

% students receiving aid	80
Average grant	NR
Average loan	NR
Average debt	NR

*Figures based on total enrollment

UNIFORMED SERVICES UNIVERSITY OF THE HEALTH SCIENCES

F. EDWARD HÉBERT SCHOOL OF MEDICINE

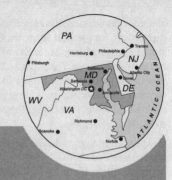

4301 Jones Bridge Road, Bethesda, MD 20814
Admission: 301-295-3101 • Fax: 301-295-3545
Email: dreston@usuhs.mil • Internet: www.usuhs.mil

The Uniformed Services University of the Health Sciences (USUHS) prepares physicians to serve in the Department of Defense and the Public Health Service, meaning that graduates understand preventive medicine, tropical medicine, disaster medicine, and survival in harsh climates. As a Federal Government institution, USUHS responds to national priorities in healthcare delivery and research. The School of Medicine is tuition-free, and attending involves a seven-year commitment of medical service with the Army, Navy, or Air Force, and up to six years commitment to the Reserves. The campus is close to the National Institutes of Health (NIH), facilitating research opportunities for students. Washington, D.C. is easily accessible on the Metro and offers ample cultural and recreational attractions.

Academics

Incoming students without prior uniformed service experience attend an Army Officer Base Course during the summer before entering the School of Medicine. Most classes and rotations are evaluated with an A–F scale. Passing both steps of the USMLE is a requirement for graduation.

BASIC SCIENCES: Lectures and labs are the primary means of instruction during the first two years, and students are in scheduled sessions for about 25 hours per week. In addition to a solid grounding in the basic sciences, students receive interdisciplinary instruction that includes sociological, historical, ethical, and legal perspectives on medicine. First-year courses are Anatomy and Physiology I; Biochemistry; Diagnostic Parasitology and Medical Zoology; Fundamentals of Epidemology and Biometrics; Head, Neck, and CNS Anatomy; Human Context in Health Care; Introduction to Clinical Medicine I; Medical Psychology; Medical History; Military Medical Field Studies-Summer; Organ System Microanatomy; and Physiology II. During the summer following the first academic year, students take part in a hands-on field experience that serves as an introduction to military operations. Students who have a background in this area use the summer for research or other activities. Second-year courses are Clinical Concepts; Clinical Pharmacology; Ethical, Legal, and Social Aspects of Medical Care; Human Behavior; Introduction to Clinical Medicine II and III; Medical Microbiology and Infectious Diseases; Military Studies II; Pathology; Pharmacology; Preventive Medicine; and Radiographic Interpretation. Instruction takes place on the grounds of the National Naval Medical Center, in Bethesda, Maryland. Educational resources include the Multidisciplinary Laboratories and the Anatomical Teaching Laboratories, both of which are open 24 hours a day. The Learning Resource Center serves as the library, and has 120,000 volumes, journals, slides, videotapes, CDs, microcomputer programs, and online informational programs.

CLINICAL TRAINING: Third-year required clerkships are Family Practice (6 weeks); Medicine (12 weeks); Ob/Gyn (6 weeks); Pediatrics (6 weeks); Psychiatry (6 weeks); and Surgery (12 weeks). During the fourth year, 20 weeks are reserved for clinical electives or research. Required fourth-year clerkships are Military Contingency Medicine; Military Emergency Medicine; Military Preventive Medicine; Neurology; and a Subinternship. The main teaching hospitals are Walter Reed Army Medical Center, National Naval Medical Center, and Malcolm Grow USAF Medical Center, which are all in the Washington, D.C., area, and the Wilford Hall USAF Medical Center, in San Antonio, Texas. In total, these hospitals provide over 3,000 beds. Electives may be fulfilled at clinical sites nationwide and overseas.

Students

In a recent class, 56 percent had no prior military experience. Others have backgrounds in service academies, ROTC activities, as active and prior duty officers and enlisted service members, and as Reservists. Students are from all over the country, and represent a large number of undergraduate institutions. The most prevalent undergraduate majors were Biology (30%); Biochemistry (12%); Chemistry (13%); and Zoology (4%). About 10 percent of students are underrepresented minorities. The average age of entering students is about 24. Class size is 165.

STUDENT LIFE: USUHS student groups include chapters of national organizations in addition to organizations focused on professional or service-oriented goals. These organizations are devoted to activities such as journalism, providing support to women medical students or spouses of medical students, and recreational pursuits. The school sponsors intramural athletic programs for men and women, and offers comprehensive athletic facilities.

Nearby military posts and bases provide recreational and social activities for students and their families. Washington, D.C., with its museums, sites, parks, events, and diverse population, is an important resource and enriches the lives of medical students. All students live off campus, most in the immediate vicinity of the school or in Metro-accessible areas.

GRADUATES: Graduates must select residency programs at military hospitals, and often enter programs at the hospitals where they performed clerkships. Residencies vary in length, depending on the medical specialty. The residency period does not fulfill the seven-year commitment involved in attending USUHS. The military branch in which a graduate will serve is determined when he or she enters the School of Medicine and reflects both the student's preference and the needs of the organization.

Admissions

REQUIREMENTS: Applicants must be citizens of the United States; be at least 18 years old at the time of matriculation (but no older than 30 as of June 30) in the year of admission; meet military regulations related to physical health; possess a B.A. degree by June 15 in the year of admissions; and fulfill academic prerequisites. These are one year each of Biology, Physics, General Chemistry, and Organic Chemistry with lab. One year of English Composition and/or Literature and one semester of Calculus are required. The MCAT is required, and scores must be from within three years of desired matriculation. For applicants who have retaken the exam, the best set of scores is used.

SUGGESTIONS: A broad undergraduate background, with courses in History, Philosophy, Literature, Economics, Political Science, Foreign Languages, Sociology, and Psychology, is considered valuable. Applicants must be dedicated both to the medical profession and to the idea of serving the country.

PROCESS: About 80 percent of AMCAS applicants are sent secondary applications. Of those returning secondaries, about 15 percent are invited to interview. Interviews take place between October and February and consist of two 30-minute sessions with practicing physicians. About one-third of interviewees are accepted, with notification occurring on a rolling basis. Wait-listed candidates may send supplementary material to enhance their files.

Costs

The cost of attending USUHS is not really an issue because there is no tuition, and a living allowance is provided to all students. All fees, travel expenses, insurance, and costs associated with uniforms are covered. Although Bethesda and Washington, D.C., can be expensive, students are able to live comfortably on the prescribed budget. Students with dependents receive a higher stipend. Students are commissioned officers receiving the pay and allowances of an Ensign in the Navy or Second Lieutenant in the Army and Air Force.

Financial Aid

All medical students are commissioned in the armed services and receive the salary and benefits of a Second Lieutenant in the Army and Air Force, or an Ensign in the Navy. Salary and benefits total $32,000 per year. In turn, students have a seven-year obligation following their residency.

UNIFORMED SERVICES UNIVERSITY OF THE HEALTH SCIENCES

STUDENT BODY

Type	Federal
*Enrollment	670
*% male/female	74/26
*% underrepresented minorities	10
# applied (total/out)	2,452/NR
% interviewed (total/out)	20/NR
% accepted (total/out)	11/NR
% enrolled (total/out)	60/NR
Average age	24

ADMISSIONS

Average GPA and MCAT Scores

Overall GPA	3.53	Science GPA	3.47
MCAT Bio	10.2	MCAT Phys	10.2
MCAT Verbal	9.8	MCAT Essay	0

Score Release Policy

The Admissions Committee generally reacts unfavorably to withheld scores. An explanation should accompany the application.

Application Information

Regular application	11/1
Regular notification	Rolling
Transfers accepted?	No
Admissions may be deferred?	Yes
AMCAS application accepted?	Yes
Interview required?	Yes
Application fee	$0

COSTS AND AID

Tuition & Fees

Tuition (in/out)	$0/$0
Cost of books	$0
Fees	$0

Financial Aid

% students receiving aid	100
Average grant	NR
Average loan	NR
Average debt	NR

*Figures based on total enrollment

UNIVERSITY OF UTAH

SCHOOL OF MEDICINE

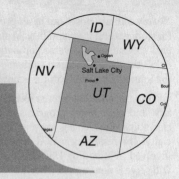

50 North Medical Drive, Salt Lake City, UT 84132
Admission: 801-581-7498 • Fax: 801-585-3300
Email: deans.admissions@hsc.utah.edu
Internet: medstat.med.utah.edu/som

The School of Medicine was founded as a two-year school in 1904 and expanded to a four-year program in 1942. It is one of the 17 colleges of the University of Utah. The medical school is a component of the University of Utah Health Sciences Center, which also includes colleges of pharmacy, nursing, health, and health sciences library; the Howard Hughes Medical Institute, the Eccles Program in Human Molecular Biology and Genetics, the Utah Genome Center, the Utah Cancer Center, the Huntsman Cancer Institute, and several other centers for special studies; the Moran Eye Center; and the University of Utah Hospitals and Clinics.

Academics

The University of Utah School of Medicine implemented a new curriculum during the 1997–1998 academic year that emphasizes active learning approaches, critical thinking skills, and information management techniques. The new curriculum builds upon the strengths of the traditional one and, in addition, explores areas of study opened up by the explosion of biomedical knowledge and the transformation of America's health care delivery system. The goal of the curriculum is to produce highly skilled physicians who are technically proficient, caring and compassionate, and flexible enough to adapt to the changing demands they will face in the 21st century medical environment.

In the first two years of medical school, students will receive a solid foundation in the sciences basic to medicine, including Gross Anatomy, Embryology, Histology, Psychiatry, Biochemistry, Pharmacology, Immunology, Microbiology, Genetics, Physiology, Pathology, and Organ System Pathophysiology. Courses cover such topics as Health Care Financing and Delivery, Community and Public Health, Research Methodology and Medical Literature Analysis, Biostatistics, and Epidemiology. The critical skills of communicating with, examining, and diagnosing patients are also covered in depth.

The third year of the curriculum centers on clinical clerkships in Internal Medicine, Surgery, Obstetrics and Gynecology, Pediatrics, Family Practice, Psychiatry, and Neurology.

During the fourth year a preceptorship in Primary Care Medicine gives students a broader perspective on the health care issues facing medically underserved rural and urban areas; students generally live in the underserved area during the six-week preceptorship. Ample elective time is available for students to pursue areas of particular interest. Finally, a required sub-internship will serve as a transition to residency. Students, with the help of faculty advisors, will apply to various post-graduate residency-training programs through the National Resident Matching Program.

Students

Almost all students are from Utah or neighboring states. About 9 percent of entering students are typically from underrepresented ethnic groups. The age range of entering students is typically from 19 to 40. A significant number of medical students at Utah are married by the fourth year. Class size is 100.

STUDENT LIFE: Medical students take advantage of the campus and the surrounding areas. The University of Utah is situated on a 1,500-acre campus that offers indoor and outdoor recreational activities. Salt Lake City is at the base of spectacular mountains and is only short drive from excellent skiing or hiking, depending on the season. Several national parks are accessible to the city. The city is relatively safe and student-friendly, with cultural activities as well as the basic amenities, such as malls, movie theaters, and restaurants. On-campus housing is available for married couples and single parents in the University Village, for all students in the Medical Plaza Towers (apartments and townhouses), and for single students in University Residence Halls. There are organizations that unite medical students around common interests or that promote interaction with students from medical schools in neighboring states.

GRADUATES: Graduates are usually successful at obtaining their first choice of residencies. Typically, more than half of graduates enter primary care fields.

Admissions

REQUIREMENTS: The MCAT is required and must be taken within three years of application. The Admissions Committee is eager to admit students with a broad perspective of life. The school believes that a true physician is not only skilled in medicine and the allied sciences, but also is a person of culture and broad intelligence. In addition to a bachelor's degree, the applicant must have subject matter competence in the following course work: 2 years of chemistry, the general chemistry series including quantitative and qualitative analysis (AP credit accepted if at a level 4 or 5), and the organic series (AP credit not accepted), both with a laboratory; 1 year of physics with a laboratory (AP credit not accepted); 1 year of English writing/speech courses that must fulfill the institution writing/composition classification (AP credit not accepted); 2 college courses of biology, one in cellular biology or biochemistry (no substitutions, AP credit not accepted); a college course in social science (AP credit not accepted); and a college course in humanities (AP credit not accepted). With the exception of Advanced Placement credit for General Chemistry at a level of 4 or 5, CLEP, Advanced Placement, and home study credit will not be accepted for completion of required course work. All premedical courses must be completed at an accredited college or university in the United States or Canada. Completion of four years of college work and a bachelor's degree are required before entering the School of Medicine. Only those students who have completed most of their undergraduate training in a U.S. or Canadian school will be considered.

SUGGESTIONS: Taking on independent research projects while in college is encouraged. Demonstration of writing skills and computer literacy is also important. Applicants should have participated in both health-related and volunteer work. For applicants who graduated college several years ago, some recent course work is required.

PROCESS: Many Utah residents are asked to submit secondary applications, and 50 percent of those who submit them are invited to interview. Approximately one-third of Utah interviewees are accepted. About one-third of out-of-state applicants are sent secondary applications, and of those who submit them, 30 percent are invited to interview. Fifteen percent of out-of-state interviewees are accepted. Interviews take place from September through February and consist of two one-hour sessions with members of the faculty or administration, or with students. Candidates are notified on a rolling basis after they interview. A ranked wait list is created.

Costs

The estimated yearly cost of living for a single student is about $10,000. This budget assumes on-campus or shared, off-campus living and car ownership.

FINANCIAL AID: In addition to the Federal Subsidized and Unsubsidized Stafford Loans and Federal Perkins Loan, a limited number of institutional loans and scholarships are awarded each year. All awards are based on the student's need as determined by the University's Financial Aid Office. However, it must be remembered that financial aid is supplementary to the contribution that can be made by the student and/or family. The student and family are expected to provide the maximum assistance possible.

VANDERBILT UNIVERSITY
SCHOOL OF MEDICINE

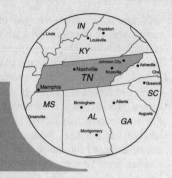

Office of Admissions, 209 Light Hall, Nashville, TN 37232

Admission: 615-322-2145 • Fax: 615-343-8397

Email: medsch.admis@mcmail.vanderbilt.edu

Internet: www.mc.vanderbilt.edu/medschool

Vanderbilt University Medical Center (VUMC) is comprised of the Schools of Medicine and Nursing, the Vanderbilt Clinic, the University Hospital, and the Children's Hospital. VUMC is an important health care provider for both the state and region, with at least one-quarter of the patient population coming from states other than Tennessee. Vanderbilt is among the nation's top-ranked medical schools, with a strong reputation for research, teaching, and clinical care. As a result, Vanderbilt attracts outstanding faculty and students from virtually all states. The School of Medicine is an integral part of Vanderbilt University, situated on a large, park-like campus less than two miles from downtown Nashville.

Academics

Most students complete a four-year curriculum leading to an M.D. degree. Some students opt to take an additional year for research or independent projects. A few students each year enter a combined M.D./Ph.D. program, leading to the doctorate degree in Cell Biology, Biochemistry, Biomedical Engineering, Microbiology and Immunology, Molecular Biology, Pathology, Pharmacology, or Molecular Physiology and Biophysics. Many joint-degree candidates are sponsored and supported by the Medical Scientist Training Program. Medical students are evaluated with letter grades of A, B, C, and F, with the exception of first- and second-year electives, which are Pass/Fail.

BASIC SCIENCES: During the first year, students focus on the basic sciences, which are taught primarily through lectures and labs. Courses are Biochemistry, Gross Anatomy, Microbiology, Cell and Tissue Biology, Introduction to Biomedical Research, Physiology, and Behavioral Science. Several afternoons each week are reserved for electives, many of which are problem-based. During the second year, introductory clinical training is integrated into basic science instruction, and small-group discussions complement the lecture/lab format. Second-year courses are Pathology, Neurobiology, Laboratory Diagnosis, Radiology, Pharmacology, Preventive Medicine, Psychiatry, and Physical Diagnosis. During the first two years, students are in class or other scheduled sessions for about 34 hours per week. Most instruction takes place in Light Hall, which is connected by tunnels to clinical and research facilities. For research and study purposes, students and faculty use the Eskind Biomedical Library, which houses more than 200,000 volumes and 2,000 periodicals, in addition to computer-based informational resources. The Vanderbilt University Computer Center provides a full range of computing services and resources to faculty, staff, and students.

CLINICAL TRAINING: Required third-year clerkships are Medicine (10 weeks); Surgery (10 weeks); Pediatrics (8 weeks); Psychiatry-Neurology (8 weeks); and Ob/Gyn (8 weeks). During their fourth year, students must also complete advanced clerkships selected from medical, surgical, primary care, and emergency medicine fields. Sixteen weeks of electives are also required. Most clinical training takes place at the Vanderbilt University Hospital (660 beds), at other VUMC institutions, and at clinical affiliates such as Veterans Administration Medical Center (439 beds); Howard Hughes Medical Institute; Saint Thomas Hospital; Baptist Hospital; and Middle Tennessee Mental Health Institute. With permission, some elective requirements may be fulfilled at other academic or clinical institutions.

Students

The 1999 entering class came from 29 states and six foreign countries. Fifty-two undergraduate institutions were represented. The age range was 20–30, 6 percent of students were underrepresented minorities, and 42 percent were females.

STUDENT LIFE: Vanderbilt's attractive campus provides a focal point for student life and promotes cohesiveness within the student body. Students interact in common areas, such as dining halls, cafes, study areas, and the student center. Athletic facilities include fitness centers, indoor and outdoor tracks, a tennis center, playing fields, a swimming pool, basketball, racquetball and squash courts, and a rock-climbing wall. Medical students join other graduate and professional students for intramural sports, fitness classes, and recreational clubs. In addition to being a world-renowned hub for live music, Nashville offers many attractions including a historic riverfront district, many restaurants, brew pubs, coffeehouses, nightclubs, bookstores, seasonal street fairs, farmers markets, museums, and a large performing arts center.

Nashville is also an academic center and is home to more than a dozen colleges and universities. Conveniently located, University-owned apartments are available to single and married students and to students with larger families. In addition, off-campus housing is readily available.

GRADUATES: Students perform exceptionally well on the USMLE, contributing to their success in securing residency positions at prestigious institutions nationwide.

Admissions

REQUIREMENTS: Prerequisites are 8 semester hours each of Biology, Chemistry, Organic Chemistry, and Physics. Six semester hours of English are also required. The MCAT is required, and scores should be from within the past five years. For applicants who have taken the exam on multiple occasions, the most recent set of scores is weighed most heavily. Thus, there is no real advantage in withholding scores.

SUGGESTIONS: Students with strong backgrounds in both the sciences and liberal arts are sought. The spring, rather than fall, MCAT is advised. Extracurricular activities, particularly those that involve hospital and medical exposure, are important.

PROCESS: About 22 percent of AMCAS applicants are sent secondary applications and are interviewed. Interviews are conducted between September and March and consist of one session with a faculty member or administrator. On interview day, applicants also take part in a group orientation session, lunch with students, and a tour of the campus. About 30 percent of interviewees are accepted with notification occurring on a rolling basis. Wait-listed candidates may send supplementary information to update their files.

Costs

Tuition for the 1999–2000 academic year is $25,200. The estimated yearly cost of living for a single student is about $12,000. This budget allows for either on- or off-campus housing and car maintenance.

FINANCIAL AID: Most aid is granted on the basis of need, as determined by the FAFSA and institutional forms. Each year, a few scholarships are granted on the basis of academic merit or other special qualifications.

VANDERBILT UNIVERSITY

STUDENT BODY

Type	Private
*Enrollment	427
*% male/female	61/39
*% underrepresented minorities	5
# applied (total/out)	4,424/4,151
% interviewed (total/out)	19/95
% accepted (total/out)	7/95
% enrolled (total/out)	31/90
Average age	23

ADMISSIONS

Average GPA and MCAT Scores

Overall GPA	3.73	Science GPA	3.72
MCAT Bio	11.5	MCAT Phys	11.5
MCAT Verbal	10.5	MCAT Essay	Q

Score Release Policy

We inform applicants that we have no MCAT scores from which to screen. At this point many then release their scores.

Application Information

Regular application	10/15
Regular notification	10/15 until filled
Early application	6/1–8/1
Early notification	10/1
Transfers accepted?	Yes
Admissions may be deferred?	Yes
AMCAS application accepted?	Yes
Interview required?	Yes
Application fee	$50

COSTS AND AID

Tuition & Fees

Tuition	$25,200
Cost of books	$500
Fees	$1,360

Financial Aid

% students receiving aid	75
Average grant	$16,255
Average loan	$23,474
Average debt	$87,308

*Figures based on total enrollment

University of Vermont

COLLEGE OF MEDICINE

C-225 Given Building, Burlington, VT 05405

Admission: 802-656-2154

Internet: www.med.uvm.edu

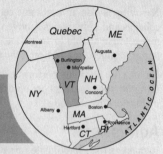

The University of Vermont (UVM) trains skilled and caring primary care physicians and specialists in a variety of fields. The curriculum is unique among medical schools, introducing clinical rotations during year two. In addition to basic sciences and clinical instruction, community service is emphasized. Although UVM is a state university, almost half of the students are out-of-state residents. The Medical School, along with the rest of the University, is situated in picturesque Burlington. The city is safe, affordable, and comfortable.

Academics

The four years are organized into three academic periods. Basic sciences cover 57 weeks and are completed half way through year two. Required clerkships occupy the second academic period, which follows the period of basic-science instruction and lasts one year. The final year and a half, the third academic period, is composed of rotations chosen from broadly specified fields in addition to general electives. Joint M.D./Ph.D. programs can be arranged with the appropriate graduate departments in the following fields: Anatomy, Biochemistry, Biophysics, Cell Biology, Genetics, Microbiology, Molecular Biology, Neuroscience, Pathology, Pharmacology, Physiology, and some nonscience disciplines. A revised curriculum, implemented by fall 2002, will fully integrate basic science instruction and clinical sciences. It will weave genetics, epidemiology, ethics, and information technology throughout the course of study, and provide a system of frequent assessment and competency review.

BASIC SCIENCES: The core sciences are taught primarily through lectures, and learning is enhanced through labs. Basic sciences are Biochemistry, Anatomy, Neuroscience, Physiology, Microbiology, Pathology, Pharmacology, and Psychopathology. Basic-science courses are complemented by the Generalist Curriculum, which consists of three courses. Doctoring in Vermont places each student in the office of a local primary care physician for four hours every other week. In addition, as part of this course, all medical students in a class take on a community service project together. The Physician and Society is a course that addresses relevant social/public health issues. Doctoring Skills introduces students to clinical techniques. During the first year and a half, students spend about 25 hours per week in a structured learning environment. Evaluations use an Honors/Pass/Fail system. Medical Students use Dana Medical Library to study in and to conduct research.

Computer technology is widely used by the Medical School, and computers are accessible to students. Students use a Web-based, UVM-designed computer assisted teaching system to aid their learning of Pathology, Anatomy, and Neurobiology. UVM is known for the health information systems that it has developed, such as the Vermont Oxford Neonatal Network Database, which is in operation nationwide.

CLINICAL TRAINING: Patient contact begins in year one, with the Generalist Curriculum. In January of year two, the following required clerkships begin: Medicine (12 weeks); Surgery (8 weeks); Pediatrics (8 weeks); Psychiatry (8 weeks); Ob/Gyn (8 weeks); and Family Practice (4 weeks). Clinical training takes place primarily at Fletcher Allen Health Care, a conglomerate formed in 1995 of the former Fanny Allen Hospital, the Medical Center Hospital of Vermont, and the University Health Center, a specialty service provider. Fletcher Allen serves the State of Vermont and beyond, attracting patients from New York and around New England. The merging of these institutions improved economic efficiency and suggests financial stability for the future. The patient population is largely rural, and rural medicine is considered a strength of UVM. Health Centers in Maine and New York are also used for clinical rotations, as are the offices of local generalist physicians. For two of their final 15 months, medical students are fully responsible for patients when serving as Acting Interns. Taking on this role is one of the few requirements of the "elective" portion of UVM's medical education. Another requirement is that students complete basic-science course work with one month each of Genetics and Epidemiology. For the most part, there is tremendous flexibility in how students may earn elective credit. Many rotate to hospitals outside of the state, some work on Indian reservations, and others head overseas. Evaluation of clinical skills uses a Honors/Pass/Fail scale, augmented with written narratives. The USMLE Step 2 is not required for graduation.

Students

Approximately one-half of medical students are Vermont residents. The vast majority of students took time off between college and medical school, and usually over one-third of entering students are older than 25. Almost half of matriculates majored in disciplines other than sciences. Class size is 93.

STUDENT LIFE: Students have access to all of the University's athletic facilities. In addition, Burlington and the surrounding area offers excellent skiing, hiking, and mountain biking. The campus is integrated into the city, which is safe, friendly, and student-oriented. Housing options on- and off-campus are good. On-campus choices include UVM's married-student housing, about four miles from campus, and nearby apartments and residence halls. Group houses or shared apartments in walking or biking distance from school are popular off-campus choices. Student organizations are numerous and include Cyberdocs, a medical computer interest group, and Mundus, a club that promotes multicultural awareness through social activities.

GRADUATES: Graduates are successful in obtaining residencies at strong programs nationwide. In 1997, more than half of the graduates entered primary care residencies. Over the past fifteen years, favored specialties were Internal Medicine (28%); Family Practice (14%); Pediatrics (12%); Surgery (18%); Ob/Gyn (7%); Transitional (7%); and Psychiatry (3%).

Admissions

REQUIREMENTS: One year each of Biology, Chemistry, Organic Chemistry, and Physics, all with associated labs are required. Students who have taken time off after college must present some recent course work. The MCAT is required, and all sets of scores are considered.

SUGGESTIONS: Balance in undergraduate course work is suggested. Applicants should have strong writing skills, as well as the ability to communicate orally. Applicants are expected to have experience in a health care setting, or in some alternate environment that demands interpersonal skills and demonstrates a commitment to community service. The MCAT should be taken in April to facilitate timely review of the entire application file.

PROCESS: All AMCAS applicants receive a secondary application. All well-qualified residents who apply are interviewed. On the other hand, less than 10 percent of out-of-state applicants are interviewed. Interviews take place from September through March, and consist of an hour-long session with a faculty member and third- or fourth-year medical student, if possible. Of Vermont residents interviewed, about half are offered places in the class. For out-of-state interviewees, less than 10 percent are admitted. However, owing to the small absolute number of in-state applicants, Vermonters make up just under one-half of a typical class. Decisions are made on a rolling basis, and applicants are notified of their status—accept, reject, or wait list—shortly after the interview. Wait-listed candidates should indicate if UVM is their first choice.

Costs

Yearly cost of living is estimated at $16,000, which includes all fees and expenses other than tuition. This presumes car ownership and either on- or off-campus housing.

FINANCIAL AID: Applicants and their parents must submit documentation of financial resources. All aid is based upon financial need.

UNIVERSITY OF VERMONT

STUDENT BODY

Type	Public
*Enrollment	380
*% male/female	50/50
*% underrepresented minorities	2
# applied (total/out)	6,262/6,157
% interviewed (total/out)	8/6
% accepted (total/out)	2/1
% enrolled (total/out)	67/60
Average age	25

ADMISSIONS

Average GPA and MCAT Scores

Overall GPA	3.28	Science GPA	3.23
MCAT Bio	10.0	MCAT Phys	9.0
MCAT Verbal	10.0	MCAT Essay	NR

Score Release Policy

The school has not responded to our inquiry regarding withheld MCAT scores. Therefore, we advise caution. Contact the Admissions Office before withholding any scores.

Application Information

Regular application	11/15
Regular notification	12/4 until filled
Early application	6/1–8/1
Early notification	10/1
Transfers accepted?	Yes
Admissions may be deferred?	Yes
AMCAS application accepted?	Yes
Interview required?	Yes
Application fee	$85

COSTS AND AID

Tuition & Fees

Tuition (in/out)	$18,150/$31,770
Cost of books	$800
Fees	$681

Financial Aid

% students receiving aid	87
Average grant	$9,000
Average loan	$31,000
Average debt	$110,000

*Figures based on total enrollment

VIRGINIA COMMONWEALTH UNIVERSITY

SCHOOL OF MEDICINE

PO Box 980565, Richmond, VA 23298
Admission: 804-828-9629 • Fax: 804-828-1246
Email: mack@som1.som.vcu.edu • Internet: views.vcu.edu/html/mcuhome.cgi

The School of Medicine is part of Virginia Commonwealth University, a comprehensive state university located in the historic city of Richmond. The MCV campus is in downtown Richmond; other parts of the university are two miles away in Richmond's Fan District. The Medical School curriculum is geared towards training physicians who are capable of meeting today's complex health care needs. As part of a statewide generalist physician initiative, the School of Medicine is dedicated to training primary care physicians. In support of this goal, a Foundations of Clinical Medicine course is taught during the first two years, and an off-campus, family-practice clerkship is required during the clinical training year.

Academics

The M.D. Degree program is four years in length. A combined M.D./Ph.D. program is also offered and generally takes seven years to complete. Medical students interested in public health can earn an M.P.H. concurrently with the M.D. degree. A fellowship program gives medical students the opportunity to participate in research projects, either during summers or throughout the school year. Medical students are graded with Honors, High Pass, Pass, Marginal, and Fail.

BASIC SCIENCES: Although the emphasis is on the basic sciences, behavioral science, preventive medicine, epidemiology, and public health are also taught during the first two years. Laboratory and classroom time is supplemented by a longitudinal experience designed to give students early clinical exposure. First-year courses are the following: Cell Biology; Biochemistry; Anatomical Sciences; Physiology; Behavioral Sciences; Human Genetics; Population Medicine/Biostatistics; Neuroscience; Pathogenesis; Immunology; Ethics; and Foundations of Clinical Medicine, which meets two half-days per week, uses community physicians as mentors, and teaches the basics of patient interviewing and physical diagnosis. The second-year curriculum is organized largely by body/organ systems. Courses are the following: Autonomic Pharmacology; Microbiology/Infectious Diseases; Preventive Medicine; Hematology/Oncology; Central Nervous System; Gastroenterology; Behavioral Science; Respiratory; Cardiovascular; Musculoskeletal/Dermatology; Renal; Endocrine; Reproduction; and continuation of Foundations of Clinical Medicine. Two libraries, the University Library and the Tompkins-McCaw Library, support the research needs of students and faculty. Another important educational resource is the computer-based instructional laboratory, which features computer workstations and audiovisual equipment.

CLINICAL TRAINING: Third-year required clerkships are the following: Medicine (12 weeks); Surgery (8 weeks); Psychiatry (6 weeks); Ob/Gyn (6 weeks); Pediatrics (8 weeks); Family Practice (4 weeks); and Neurology (4 weeks). An additional requirement is one week of a workshop that covers topics such as nutrition, ethics, legal medicine, health economics, and clinical pharmacology. Fourth-year requirements are an acting internship, a board review course, a clinical update course, and 24 weeks of electives. For training purposes, medical students have access to over 1,050 beds at MCV hospitals. A Level I trauma center, a transplant center, and one of the nation's most prominent head injury centers are among MCV's clinical facilities. Students also have contact with outpatients at McGuire Veterans Administration Medical Center.

Students

Approximately 70 percent of students are Virginia residents. The average age of incoming students is usually 23, and each year about 30 students in their late twenties and thirties enter MCV. Underrepresented minorities account for about 10 percent of the student body. Class size is 172.

STUDENT LIFE: MCV has at least 20 student organizations. These include groups focused on professional pursuits, community service, and religious interests. A variety of facilities, services, and programs designed to meet the leisure and health needs of students are coordinated by the recreational sports staff. The Cary Street Recreation complex and the main MCV gym offer fitness facilities including a pool, weight rooms, areas for fitness classes and squash, tennis, and basketball courts. Students have the opportunity to interact outside of class in the new student lounge and in other common areas. Richmond offers many recreational attractions such as parks, museums, historical centers, and shopping areas. While some medical students live in campus residence halls, most live in nearby restored neighborhoods or in surrounding suburban areas.

GRADUATES: MCV students score above the national average on the USMLE, contributing to their success in obtaining post-graduate positions. About 25 percent of each graduating class enters residency programs administered by MCV, while others are successful at securing positions in other parts of the state and country. MCV alumni sponsor a unique "bed-and-breakfast" program, whereby members of the alumni host medical students when they travel for residency interviews.

Admissions

REQUIREMENTS: Prerequisites are eight semester hours each of Biology, Chemistry, Organic Chemistry, and Physics all with associated labs. Two semesters of English and two semesters of college-level Math are also required. The MCAT is required and must have been taken in 1996, 1997, or 1998. For applicants who have taken the exam more than once, the best set of scores is considered.

SUGGESTIONS: Students are encouraged to pursue their own intellectual interests in college. MCV recognizes that studying medicine requires commitment, strong analytical abilities, good judgment, and sound communication skills. In addition to academic abilities, the Admissions Committee looks for important attributes of character and personality.

PROCESS: About 75 percent of AMCAS applicants who are Virginia residents are sent secondary applications, and about 40 percent of nonresidents are sent secondaries. Applicants returning secondary applications are further screened, and some are invited to interview on campus. Interviews take place between August and March, and consist of one session with a faculty member, medical student, or administrator. On interview day, students also attend group informational sessions, have lunch with current medical students, and tour the campus. Notification occurs on October 15, in mid-December, and in mid-March.

Costs

In addition to tuition, the estimated yearly cost of living is about $16,000. This budget is for a single student. It allows for either on- or off-campus housing and car maintenance.

FINANCIAL AID: Financial assistance is available to eligible medical students with financial need, as determined by federal and institutional forms. Aid is in the form of loans, grants, scholarships, and employment. The Virginia Primary Care Medicine Scholarship pays $10,000 per year to students in exchange for each year of service in a state health department or underserved area after graduation and post-graduate training. Some scholarships are offered on the basis of academic merit or other special criteria.

VIRGINIA COMMONWEALTH UNIVERSITY

STUDENT BODY

Type	Public
*Enrollment	675
*% male/female	60/40
*% underrepresented minorities	10
# applied (total/out)	4,586/3,615
% interviewed (total/out)	14/9
% accepted (total/out)	8/3
% enrolled (total/out)	48/39
Average age	23

ADMISSIONS

Average GPA and MCAT Scores

Overall GPA	3.48	Science GPA	NR
MCAT Bio	9.90	MCAT Phys	9.80
MCAT Verbal	9.50	MCAT Essay	NR

Score Release Policy
The School has not responded to our inquiry regarding withheld MCAT scores. Therefore, we advise caution. Contact the Admissions Office before witholding any scores.

Application Information

Regular application	11/15
Regular notification	10/15 until filled
Early application	6/1–8/1
Early notification	10/1
Transfers accepted?	Yes
Admissions may be deferred?	Yes
AMCAS application accepted?	Yes
Interview required?	Yes
Application fee	$75

COSTS AND AID

Tuition & Fees

Tuition (in/out)	$10,085/$25,932
Cost of books	$3,370
Fees	$1,159

Financial Aid

% students receiving aid	91
Average grant	$4,500
Average loan	$26,000
Average debt	$74,600

*Figures based on total enrollment

UNIVERSITY OF VIRGINIA
SCHOOL OF MEDICINE

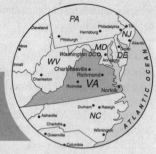

Medical School Admissions Office, Box 235, Charlottesville, VA 22908

Admission: 804-924-5571 • Fax: 804-982-2586

Internet: www.med.virginia.edu/home.html

The University of Virginia (UVA) School of Medicine is among the top-ranked medical schools. UVA enjoys a national reputation for both research and clinical care. In response to recent health care trends, UVA offers enhanced opportunities for students interested in pursuing careers in primary care but is still committed to the education of physician scientists and academic physicians. Fundamental to UVA's approach to learning are the notions that problem solving is more important than retention of isolated facts and that learning is facilitated by the presence of the patient. Thus, patient-contact is incorporated into the first- and second-year curriculum.

Academics

Most medical students follow a four-year, highly integrated curriculum leading to the M.D. Each year six students enter a combined M.D./Ph.D. curriculum. Training for the Ph.D. degree is usually in one of the Biomedical Science programs, which include Anatomy, Biochemistry, Microbiology, Pharmacology, Physiology, Biophysics, and Neuroscience. A Generalist Scholars Program supplements the medical education of students with special opportunities in the area of primary care. Students who participate in this program work closely with a faculty mentor and complete a thesis as part of their graduation requirements. Medical students are evaluated in a variety of ways including both Pass/Fail and letter grades.

BASIC SCIENCES: First-year courses are Biochemistry; Cell and Tissue Structure; Gross Anatomy; Physiology; Human Behavior; Neuroscience; Genetics; Physical Diagnosis; Medical Ethics; and The Practice of Medicine, in which topics such as human behavior and medical ethics are discussed. Basic clinical skills such as the patient interview are also introduced. Second-year courses are Microbiology; Pathology; Pharmacology; Psychiatric Medicine; Psychopathology; Clinical Epidemiology; Community Preceptorship; and Introduction to Clinical Medicine (ICM). Basic-science concepts are coordinated with the ICM course, which involves discussion of clinical cases in small-group tutorials. In the spring of the second year, each student completes a one-month community medicine preceptorship that provides hands-on primary care experience and serves as a transition to third-year clinical rotations. Instruction takes place at the Harvey E. Jordan Hall, a seven-story structure that houses lecture halls and laboratories. First- and second-year students also use the School of Medicine Learning Center, which contains conference rooms, tutorial rooms, and a student lounge. The Claude Moore Health Sciences Library is a modern, fully computerized facility with almost 79,000 books, 3,000 periodicals, and 4,000 audiovisual titles.

CLINICAL TRAINING: Third-year required rotations are Medicine (12 weeks); Surgery (12 weeks); Psychiatry (6 weeks); Family Medicine (4 weeks); Pediatrics (8 weeks);

and Obstetrics (6 weeks). During the fourth year, a four-week Neurology clerkship is required as are 28 weeks of electives. Clinical training takes place primarily at the University of Virginia Medical Center University Hospital (552 beds); Kluge Children's Rehabilitation Center; and at 40 outpatient clinics associated with the Medical Center. Students also train at affiliated hospitals, which include The Community Hospital of Roanoke Valley (400 beds); Roanoke Memorial Hospital (677 beds); and the Veterans Affairs Medical Center (750 beds). Electives may be taken at other academic or clinical institutions in other parts of the country or abroad.

Students

About 90 of the 139 students in each class are Virginia residents. Underrepresented minorities account for approximately 10 percent of the student body. There is typically a wide age range among incoming students, with at least a few students in their thirties.

STUDENT LIFE: Students are highly active in on-campus activities and events. Many are involved in community activities such as Service, Humanity, Action, Responsibility, Education (SHARE), which initiates health education projects and other service-oriented activities. Support groups for minority students are available, as are clubs focused on professional interests and recreational pursuits, such as singing. UVA also has local chapters of national medical student organizations. Medical students enjoy Charlottesville, a thriving tourist and cultural center located at the foot of the Blue Ridge Mountains and close to the Shenandoah Valley. The city of Richmond, Virginia, is an hours drive, and Washington, D.C. is just two hours away.

GRADUATES: Graduates are successful in securing top residency positions in all regions of the country. A significant number stay on to do post-graduate training at UVA-affiliated hospitals.

Admissions

REQUIREMENTS: Prerequisites are one year each of Biology, General Chemistry, Organic Chemistry, and Physics, all with associated labs. The MCAT is required, and scores must be no more than three years old at the time of matriculation. For applicants who have taken the exam more than once, the best scores are considered. Thus, there is no advantage to withholding scores.

SUGGESTIONS: State residency is a factor in admissions decisions as about 65 percent of positions in a class are reserved for Virginia resident applicants. The Admissions Committee looks for students who will make significant contributions to society as members of the medical profession. Factors such as depth of motivation and commitment to medicine are evaluated. Some medically related experience that involves patient contact is considered important.

PROCESS: AMCAS applicants are sent secondary applications. About 25–30 percent of Virginia resident applicants are interviewed, while only about 8 percent of nonresidents make it to the interview stage. On interview day, applicants have two interviews, each with a member of the Admissions Committee. Candidates also attend a group orientation session and have the opportunity to tour the campus and eat lunch with current medical students. Notification begins after October 15, and continues on a rolling basis until the class is filled. Wait-listed candidates may send additional information to update their files.

Costs

The estimated yearly budget for a single student is about $12,000–$15,000. This does not include tuition but covers all other expenses.

FINANCIAL AID: Financial aid comes from several sources including school-administered scholarships and loans, federal loans, supplemental loans and Virginia Medical Scholarships, which are generally awarded in exchange for a commitment to service in an underserved part of the state. Most assistance is awarded on the basis of financial need, as determined by the FAFSA and other forms.

UNIVERSITY OF VIRGINIA

STUDENT BODY

Type	Public
*Enrollment	550
*% male/female	58/42
*% underrepresented minorities	10
# applied (total/out)	4,151/3,355
% interviewed (total/out)	12/8.5
% accepted (total/out)	8.2/5.7
% enrolled (total/out)	41/24

ADMISSIONS

Average GPA and MCAT Scores

Overall GPA	3.67	Science GPA	NR
MCAT Bio	11.11	MCAT Phys	10.86
MCAT Verbal	10.22	MCAT Essay	Q

Score Release Policy

The Admissions Committee says that the decision to withhold scores is entirely up to the student. They will assume only that the student was not happy with the score.

Application Information

Regular application	11/1
Regular notification	10/15 until filled
Transfers accepted?	Yes
Admissions may be deferred?	Yes
AMCAS application accepted?	Yes
Interview required?	Yes
Application fee	$60

COSTS AND AID

Tuition & Fees

Tuition (in/out)	$12,466/$25,146
Cost of books	$950 (4-yr. avg.)
Fees	$1,220

Financial Aid

% students receiving aid	85
Average grant	$9,728
Average loan	$17,108
Average debt	$60,330

*Figures based on total enrollment

WAKE FOREST UNIVERSITY

SCHOOL OF MEDICINE

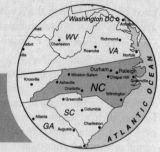

Medical Center Boulevard, Winston-Salem, NC 27157

Admission: 336-716-4264 • Fax: 336-716-5807

Email: medadmit@wfubmc.edu • Internet: www.wfubmc.edu

Wake Forest has three primary missions—education, clinical service, and research. The School continuously re-evaluates its curriculum to keep pace with the demands of the medical profession, the needs of its patient population, and the national trends in health care. Wake Forest is a private institution with a national reputation that attracts students from all over the country. However, it is active within the local community and is geared to respond to health care priorities of the state. The school is located in a residential area of Winston-Salem, a historic city of 165,000.

Academics

A new curriculum which combines features of traditional and problem-based learning methodologies was implemented in 1998. For details about the new curriculum, contact the admissions office. Joint-degree programs include the M.D./M.B.A. in conjunction with The Babcock Graduate School of Management, the M.D./M.S. (Epidemiology); and the M.D./Ph.D. The Ph.D. degree is offered in the following fields: Anatomy, Biochemistry, Genetics, Immunology, Microbiology, Molecular Biology, Neuroscience, Pathology, Pharmacology, and Physiology. Students are evaluated using a 0–4 scale, and both steps of the USMLE are required for graduation.

BASIC SCIENCES: The pre-clinical curriculum emphasizes self-directed and lifelong learning skills, core biomedical science knowledge, problem-solving/reasoning, interviewing and communication skills, information management, and professional attitudes and behavior. The course Foundations of Clinical Medicine is taken throughout years one and two, and correlates clinical experiences with basic-science instruction. Science courses are organized around body/organ systems. The course Medicine as Profession is an interdisciplinary course that touches on a range of issues related to the practice of medicine. Most pre-clinical instruction takes place in the Hanes Research Building. The James A. Gray Building houses the library, which contains more than 120,000 volumes and 3,800 medical and scientific journals, in addition to audiovisual and computer-based educational aids.

CLINICAL TRAINING: Third-year required rotations are: Medicine (8 weeks); Surgery (8 weeks); Ob/Gyn (4 weeks); Pediatrics (4 weeks); Neurology (3 weeks); Psychiatry (3 weeks); Anesthesiology (1 week); Radiology (1 week); and Family Medicine (3 weeks). During the fourth year, students fulfill the remaining requirements, which are Community Medicine (4 weeks); Emergency Medicine (4 weeks); Critical Care (4 weeks); 12 weeks of required Advanced Patient Management Clerkships; and Electives (16 weeks). Training takes place at the North Carolina Baptist Hospital (806 beds), which includes a Children's Hospital and a rehabilitation unit, among other specialty facilities. Other sites used for instruction, located in both rural and urban areas, are Forsyth Memorial Hospital; Reynolds Health Center; Moses Cone Hospital; Forsyth County Health Clinic; Umstead Hospital; Catawba Memorial Hospital; Rowan Memorial Hospital; and Watuaga County Hospital.

Students

Approximately 60 percent of each class is made up of North Carolina residents, and about 10 percent are from Wake Forest's undergraduate program. The remainder represent up to 100 different colleges. About 10 percent of students are underrepresented minorities, most of whom are African American. Class size is 108.

STUDENT LIFE: A Student Life and Fitness Center gives students the opportunity to work out, study, gather, or simply relax. The fitness center includes nautilis equipment, free weights, showers and a sauna. Other features are a quiet, 24-hour study area, vending machines, a TV lounge, and rooms suitable for small-group discussions. The School of Medicine is located on the Bowman Gray campus, about four miles from the Reynolds campus of Wake Forest, where many academic and cultural events take place. Two state parks are within an hour's drive of Wake Forest, and the Carolina beaches are about four hours away. There is no campus housing, but apartments and rooms are readily available in the surrounding area.

GRADUATES: Wake Forest's reputation, coupled with its students above-average scores on national boards, allows graduates to enter competitive residency programs all over the country.

Admissions

REQUIREMENTS: Requirements are eight semester hours in Biology, Chemistry, Organic Chemistry, and Physics. The MCAT is required and scores must be no more than three years old. For applicants who have retaken the exam, the best set of scores is considered.

SUGGESTIONS: A well-rounded academic experience, including courses in the humanities, is strongly advised. For students who have taken significant time off after college, recent course work is suggested. The April, rather than August, MCAT is recommended, as it allows applicants to retake the exam if necessary. Medically related or community-service experiences are considered valuable. North Carolina residency is a slight advantage in the admissions process.

PROCESS: Approximately half of AMCAS applicants are sent secondary application materials. About 15 percent of those returning secondary applications are invited to interview sometime between October and March. Interviews are one on one, and consist of three 15–20 minute sessions with faculty and/or Admissions Committee members. On interview day, candidates also receive a tour and a group orientation. Notification occurs on a rolling basis, the possible outcomes being accept, reject, or wait list. Wait-listed candidates are generally not encouraged to submit supplementary materials. An alternate path to admissions is through an early assurance program which accepts college juniors who are North Carolina residents without the MCAT. If successful, these students complete their senior year knowing that they have been admitted to medical school for the year following college graduation.

Costs

The annual cost of living for a single student, beyond tuition, is about $15,000. On this budget, students are able to live off campus and own cars.

FINANCIAL AID: Eighty-five percent of students receive financial aid. Assistance is awarded on the basis of need and/or scholastic achievement. Three merit-based awards covering the cost of tuition are offered to incoming North Carolina residents, while other scholarships are available to students who commit to serving in certain parts of the state.

WAKE FOREST UNIVERSITY

STUDENT BODY

Type	Private
*Enrollment	447
*% male/female	59/41
*% underrepresented minorities	11
# applied (total/out)	5,859/5,153
% interviewed (total/out)	9/5
% accepted (total/out)	3/2
% enrolled (total/out)	53/47
Average age	23

ADMISSIONS

Average GPA and MCAT Scores

Overall GPA	3.40	Science GPA	3.40
MCAT Bio	10.0	MCAT Phys	9.9
MCAT Verbal	10.2	MCAT Essay	P

Application Information

Regular application	11/1
Regular notification	10/15 until filled
Early application	6/1–8/1
Early notification	10/1
Transfers accepted?	Yes
Admissions may be deferred?	Yes
AMCAS application accepted?	Yes
Interview required?	Yes
Application fee	$55

COSTS AND AID

Tuition & Fees

Tuition	$27,500
Cost of books	$1,400
Fees	NR

Financial Aid

% students receiving aid	85
Average grant	$5,500
Average loan	$21,800
Average debt	$83,872

*Figures based on total enrollment

WASHINGTON UNIVERSITY

SCHOOL OF MEDICINE

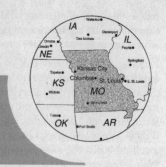

660 South Euclid Avenue, #8107, St. Louis, MO 63110

Admission: 314-362-6857 • Fax: 314-362-4658

Email: wumscoa@msnotes.wustl.edu

Internet: medschool.wustl.edu/admissions

Washington University is a private school with an international reputation that draws outstanding students from across the country and around the world. The School of Medicine offers outstanding basic-science instruction alongside cutting-edge clinical care and research. Graduates enter careers in all areas of medicine, from primary care to basic science research. The School of Medicine is situated in such a way that students are able to learn from a diverse patient population, representing both urban and rural areas. Wash U. is located in the Central West End of St. Louis, a neighborhood filled with coffee houses, bookstores, and students.

Academics

In addition to the four-year M.D. program, students may apply for a five-year combined M.A./M.D. program, which involves a year of funded research and the completion of a thesis. The MSTP-sponsored M.D./Ph.D. program is one of the largest in the country, with up to 23 positions available each year. During the first year, students are graded using a Pass/Fail system, but grades of Honors/High Pass/Pass/Fail are used from the second year onward.

BASIC SCIENCES: During the first two years, students are in class for about 20 hours per week. Scheduled sessions are divided among lectures, labs, and problem-based sessions conducted in small groups. Topics covered in lectures are documented by a transcript service, to which most students subscribe. Most first-year courses address normal human structure and function. They are Anatomy, the Molecular Foundations of Medicine, Cell and Organ Systems Biology, Immunology, Genetics, and Neuroscience. The course Physicians, Patients, and Society offers first-year students a multidisciplinary perspective on practicing medicine, and continues into the second year. Patient contact begins in the first year, in Introduction to Clinical Medicine. Second-year courses focus on the effects of disease and are organized into blocks, most of which are defined by body systems or physiological concepts. These are Cardiovascular; Clinical Epidemiology; Dermatology; Nervous System; ENT; Endocrinology and Metabolism; Gastrointestinal and Liver Disease/Nutrition; Hematology and Oncology; Infectious Disease; Ob/Gyn; Ophthalmology; Pathology; Pediatrics; Nervous System; Pulmonary; Renal and Genitourinary; and Rheumatology. Clinical experience is expanded and integrated into Pathology, Pathophysiology, and Pharmacology. Students have significant input in curriculum development and revision. The library is extensive, housing about 300,000 volumes and equipped with computer and Internet facilities. The gross anatomy lab is particularly renowned.

CLINICAL TRAINING: The third year is reserved for core, required clerkships, which are: Medicine (12 weeks); Surgery (12 weeks); Neurology (4 weeks); Psychiatry (4 weeks); combined Ob/Gyn and Pediatrics (12 weeks); and Ambulatory Care, which involves Emergency Medicine, Family Practice, and Psychiatric Consultation (12 weeks). The fourth year (44 weeks) is reserved entirely for electives, which may be in clinical and/or basic science departments. Students are permitted to fulfill up to 12 weeks of clinical clerkships at nonaffiliated institutions. While many other academic health care institutions are struggling, Washington University's Medical Center and their other Barnes-Jewish associated hospitals and clinics are thriving and expanding. Children's Hospital ranks as one of the premier pediatric hospitals in the country. In total, affiliated hospitals provide over 2,000 patient beds. Students are exposed to a local population in need of basic care and to patients who have come from around the world for the most advanced treatments. The School of Medicine expects students to play important roles in the provision of patient care.

Students

The current student body represents 43 states and 21 foreign countries. Although most are recent college graduates with degrees in one of the hard sciences, there is tremendous diversity in terms of age and undergraduate background. Class size is 120.

STUDENT LIFE: Since most students come from out-of-state (and country), they are eager to get to know each other and tend to form a coherent group quickly. An extensive orientation session at the beginning of the year aids in this process. Student groups are extremely active, and range from those that focus on community service projects, such as operating a free clinic on weekends, to intramural sports clubs, to Hot Docs (a musical group). Well-used, on-campus facilities include the Hilltop Campus Athletic Facility, which is a comprehensive gym and sports center.

Social life often centers on the restaurants and bars of the Central West End and the tree-lined paths of Forest Park. Campus housing is available adjacent to the Medical School, but many students prefer to live in the surrounding areas, where housing is affordable and attractive.

GRADUATES: Graduates gain acceptance to the nation's most competitive residency programs. About half enter a primary care field.

Admissions

REQUIREMENTS: Washington University expects applicants to have completed one year of Biology, General Chemistry, Organic Chemistry, and Physics, in addition to Math through the Calculus level. The MCAT is required, and scores must be no more than three years old.

SUGGESTIONS: The Admissions Committee looks favorably on those who have pursued in-depth study of a particular subject, whether in the natural sciences, social sciences, or humanities. Successful applicants also demonstrate commitment and leadership through their extracurricular activities. Since the Medical School offers rolling admissions beginning October 15, applicants should make every attempt to complete materials early.

PROCESS: About 20 percent of AMCAS applicants are interviewed, with interviews taking place between September and March. Interviews consist of one session with a member of the School's Faculty or Administration. Notification occurs on a rolling basis, and about one-third of interviewees are accepted. Wait-listed candidates are not ranked and are generally not encouraged to send supplementary material.

Costs

For an urban area, St. Louis is relatively inexpensive. Estimated costs for a single student, beyond tuition, amount to less than $10,000 per year.

FINANCIAL AID: Students' and parents' resources are considered when determining institutional financial aid. In addition to need-based loans and grants, Washington University offers 11 merit-based, full-tuition scholarships each year without regard to need.

WASHINGTON UNIVERSITY

STUDENT BODY

Type	Private
*Enrollment	548
*% male/female	51/49
*% underrepresented minorities	9
# applied (total/out)	4,376/4,197
% interviewed (total/out)	17/17
% accepted (total/out)	NR/NR
% enrolled (total/out)	12/12
Average age	24

ADMISSIONS

Average GPA and MCAT Scores

Overall GPA	3.83	Science GPA	3.80
MCAT Bio	12.46	MCAT Phys	12.26
MCAT Verbal	11.30	MCAT Essay	NR

Score Release Policy

The Admissions Committee cautions that withholding scores may be viewed negatively, depending on circumstances.

Application Information

Regular application	12/15
Regular notification	10/15 until filled
Non-fall registration?	Yes
Transfers accepted?	Yes
Admissions may be deferred?	Yes
AMCAS application accepted?	Yes
Interview required?	Yes
Application fee	$50

COSTS AND AID

Tuition & Fees

†Tuition	$32,960
Cost of books	NR
Fees	$0

Financial Aid

% students receiving aid	NR
Average grant	NR
Average loan	NR
Average debt	$79,201

† Tuition is fixed at entry to medical school and does not increase.

*Figures based on total enrollment

UNIVERSITY OF WASHINGTON

SCHOOL OF MEDICINE

Health Sciences Center A-300, Box 356340, Seattle, WA 98195

Admission: 206-543-7212

Email: askuwsom@u.washington.edu

Internet: www.washington.edu/medical/som

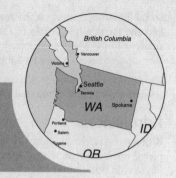

The University of Washington (UW) has 16 major schools and colleges. Within the UW Warren G. Magnson Health Sciences Center is the School of Public Health and Community Medicine, in addition to the Schools of Medicine, Nursing, Pharmacy, and Dentistry. The School of Medicine is known both for its achievements in biomedical research and for its commitment to training primary care physicians. UW ranks among the top 10 medical schools in receipt of federal research funding and is sixth in the nation in the number of graduates practicing in primary care fields.

Academics

Students who enter UW as residents of Wyoming, Alaska, Montana, and Idaho spend their first year at the University site in their home state. Twenty Washington students begin medical studies at Washington State University in Pullman and then transfer to the UW campus after completion of their first year. Other students complete a four-year program based in Seattle. From 8 to 10 students each year enter the M.S.T.P. M.D./Ph.D. program. The doctorate degree may be earned in Biochemistry, Bioengineering, Biomathematics/Biostatistics, Biological Structure, Epidemiology, Environmental Health, Genetics, Immunology, Microbiology, Molecular Biotechnology, Pathology, Pharmacology, Physiology, Biophysics, and Zoology. Medical students are evaluated with Honors, Satisfactory, and Not Satisfactory. Passing Step 1 of the USMLE is a requirement for promotion to year three and passing Step 2 is a requirement for graduation.

Basic Sciences: First-year courses at the UW campus are Microscopic Anatomy; Gross Anatomy and Embryology; Mechanisms in Cell Physiology; Biochemistry; Cell and Tissue Response to Injury; Natural History of Infectious Diseases and Chemotherapy; Introduction to Immunology; Systems of Human Behavior; Epidemiology; Head, Neck, Ear, Nose and Throat; and Nervous System. Most second-year topics are organized around body/organ systems, which are Cardiovascular; Complementary Medicine; Respiratory; Pharmacology; Endocrine; Systemic Pathology; Gastrointestinal; Hematology; Musculoskeletal; Genetics; Urinary; Reproduction; Skin; and Nutrition. Other courses are Introduction to Clinical Medicine and Medicine, Health, and Society. The Rural/Underserved Opportunities Program enables first-year medical students to work with practicing physicians in small towns or inner-city neighborhoods and to learn first-hand about working with underserved communities.

Clinical Training: The clinical curriculum covers the third and fourth years and includes clerkships in Medicine (12 weeks); Ob/Gyn (6 weeks); Pediatrics (6 weeks); Psychiatry (6 weeks); Surgery (6 weeks); Family Medicine (6 weeks); Emergency Medicine (4 weeks); and Rehabilitation (2 weeks). An additional 24 weeks of electives are required. Selected third-year students participate in an alternate, rural training program, which involves six months in a rural, primary care practice. In its teaching, patient care, and research programs, the School of Medicine is affiliated with Children's Hospital, Harborview Hospital (411 beds), UW Medical Center (450 beds), Seattle Veterans Affairs Hospital, Fred Hutchinson Cancer Research Center, Boise Veterans Affairs Hospital, Providence Hospital, Swedish Hospital, Madigan Hospital, and the Group Health Cooperative. Additional affiliations across the Pacific Northwest enable medical students to train in more than 75 communities in Washington, Alaska, Montana, and Idaho. The International Medical Education Office organizes a range of activities including exchange programs that allow UW medical students to participate in clinical electives overseas.

Students

About 93 percent of the 176 students in each class are residents of Washington, Alaska, Montana, Wyoming or Idaho. Out-of-region students, who comprise a total of about 10 percent of the student body, which includes M.D./Ph.D. students. There is a wide age range among medical students, with significant numbers of entrants in their late twenties and thirties.

Student Life: UW offers countless extracurricular opportunities and attractions, including cultural programs, student groups, intercollegiate sporting events, and social functions. Medical students take advantage of these opportunities and the tremendous resources afforded by UW and its student community. Seattle is an ideal city for students, offering outstanding daytime and outdoor activities and an excellent nightlife. Around the city are beautiful areas suitable for hiking, camping, mountain climbing, running, biking, swimming, and skiing. Most students live off campus.

Graduates: Of the roughly 5,000 UW School of Medicine alumni, about 50 percent are practicing or training in fields designated as physician-shortage specialties, which include family physicians, general internists, general pediatricians, psychiatrists, general surgeons, and general practitioners. Among students in the 1996 graduating class, 62 percent entered residency programs in primary care fields, which encompass family medicine, internal medicine, and pediatrics.

Admissions

REQUIREMENTS: Prerequisites are Biology (8 semester hours), Chemistry (12 semester hours, which can be satisfied by any combination of Inorganic, Organic, Biochemistry, or Molecular Biology courses), and Physics (4 semester hours). In addition the understanding of basic biochemistry molecular biology concepts is required. An additional 8 semester hours of unspecified science course work is required. This requirement can be met by taking other courses in any of the above three categories. The MCAT is required, and scores must be from within three years of application.

SUGGESTIONS: Preference is given to legal residents of Washington, Wyoming, Alaska, Montana, and Idaho. Applicants from disadvantaged backgrounds or who are willing to serve the underserved are also considered. Candidates should be proficient in the use of the English language and in basic mathematics and are expected to have an understanding of personal computing and information technologies. Some Biochemistry or Molecular Biology is also recommended.

PROCESS: All Washington residents and a limited number of highly qualified, nonresidents are sent secondary applications and invited to interview. Interviews take place between October and April and consist of one session with a panel of interviewers. Also on interview day, candidates have the opportunity to meet with current students and to tour the campus. About 30 percent of interviewed candidates are accepted. Others are rejected or put in a hold category.

Costs

The estimated yearly budget for a single student is about $15,000. Included in the first-year student budget is the cost of a computer, considered mandatory for medical students.

FINANCIAL AID: All financial aid is based on demonstrated need as determined by the FAFSA form. Full disclosure of parental financial resources is required. In addition to federal sources of funds, partial scholarships are available through the School of Medicine Scholarship Fund.

UNIVERSITY OF WASHINGTON

STUDENT BODY

Type	Public
*Enrollment	734
*% male/female	52/48
*% underrepresented minorities	10
# applied (total/out)	3,188/2,141
% interviewed (total/out)	25/4
% accepted (total/out)	NR/NR
% enrolled (total/out)	23/13

ADMISSIONS

Average GPA and MCAT Scores

Overall GPA	3.59	Science GPA	3.69
MCAT Bio	10.30	MCAT Phys	10.00
MCAT Verbal	10.10	MCAT Essay	P

Application Information

Regular application	11/1
Regular notification	11/1 until filled
Admissions may be deferred?	Yes
AMCAS application accepted?	Yes
Interview required?	Yes
Application fee	$35

COSTS AND AID

Tuition & Fees

Tuition (in/out)	$8,490/$21,404
Cost of books	NR
Fees	NR

Financial Aid

% students receiving aid	83
Average grant	NR
Average loan	NR
Average debt	NR

*Figures based on total enrollment

WAYNE STATE UNIVERSITY
SCHOOL OF MEDICINE

540 East Canfield, Detroit, MI 48201
Admission: 313-577-1466 • Fax: 313-577-1330
Internet: med.wayne.edu/admiss.htm

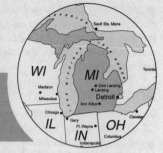

Wayne State is a large, urban university with approximately 33,000 enrolled students and hundreds of undergraduate and graduate degree programs. The School of Medicine is the only medical school in Detroit and is directly affiliated with the Detroit Medical Center. As a result, students are exposed to a diverse patient population and intensive clinical training. Medical students often gain additional clinical and interpersonal experience through volunteer work and community outreach efforts.

Academics

The School of Medicine administers academic programs leading to the M.D., M.S., and Ph.D. Some medical students pursue a combined M.D./Ph.D., leading to the doctorate degree in Anatomy and Cell Biology, Cellular and Clinical Neurobiology, Immunology/Microbiology, Medical Physics, Molecular Biology and Genetics, Pathology, Pharmacology, and Physiology. Other students earn an M.S. in biomedical or behavioral sciences along with the M.D. The standard medical curriculum consists of two years of basic sciences, a year of clinical clerkships, and a year of clinical electives. Evaluation of medical student performance uses Honors, Pass, and Fail. Promotion to year three requires passing Step 1 of the USMLE. In order to graduate, all students must record a score on Step 2 of the USMLE.

BASIC SCIENCES: Basic-science courses are taught primarily in a lecture/lab format, with some use of small-group sessions. Students are in class for about 20 hours per week. This schedule gives students the time they need to study, pursue independent projects, and take part in community service or other extracurricular activities. During year one, students learn about the normal functions of the human body. Courses are Anatomy, Histology, Embryology, Evidence Based Medicine, Physiology, Biochemistry, Genetics, Neuroscience, Clinical Nutrition, Introduction to the Patient, Human Sexuality, and Behavioral Medicine. Second-year courses focus on the effects of disease and the principles of drug action and therapy. The Pathophysiology course is organized by body/organ systems, which are Connective Tissue, Cardiovascular, Hematology, Pulmonary, Renal, Endocrine, Gastrointestinal, and Neuroscience. Other courses are Pathology, Microbiology, Psychiatry, Pharmacology, Public Health and Preventive Medicine, Physical Diagnosis/Interviewing, Introduction to the Patient, Medical Ethics, and Human Sexuality. The majority of first- and second-year classes are conducted in Scott Hall, a modern building that houses laboratories, lecture halls, and faculty offices. The Shiffman Medical Library has more than 150,000 volumes, computer facilities, and ample space for studying. Students can view recorded lectures and take advantage of other audio-visual study aids in the Self-Instruction Center.

CLINICAL TRAINING: During the third year, students complete 8-week, required clerkships in Internal Medicine, Surgery, Pediatrics, and Ob/Gyn. There are also 4-week clerkships in Family Medicine, Neurology, and Psychiatry. During the fourth year, Selectives in Ambulatory Medicine (4 weeks) and Emergency Medicine (4 weeks), in addition to a Subinternship (4 weeks), are required. Five months of electives are also required, a significant portion of which may be taken at other institutions. Clinical training takes place at the Detroit Medical Center (DMC) which is comprised of numerous hospitals, institutes, and care centers and has, in total, over 2,400 beds. DMC includes Harper Hospital; Grace Hospital; Hutzel Hospital; Children's Hospital of Michigan; Rehabilitation Institute of Michigan; Detroit Receiving Hospital/University Health Center; Gershenson Radiation Oncology Center; Kresge Eye Institute; and Huron Valley Hospital. Medical students also rotate to affiliated hospitals in suburban areas.

Students

About 90 percent of the 256 students in each class are Michigan residents. Approximately 12 percent of students are underrepresented minorities, most of whom are African American. Although a few students are older or nontraditional, most entering students are in their early twenties.

STUDENT LIFE: Medical students are involved in chapters of national organizations such as the American Medical Student Association, professionally oriented groups such as the Family Medicine Interest Group, production of a student newspaper, and numerous community service projects. Volunteer activities involve working with the city's youth, elderly, under- and non-insured populations. Medical students also enjoy the extensive extracurricular offerings of Wayne State University, as well as the diverse culture of Detroit. Students live off campus, usually in apartments in the Detroit metropolitan area or in surrounding suburbs. Parking is available on campus, and most students own cars.

GRADUATES: About 65 percent of graduates chose residency programs in Michigan hospitals, with more than 50 percent staying in the Detroit area. In recent years, more than half of graduates entered primary care fields.

Admissions

REQUIREMENTS: One year each of Biology, Chemistry, Organic Chemistry, and Physics, all with associated labs, is required. The MCAT is required, and scores should be from the spring or fall of the year prior to entrance. For applicants who have retaken the exam, the most recent set of scores is weighed most heavily. Thus, there is no advantage in withholding scores.

SUGGESTIONS: Although most positions are reserved for Michigan residents, well-qualified, nonresidents are also considered. In addition to academic credentials, the Admissions Committee is interested in extracurricular activities and work. Health-related volunteer work and research are valuable.

PROCESS: About 50 percent of AMCAS applicants are sent secondary applications. Of those returning secondaries, about 20 percent are interviewed between September and April. The interview consists of one session with a member of the Admissions Committee. Candidates also receive a tour and have the opportunity to meet with current students. About one-third of interviewed candidates are accepted and are notified shortly after the interview. Wait-listed candidates are generally not encouraged to send additional information.

Costs

Beyond tuition, the estimated yearly cost of living for a single student is $14,000. This budget allows for off-campus housing and car maintenance.

FINANCIAL AID: All financial aid recipients must apply for federal loans before being considered for institutional funds. Most aid is awarded on the basis of need, as determined by the student's and his or her family's resources. A limited number of full-tuition merit scholarships are awarded each year.

WAYNE STATE UNIVERSITY

STUDENT BODY

Type	Public
*Enrollment	1,049
*% male/female	59/41
*% underrepresented minorities	12
# applied (total/out)	3,655/2,162
% interviewed (total/out)	21/4
% accepted (total/out)	NR/NR
% enrolled (total/out)	33/27

ADMISSIONS

Average GPA and MCAT Scores

Overall GPA	3.50	Science GPA	NR
MCAT Bio	8.80	MCAT Phys	9.10
MCAT Verbal	8.80	MCAT Essay	NR

Score Release Policy

The school has not responded to our inquiry regarding withheld MCAT scores. Therefore, we advise caution. Contact the Admissions Office before withholding any scores.

Application Information

Regular application	11/15
Regular notification	10/15 until filled
Early application	6/1–8/1
Early notification	10/1
Admissions may be deferred?	Yes
AMCAS application accepted?	Yes
Interview required?	Yes
Application fee	$30

COSTS AND AID

Tuition & Fees

Tuition (in/out)	$10,149/$20,222
Cost of books	NR
Fees	$350

Financial Aid

% students receiving aid	NR
Average grant	NR
Average loan	NR
Average debt	NR

*Figures based on total enrollment

WEST VIRGINIA UNIVERSITY

SCHOOL OF MEDICINE

PO Box 9111, Morgantown, WV 26506

Admission: 304-293-3521 • Fax: 304-293-7814

Email: rmoore@wvuhsc1.hsc.wvu.edu

Internet: www.hsc.wvu.edu

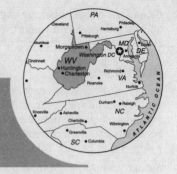

The Health Sciences Center at West Virginia University (WVU) includes Schools of Dentistry, Medicine, Nursing, and Pharmacy. Together, these academic institutions offer a comprehensive range of undergraduate, graduate, and professional degrees in health care and bio-sciences. The School of Medicine is highly committed to the surrounding community, illustrated by the fact that all medical students must complete 100 hours of community service prior to graduation. A two-month, required clinical rotation in a rural, primary care setting is among the features that demonstrate WVU's focus on generalist and community-oriented medicine.

Academics

While most medical students follow a four-year curriculum and earn the M.D. degree, about two medical students each year pursue joint M.D./Ph.D. degrees, leading to the doctorate in Anatomy, Biochemistry, Medical Technology, Microbiology, Pathology, Pharmacology and Toxicology, and Physiology. Medical students are graded with Honors, Satisfactory, or Unsatisfactory for all courses and clerkships. All students must pass Step 1 of the USMLE to be promoted to year three. Passing Step 2 is a graduation requirement.

BASIC SCIENCES: First-year courses are Physiology; Gross Anatomy; Biochemistry; Genetics; Histology; Embryology; Microanatomy; and Problem Based Learning, which integrates clinical correlation to the basic sciences. Second-year courses are Pathology; Microbiology; Behavioral Medicine and Psychiatry; Pharmacology and Toxicology; Genetics; Community Medicine; and Introduction to Clinical Medicine (ICM). The ICM courses uses faculty mentors as teachers and trains students in basic clinical techniques, such as the physical examination and patient interview. Instructional aids include computer-assisted learning programs. For research purposes and for studying, students use the Health Sciences Library, which has a collection of more than 205,000 volumes, in addition to extensive holdings of audio-visual equipment.

CLINICAL TRAINING: Third-year, required clerkships are eight weeks each of Medicine; Surgery; Behavioral Medicine and Psychiatry; Ob/Gyn; Pediatrics; and Family Medicine, which includes a rural rotation. Fourth-year requirements include one month of a subinternship in Internal Medicine, Pediatrics, or Family Medicine, a one-month Critical Care Clerkship, an additional one-month Surgery clerkship, and two months of a Rural Primary Care experience. Half of the fourth year is reserved for electives. Five months of fourth-year clerkships must be taken at WVU sites, leaving ample opportunity for students to rotate to other academic and clinical institutions. Clinical training takes place primarily at the Ruby Memorial Hospital (376 beds), which is part of the West Virginia University Robert C. Byrd Health Sciences Center Complex. The Complex also includes the Physicians Office Center, the Mary Babb Randolph Cancer Center, Chestnut Ridge Psychiatric Hospital (70 beds), Southview Regional Rehabilitation Hospital (60 beds), and the National Institute of Occupational Safety and Health (NIOSH). About one-third of third year students enter a clinical training program at University-affiliated hospitals in Charleston. All students also have the opportunity to rotate to facilities that are part of a large network of hospitals and physicians in rural areas of the state.

Students

At least 95 percent of students are West Virginia residents, and more than one-third attended WVU for undergraduate studies. About 40 other undergraduate institutions are represented in a typical class. Approximately 68 percent of students were Biology or Chemistry majors in college. In a recently admitted class of 88 students, 25 were 20 or 21 years of age, 56 were 22 or 23, and 7 were 24 or older.

STUDENT LIFE: With more than 1,700 students enrolled in programs at the Health Sciences Center, a camaraderie exists among WVU students. The small class size of the medical school also promotes class cohesion and cooperation. Student organizations include local chapters of national medical student organizations, community service-based groups, and clubs focused on professional interests. University-owned housing is available to medical and graduate students.

GRADUATES: About one-third of the practicing physicians in the state of West Virginia are graduates of WVU. At least half of graduates enter primary care fields, considered as Family Medicine, Internal Medicine, Pediatrics, and Ob/Gyn.

Admissions

REQUIREMENTS: Prerequisites are one year each of English, Social Sciences, Biology, General Chemistry, Organic Chemistry, and Physics. All science courses should include lab work. The MCAT is required and is used, along with undergraduate transcripts, to assess academic achievement. For applicants who have taken the exam on multiple occasions, all scores are considered.

SUGGESTIONS: State residents are given strong preference in admission. However, a limited number of highly qualified nonresidents may also be admitted. Beyond required course work, recommended courses are Biochemistry, Cell and Molecular Biology, and Calculus. The Committee on Admissions expects strength in the sciences but gives no preference to any particular major. Demonstration of an understanding of the medical profession is important.

PROCESS: All qualified West Virginia resident applicants and highly qualified nonresidents are sent secondary applications. Of those returning secondaries, about 50 percent of residents and 10 percent of nonresidents are interviewed between September and February. Interviews generally consist of one two-on-one session, usually with medical school faculty, fourth-year students, or administrators. On interview day, students also have the opportunity to tour the campus and meet current students. Approximately one-third of interviewed candidates are accepted on a rolling basis. Others are either rejected or wait-listed. West Virginia residents on the wait list have a reasonable chance of being accepted later in the spring.

Costs

The estimated yearly cost of living for a single student is about $14,000. This budget allows for either on- or off-campus living and car maintenance.

FINANCIAL AID: Most financial aid is awarded on the basis of need, as determined by the FASA form. In addition to federal sources of aid there are state-sponsored scholarships, loans, and loan-repayment programs aimed at increasing the number of primary care physicians in rural areas.

WEST VIRGINIA UNIVERSITY

STUDENT BODY

Type	Public
*Enrollment	348
*% male/female	61/39
*% underrepresented minorities	3
# applied (total/out)	1,146/832
% interviewed (total/out)	22/2
% accepted (total/out)	10/1
% enrolled (total/out)	79/80
Average age	23

ADMISSIONS

Average GPA and MCAT Scores

Overall GPA	3.66	Science GPA	3.61
MCAT Bio	9.7	MCAT Phys	9.2
MCAT Verbal	9.1	MCAT Essay	NR

Score Release Policy

The Admissions Committee strongly discourages withholding scores.

Application Information

Regular application	11/15
Regular notification	Rolling
Early application	8/1
Early notification	10/1
Transfers accepted?	Yes
Admissions may be deferred?	Yes
AMCAS application accepted?	Yes
Interview required?	Yes
Application fee	$45

COSTS AND AID

Tuition & Fees

Tuition (in/out)	$1,640/$4,550
Cost of books	$4,450
Fees (total/out)	$7,384/$17,974

Financial Aid

% students receiving aid	79
Average grant	$1,500
Average loan	$26,000
Average debt	NR

*Figures based on total enrollment

Medical College of Wisconsin

Office of Admissions, 8701 Watertown Plank Road, Milwaukee, WI 53226

Admission: 414-456-8246

Internet: www.mcw.edu/medschool

The Medical College of Wisconsin (MCW) was ranked the top private medical school for primary care education in *U.S. News & World Report*'s 1996 guide. Although MCW attracts a nationally represented student body, one of its main priorities is contributing to the local community through patient care, relevant research, and student-led volunteer activities. Prominent areas of faculty research include cancer, cardiovascular studies, neuroscience, AIDS behavioral intervention, aging, arthritis, and health policy. Students at MCW enjoy proximity to a major urban center as well as to beaches and other outdoor attractions.

Academics

Although most students earn the M.D. degree in four years, an Extended Curriculum allows students to complete first-year course work over a two-year period and to graduate in five years. This enables students to pursue research, employment, or personal activities. Medical students interested in research are also encouraged to take part in research projects during summers and as part of electives. Other degrees offered by MCW are the Ph.D., M.S., M.A., and M.P.H. Qualified students may enter a combined M.D./Ph.D. degree program, and two students each year do so through the M.S.T.P. The Graduate School of Biomedical Sciences offers programs in Bioethics, Biostatistics, Biochemistry, Biophysics, Cellular Biology, Medical Informatics, Microbiology, Pathology, Pharmacology and Toxicology, and Physiology. Medical students are evaluated by use of a five-interval grading system. Passing Step 1 of the USMLE and sitting for Step 2 are requirements for graduation.

BASIC SCIENCES: Basic sciences are taught through a combination of lectures, labs, tutorials, and small-group discussions along with computer aided instructing (CAI), problem-based learning (PBL), and independent study options. On average, students are in class or other scheduled sessions for 23 hours per week. First-year courses are Clinical Human Anatomy, Medical Microanatomy, Integrated Medical Neuroscience, Human Development, Biochemistry, Physiology, and Clinical Continuum I. Second-year courses are Pathology, Pharmacology, Microbiology, Foundations of Clinical Psychiatry, and Clinical Continuum II. In the Clinical Continuum sequence, a local physician is assigned as a personal mentor who guides the students through clinical studies in one of the primary care specialties. In addition to learning physical examination and evaluation skills, topics of discussion include the doctor-patient relationship, medical ethics, and health care systems. As part of the course, students follow individual patients for the two-year period, observing their treatment and progress. Support services for medical students include individual and group advising, tutorials, preparation for USMLE exams, and career counseling. Educational facilities include the new Health Research Center completed in the fall of 1998. The HRC features an auditorium with modern electronic capabilities, rooms designated for small-group instruction, and an expanded library. In total, MCW libraries house more than 240,000 volumes and 1,800 journal titles.

CLINICAL TRAINING: Third-year required rotations are Introductory Clinical Skills (1 week); Ambulatory Medicine (1 month); Medicine (2 months); Surgery (2 months); Pediatrics (2 months); Ob/Gyn (2 months); Psychiatry (6 weeks); and Anesthesiology (2 weeks). The fourth year consists of a Medicine or Pediatric Subinternship (1 month); a Medicine Selective rotation (1 month); a Surgery Selective (1 month); and six months of electives. MCW is one of six components of the Milwaukee Regional Medical Center (MRMC), a campus that includes Froedtert Memorial Lutheran Hospital, Children's Hospital of Wisconsin, Curative Rehabilitation Center, Milwaukee County Mental Health Complex, and the Blood Center of Southeastern Wisconsin Research Institute and Eye Institute. MCW is affiliated with over 15 additional hospitals and clinics in and around Milwaukee, and with rural care centers in other parts of the state. Up to four months of electives may be taken at other academic medical centers and in foreign countries.

Students

Of the 204 students in a typical class, 100 are Wisconsin residents. Underrepresented minorities account for about 10 percent of the student body. About one-quarter of students took significant time off between college and medical school.

STUDENT LIFE: Student organizations focus on professional and leadership development, community service, support for minority students, and recreational pursuits. The Medical College is involved with over 30 community service activities, including a student-run clinic for uninsured patients, an AIDS intervention research center, and a health education program in high schools. Medical students take part in organized social events, such as parties and dinners, and ongoing activities, such as intramural sports. Located in the medical education building are an expanded fitness center and a lounge. These facilities allow students to relax and socialize or exercise between scheduled classes. The MCW campus is park-like, covering 248 acres. However, it is an easy drive to downtown Milwaukee, a city of over one million. Milwaukee has a wide variety of cuisine, performing arts and musical groups, several professional sports teams, and outdoor sites like Lake Michigan. Most students live off campus.

GRADUATES: In June, 1996, MCW was one of only six medical schools nationwide in which 100 percent of second-year students passed the USMLE. This type of performance, coupled with the school's reputation for excellent clinical training, results in excellent placement records for graduates.

Admissions

REQUIREMENTS: Prerequisites, which must be taken for graded credit, are eight semester hours including lab each of Biology, General Chemistry, Organic Chemistry, and Physics. In addition, six semester hours of English, and one high school or college course in Algebra, are required. AP credit is only accepted for 3 graded credits of English. The MCAT is required and must be taken no more than three years prior to matriculation. For applicants who have taken the exam on more than one occasion, the most recent set of scores is considered.

SUGGESTIONS: Beyond required courses, applicants are encouraged to study public speaking, literature, history, music, philosophy, and social sciences. In addition to academic credentials, qualities such as a mature sense of values, sound motivation, and the willingness to assume responsibility are important.

PROCESS: MCW uses a secondary application. Interviews consist of two half-hour sessions, each with a faculty member or medical student. On interview day, applicants hear group presentations, receive a campus tour, and have the opportunity to talk with current students. Notification of decision is on a rolling basis.

Costs

The estimated yearly cost of living for a single student is about $10,000. This budget allows for off-campus living and car ownership.

FINANCIAL AID: All aid is need-based, with financial need determined by the FAFSA and other forms. Most assistance is in the form of loans.

MEDICAL COLLEGE OF WISCONSIN

STUDENT BODY

Type	Private
*Enrollment	810
*% male/female	62/38
*% underrepresented minorities	10
# applied (total/out)	5,335/4,795
% interviewed (total/out)	11/7
% accepted (total/out)	9/5
% enrolled (total/out)	44/37

ADMISSIONS

Average GPA and MCAT Scores

Overall GPA	3.71	Science GPA	3.67
MCAT Bio	10.00	MCAT Phys	10.00
MCAT Verbal	10.00	MCAT Essay	0

Score Release Policy

The school has not responded to our inquiry regarding withheld MCAT scores. Therefore, we advise caution. Contact the Admissions Office before withholding any scores.

Application Information

Regular application	11/1
Regular notification	10/15 until filled
Early application	6/1–8/1
Early notification	10/1
Transfers accepted?	No
Admissions may be deferred?	Yes
AMCAS application accepted?	Yes
Interview required?	Yes
Application fee	$60

COSTS AND AID

Tuition & Fees

Tuition (in/out)	$17,359/$27,450
Cost of books	$1,235
Fees	45

Financial Aid

% students receiving aid	95
Average grant	$5,492
Average loan	$26,123
Average debt	$101,631

*Figures based on total enrollment

UNIVERSITY OF WISCONSIN
MEDICAL SCHOOL

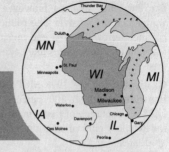

1300 University Avenue, Madison, WI 53706
Admission: 608-263-4925 • Fax: 608-262-2327
Internet: www.biostat.wisc.edu

In 1994 the University of Wisconsin Medical School implemented a new curriculum that emphasizes active learning, generalist training, integrated courses, and an interdisciplinary approach, which includes topics such as ethics, health policy, and women's health. The Medical School's focus on primary care is longstanding: UW was the first school in the country to offer a community-physician preceptorship program. Established in 1926, this program continues to provide invaluable hands-on training to medical students.

Academics

While most students earn the M.D. degree in four years, UW also offers a M.D./Ph.D. Integrated Degree Program, which prepares students for careers in academic medicine and biomedical research. Participants are financially supported by the program or through research training grants. The doctorate may be earned in Anatomy, Biochemistry, Cell Biology, Genetics, Immunology, Microbiology, Molecular Biology, Neuroscience, Pathology, Pharmacology, and Physiology. Medical students are evaluated with letter grades. Students must pass Step 1 of the USMLE for promotion to year three and Step 2 for graduation.

BASIC SCIENCES: The revised curriculum features fewer lectures and instead relies on small-group discussions, practical laboratories, multimedia computer programs and videos, and significant opportunities to learn through real-life clinical examples. An important component of the new curriculum is the Generalist Partners Program (GPP) which matches first-year medical students with primary care physicians who practice in the community and who serve as teachers and mentors to students. Through GPP, students learn first-hand about generalist medicine, and enjoy early patient-care opportunities. Also during the first and second years, students take an interdisciplinary course that addresses practicing medicine in a variety of modern-day environments. Other first-year courses are Gross Anatomy, Biomolecular Chemistry, Genetics, Histology, Human Sexuality, Neuroscience, Pathology, and Physiology. The second-year Pathophysiology course is organized around body/organ systems, which are Hematology, Cardiovascular, Renal/Hypertension, Respiratory, Neoplastic Disease, Endocrine, Gastrointestinal, and Hepatic. Other courses are Infection and Immunity, Pharmacology, Psychiatry, and Nutrition. The William S. Middleton Medical Library is used by students for research and for studying. It houses 150,000 volumes and 2,000 publications.

CLINICAL TRAINING: The third- and fourth-year clerkships expose students to a wide variety of clinical settings (outpatient, inpatient, community based, rural, and inner city). Training takes place at University hospitals in Madison as well as in affiliated sites in Milwaukee, La Crosse, Marshfield, two preceptor sites, and at area health education centers. Third-year required clerkships are Transition (1 week); Medicine (8 weeks); Primary Care (8 weeks); Surgery (8 weeks); Pediatrics (6 weeks); Ob/Gyn (6 weeks); Anesthesia (2 weeks); Neurology (3 weeks); Psychiatry (4 weeks); Ophthalmology (1 week); and Selectives (2 weeks). During the fourth year, students complete an Acting Internship in Medicine (4 weeks); an advanced Surgery Clerkship (4 weeks); a Preceptorship (8 weeks); and 16 weeks of electives. A portion of electives may be taken at other academic and clinical institutions, both in the United States and overseas. The UW International Health Exchange is an affiliated nonprofit foundation that increases awareness of international health issues through a range of activities including promoting overseas clinical experiences for students.

Students

Each class is comprised of 143 students. Approximately 80–85 percent of students are Wisconsin residents, and during the past four years, about 50 percent of students attended UW for their undergraduate education. About 14 percent of students are underrepresented minorities. Typically, about one-quarter of entering students took some time off between college and medical school, and about 10 students in each class are in their late twenties or thirties.

STUDENT LIFE: The Medical School benefits from the resources of one of the nation's top public universities. Medical students have access to the facilities of the large campus and enjoy the lively environment of a popular college city. Students are active in community service projects, volunteering at homeless shelters and clinics, and organizing AIDS or other education projects. On-campus housing, including married-student facilities, is available. However, most students prefer to live in shared apartments off campus. Madison is a medium-sized city, organized around three lakes, which provide many opportunities for outdoor recreation.

GRADUATES: Graduates are successful in securing residency positions at prestigious institutions nationwide.

Admissions

REQUIREMENTS: Minimum science requirements are General Biology with lab (1 semester); Advanced Biology/Zoology with lab (1 semester); General Chemistry with lab (1 year); Organic Chemistry with lab (1 year); General Physics with lab (1 year); and Mathematics (1 semester). The MCAT is required, and for the 1999 entering class, scores must be from 1995 or later. Where more than one MCAT has been taken, the higher values of the two most recent scores are used.

SUGGESTIONS: UW gives preference to residents of Wisconsin, but about 25 out-of-state applicants are accepted each year. A sound liberal arts education, including both humanities and social sciences, is considered important. While specific courses are not required, the applicant's preparation should include courses in those areas that prepare for the social, psychological, and economic aspects of medical practice. The Admissions Committee members rely heavily on the applicants' essays, letters of recommendation, and the personal interview to assess motivation and personal character.

PROCESS: Upon receipt of the AMCAS application, the UW Supplemental Application, is automatically sent to Wisconsin resident applicants and to highly qualified nonresidents. Although all applications are reviewed by committee members, a formula that weights all sections of the MCAT (including the essay) and the overall GPA helps with decisions about whether or not a candidate will be invited to interview. About half of residents and one-third of nonresidents are interviewed. Interviews take place between December and April and consist of one session with a faculty member or medical student. Interview-day activities include group informational sessions, a tour, and lunch with medical students. About 75 percent of interviewed candidates are accepted on a rolling basis. An alternate route to admissions is through the Medical Scholars Program, which offers early admission to medical school for outstanding Wisconsin high school graduates.

Costs

The estimated yearly cost of living for a single student is about $11,700. This budget allows for book purchases, off-campus housing, and possibly car maintenance.

FINANCIAL AID: All financial aid is awarded on the basis of documented need. Although some scholarships are available, most assistance is in the form of loans.

UNIVERSITY OF WISCONSIN

STUDENT BODY

Type	Public
*Enrollment	605
*% male/female	53/47
*% underrepresented minorities	14
# applied (total/out)	2,299/1,680
% interviewed (total/out)	11/2
% accepted (total/out)	NR/NR
% enrolled (total/out)	56/36

ADMISSIONS

Average GPA and MCAT Scores

Overall GPA	3.67	Science GPA	NR
MCAT Bio	10.10	MCAT Phys	9.90
MCAT Verbal	9.80	MCAT Essay	P

Score Release Policy

The school has not responded to our inquiry regarding withheld MCAT scores. Therefore, we advise caution. Contact the Admissions Office before withholding any scores.

Application Information

Regular application	10/15
Regular notification	11/15–varies
Early application	6/1–8/1
Early notification	10/1
Admissions may be deferred?	Yes
AMCAS application accepted?	Yes
Interview required?	Yes
Application fee	$45

COSTS AND AID

Tuition & Fees

Tuition (in/out)	$15,106/$22,240
Cost of books	NR
Fees	$406

Financial Aid

% students receiving aid	NR
Average grant	NR
Average loan	NR
Average debt	NR

*Figures based on total enrollment

WRIGHT STATE UNIVERSITY

SCHOOL OF MEDICINE

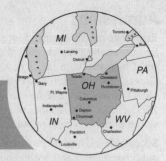

PO Box 1751, Dayton, OH 45401

Admission: 937-775-2934 • Fax: 937-775-3322

Email: som_saa@desire.wright.edu • Internet: www.med.wright.edu

Wright State was among the first medical schools to develop a comprehensive, community-based education program. Clinical training takes place at more than 20 small, Miami Valley health care facilities as well as at eight major teaching hospitals. Primary care is emphasized, and the percentage of graduates who enter primary care practices ranks in the top 5 percent of medical schools nationwide. Patient contact experiences are integrated with basic science instruction during the first two years.

Academics

Although most students complete the M.D. curriculum in four years, a few enter the M.D./Ph.D. program, which requires additional course work. Graduate degrees are offered in most Biomedical Sciences including Anatomy, Physiology, Biochemistry, Pathology, and Pharmacology. Medical students are evaluated with percentile scores and ratings of Pass/Fail. Students take the USMLE Step 1 after completion of year two and Step 2 after the completion of year three.

BASIC SCIENCES: Basic-science instruction includes use of small-groups, clinical case studies, problem-based learning, and computer-aided instruction. First-year courses are Human Structure, Human Development, Introduction to Clinical Medicine I (ICM I), Molecular, Cellular, and Tissue Biology, Social and Ethical Issues in Medicine, Principles of Disease, and Evidence-Based Medicine. The second year is organized around organ/body systems. These are Blood, Cardiology, Endocrine, GI, Integument, Musculoskeletal, Neuroscience, Renal, Reproductive, and Respiratory. Students also learn about Infectious Diseases and continue clinical training in ICM II. The ICM course provides clinical contact from the very first week of class. In this series, students learn to take medical histories, conduct physical exams and identify common diseases. Three two-week elective periods during the first two years give students the opportunity to pursue intensive research or clinical projects. Students are also encouraged to participate in faculty-guided research during the summer in between the first and second years. The Fordham Health Sciences Library is fully computerized and provides 106,000 volumes, in addition to journals and special collections. Students also study in the Student Lounge and the main university's libraries. The Interdisciplinary Teaching Laboratory enhances learning through the use of audio-visual equipment, hard-wired labs, and medical software.

CLINICAL TRAINING: Third-year required rotations are: Family Medicine (6 weeks); Internal Medicine (12 weeks); Women's Health (8 weeks); Pediatrics (8 weeks); Psychiatry (6 weeks); and Surgery (8 weeks). Fourth-year requirements are Emergency Medicine (4 weeks), Neurology (4 weeks), Surgical Specialties (4 weeks), and a variety of Selectives (5 months). Students also participate in a Senior Seminar Program. Training takes place at Children's Medical Center (155 beds); Dayton Veterans Affairs Medical Center; Franciscan Medical Center Dayton Campus (622 beds); Good Samaritan Hospital and Health Center (560 beds); Green Memorial Hospital (210 beds); Kettering Medical Center (486 beds); Miami Valley Hospital (811 beds); and Wright-Patterson Air Force Base Medical Center (301 beds). Some students rotate overseas as part of individually designed or faculty-led experiences.

Students

About 90 percent of entering students are Ohio residents. In the class that will graduate in 2000, 21 percent of students are underrepresented minorities. Typically, about 10 percent of entering students took significant time off between college and medical school. Class size is 90.

STUDENT LIFE: Medical students have active extracurricular lives, taking advantage of the offerings of the Medical School, the main University, and the greater community. Students are involved in community service organizations and projects such as the Center for Healthy Communities, which provides health education services to the Dayton community. Other student organizations are chapters of state and national medical organizations, honor societies, support groups and clubs focused on professional or recreational interests. Athletic facilities on campus include racquetball, squash, basketball and tennis courts, indoor and outdoor tracks, and several fitness centers. The University's 200 acres of woods are used for walking and jogging. The University is located 12 miles northeast of Dayton, a city of nearly 1 million residents. Students live in privately owned apartments and houses, which are generally affordable and conveniently located.

GRADUATES: Among students who graduated in 1998, 72 percent entered primary care residencies, which are defined as Family Medicine, Internal Medicine, and Pediatrics. About 63 percent choose residency programs in Ohio.

Admissions

REQUIREMENTS: Prerequisites are one year each of Biology, Chemistry, Organic Chemistry, and Physics, all with associated labs. In addition, one year each of English and Mathematics are required. The MCAT is required, and scores should be from within the past three years. For applicants who have retaken the exam, all scores are considered.

SUGGESTIONS: Ohio residents are given strong preference, making admission for nonresidents very competitive. The April, rather than August, MCAT is advised. In addition to academic strength, selection is based on dedication to human concerns, communication skills, maturity, and motivation. Some hospital or other medically related experience is recommended.

PROCESS: All AMCAS applicants receive secondary applications. About 10 percent of those returning secondaries are invited to interview between September and March. Interviews consist of two sessions, each with a faculty member. On interview day, students also attend group information presentations, have lunch with faculty and students, and tour the campus and hospital. About 45 percent of interviewed candidates are accepted on a rolling basis. Others are rejected or put on a wait list. Waitlisted candidates are not encouraged to send additional information.

Costs

The estimated yearly cost of living for a single student is about $15,034. This budget allows for off-campus housing and car maintenance.

FINANCIAL AID: Although the majority of financial aid programs consider students independent, parental financial disclosure is generally required. Most financial aid is awarded on the basis of demonstrated financial need. However, a limited number of scholarships are based on academic merit or other special criteria.

WRIGHT STATE UNIVERSITY

STUDENT BODY

Type	Public
*Enrollment	372
*% male/female	45/55
*% underrepresented minorities	30
# applied (total/out)	3,123/1,894
% interviewed (total/out)	13/4
% accepted (total/out)	6/1
% enrolled (total/out)	48/70
Average age	23

ADMISSIONS

Average GPA and MCAT Scores

Overall GPA	3.50	Science GPA	3.42
MCAT Bio	8.90	MCAT Phys	8.30
MCAT Verbal	8.50	MCAT Essay	NR

Application Information

Regular application	11/15
Regular notification	10/15 until filled
Early application	6/1–8/1
Early notification	10/1
Transfers accepted?	Yes
Admissions may be deferred?	Yes
AMCAS application accepted?	Yes
Interview required?	Yes
Application fee	$30

COSTS AND AID

Tuition & Fees

Tuition (in/out)	$10,326/$14,616
Cost of books	$1,100
Fees	$723

Financial Aid

% students receiving aid	NR
Average grant	NR
Average loan	NR
Average debt	NR

*Figures based on total enrollment

YALE UNIVERSITY
SCHOOL OF MEDICINE

367 Cedar Street, New Haven, CT 06510
Admission: 203-785-2643 • Fax: 203-785-3234
Email: medicalschool.admissions@quickmail.yale.edu
Internet: info.med.yale.edu/medadmit

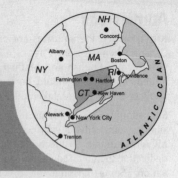

Yale is widely regarded as one of the top medical schools in the country. Hallmarks of the Yale curriculum are the tremendous amount of autonomy given to students during the first two years, the close cooperation between faculty and students, and the thesis requirement. The thesis exposes students to academic medicine and allows them to focus on a particular area of interest while in medical school. The patient population of New Haven and the surrounding areas is diverse, giving students a comprehensive clinical experience.

Academics

Although most students complete courses, clerkships, and a thesis in four years, about 30–50 percent of students extend their studies over a five-year period at no extra cost. Some students take an extra year to earn a M.P.H. along with the M.D. Other combined degree programs offered are the M.D./J.D., M.D./M.Div, and M.D./Ph.D. Entering students are assigned a clinical tutor who serves as a mentor during all four years. Also throughout all four years, students take a series of lectures, workshops, and clinical discussion under the broad topic of Medicine, Society and Public Health. Evaluation of students is strictly Pass/Fail. Passing Steps 1 and 2 of the USMLE is a graduation requirement.

BASIC SCIENCES: The first two years are spent building a foundation in the basic sciences as well as learning skills and techniques for training in clinical responsibilities. Year one is devoted to understanding normal relevant biological form and function. Year two concentrates on the study of disease. Formats include lecture, small group discussion, laboratories, demonstrations, and individual tutorials; many of these involve patients, both at the bedside and in the classroom. First year students must pass the following courses: Cellular and Physiologic Basis of Medicine (Physiology and Cell Biology), Human Genetics, Human Anatomy and Development, Molecular Foundations of Medicine (Biochemistry), Neurobiology, Psychological Basis of Medical Practice, Biological Basis of Behavior, and Aspects of Child and Adolescent Development. In addition there is an umbrella course called Medicine, Society and Public Health that includes related but distinct subcourses: Biostatistics, History of Medicine, Professional Responsibility, and Health Policy. Pre-clinical training is included in the course The Doctor/Patient Encounter. The major, second-year course is called Mechanisms of Disease and is organized into two segments. The initial offering, called Basic Principles, includes Immunobiology, Pathology, Pharmacology, Microbiology, and Basics of Diagnostic Radiology, and Laboratory Medicine. The second segment is called Mechanisms of Disease: Organs/Systems. Each integrated module, organized around body systems or organs, includes Pathology, Pharmacology, Pathophysiology, Diagnostic Radiology, Laboratory Medicine, and Prevention. The modules are Blood/Hematology; Neoplasias/Oncology; Cardiovascular System; Respiratory System; Digestive System; Musculoskeletal System; Renal, Urinary Tract and Male Reproductive System; Female Reproductive System; Endocrine Systems; Skin; Clinical Neuroscience; and Psychiatry. Medicine, Society and Public Health continues, offering Epidemiology and Public Health in the first semester, and relevant Prevention during the modules. The Doctor/Patient Encounter course also continues, building as it progresses.

CLINICAL TRAINING: There are seven required clerkships in the third year, one of which may be completed early in the fourth year. These are Internal Medicine (12 weeks); General Surgery/Surgical Subspecialties (12 weeks); Pediatrics (8 weeks); Psychiatry (6 weeks); Ob/Gyn (6 weeks); and Clinical Neuroscience (4 weeks). During the fourth year, an Integrated Clinical Medicine Clerkship (3 weeks) and a Primary Care Clerkship (4 weeks) are required. The Primary Care Clerkship takes place in a variety of community- and practice-based sites. Most clinical rotations are completed at the Yale New Haven Hospital and the West Haven Veteran's Administration Hospital. Other affiliated hospitals are Bridgeport Hospital; Danbury Hospital; Greenwich Hospital; Griffin Hospital in Derby; Hospital of Saint Raphael; Lawrence and Memorial Hospital; Norwalk Hospital; Saint Mary's Hospital in Waterbury; Saint Vincent's Medical Center in Bridgeport; and Waterbury Hospital. Several clinics and mental health centers are also used for training. Although some students begin working on their thesis early in medical school, the majority of research and writing takes from four to seven months and is completed in the fourth year. Some students publish their work, while others continue developing their research post-graduation.

Students

Yale attracts students from all regions of the country. Approximately 15–20 percent of entering students are underrepresented minorities. Among students in the 1997 entering class, the average age was 24, with a considerable age range. Class size is 100.

STUDENT LIFE: The School of Medicine is a short walk from the University's main campus. This gives medical students access to athletic facilities, student meeting areas, libraries, and university-sponsored events. Medical students participate in intramural sports, competing against other graduate and professional school teams. About three-quarters of medical students are involved in community service activities such as STATS (Students Teaching AIDS to Students), the Prenatal Care Project, and ASAP (the Adolescent Substance Abuse Prevention Project). The Office for Women in Medicine is the oldest of its kind in the nation and provides support, guidance, and special programs of interest for women medical students. The Office for Multicultural Affairs recruits and supports minority students, serves as a link between the school and its surrounding community, and sponsors various cultural events and centers. The Edward S. Harkness Memorial Hall is a residence hall for medical, physician associate, nursing, public health, and other graduate students. Both dormitory-style rooms and apartments are available.

GRADUATES: Among 1998 graduates, the most popular areas for residency training were Internal Medicine (40%); Pediatrics (12%); Surgery (5%); Diagnostic Radiology (1%); Orthopedics (8%); Plastic Surgery (4%); Dermatology (3%); and Otolaryngology (5%).

Admissions

REQUIREMENTS: Prerequisites are one year each of General Biology or Zoology, General Chemistry, Organic Chemistry, and General Physics, all taken with associated labs. The MCAT is required, and scores should be from within the past four years. For applicants who have retaken the exam, the best set of scores is considered.

SUGGESTIONS: In addition to academic credentials, the Committee on Admissions looks for intelligent, mature, and highly motivated students who possess integrity, common sense, personal stability, dedication to service, and the ability to inspire and maintain confidence.

PROCESS: Yale does not participate in AMCAS. Applications should be requested from the address above, or downloaded from info.med.yale.edu/medadmit. About 25 percent of applicants are interviewed between October and February. Interviews consist of two sessions, each with a faculty member or medical student committee member. Candidates attend group information sessions and have the opportunity to eat lunch and tour the campus with current medical students. About 15 percent of interviewed candidates are accepted. Notification occurs in mid-March.

Costs

The anticipated first-year budget for a single student is about $43,925. This includes tuition, books, required fees, and living expense of $14,725. This allows for on-campus or shared off-campus housing and use of public transportation.

FINANCIAL AID: All aid is need-based. Generally, students borrow $18,500 in Stafford loans before becoming eligible for institutional grants and loans. Parental financial disclosure is required for students younger than 30.

YALE UNIVERSITY

STUDENT BODY

Type	Private
*Enrollment	479
*% male/female	51/49
*% underrepresented minorities	18
# applied (total/out)	3,093/NR
% interviewed (total/out)	26/NR
% accepted (total/out)	NR/NR
% enrolled (total/out)	NR/NR
Average age	24

ADMISSIONS

Average GPA and MCAT Scores

Overall GPA	3.70	Science GPA	3.71
MCAT Bio	11.81	MCAT Phys	11.78
MCAT Verbal	10.68	MCAT Essay	P–Q

Score Release Policy

The Admissions Committee considers only the best score, but all scores must be reported and verified. The Committee does not penalize a student for withholding scores, but it's in the best interest of the student to reveal all scores.

Application Information

Regular application	10/15
Regular notification	3/15 until filled
Early application	6/1–8/1
Early notification	10/1
Transfers accepted?	Yes
Admissions may be deferred?	Yes
AMCAS application accepted?	Yes
Interview required?	Yes
Application fee	$60

COSTS AND AID

Tuition & Fees

Tuition	$29,200
Cost of books	$1,450
Fees	$200

Financial Aid

% students receiving aid	58.5
Average grant	$11,586
Average loan	$22,665
Average debt	$92,613

*Figures based on total enrollment

Canadian Medical School Profiles

UNIVERSITY OF ALBERTA
FACULTY OF MEDICINE AND DENTISTRY

2-45 Medical Sciences Building, Edmonton, Alberta T6G 2H7

Admission: 780-492-6350

Internet: www.med.ualberta.ca

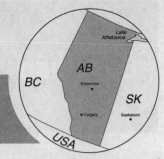

The Faculty of Medicine and Dentistry is a part of the University of Alberta, an institution with nearly 30,000 graduate and undergraduate students. Located in Edmonton, the Medical School benefits from access to both rural and urban patient populations through a network of affiliated teaching hospitals. In addition to the M.D., the Faculty awards graduate degrees in Public Health, Dentistry, Health Sciences, and a range of Biological and Biomedical fields. Other graduate schools at the university include Faculties of Nursing, Law, Education, Pharmacy, and Rehabilitative Medicine. Only Canadian applicants are considered for admission.

Academics

Alberta's curriculum reflects the School's emphasis on clinical care and research. The preclinical curriculum has been revised, and is largely centered on organ systems. It is multidisciplinary, including both biological and social science perspectives. Although basic sciences are the focus of study during the first two years, courses are taught with clinical applications in mind. The second two years integrate classroom and hospital-based instruction. While most medical students earn an M.D. degree in four years, qualified students may pursue joint degrees such as the M.D./Ph.D. or M.D./M.P.H in a longer period of study.

BASIC SCIENCES: Basic sciences are taught in a variety of forums, including lectures, small group discussions, laboratories, problem-based learning, independent study, and computer-based instruction. The academic period begins in August, covers 35 weeks, and includes courses in Introduction to Medicine; Immunity, Infection and Inflammation; Practice of Medicine (Part I); Cardiology, Renal, and Pulmonary; and Endocrine and Metabolism. On average, students are in class or other scheduled sessions for about twenty-five hours per week. The second academic period also begins in August and includes Gastroenterology, Reproduction and Urology, Musculoskeletal, Neuroscieces, Oncology, and Practice of Medicine (Part II) in addition to a systems-based curriculum. Systems studied are Cardiovascular, Endocrinology, Gastrointestinal, Hematology, Medical Ethics, Nephrology, Ophthalmology, Pediatrics, Pulmonary, Surgery, and Urology. Basic science instruction takes place mainly at the Medical Sciences Building and uses the resources of the John W. Scott Health Sciences Library. Medical students may use all university libraries and computer facilities. All enrolled students have access to free online service.

CLINICAL TRAINING: The third and fourth academic periods primarily teach clinical skills and are comprised of classroom instruction, required rotations, electives, and selectives. Required clerkships are: Anesthesia (2 weeks), Geriatrics (2 weeks), Medicine (10 weeks), Ob/Gyn (8 weeks), Pediatrics (8 weeks), Psychiatry (8 weeks), Radiology (2 weeks), Rural Family Medicine (4 weeks), and Surgery (10 weeks). Selectives include two weeks in Internal Medicine and two weeks in Surgery. Training takes place at University of Alberta hospitals, the Royal Alexandra Hospital, Edmonton General Hospital, Misericordia Hospital, Alberta Hospital, Glenrose Hospital, Cross Cancer Institute, and Grey Nuns Hospital. A certain number of electives may be taken at non-affiliated institutions.

Students

Among 102 students in the 1998 entering class, 42 percent are female. About 15 percent are from outside of Alberta. A total of 81 students completed at least four years of university.

STUDENT LIFE: Campus housing is available, though most students opt to live off campus in the surrounding area. The Students' Union provides a registry informing students of available housing. Medical students participate in clubs, events, and recreational activities geared toward medical students and the student body in general. Counseling and other support services are available to students, as are groups focused on special interests and minority groups. Edmonton is a medium-sized city, offering plenty of restaurants, shops, parks, theaters, sporting events, and outdoor activities. Though public transportation is available, most medical students own cars.

GRADUATES: Graduates enter both clinical medicine and research-oriented careers.

Admissions

REQUIREMENTS: Only applications from Canadians are accepted. All applicants should have completed at least sixty units of university course work (approximately two years of full-time studies). Requirements are six units each of General Chemistry, Organic Chemistry, Biology, Physics, and English, along with three units each of Statistics and Biochemistry. The MCAT is required and scores are valid for three years after the exam is taken. In addition to an application form, an autobiographical essay and two letters of reference are required.

SUGGESTIONS: Residency is an important consideration in admissions decisions. For admissions purposes, a resident of Alberta is defined as a Canadian Citizen or Permanent Resident who has lived in the Province of Alberta or Yukon or Northwest Territories for at least one continuous year immediately prior to the date of intended matriculation. At least 85 percent of available positions in an entering class are reserved for Alberta residents. The remaining 15 percent are available to other Canadians. Typically, successful applicants have completed four years of university with a grade point average of 7.0 on the University of Alberta's nine-point grading system. An MCAT score of less than 7 in any category is not accepted.

PROCESS: Requests for applications should be directed to the address above. Applications are accepted between July 1 and November 1 in the year preceding anticipated matriculation. The essay and reference letters must be received by January 15, and transcripts must be submitted by January 31. Interviews are conducted between February and March, and admissions decisions are made between May and July. For the 1998 entering class, 1011 students applied for 102 positions. Applicants who feel that they may merit special consideration (because of studies in a nontraditional area or unusual pattern) should write to the Admissions Officer outlining their situation and goals. All Native (Aboriginal) students interested in medical studies are encouraged to contact: Coordinator, Native Health Care Careers Program in care of the address above.

Cost

Tuition is approximately $5,000 per year for full-time medical students. Living expenses are around $12,000 per year, but vary considerably depending on lifestyle. (Note: All amounts are listed in Canadian dollars.)

FINANCIAL AID: Students finance their education with a combination of personal resources, earnings while in school, loans, research fellowships, and grants. About 70 percent of students receive some sort of financial aid.

UNIVERSITY OF ALBERTA

STUDENT BODY

Type	Public
# applied (total/out)	1,095
% interviewed	4/2

ADMISSIONS:

Average GPA and MCAT Scores

Overall GPA	10.6	Science	NR
MCAT Bio	10.8	MCAT Phys	11.3
MCAT Verba	9.7	MCAT Essays	NR

Application Information

Regular application	11/1
Regular notification	7/1
Transfer's accepted	NR
Admissions may be deferred	Yes
Interview required	Yes
Application fee	$60

COSTS AND AID

Tuition & Fees

Tuition	$7,289
Cost of books	$900
Fees	NR

Note: All fees and expenses are listed in Canadian dollars

UNIVERSITY OF BRITISH COLUMBIA

FACULTY OF MEDICINE

Admissions 317-2194 Health Sciences Mall

Vancouver, British Columbia V67 1Z3

Admissions: 604-822-4482

Internet: www.med.ubc.ca

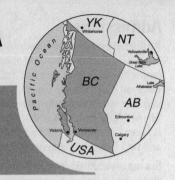

The University of British Columbia enrolls over 30,000 undergraduate, graduate, and professional students. The clinical and educational facilities of the Health Science Center are important components of the University. The Faculty of Medicine is situated within the Health Science Center, allowing medical students—even those in their first and second years—ongoing and consistent exposure to clinical medicine. The Faculty of Medicine is committed to the provision of educational programs characterized by strong scientific and clinical rationales, future-oriented content and technology, innovation, and relevance.

Academics

The four-year curriculum leading to the M.D. degree is integrated and comprehensive, designed to take advantage of the vast resources of the Faculty of Medicine. A new case-based curriculum that emphasizes problem solving and lifelong learning was introduced during the Fall of 1998. In addition to the M.D. program, graduate programs leading to Masters, Doctorate, and combined degrees are available.

BASIC SCIENCES: Basic sciences are taught along with introductory clinical concepts during the first two years. First-year courses include Introductory Clinical Skills and Systems 1; Doctor/Dentist; Patient & Society; Family Practice Continuum; Principles of Human Biology; Host Defenses &Infection; Cardiovascular System; Pulmonary; and Fluids, Electrolytes & Renal. Second-year courses include Clinical Skills & Systems II; Doctor/Dentist, Patient & Society; Family Practice Continuum; Blood and Lymphatic; Musculoskeletal and Locomotor; GI/Nutrition; Metabolism and Endocrine; Integument; Brain and Behavior and Reproduction; and Growth and Development. Basic sciences are taught primarily through small group forums, though lectures, computer-based instruction and labs are also utilized.

CLINICAL TRAINING: The third academic period begins with courses in Health Care and Epidemiology, Radiology, and Therapeutics. Following these three courses, students enter a sequence of required clerkships. These are: Orientation (4 weeks), Anesthesia (2 weeks), Dermatology (1 week), Emergency Medicine (4 weeks), Medicine (10 weeks), Ob/Gyn (8 weeks), Ophthalmology (1 week), Orthopedics (2 weeks), Pediatrics (8 weeks), Psychiatry (8 weeks), and Surgery (8 weeks). Six weeks are left open for electives during the third academic period. Sixteen weeks are left open for electives during the fourth academic period. A portion of electives may be completed at sites outside of the network of affiliates. Most clinical training takes place at affiliated institutions including the University Hospital, St. Paul's Hospital, British Columbia Children's Hospital, Vancouver General Hospital, British Columbia Women's Hospital and Health Center, British Columbia Cancer Agency, G.F. Strong Rehabilitation Center, and the Canadian Arthritis and Rheumatism Society Center.

Students

Each entering class has about 120 students. Approximately 50 percent of students are women. Typically, all but a handful of students in each class are from British Columbia.

STUDENT LIFE: Beyond a rich academic life, medical students enjoy the resources, facilities, and surroundings of the Health Science Center, the University of British Columbia, and the city of Vancouver. The Faculty of Medicine and the greater University offer a wide range of support services including counseling, special interest clubs and organizations, resources for minorities and international students, and day-care. There are ample opportunities for athletic, social, and recreational activities on campus. Students also enjoy the cultural and recreational aspects of Vancouver.

GRADUATES: A significant number of graduates enter residency programs at hospitals affiliated with the University of British Columbia. Though most graduates enter clinical medicine, others successfully pursue research and academic medicine.

Admissions

REQUIREMENTS: Applicants should have successfully completed a minimum of 90 credits or the equivalent of three years of full-time course work in any degree program at an accredited university. A minimum of a 70 percent academic average is required, and all undergraduate courses are included in this average. Prerequisites are one year each of university-level Biology, Biochemistry, Chemistry, Organic Chemistry, and English Literature and Composition. The MCAT is required. The exam should be taken no later than August of the year of application.

SUGGESTIONS: There is no preferred program of study for preparation for medical school. Often, due to the large number of applicants, the competitive average for successful applicants is much higher than 70 percent. MCAT scores of a recently admitted class averaged about 10. In addition to excellent academic qualifications, admission decisions are based on applicants' personal characteristics such as motivation and integrity. Last year, 695 applications were received for 120 positions.

Cost

Yearly tuition for Canadian residents is about $5,500 (Canadian dollars) per year.

FINANCIAL AID: A number of sources of financial assistance are available. Loans and some grants are available through government entities, typically offered on the basis of financial need. The Faculty offers fellowships, research assistantships, teaching assistantships, loans, and paid internships. Institutionally sponsored aid is offered on the basis of need, merit, and other criteria such as area of professional interest.

UNIVERSITY OF BRITISH COLUMBIA

STUDENT BODY

Type	Public
*Enrollment	120
*% male/female	NR
*% underrepresented minorities	NR
# applied (total/out)	621/145
% interviewed (total/out)	63/1
% accepted (total/out)	NR/NR
% enrolled (total/out)	NR/NR
Average age	23

ADMISSIONS

Average GPA and MCAT Scores

Overall GPA	82%	Science GPA	80%
MCAT Bio	10.4	MCAT Phys	10.1
MCAT Verbal	9.5	MCAT Essay	Q

Score Release Policy

The school has not responded to our inquiry regarding withheld MCAT scores. Therefore, we advise caution. Contact the Admissions Office before withholding any scores.

Application Information

Regular application	10/1
Regular notification	3/1
Transfers accepted?	Yes
Admissions may be deferred?	Yes
Interview required?	Yes
Application fee (in/out)	$105/$155

COSTS AND AID

Tuition & Fees

Tuition (in/out)	$4,000
Cost of books	$1,200
Fees	$256

Note: All fees and expenses are listed in Canadian dollars
*Figures based on total enrollment

University of Calgary

FACULTY OF MEDICINE

3330 Hospital Drive NW, Calgary, Alberta T2N 4N1
Admission: 403-220-4262
Internet: www.ucalgary.ca

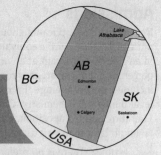

The Faculty of Medicine at the University of Calgary is known internationally for both research and teaching. It is somewhat unique in offering a three-year program leading to the M.D. degree. The curriculum emphasizes problem solving, lifelong learning skills, clinical medicine, and flexibility such that students may tailor their education to suit particular talents and interests. Though priority is given to Canadian citizens who are residents of Alberta, applications are accepted from residents of other Canadian provinces and international students.

Academics

Medical students follow an intensive, eleven-month curriculum for a period of three years. Learning is based in part on clinical case presentations. In addition to the standard M.D. course of study, programs are offered in conjunction with the Faculty of Graduate Studies in Biomedical and Health Sciences with the objective of training clinician-scientists for academic medical research and those who will design, manage, and implement health care delivery programs. M.D./Ph.D. and M.D./M.Sc. programs are available in Biochemistry and Molecular Biology, Cardiovascular/Respiratory Sciences, Community Health Sciences, Gastrointestinal Sciences, Medical Science, Microbiology and Infectious Diseases, and Neuroscience.

BASIC SCIENCES: First-year courses are based on organ systems and are taught primarily through lectures and small group discussions. Subjects are: Principles for Medicine, Blood, Musculoskeletal and Skin, Cardiovascular, Respiratory, Renal-Electrolyte, Endocrine Metabolic, Medical Skills Program, and Integrative. The second academic period begins in July. Subjects are: Neuroscience, The Mind, Gastrointestinal, Reproduction, Human Development, and Medical Skills Program. Throughout the first and second years, students also take part in independent research projects. Courses are taught in the Calgary Health Sciences Center, about 1.5 km from the main campus of the University of Calgary. The medical library is fully computerized, receives more than 1,000 serials, and houses approximately 130,000 books. It serves medical and nursing students as well as the greater university and the medical community. Other important facilities include the Medical Learning Resource Center that houses instructional tools geared towards learning anatomical systems, and the Medical Skills Center for improving clinical skills and techniques.

CLINICAL TRAINING: Required clerkships are Anesthesia (2 weeks), Family Medicine (4 weeks), Internal Medicine (12 weeks), Ob/Gyn (6 weeks), Pediatrics (6 weeks), Psychiatry (6 weeks), and Surgery (8 weeks). Ten weeks are available for clinical electives. Training takes place primarily at the facilities of the Foothills Hospital, the Peter Lougheed Center, the Alberta Children's Hospital, and the Rockyview Hospital. In addition, the University of Calgary Medical Clinic allows medical students to learn about outpatient service delivery, preventative programs, and travel medicine.

Students

While medical students are primarily Canadian, the student body at the University of Calgary includes several hundred international students. Within the Faculty of Medicine, women comprise about 50 percent of students. The majority of medical students are from within the province of Alberta.

STUDENT LIFE: Student life is enhanced by campus activities, the resources of the community and city of Calgary, and the wide range of outdoor activities available. Nearby national parks, such as Banff and Jasper, offer skiing and hiking. The region also has vibrant wildlife and areas for fishing, swimming, and canoeing. In addition to its academic facilities, the Health Sciences Center includes a medical bookstore, exercise room, student lounge, cafeteria, and mall area. Medical students also have access to the resources of the greater university, including complete athletic and recreational facilities, intramural sports programs, outdoor programs, arts, and theater. The university student union organizes events and activities and operates a bookstore, café, and bar, along with other services. On-campus housing is available for single and married students. An off-campus housing registry is managed by the student union.

Graduates: Though most graduates enter postgraduate training that leads to careers in clinical medicine, some go on to pursue research and academic medicine. Increasingly, graduates are entering primary care fields.

Admissions

Requirements: Students must have completed at least two full years of university education before being considered for admission. The minimum grade requirement is an average of 3.0/4.0, which translates to a grade of B or at least 78 percent for each year of study. The MCAT is required, and applicants should have at least an average score of 8. In addition to transcripts and a completed application form, three letters of reference are required.

Suggestions: Although the Faculty has no prescribed prerequisites, the one year of each of the following courses is strongly recommended: English, Biology, General Chemistry, Organic Chemistry, Biochemistry, Physics, Physiology, Calculus, and Psychology/Sociology. Presently, spaces for international students are limited to those students who come from institutions and/or countries with which the Faculty of Medicine at the University of Calgary has a formal, contractual agreement. All international students must sign an acknowledgment that the M.D. program would not lead to an opportunity for postgraduate training through the Canadian Resident Matching Service.

Process: The application is in the form of a computer disk. It requires information about all university courses taken, MCAT test dates/results, employment history, extracurricular activities, and an essay. The completed application is due November 15. The deadline for receipt of the three letters of reference, all official transcripts, and official MCAT scores is January 4. Applicants will be notified by March 15 whether or not they will be invited for an interview. In a recent year, there were 1,300 applicants for 69 positions.

Cost

(Note: all figures in Canadian dollars) Tuition for residents is $6,332 per year, and for international students is $30,000 per year. The annual cost of living is about $10,000 per year.

Financial Aid: Alberta government loans and grants are available only to Canadian citizens who have lived for twelve consecutive months in Alberta. A number of awards are offered by the Faculty and private donors based on financial need, merit, field of study, or a combination of these conditions.

UNIVERSITY OF CALGARY

STUDENT BODY

Type	Public
*Enrollment	234
*% male/female	48/52
*% underrepresented minorities	NR
# applied (total/out)	1,314/784
% interviewed (total/out)	17/17
% accepted (total/out)	5/3
% enrolled (total/out)	5/3
Average age	25

ADMISSIONS

Average GPA and MCAT Scores

Overall GPA	3.50	Science GPA	NR
MCAT Bio	10.67	MCAT Phys	10.48
MCAT Verbal	9.77	MCAT Essay	Q

Score Release Policy

The school has not responded to our inquiry regarding withheld MCAT scores. Therefore, we advise caution. Contact the Admissions Office before withholding any scores.

Application Information

Regular application	11/15
Regular notification	5/14
Transfers accepted?	Yes
Admissions may be deferred?	Yes
Interview required?	Yes
Application fee	$65

COSTS AND AID

Tuition & Fees

Tuition (in/out)	$6,519/$30,000
Cost of books	$1,200
Fees	$333

Note: All fees and expenses are listed in Canadian dollars
*Figures based on total enrollment

DALHOUSIE UNIVERSITY
FACULTY OF MEDICINE CLINICAL RESEARCH CENTER

5849 University Ave. Room C–132, Halifax, Nova Scotia B3H 4H7

Admission: 902-494-1083

Internet: www.dal.ca

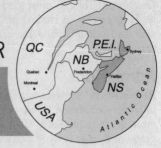

The Medical School of Dalhousie University was founded over 125 years ago. It is located near Dalhousie's other health professional faculties and schools, such as the schools of Dentistry, Nursing, and Occupational Therapy. The Medical School at Dalhousie is the sole academic medical institution serving Nova Scotia, New Brunswick, and Prince Edward Island. It plays a leading role in national and international medical research and is active in community and economic development as well as clinical care.

Academics

The progressive Case-Oriented Problem-Stimulated (COPS) curriculum, which was introduced in 1992, prepares students for the pressures and problems facing physicians today. The COPS curriculum uses real-life patient cases and is based on a tutorial system that emphasizes group learning, contextual learning, communication skills, and clinical interaction with patients. In addition to the M.D. curriculum, programs leading to Masters and Ph.D. degrees are offered. Some students opt for a combined degree program, earning both an M.D. and a graduate degree in a biomedical or related field.

BASIC SCIENCES: In their first two years, students are organized into small groups and build their basic science knowledge by examining matter relevant to patient cases. Faculty/staff tutors guide the group's learning process. Students also choose specific areas of medicine for an elective period and begin to acquire clinical skills in the first month of school. The first academic period lasts 40 weeks and covers the following subjects: Human Body; Metabolism and Function; Pathology, Immunology and Microbiology; Genetics, Embryology and Reproduction; Pharmacology; and Population Health. During the second academic period, students learn Brain and Behavior; Skin, Glands, and Blood; Respiratory and Cardiovascular; Genitourinary, Gastrointestinal, and Musculoskeletal; and Clinical Epidemiology and Biostatistics. Throughout the first and second years, students have ongoing patient contact through the Patient-Doctor unit and have the opportunity to take elective courses. Teaching, research, and administration take place within two buildings, the Sir Charles Tupper Medical Building and the Clinical Research Center. The Patient-Doctor sessions are organized within the hospitals and pair the students with a clinical preceptor each week. The students gain exposure to pediatrics, psychiatry, and various disciplines of medicine.

The Kellogg Health Sciences Library houses more than 150,000 books and journals. The library is fully computerized and provides links to other libraries on campus.

CLINICAL TRAINING: Beginning in September 1999, a new clerkship will be implemented. The clerkship is organized into two phases, each of which has a central theme. All clerks will begin in a one-month Introduction to Clerkship unit in which clinical skills, procedures, history-taking, and physical-taking skills will be reviewed for all students. Phase 1 includes Medicine, Surgery, Obstetrics and Gynecology, Pediatrics, Family Medicine, and Psychiatry. Each unit will be accountable for integrating objectives from other disciplines, and ambulatory and community experiences will be expected. Phase 2 begins with rotations offering the clerks maximum choice or remediation depending on their performance. In the final unit, Continuing and Preventive Care, clerks are required to complete three-week rotations in Long Term Care of the Elderly and again have an opportunity for a choice of rotations. Clerks will be evaluated frequently to receive feedback on their progress to guide self-directed learning. The major teaching hospitals are within walking distance of the school. They include a 202-bed pediatric hospital, a 254-bed obstetrics hospital, a psychiatric hospital, a rehabilitation center, and two large tertiary care adult hospitals. Other affiliated hospitals, clinics, and outpatient facilities also provide important training sites for medical students.

Students

Each entering class has 82 students. In a recent class, 74 students were from the Maritime provinces and 8 were from non-Maritime regions. At least 50 percent of students are women.

STUDENT LIFE: Although the academic workload is heavy, students are encouraged to pursue nonacademic interests. All students belong to the Dalhousie Medical School Society (DMSS), which promotes the interests of medical undergraduates. The DMSS organizes social and sporting events and raises money to support various nonprofit organizations. Through the Student Advisory, students have access to informal counseling, activities, and organized discussions that are coordinated and sponsored by other students. Dalhousie offers a variety of housing options on campus including residencies, singles rooms, and shared apartments. Outside of the campus, the city of Halifax offers a wide variety of entertainment, leisure, and shopping activities.

GRADUATES: Many graduates choose to enter postgraduate training at Dalhousie. Areas of training include Family Practice, numerous surgical and medical specialties, and laboratory medicine.

Admissions

REQUIREMENTS: The MCAT is required, and scores cannot be more than five years old. A baccalaureate degree is required for entrance to Dalhousie. There are no absolute prerequisite courses, though a minimal science background is advisable for success on the MCAT. Maritime applicants (those from Nova Scotia, New Brunswick, and Prince Edward Island) should have a minimum academic average of a B+, while non-Maritime applicants should have at least an A– average.

SUGGESTIONS: Applicants from non-Maritime provinces and countries other than Canada should be exceptionally qualified. In addition to place of residence and academic credentials, the Admissions Committee reviews recommendations, results of personal interviews, and the applicant's extracurricular interests and activities.

PROCESS: For applications and details on the admissions cycle, contact the Admissions Coordinator at the phone number and/or address above.

Cost

(Note: All amounts are listed in Canadian dollars.) Annual tuition and fees amount to about $6,575. Textbooks and instruments cost about $1,000 during the first year, and slightly less thereafter.

FINANCIAL AID: Assistance is available in the form of bursaries, prizes, and interest-free loans. Some financial aid is awarded solely to residents of Maritime provinces. Summer research grants are available, offering support of approximately $4,000 for the twelve-week period.

DALHOUSIE UNIVERSITY

STUDENT BODY

Type	Private
*Enrollment	NR
*% male/female	NR
*% underrepresented minorities	NR
# applied (total/out)	551/317
% interviewed (total/out)	37/6
% accepted (total/out)	NR/NR
% enrolled (total/out)	NR/NR

ADMISSIONS

Average GPA and MCAT Scores

Overall GPA	NR	Science GPA	NR
MCAT Bio	NR	MCAT Phys	NR
MCAT Verbal	NR	MCAT Essay	NR

Score Release Policy

The Admissions Office says that withholding scores is not recommended.

Application Information

Regular application	11/15
Regular notification	2/1
Transfers acceped	NR
Admissions may be deferred?	Yes
†Interview required?	Yes
Application fee	$60

COSTS AND AID

Tuition & Fees

Tuition (in/out)	$6,575/$9,300
Cost of books	$1,000
Fees	$225

† Selected applicants only

Note: All fees and expenses are listed in Canadian dollars

*Figures based on total enrollment

Université Laval

FACULTY OF MEDICINE

Sainte-Foy, Quebec GlK 7P4
Admissions: 418-656-2131
Internet: www.ulaval.ca

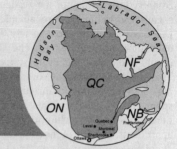

Laval is a comprehensive university with over 30,000 undergraduate, graduate, and professional students. The Faculty of Medicine is the oldest of the Francophone medical schools in North America. Students at the Faculty of Medicine enjoy the resources of the medical school, Laval's health science departments, the greater university, and the surrounding community. Important goals of the Faculty of Medicine include advancing research, promoting leadership, and providing clinical care to the people of Quebec. Fluency in French is a prerequisite for admission.

Academics

Laval offers a four-year curriculum leading to the M.D. degree. In addition, academic programs are available in a number of health and medical science fields including Molecular Biology, Community Health, Epidemiology, Occupational Health and Safety, and Physiology. Research is an important part of the academic experience at Laval, and students are encouraged to pursue research during summers and throughout the academic year.

BASIC SCIENCES: The first two years involve basic science instruction and opportunities for addressing clinical problems. The first year includes courses in Biochemistry, Physiology, Pharmacology, Microbiology-Immunology, Histology-Pathology, and Introduction to Problems. During the second part of the first year, instruction is organized around anatomical systems and medical concepts. These are Cardiovascular System, Respiratory System, Uro-nephrology, Microbiology/Infectious Disease, and Physiological/Sociological. Introduction to Problems continues during the second semester. Students also study Endocrinology, Ob/Gyn, and Growth/Development during their first year. Year two subjects are Nervous System, Locomotor System, Medical Ethics, Problem Discussion, The Art of Interviewing, ENT, Ophthalmology, Hematology, Gastroenterology, Psychopathology, Preventive Medicine, and Skin. Laval's library system is an important academic resource for students, holding millions of volumes and periodicals.

CLINICAL TRAINING: Years three and four are devoted to clinical rotations. Required clerkships are Introduction to Clinical Medicine (9 weeks), Medicine (8 weeks), Surgery (8 weeks), Pediatrics (8 weeks), Psychiatry (8 weeks), Ob/Gyn (8 weeks), Preventive Medicine (4 weeks), Geriatrics/Rehabilitation Medicine (4 weeks), Family Practice (4 weeks), and Emergency Medicine (4 weeks). In addition, up to 20 weeks are open for various clinical and basic science electives. Training takes place at a number of affiliated hospitals including Centre Hospitalier de l'Universite Laval, Hopital Laval, Hopital de l'Enfant-Jesus, Hotel-Dieu de Levis, Hotel-Dieu de Quebec, Hopital du Saint-Sacrement and Hopital Saint-Francois d'Assie.

Students

Each entering class at the Faculty of Medicine is comprised of about 112 students. Typically, all but a few are from within the province of Quebec. Students from other provinces must be French speakers. Within the student body are a limited number of international, French-speaking students. Women make up about 60 percent of the students.

STUDENT LIFE: Laval supports medical students both inside and outside the classroom. Programs offered include orientation and counseling services, religious organizations, career placement services, social and athletic organizations, childcare, and attractive, low-cost student housing. The Laval campus is situated in an urban environment.

GRADUATES: Graduates of Laval Faculty of Medicine enter both clinical and academic medicine. The teaching hospitals affiliated with Laval offer many programs for graduate medical training.

Admissions

REQUIREMENTS: Generally, all applicants must have completed at least two years of college to be considered for admission. Required undergraduate courses are Biology (8 semester hours), General Chemistry (8 semester hours), Organic Chemistry (8 semester hours), General Physics (2 hours), and Mathematics including Calculus (2 hours). In addition, some course work in French, Humanities, and Social Sciences is required. Fluency in French is a requirement for admission.

Suggestions: Priority is given to residents of the province of Quebec. Candidates are evaluated on the basis of academic achievement, interpersonal skills, experience, and personal characteristics. Although two years of college is the minimum requirement, additional schooling serves to strengthen applications.

Process: Applications are coordinated in part by the organization of Quebec Colleges and Universities. For entrance in the Fall, the application deadline is March 1. In addition to a written application, interviews are an important part of the selection process. Generally, about 10 to 15 percent of applicants are accepted in a given year.

Cost

(Note: All amounts are listed in Canadian dollars.) Yearly tuition for residents of Canada is very low compared to that of other medical schools. It is about $2,000. For nonresidents, the rate is about $9,000. Student housing helps to reduce the cost of living for medical students.

Financial Aid: Financial aid in the form of bursaries is available from the province. Other grants and loans may be funded by the University and occasionally by private sources. Some students are eligible for special scholarships offered on the basis of academic merit. Others receive funding in the form of small stipends or grants for summer research projects.

UNIVERSITÉ LAVAL

STUDENT BODY

Type	Public
*Enrollment	NR
*% male/female	NR
*% underrepresented minorities	NR
# applied (total/out)	1,525/123
% interviewed (total/out)	21/1
% accepted (total/out)	NR/NR
% enrolled (total/out)	NR/NR
Average age	NR

ADMISSIONS

Average GPA and MCAT Scores

Overall GPA	NR	Science GPA	NR
MCAT Bio	NR	MCAT Phys	NR
MCAT Verbal	NR	MCAT Essay	NR

Score Release Policy

The Admissions Committee will suspect that student did poorly if they withhold scores, so they do not recommend doing so.

Application Information

Regular application	3/1 in Quebec
	2/1 others
Regular notification	5/15
Transfers accepted	NR
Admissions may be deferred?	No
Interview required?	Yes
Application fee	$65

COSTS AND AID

Tuition & Fees

Tuition (in/out)	$1,964/7,927
Cost of books	NR
Fees	$200

Note: All fees and expenses are listed in Canadian dollars
*Figures based on total enrollment

UNIVERSITY OF MANITOBA

FACULTY OF MEDICINE

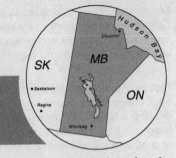

753 McDermot Avenue, Winnipeg, Manitoba R3E 0W3

Admissions: 204-789-3569 • Fax: 204-789-3929

Email: registrar_med@umanitoba.ca

Medical education began in Manitoba in 1883 when the Manitoba Medical College was established. Shortly thereafter, the College became a Faculty of the University of Manitoba. The Faculty is located at the Bannatyne Campus of the University, in the heart of Winnipeg and adjacent to the Health Sciences Centre, the major tertiary care facility in Manitoba and a major clinical teaching facility. The mission of the Faculty is to assist students to become competent, caring, ethical physicians with the ability to think critically and ultimately to meet their responsibility to their patients and society.

Academics

Medical students complete a four-year curriculum leading to the M.D. degree. Classes during the first two years are largely systems-based. Small groups are the predominant format for instruction, though lectures, labs, computer-based learning, and early clinical exposure are also important educational tools. The second two years are spent in clinical clerkships.

BASIC SCIENCES: The first academic period begins in September and lasts 35 weeks. It is divided into Core Concepts (Health and Medicine, Structure and Function and Survival Mechanisms); Human Development; Systems (Cardiovascular, Respiratory, Dermatology, ENT); Clinical/Communications Skills; and Medical Humanities. The second academic period is organized around anatomical and physiological systems. These are: Reproduction, Endocrine, Renal, Neuroscience, Musculoskeletal, Ophthalmology, Gastrointestinal, Liver, and Blood/Lymphoid. Students also continue first year studies in Clinical/Communication Skills and Medical Humanities.

CLINICAL TRAINING: During their third and fourth years, students complete required clinical clerkships. These are: Family/Community Medicine (7 weeks), Internal Medicine (12 weeks), Ob/Gyn (7 weeks), Pediatrics (7 weeks), Psychiatry (7 weeks), Surgery (9 weeks), Anesthesia (2 weeks), Emergency Medicine (4 weeks), and Ophthalmology/ENT (1 week). Fifteen weeks are available for clinical electives. Teaching hospitals include those of the Health Sciences Centre (comprised of the Children's, Adult's, Women's, and Respiratory and Rehabilitation Hospitals with a total of over 1,000 beds), St. Boniface General Hospital (900 beds), Deer Lodge Veterans Hospital (500 beds), Grace Hospital (306 beds), Steven Oaks Hospital (336 beds), Victoria Hospital (254 beds), Misericordia Hospital (409 beds), and the Diabetes Research and Treatment Center.

Students

In the entering class of 1998, approximately 40 percent of students are women. The average age of incoming students was 23.4 years. All students have Bachelors degrees.

STUDENT LIFE: Medical students often choose to live in an apartment complex operated by the Health Sciences Centre. Other options include dormitories and off-campus housing which is facilitated by listings available through the off-campus housing office. Recreational activities and events are sponsored by the student union. In addition, numerous student groups and organizations offer medical students a wide range of social and community-based activities.

Admissions

REQUIREMENTS: Applicants must have or be eligible to receive their Bachelor's degree by June 30, 1999 from a university recognized by the University of Manitoba. Applicants must have completed a full course of English or French and a full course of Biochemistry at the university level and received a grade of C or higher. Two full courses in Humanities/Social Sciences are also required. The MCAT is required and should be taken within the past three years but no later than August of the year of application. Students usually prepare for the MCAT by taking university courses in Physics, Organic and Physical Chemistry, and Biology.

SUGGESTIONS: Priority is given to residents of Manitoba who are Canadian citizens or Permanent Residents. The most successful applicants have grade point averages between 3.8–4.2 on a 4.5 scale and at least an 8 on each scored section of the MCAT. In addition to academic and intellectual credentials, the Admissions Committee selects applicants who demonstrate social skills, maturity, and a sense of responsibility. The Admissions Committee selects

70 students for admission out of about 400 applicants. Typically, about seven places are offered to applicants from outside Manitoba.

PROCESS: For application material, contact the Faculty at the following email: admissions@umanitoba.ca or call: (204) 474-8808. The application deadline is November 16. Applicants who meet scholastic and MCAT requirements will be invited to interview and submit a personal statement. About 150 applicants are interviewed, and from this group the class is selected in early June. There is a special consideration category for some Manitoba residents who fall into one of the following three groups: those who are sponsored by Faculty-approved agencies, those who are from native populations of Manitoba, and those who have been employed for two or more years in the areas of health, social welfare, or health education.

Cost

(Note: All amounts are listed in Canadian dollars.) Tuition for 1998/99 was $6,780. Books and supplies amounted to $3,100. Room and board in campus residences is about $4,000 for an eight-month period.

FINANCIAL AID: Over 60 percent of medical students receive financial aid from the Canada Student Loan Program and the Manitoba Government Loan Program. Eligible applicants may receive up to $275 per week for the 39-week study period. In addition, the Faculty provides bursaries and scholarships to eligible applicants. Loans from several sources are also available.

UNIVERSITY OF MANITOBA

STUDENT BODY

Type	Public
*Enrollment	NR
*% male/female	NR
*% underrepresented minorities	NR
# applied (total/out)	385/230
% interviewed (total/out)	39/8
% accepted (total/out)	7/54
% enrolled (total/out)	43/50
Average age	23

ADMISSIONS

Average GPA and MCAT Scores

Overall GPA	NR	Science GPA	NR
MCAT Bio	NR	MCAT Phys	NR
MCAT Verbal	NR	MCAT Essay	NR

Score Release Policy

The school has not responded to our inquiry regarding withheld MCAT scores. Therefore, we advise caution. Contact the Admissions Office before withholding any scores.

Application Information

Regular application	11/15
Regular notification	6/6
Transfers accepted?	Yes
Admissions may be deferred?	Yes
AMCAS application accepted?	No
Interview required?	Yes
Application fee	$50

COSTS AND AID

Tuition & Fees

Tuition	$6,981
Cost of books	NR
Fees	$41

Note: All fees and expenses are listed in Canadian dollars
*Figures based on total enrollment

MCGILL UNIVERSITY
FACULTY OF MEDICINE

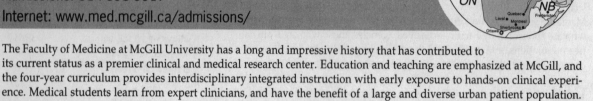

3655 Drummond Street, Montreal, Quebec H3G IY6
Admissions: 514-398-3517
Internet: www.med.mcgill.ca/admissions/

The Faculty of Medicine at McGill University has a long and impressive history that has contributed to its current status as a premier clinical and medical research center. Education and teaching are emphasized at McGill, and the four-year curriculum provides interdisciplinary integrated instruction with early exposure to hands-on clinical experience. Medical students learn from expert clinicians, and have the benefit of a large and diverse urban patient population.

Academics

The curriculum recognizes the importance of a solid database and a multidisciplinary approach to medical education with integration of clinical and basic science experience. It is designed to permit a variety of teaching and evaluation methods recognizing the importance of small-group teaching and clinical relevance of material. Flexibility in the program permits opportunities for research and for a range of ongoing clinical inpatient and ambulatory care experience. The curriculum is composed of four components entitled Basis of Medicine, Introduction to Clinical Medicine, Practice of Medicine, and Back to Basics. Though most students complete a four-year program leading to the M.D. degree, joint degree programs are also offered. An M.D./Ph.D. program is open to qualified students interested in a research career in academic medicine. For students interested in both medicine and health management, the faculties of Medicine and Management offer a five year program leading to an M.D./M.B.A. degree.

BASIC SCIENCES: The first academic period begins in September and continues through December of the second year. The theme of the first academic period is Basis of Medicine, and courses are organized into blocks. These are: Molecules, Cells, and Tissues (4 weeks); Gas, Fluids, and Electrolytes (9 weeks); Life Cycle (3 weeks); Endocrinology, Metabolism, and Nutrition (7 weeks); Musculoskeletal and Blood (4 weeks); Nervous System and Special Senses (8 weeks); Host Defense and Host Parasite (8 weeks); and Pathobiology, Treatment and Prevention of Disease.

CLINICAL TRAINING: The second academic period, Introduction to Clinical Medicine (ICM), begins in January of the second year and goes through September of the third year. ICM takes place in hospitals and outpatient clinical settings. Topics covered are Introduction to Clinical Sciences, Medical Ethics, Health Law, Medicine, Family Medicine, Geriatric Medicine, Neurology, Surgery, Emergency

Medicine, Anesthesia, Radiology, Introduction to Hospital Practice, Pediatrics, Psychiatry, Ob/Gyn, and an elective. During the third academic period, Practice of Medicine, students rotate through required clerkships. These are Medicine (8 weeks), Surgery (8 weeks), Psychiatry (8 weeks), Psychiatry (8 weeks), Ob/Gyn (8 weeks), Pediatrics (8 weeks), Family Medicine (4 weeks), and Electives/Selectives (16 weeks). The final academic period is Back to Basics. During this 16-week session, students take Medicine and Society, Topics in Medical Science, and Ambulatory Care. Teaching hospitals include Montreal General Hospital, Montreal Children's Hospital, Montreal Neurological Hospital, Sir Mortimer B. Davis-Jewish General Hospital, Douglas Hospital, and Royal Victoria Hospital. Training also takes place at a number of affiliated hospitals and other clinical care centers.

Students

Each entering class has about 110 students. Typically, 25 percent of students are non-Canadians, most of whom are from the U.S. About 50 percent of students are women.

STUDENT LIFE: McGill is a large and active campus that offers social and recreational activities to a diverse student body. In addition, the city of Montreal itself is an interesting and exciting place for students to live. McGill has four co-educational residences and one women's residence located on the main campus, which are open to medical students. Information concerning apartments or flats located in the vicinity of the campus can be obtained from the Off-Campus Housing Office.

Admissions

The Faculty of Medicine offers a four-year undergraduate medical curriculum. Students are ordinarily admitted into the first year of this program, but admission is also available by means of a Med-P program directly after CEGEP. The faculty does not accept students for part-time medical studies.

An M.D.-Ph.D. program is offered for students interested in a research career in academic medicine. For students interested in both medicine and management, the faculties of medicine and management offer a five-year program leading to an M.D.-M.B.A. degree. The language of instruction is English.

REQUIREMENTS: Applicants must have received an undergraduate degree or be in the final year of a course of study at a recognized college or university leading to an undergraduate degree with at least 120 academic credits. Prerequisites include one year with laboratory work in each of General Biology, General Chemistry, Organic Chemistry, and Physics. The MCAT is required and applicants must have taken the exam no later than August 1999.

SUGGESTIONS: In addition to prerequisite science courses, some course work in Biochemistry or Molecular Biology is strongly recommended. Applicants to the four-year program should have undergraduate GPAs of 3.5 or better and a total of 30 or more in the MCAT scores. In a recent entering class, the average GPA was a 3.7 and the average overall MCAT score was 31.10.

PROCESS: The deadline for receipt of applications to the regular M.D. program is January 15 for Quebec residents and November 15 for all others. Applicants with strong academic qualifications submit an application that includes an autobiographical letter used to assess personal qualities and achievements. Selection for interview is based on grades, MCAT scores, letters of reference, and autobiographical letter. Once interviews have been completed, all the components of the application are considered in making admissions decisions. Residents of Quebec will be notified after May 1. Nonresidents will be notified as soon as possible after March 31.

Cost

(Note: Amounts are listed in Canadian dollars.) Tuition and fees for first year medical students amounts to $4,565 for Quebec residents, $7,125 for other Canadians, and $20,497 for international students.

FINANCIAL AID: Eligible medical students may receive grants, loans and/ or research assistantships. Students who achieve high academic standing in the course of their studies may be considered for university scholarship and awards.

McGILL UNIVERSITY

STUDENT BODY

Type	Public
*Enrollment	NR
*% male/female	NR
*% underrepresented minorities	NR
# applied (total/out)	946/382
% interviewed (total/out)	34/13
% accepted (total/out)	NR/NR
% enrolled (total/out)	NR/NR
Average age	NR

ADMISSIONS

Average GPA and MCAT Scores

Overall GPA	3.7	Science GPA	NR
MCAT Bio	NR	MCAT Phys	NR
MCAT Verbal	NR	MCAT Essay	NR

Score Release Policy

Withholding scores is not recommended. The school needs to see all MCAT scores.

Application Information

Regular application	11/15
Regular notification	3/31
Transfers accepted?	No
Admissions may be deferred?	Yes
Interview required?	Yes
Application fee	$60

COSTS AND AID

Tuition & Fees

Tuition (in/out)	$4,565/$7,125
Tuition (US and International)	$20,497
Cost of books	NR
Fees	$799

Financial Aid

% students receiving aid	100
Average grant	$16,085
Average loan	$14,956
Average debt	$56,485

Note: All fees and expenses are listed
in Canadian dollars
*Figures based on total enrollment

MCMASTER UNIVERSITY

SCHOOL OF MEDICINE

HSC 1B7-Health Sciences Centre, 1200 Main Street West
Hamilton, Ontario L8N 325
Admissions: 905-525-9140 • Fax: 905-527-2707 ext. 22235
Email: mdadmit@fhs.csu.mcmaster.ca • Internet: www-fhs.mcmaster.ca/mdprog

The School of Medicine is part of the Faculty of Health Sciences, which also offers educational programs in nursing, health sciences, occupational therapy, physiotherapy, and midwifery. The aim of the undergraduate medical program is to provide students with a general professional education as physicians that is applicable to careers in both clinical and academic medicine. The overriding objective is to teach students to identify, analyze, and manage clinical problems in order to provide effective, efficient, and humane patient care. McMaster was the first school to introduce problem-based learning, a successful and popular teaching methodology currently used by many top-ranking medical schools. The medical school is fully accredited by the Committee on Accreditation of Canadian Medical Schools (CACMS) of the Association of Canadian Medical Colleges and the Liaison Committee on Medical Education (LCME) of the Association of American Medical Colleges. These accreditations mean that the medical school is equivalent in every respect to other schools in Canada and the United States.

Academics

The three-year program in Medicine uses a problem-based approach to learning that emphasizes skills, knowledge, critical thinking, independent study, professional behavior, and lifelong learning. The components have been organized in sequential units with early exposure to patients and case management. Flexibility is ensured to allow for the variety of student backgrounds and career goals. In addition to required units, electives form an integral part of the curriculum. Full-time elective blocks, ongoing horizontal electives, and special enrichment electives are all important components of the medical education.

The three-year program (130 weeks of instruction) uses an approach to learning that will apply throughout the physician's career. The components have been organized in a relevant and logical manner with early exposure to patients. Flexibility is ensured to allow for the variety of student backgrounds and career goals. The graduates of McMaster's Undergraduate Medical Programme will have developed the knowledge, ability, and attitudes necessary to qualify for further education in any medical career. The general goals for students in the program include the following: the development of competency in problem-based learning and in problem solving; the development of the personal characteristics and attitudes compatible with effective health care; the development of clinical and communication skills; and the development of the skills to be a lifelong, self-directed learner. To achieve the objectives of the Undergraduate Medical Programme, students are introduced to patients and their problems within the first unit. They are presented with a series of health care problems and questions requiring the understanding of principles and data collection. Much of the students' learn-

ing occurs within the setting of the small-group tutorial. Faculty members serve as tutors/facilitators or as sources of expert knowledge. The Undergraduate Medical Programme is arranged as a four-unit pre-clerkship sequence followed by a clerkship; there are additional elective opportunities, both in block periods (totaling 26 weeks) and horizontal electives taken concurrently with ongoing units. Unit 1 is a 12-week introduction to concepts and information from three knowledge perspectives: population, behavior, and biology. In addition, a major theme of the entire curriculum, the life cycle, is developed as a perspective and anchors the three subunits of Unit 1: Early Development, Maturation, and Aging. Units 2, 3, and 4 are 14-week units organized on the basis of organ systems, where biomedical and health care problems are analyzed in depth. The clerkship emphasizes the clinical application of concepts learned in the earlier units and consists of experience in inpatient and ambulatory settings. These concepts include internal medicine, family medicine, surgery, psychiatry, obstetrics-gynecology, and pediatrics. Unit 6, which follows the clerkship, will be an interactive unit in which students will tackle issues derived from societal expectations of a practicing physician.

Students

Each entering class has 100 students. In a recent entering class, 94 were from Ontario, and 6 were from the rest of Canada. About one third of the class is over 25, with an age range of 20–40. In this class, the male/female ratio was 33/62. Beginning in the fall of 2000, McMaster will also admit up to 10 students from a new international applicant pool.

STUDENT LIFE: The teaching methodology and general approach at McMaster fosters student interaction, which carries over outside of the classroom. Medical students take part in extra-curricular activities including clubs, athletics, and community service. Off-campus housing is available.

GRADUATES: Postgraduate programs are offered at McMaster in Anesthesia, Community Medicine, Critical Care, Emergency Medicine, Family Medicine, Internal Medicine, Laboratory Medicine, Ob/Gyn, Pediatrics, Psychiatry, Radiology, and Surgery.

Admissions

Regular Applicant Pool

REQUIREMENTS: At the time of entrance, students must have completed a minimum of three years of undergraduate work. Only degree credit courses taken at an accredited university are considered. Applicants must have achieved an overall simple average of at least a 3.0 on a 4.0 scale in their academic work at the time of application. There are no specific prerequisite courses and the MCAT is not required. Students granted admission must be proficient in spoken and written English. All students are required to have obtained a current certificate in Basic Cardiac Life Support prior to registration in the medical program.

GEOGRAPHICAL STATUS: Priority is given to residents of Ontario and then to applicants from the rest of Canada. International students through this applicant pool are invited for interview only if judged superior to other applicants in each selection criterion.

PROCESS: The application and transcript deadline for submission to OMSAS is October 16. Approximately 400 applicants are invited for interviews at McMaster in March or April. All applicants are notified in writing on the last day of May as to the results of their application.

International Applicant Pool

McMaster has developed an international applicant pool to admit up to 10 students (in addition to the 100 in the regular pool) with its first intake in the fall of 2000.

REQUIREMENTS: Applicants must have completed and undergraduate university degree from a recognized university. An associate or technical degree is not acceptable. Each academic record will be assessed individually. The academic work must be comparable to at least an overall B+ average. No preference will be given to one university over another or one programme over another. By June 30 of the year of possible admission, applicants must have completed an undergraduate degree. A minimum of three years of university undergraduate work is required and two of the three years must be above the year-one level of courses. A "year" is the full block of work specified for a year or level of the programme as indicated on the university transcript and in the appropriate university calendar. If requested, applicant must provide evidence that the requirement has been met.

PROCESS: The application deadline is June 15 for possible admission in the fall of the following year.

Cost

(Note: Amounts are listed in Canadian dollars.) Academic fees and tuition for first-year students amount to $14,023. The cost of books and diagnostic equipment for a first-year student is approximately $1,900.

FINANCIAL AID: Financial aid is available for Canadian students only from a variety of sources. A large number of bursaries are allocated each year for medical students in financial need. Academic awards are also offered to students who distinguish themselves by virtue of their scholarship.

MCMASTER UNIVERSITY

REGULAR ADMISSION POOL

STUDENT BODY

Type	Public
*Enrollment	NR
*% male/female	38/62
*% underrepresented minorities	NR
# applied (total/out)	2,507/840
% interviewed (total/out)	14/6
% accepted (total/out)	NR/NR
% enrolled (total/out)	NR/NR
Average age	NR

ADMISSIONS

Average GPA and MCAT Scores

Overall GPA	NR	Science GPA	NR
MCAT Bio	NR	MCAT Phys	NR
MCAT Verbal	NR	MCAT Essay	NR

Score Release Policy

Withholding scores is not recommended. The school needs to see all MCAT scores.

Application Information

Regular application	10/16
Regular notification	5/31
Transfers accepted?	NR
Admissions may be deferred?	Yes
Interview required?	Yes
Application fee	$175 OMSAS, plus $75 for each additional school (subject to change)

COSTS AND AID

Tuition & Fees

Tuition (in/out)	$13,500
Cost of books	$1,900
Fees	$523

INTERNATIONAL ADMISSION POOL

Application fee	$400
Tuition	$38,970

Note: All fees and expenses are listed in Canadian dollars
*Figures based on total enrollment

MEMORIAL U. OF NEWFOUNDLAND

FACULTY OF MEDICINE

Room 1751, St. John's, Newfoundland, AlB 3V6

Admissions: 709-737-6615

Internet: www.med.mun.ca

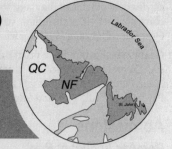

The Faculty of Medicine at the Memorial University of Newfoundland emphasizes clinical medicine and is geared toward training primary care physicians. The curriculum, physical structure, and administration promote maximum cooperation between the various basic sciences and clinical disciplines. As it is a relatively small school, Memorial is able to offer a personalized learning environment to its medical students. Acknowledging the special geography of the province, part of the Faculty's mission is to train physicians with exemplary skills for rural medical practice.

Academics

Each of the first two years is organized into three terms. Although the emphasis of the course work is on basic science, clinical medicine is also introduced. During the second two years, students perform clerkships in affiliated hospitals that provide both undergraduate and graduate medical education. In addition to the four-year M.D. degree, M.Sc. and Ph.D. degree programs are also open to qualified students. Areas of academic strength include Endocrinology and Metabolism; Gastroenterology, Human Genetics; Immunology; Molecular Biology; Neurosciences, and Cardiovascular Sciences including Epidemiology; and Community Medicine.

Basic Sciences: An important component of the first year is Basic Science of Medicine. This course introduces students to the biology of the normal human and integrates Biochemistry, Physiology, Immunology, Cell Biology, Genetics, Microbiology, Nutrition, Pharmacology, Pathology, and Anatomy. Teaching methods include lectures, small group sessions, laboratories, seminars, and open discussions. Students have the opportunity to initiate basic science research, which can be pursued throughout medical school. First-year students also take Integrated Study of Disease, which teaches Pathology and Pharmacology through the study of diseases of the major organ systems. In Clinical Skills, students are first introduced to the medical interview and techniques of counseling. The physical exam and important ethical issues are also part of the course. Community Medicine is a unique course, which focuses on the contextual aspects of disease and introduces Preventive Medicine, Biostatistics, Epidemiology, Social and Organizational Factors in Health, Environmental and Occupational Health, Community Nutrition, and Behavioral Sciences. The course includes visits to community-based hospitals and clinics. All courses continue in the second year, building on principles learned during the first year. On average, preclinical students are in class or other scheduled sessions for twenty-three hours per week.

Clinical Training: Year three is of twelve months duration beginning in September and continuing to the following Fall. It is composed of the core clerkships and some electives. Core clerkships, typically eight weeks in length, are Internal Medicine, Surgery, Psychiatry, Pediatrics and Ob/Gyn. A four-week Rural Family Medicine rotation is also required. The fourth year consists of electives and selectives, some of which may be completed at institutions other than those affiliated with the University. Teaching hospitals include General Hospital (531 beds), Grace General Hospital, Dr. Charles A Janeway Child Health Centre, St. Clare's Mercy Hospital, Waterford Hospital, and a number of institutions that are not under the Health Care Corporation of St. Johns.

Students

The school's class size is relatively small at 60 students. The male/female ratio within the student body is about 50/50.

Student Life: On-campus housing is available for both single and married students. In addition, the University provides assistance in locating off-campus housing. Medical students benefit from an active counseling center, childcare services, learning enhancement programs, a career planning office, and a student health service. The Student's Union promotes artistic, educational, charitable, and social activities, and the graduate student union provides common areas for social and other activities. Medical students have access to the services and resources of the greater university.

Graduates: A significant proportion of graduates enter residencies at affiliated hospitals in areas such as Anesthesia, Internal Medicine, Neurology, Ob/Gyn, Orthopedics, Anatomic Pathology, General Pathology, Pediatrics, Psychiatry, Radiology, and Surgery. Most graduates enter clinical medicine, often in primary care fields.

Admissions

Requirements: To be eligible for admission, a bachelor's degree is required in almost all circumstances. Requirements include two courses in English. The MCAT is also required, and must be taken prior to the application deadline, which is normally November 15. Transcripts and letters of reference must be submitted by November 29. Interviews are required of some candidates. The majority of places in each class are reserved for applicants who are residents of Newfoundland and Labrador. There are a limited number of places available for applicants from New Brunswick, from other Canadian provinces, and non-Canadians. Non-Canadians pay higher fees.

Suggestions: There are approximately 650 applications received for 60 places each year. Therefore, competition is high. Material submitted after the stated deadlines will not be considered. Academic achievement, MCAT scores, work or other experiences, and personal traits are all reviewed in admissions decisions. Though age itself is not used as a basis for selection, time away from academic studies may be taken into consideration.

Process: Requests for applications should be directed to the address above. Applications are accepted until November 15 in the year preceding anticipated matriculation. Decisions are made in the spring. Notification of the committee's decision will be made to candidates by letter from the Admissions Committee. Applicants have 14 days in which to confirm that he/she will accept the place offered to them.

Cost

(Note: Amounts are listed in Canadian dollars.) Annual tuition is $6,250 for Canadian residents and $30,000 for international students. Living expenses are reasonable for students living on campus, with per semester rent at about $2,500 and full meal plans at about $3,000 per year.

Financial Aid: The basic source is through Canada Student Loans Program. For U.S. students, it is through Federal Stafford Loans and alternate loans. Scholarships are awarded at the end of each year of medical studies. Recipients are selected by the Promotions Committees.

MEMORIAL UNIVERSITY OF NEWFOUNDLAND

STUDENT BODY

Type	Public
*Enrollment	60
*% male/female	NR
*% underrepresented minorities	NR
# applied (total/out)	647/460
% interviewed (total/out)	30/11
% accepted (total/out)	13/9
% enrolled (total/out)	10/4

ADMISSIONS

Average GPA and MCAT Scores

Overall GPA	NR	Science GPA	NR
MCAT Bio	NR	MCAT Phys	NR
MCAT Verbal	NR	MCAT Essay	NR

Score Release Policy

The Admissions Committee requires all writings of the MCAT to be reported and scores submitted.

Application Information

Regular application	11/15
Regular notification	3/1
Transfers accepted?	Yes
Admissions may be deferred?	Yes
AMCAS application accepted?	No
Interview required?	Yes
Application fee	$75

COSTS AND AID

Tuition & Fees

Tuition (in/out)	$6,250/$30,000
Cost of books	$943
Fees (in/out)	$227/$553

Note: All fees and expenses are listed in Canadian dollars
*Figures based on total enrollment

UNIVERSITY OF MONTREAL
SCHOOL OF MEDICINE

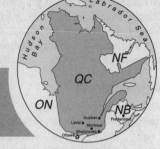

P.O. Box 6128, Station Centre-Ville, Montreal, Quebec H3C 3J7

Admissions: 514-343-6265

Internet: medes3.med.umontreal.ca

The School of Medicine at the University of Montreal has its origins in a medical school that was established in 1843. Today, the School of Medicine is a leader in both clinical medicine and medical research. It offers a revised curriculum with early clinical exposure, small-group and problem-based learning methods, and opportunities for independent research and study. Students benefit from exposure to a large and diverse patient population.

Academics

Instruction is solely in French. Some students enter a one-year Pre-Medical program that leads into the four year M.D. curriculum, while others who qualify enter the medical curriculum directly. Although clinical exposure begins during the first year of premedical or medical training, intensive clinical training begins in the third year. The Pre-Medical program is taught through lectures. On the other hand, the majority of instruction for medical students takes place in a small-group setting. In addition to the four-year M.D. curriculum, graduate degree programs are offered in all major medical science fields. Affiliated with the School of Medicine are other health science programs in areas such as Health Administration, Public Health, Social and Preventive Medicine, Nutrition, Rehabilitation, and Speech Language Therapy.

BASIC SCIENCES: Students who enter the Pre-Medical program take courses in Genetics and Embryology, Biostatistics, Cell Biology and General Histology, General Microbiology and Virology, Clinical Immersion, Introduction to Clinical Anatomy, Cell and Molecular Biology, Nutrition and Metabolism, Cell Physiology and Pharmacology, Introduction to Physiology, Psychology and Human Behavior, Introduction to Sociology, Basic Concepts in Ethics, and an elective. First-year medical school courses are Introduction to Medical Studies; Growth, Development and Aging, General Pathology and Immunology; Infectious Diseases; Hematology; Neurological Sciences; Mind; Musculoskeletal System; Introduction to Clinical Medicine; History of Medicine; Epidemiology; and an elective. Second year studies are largely organized by anatomical systems. These are Cardiovascular, Respiratory, Kidney, Digestion, Endocrinology, and Multi-system. Second year students also take an elective and continue with Introduction to Clinical Medicine.

CLINICAL TRAINING: For clinical training, students complete a series of required clerkships that provide hands-on experience in the major medical disciplines. During the third year, required clerkships are Medicine (8 weeks), Surgery (8 weeks), Pediatrics (8 weeks), Psychiatry (8 weeks), Ob/Gyn (8 weeks), and Family Medicine (4 weeks). Third-year students also have the opportunity for a four-week clinical elective. Fourth-year clerkships are Anesthesiology (2 weeks), Ophthalmology (2 weeks), Radiology (4 weeks), Geriatrics (4 weeks), Community Medicine (4 weeks), and an elective (4 weeks). Selectives are chosen from Medical or Pediatric subspecialties (8 weeks) and from Surgical subspecialties (4 weeks). Clinical training takes place at over fifteen affiliated hospitals including Hopital Maisonneuve-Rosemont, Hopital Notre-Dame, Hopital Riviere-des-Prairies, Hopital du Sacre-Coeur de Montreal, Hopital Louis-H Lafontaine, Hopital Sainte-Justine, Hopital Saint-Luc, Hotel-Dieu de Montreal, Institute de Cardiologie de Montreal, Institut de Readaptation de Montreal, Centre Hospitalier de Verdun, Cite de la Sante de Laval, Institue de Recherches Clinique de Montreal, Institut Philppe-Pinelde Montreal, and Centre Hospitalier Cote-des-Nieges.

Students

Entering class size is 143. In a recent class, all but four students were from the province of Quebec. About 60 percent of the students are women.

STUDENT LIFE: Medical students enjoy a good quality of life. The School of Medicine is committed to its students, providing academic and nonacademic support services. Outside of the classroom, medical students interact through student groups and organized social activities. The resources of the greater university, including athletic and recreational facilities, are available to medical students as well. Finally, the city of Montreal is an internationally recognized cultural center with a wealth of activities accessible to students.

GRADUATES: Graduates enter both academic and clinical medicine. At hospitals affiliated with the University of Montreal, postgraduate medical training is available in Anesthesiology, Family Medicine, Medicine, Ob/Gyn, Ophthalmology, Pediatrics, Psychiatry, Radiology, Surgery, and many other post-graduate programs.

Admissions

REQUIREMENTS: Only Canadian citizens, landed immigrants, and highly qualified French-speaking applicants from the United States are considered for admission. Fluency in French is a requirement. Two years of college is the minimum requirement for admission to the School of Medicine. Prerequisites are Philosophy, Behavioral Sciences, Social Sciences, French, English, Mathematics (through Trigonometry), Biology, Organic Chemistry, General Chemistry, and Physics.

SUGGESTIONS: Strong preference is given to applicants from the province of Quebec. Selection is based on both records of academic performance and interviews.

PROCESS: The absolute deadline for applications is March 1. About one-third of all applicants are asked to interview, with invitations based on the candidate's academic record. The strongest candidates are then selected from those interviewed. Admissions decisions are made in the Spring, with the first acceptance notices given in May. Accepted applicants have two weeks in which to confirm their place in the entering class.

Cost

(Note: All amounts are listed in Canadian dollars.) Tuition for residents is $2,575 and for nonresidents is $12,836.

FINANCIAL AID: Loans, scholarships, and stipends for summer research are available to students who qualify. Most assistance is granted on the basis of financial need, though some scholarships are offered on the basis of academic merit or other criteria.

UNIVERSITY OF MONTREAL

STUDENT BODY

Type	Public
*Enrollment	NR
*% male/female	NR
*% underrepresented minorities	NR
# applied (total/out)	1,859/270
% interviewed (total/out)	22/1
% accepted (total/out)	NR/NR
% enrolled (total/out)	NR/NR
Average age	NR

ADMISSIONS

Average GPA and MCAT Scores

Overall GPA	NR	Science GPA	NR
MCAT Bio	NR	MCAT Phys	NR
MCAT Verbal	NR	MCAT Essay	NR

Score Release Policy

The school has not responded to our inquiry regarding withheld MCAT scores. Therefore, we advise caution. Contact the Admissions Office before withholding any scores.

Application Information

Regular application	3/1
Regular notification	3/31
Transfers accepted?	NR
Admissions may be deferred?	No
Interview required?	Yes
Application fee	$45

COSTS AND AID

Tuition & Fees

Tuition (in/out)	$2,575/$12,836
Cost of books	NR
Fees	$30

Note: All fees and expenses are listed in Canadian dollars
*Figures based on total enrollment

UNIVERSITY OF OTTAWA
FACULTY OF MEDICINE

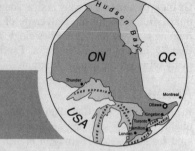

451 Smyth Road, Ottawa, Ontario K1H 8M5
Admissions: 613-562-5409 • Fax: 613-562-5420
Email: admissmd@uottawa.ca

The University of Ottawa is a public institution with over 23,000 graduate, professional, and undergraduate students. The Faculty of Medicine is part of the Faculty of Health Sciences, which also includes the School of Nursing and the School of Human Kinetics. The campus is located in an urban environment, and medical students learn through exposure to a diverse patient population. Admission is limited to Canadian residents and children of alumni.

Academics

During the four-year M.D. program, students acquire the knowledge, skills, and attitudes they need to apply effective, efficient strategies for the prevention and management of health problems ranging from the most common to the most severe. The program integrates the basic and clinical sciences throughout the four years. It also emphasizes health promotion and disease prevention, and is responsive to individual needs and abilities and to the changes occurring in society and the health care system. Instruction is available in both French and English. In addition to the M.D., Masters, and Ph.D., programs are offered in Biochemistry, Cell and Developmental Biology, Epidemiology and Community Medicine, Microbiology and Immunology, Pharmacology, and Physiology.

BASIC SCIENCES: The basic science curriculum spans 70 weeks, and emphasizes self-learning and multidisciplinary teaching. Lecture, seminars, computer applications, problem-based learning, and labs are all important teaching methodologies. During the first academic period, students complete blocks focused on Development and Homeostasis, Infection and Neoplasia, Hematology, and Immune, Cardiovascular, Respiratory, and Renal systems. The second academic period teaches Endocrinology, Human Reproduction and Sexuality, Musculoskeletal, Nervous System, Mind, Special Senses, and Gastrointestinal. Throughout the first and second years, students also take Physicians Skills Development. In addition to the Health Sciences Library, the other libraries and learning resources of the University are available to students.

CLINICAL TRAINING: During the third year, required rotations are Medicine (3 weeks), Surgery (8 weeks), Ambulatory Medicine (8 weeks), Ob/Gyn (8 weeks), Pediatrics (8 weeks), and Psychiatry (8 weeks). The fourth year is comprised of 14 weeks of electives and selectives in Medicine, Surgery, and Ambulatory Medicine. Training takes place at Ottawa General Hospital, Ottawa Civic Hospital, Children's Hospital of Eastern Ontario, Royal Ottawa Hospital, National Defense Medical Center, Brockville Psychiatric Hospital, Elisabeth Bruyere Health Center, Monfort Hospital, Pierre Janet Hospital, North Bay Psychiatric Hospital, Saint Vincent Hospital, Riverside Hospital, Sudbury Algoma Hospital, Sudbury Memorial Hospital, Grace General Hospital, and Queensway-Carleton Hospital, among other institutions. Affiliated research institutions include the Institute of Mental Health Research, The Institute for Rehabilitation Research and Development, The Loeb Medical Research Institute, The University of Ottawa Heart Institute Research Center, and the University of Ottawa Eye Institute.

Students

There are 84 students in each class. Typically, all but a few are residents of the province of Ontario. About 50 percent of members of the student body are women.

STUDENT LIFE: Medical students benefit from the resources and activities of a large university and an urban environment. Student clubs and organizations exist within the medical school and the greater university. Support services, such as counseling, child care, health care, and academic assistance are available to medical students. On-campus housing is offered.

GRADUATES: Graduates enter both clinical medicine and research-oriented careers. Graduate-level medical training is offered at Ottawa in most clinical fields.

Admissions

REQUIREMENTS: To be eligible for admissions, applicants must have successfully completed three years of full-time university studies in any undergraduate program leading to a bachelor's degree, including one year of General Biology, one year of Humanities or Social Sciences, and two years of some combination of Biochemistry, General Chemistry, and Organic Chemistry. The MCAT is no longer required. Only Canadian citizens or permanent residents are accepted, with the exception of eligible children of the University of Ottawa alumni.

SUGGESTIONS: The Admissions Committee primarily considers those eligible candidates who have maintained a weighted average of at least a B+ in the last three years of their undergraduate university studies. Priority is given in order to Franco-Ontarians, Aboriginal applicants, residents of under-serviced areas, bona fide residents of the Ottawa-Outaouais region, Ontario residents, and residents of other provinces. In recent entering classes, about 20 percent of applicants were accepted.

PROCESS: After a written application is submitted, supporting materials and an interview will be requested of applicants with acceptable academic records. The interview is used to further screen applicants. Documents for application to the first year of medicine are available through the Faculty or through OMSAS (Ontario Medical School Application Service). Kits are available in July of the preceding year from:

> OMSAS
> PO Box 1328
> 650 Woodlawn Road West
> Block C
> Guelph, Ontario N1H 7P4

Applications must be completed and returned by October 15.

Cost

(Note: Amounts are listed in Canadian dollars.) Tuition is approximately $4,266 per year for full time medical students who are Canadian residents and $8,700 for nonresidents. Food, housing and other expenses amount to around $10,000 per year but range considerably depending on lifestyle.

FINANCIAL AID: Fellowships, research and teaching assistantships are available in addition to grants and loans which are typically offered by a student's provincial government. Financial aid in the form of grants and loans is determined on the basis of need and good academic standing.

UNIVERSITY OF OTTAWA

STUDENT BODY

Type	Public
*Enrollment	NR
*% male/female	NR
*% underrepresented minorities	NR
# applied (total/out)	1,851/482
% interviewed (total/out)	24/NR
% accepted (total/out)	NR/NR
% enrolled (total/out)	NR/NR
Average age	NR

ADMISSIONS

Average GPA and MCAT Scores

Overall GPA	NR	Science GPA	NR
MCAT Bio	NR	MCAT Phys	NR
MCAT Verbal	NR	MCAT Essay	NR

Score Release Policy

The school has not responded to our inquiry regarding withheld MCAT scores. Therefore, we advise caution. Contact the Admissions Office before withholding any scores.

Application Information

Regular application	10/15
Regular notification	5/1
Transfers accepted?	NR
Admissions may be deferred?	Yes
AMCAS application accepted?	NR
Interview required?	Yes
Application fee	$75
$175 OMSAS, plus $75 for each additional school (subject to change)	

COSTS AND AID

Tuition & Fees

Tuition (in/out)	$4,266/$8,700
Cost of books	NR
Fees	$373

Note: All fees and expenses are listed in Canadian dollars
*Figures based on total enrollment

QUEEN'S UNIVERSITY

FACULTY OF HEALTH SCIENCES SCHOOL OF MEDICINE

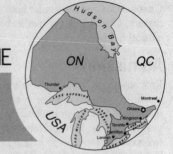

Kingston, Ontario K7L 3N6
Admissions: 613-533-2542 • Fax: 613-533-6884
Internet: meds.queensu.ca/medicine/calendar/toc.html

The Faculty of Health Sciences at Queen's University originated as the University's Department of Medicine in 1845. Since then it has grown and evolved into an important medical institution known for its research, patient care, and teaching. The major goal of the undergraduate program is the education of students as problem solvers and critical thinkers so that they will be prepared for all clinical disciplines and medical careers. In support of this goal, a problem-based, interdisciplinary curriculum has been developed. The medical school is part of the main Queen's University campus, which offers students a wide range of resources and facilities. Only Canadian citizens, permanent residents, and children of alumni are eligible for admission.

Academics

Most students follow a four-year curriculum leading to an MD degree. Masters and Doctoral degree programs are also offered in Biochemistry, Biostatistics, Environmental and Occupational Health, Epidemiology, General Community Health, Health-Care Systems, Pathology, and Preventive Medicine. Although there are no formally structured combined programs, superior students may be permitted the flexibility to work toward an M.Sc. or a Ph.D. concurrently with the M.D. Grading uses a Honours/Pass/Fail system.

BASIC SCIENCES: Most basic science instruction takes place during the first three years. First-year course starts with Phase I, Introduction to the Sciences Relevant to Medicine, an introduction to the fundamental language and concepts of medical science, and Communication/Clinical Skills. Phase IIA includes Dermatology/Musculoskeletal systems, Haematology and Oncology, Microbiology and Infectious Diseases, Allergy and Immunology, and Clinical Skills. Second year courses are Psychiatry/Neuroscience/Ophthalmology/ ENT, Genitourinary/Cardiovascular/Respirology, and Clinical Skills. In addition, eight weeks are left open for an elective. Third year courses are: Endocrine/Metabolism/ Reproduction, Gastrointestinal, and Clinical Skills. In addition to problem-based learning, teaching methods include lectures, seminars, small group discussions, laboratory experience, and computer-based instruction. Basic science instruction takes place primarily at Botterell Hall, which also houses administrative offices and Bracken Library. The Clinical Learning center is an important educational facility within the Faculty of Health Sciences specifically designed for the teaching, learning, and evaluation of important clinical skills, and is used during both preclinical and clinical years. The Health Sciences library subscribes to approximately 844 serials and its total collection consists of 156,000 volumes. In the library is the Multimedia Learning Centre, which offers both video- and computer-assisted instruction.

CLINICAL TRAINING: Clerkships begin in January of the third year. They are: Medicine (12 weeks), Surgery (8 weeks), Psychiatry (6 weeks), Ob/Gyn (6 weeks), Pediatrics (6 weeks), Family Medicine (4 weeks), Geriatrics (2 weeks), and Emergency Medicine (2 weeks). Four weeks of selectives and 12 weeks of electives are also required. Clerkships takes place at a number of affiliated hospitals including Kingston General Hospital, Hotel Dieu Hospital, St. Mary's of the Lake Hospital, Kingston Psychiatric Hospital, and Ongwanada Hospital. The provision of healthcare services in Kingston is presently being restructured and will change over the next few years.

Students

Each class has 75 students, about 50 of whom are typically from the province of Ontario. The student body is approximately 50 percent women.

STUDENT LIFE: Medical students enjoy the recreational, cultural, and social activities of the greater university and the city of Kingston. On-campus attractions include museums, concert halls, cinema, and an observatory. Student services include a child care resource center, a foundation supporting women, comprehensive health services, an international center, a physical education center and a student center. The University provides accommodations in single and double occupancy rooms for approximately 300 graduate students. In addition, the Apartment and Housing office manages University-owned rentals in the area.

Admissions

REQUIREMENTS: In order to apply, students must have completed three years of full-time study at a university. In addition, one year each of Biological sciences, Physical sciences, and Humanities/Social Sciences are required. The MCAT is required. To be eligible for admission, applicants must be Canadian citizens, Canadian permanent residents, or children of Queen's University alumni.

SUGGESTIONS: The Admissions Committee looks for both academic abilities, such as commitment, achievement, critical thinking, and self-directed learning, and personal characteristics such as communication skills, creativity, and sensitivity. No preference is given to a particular undergraduate program of studies, and college students seeking admission are encouraged to pursue studies in their area of interest.

PROCESS: Applicants seeking further information about admission should contact the School of Medicine. Applications are made through:

> Ontario Medical Schools' Application Service
> Box 1328
> Guelph, Ontario N1H 7P4

The deadline is October 15. The first admissions cutoff is based on the cumulative converted grade point average, and the second is made on the basis of MCAT scores. Those applicants who qualify are interviewed. Applicants are then ranked according to evaluation of letters of reference, autobiographic sketch, and interview results.

Cost

(Note: Amounts are listed in Canadian dollars.) Yearly tuition is $9,384 for Canadians and $16,000 for international students.

FINANCIAL AID: A number of scholarships are available on a competitive basis to incoming and other students. Generally, students are judged on the basis of academic merit or on other special critera. A limited number of summer scholarships are offered in conjunction with research projects. The University also offers loans and bursuries to students with financial need.

QUEEN'S UNIVERSITY

STUDENT BODY

Type	Public
*Enrollment	NR
*% male/female	NR
*% underrepresented minorities	NR
# applied (total/out)	1,511/397
% interviewed (total/out)	NR/NR
% accepted (total/out)	NR/NR
% enrolled (total/out)	NR/NR
Average age	NR

ADMISSIONS

Average GPA and MCAT Scores

Overall GPA	NR	Science GPA	NR
MCAT Bio	NR	MCAT Phys	NR
MCAT Verbal	NR	MCAT Essay	NR

Score Release Policy

The school has not responded to our inquiry regarding withheld MCAT scores. Therefore, we advise caution. Contact the Admissions Office before withholding any scores.

Application Information

Regular application	10/15
Regular notification	5/31
Transfers accepted?	NR
Admissions may be deferred?	Yes
AMCAS application accepted?	NR
Interview required?	Yes
Application fee	$175 OMSAS, plus $75 for each additional school

COSTS AND AID

Tuition & Fees

Tuition (in/out)	$9,384/$16,000
Cost of books	NR
Fees	$716

Note: All fees and expenses are listed in Canadian dollars
*Figures based on total enrollment

UNIVERSITY OF SASKATCHEWAN

COLLEGE OF MEDICINE

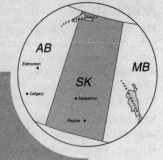

B103 Health Sciences Building, 107 Wiggins Road
Saskatoon, Saskatchewan S7N 5E5
Admission: 306-966-8554
Internet: www.usask.ca/medicine/ • Email: med.admissions@usask.ca

The College of Medicine at the University of Saskatchewan is the only medical school in the province of Saskatchewan. Although research has become increasingly important, the primary function of the institution and its faculty is to educate medical students. With the input of students, faculty, and administrators, the curriculum was recently revised to include innovative teaching methods and to reflect the rapid evolution of fields within clinical medicine.

Academics

The goal of the College of Medicine is to enable medical students to develop the knowledge, skills, values, and attitudes that will serve as a foundation for subsequent education in primary and specialty patient care and research. In its curriculum, the College promotes the integration of basic and clinical sciences. Independent learning, problem-solving, and early patient interaction are emphasized. The curriculum is divided into four phases. For the most part, basic science instruction occurs during the first three phases. However, basic science and clinical training are integrated throughout the four-year curriculum.

BASIC SCIENCES: Phase A (1 year) comprises 33 weeks and includes the introductory study of basic sciences, the History of Medicine, Professional Skills (includes two-week community experience), and Life Cycle and Humanities. Instruction in basic sciences is interdisciplinary, covering fundamental principles of Anatomy, Physiology, Biochemistry, and Microbiology. Instruction in the basic sciences continues into Phase B (1 year) which lasts 33 weeks. Subjects include Pathology, Microbiology, and Pharmacology. Also included in Phase B is Clinical Sciences, Systems, and Genetics. Phase C comprises 15 weeks only and is a continuation of Clinical Sciences and Systems, but also includes the Linking Courses, Microbiology, and Community Health and Epidemiology.

CLINICAL TRAINING: Phase D (16 months) is a discipline-based rotation clerkship that builds on the clinical training and offers students the opportunity to study clinical electives (12 weeks) and specialty fields. Teaching Hospitals are Royal University Hospital, St. Paul's Hospital, Saskatoon City Hospital, Regina General Hospital, and Pasqua Hospital.

Students

The maximum size of entering classes is 55. Typically, all but one or two students are from the province of Saskatchewan. In general, about 50 percent of students are women.

STUDENT LIFE: With a relatively small student body and a curriculum that encourages interaction, students are generally cohesive. Between the medical school and the greater University, a wide range of extra-curricular activities and events are offered. Medical students live both on and off campus.

GRADUATES: Though research is an increasingly important activity for the College of Medicine, a large number of graduates become practicing clinical physicians in the province of Saskatchewan.

Admissions

REQUIREMENTS: A minimum of two years of undergraduate work is required. In general, prerequisites are Biochemistry, Biology, Chemistry, Organic Chemistry, Physics, English, Social Sciences, and Humanities. Incoming students should also have a Standard First Aid Certification. Applicants must have an academic average of 70 percent in prerequisite courses in order to be considered for admission. Overall academic averages must be at least 78 percent. The MCAT must be taken and a minimum score of 8 in all sections is required.

SUGGESTIONS: Criteria for selection are academic performance and personal qualities. Academic performance is based on applicants' two best full undergraduate years of study. Personal qualities are assessed primarily by interview. Realistically to be competitive academically, an overall two-year average of over 80 percent is required.

Process: Application forms may be obtained from the Admissions Secretary after July 1 or from the internet at the address above. Applications from Saskatchewan residents must be post-marked no later than January 15. Applications from out-of-province residents must be post-marked no later than December 1. Interviews are approximately 45 minutes and occur during a weekend in March. The applicant is interviewed by a team of four, including a medical doctor, a faculty member, a medical student, and a community member. Three letters of reference are also considered. All candidates are notified of their acceptance by the end of June.

Cost

The estimated total cost for the first year of medical school is $12,887 (Canadian dollars). This figure includes tuition, fees and books but does not cover living expenses.

Financial Aid: Fellowships, scholarships, research assistantships, teaching assistantships and loans are available to students who qualify. Assistance is based on financial need as well as on academic merit.

UNIVERSITY OF SASKATCHEWAN

STUDENT BODY

Type	Public
*Enrollment	NR
*% male/female	NR
*% underrepresented minorities	NR
# applied (total/out)	NR/NR
% interviewed (total/out)	NR/NR
% accepted (total/out)	NR/NR
% enrolled (total/out)	NR/NR
Average age	24

ADMISSIONS

Average GPA and MCAT Scores

Overall GPA	NR	Science GPA	NR
MCAT Bio	NR	MCAT Phys	NR
MCAT Verbal	NR	MCAT Essay	NR

Score Release Policy

The school has not responded to our inquiry regarding withheld MCAT scores. Therefore, we advise caution. Contact the Admissions Office before withholding any scores.

Application Information

Regular application	1/15 in province
	12/1 out of province
Regular notification	6/25
Transfers accepted?	NR
Admissions may be deferred?	Yes
AMCAS application accepted?	NR
Interview required?	Yes
Application fee (in/out)	$40/$75
	+ transcript fee

COSTS AND AID

Tuition & Fees

Tuition	$6,450
Cost of books	NR
Fees	$150

Note: All fees and expenses are listed in Canadian dollars
*Figures based on total enrollment

UNIVERSITY OF SHERBROOKE
FACULTY OF MEDICINE

Sherbrooke, Quebec J1H 5N4
Admissions: 819-564-5208
Internet: www.usherb.ca • Email: admmed@courrier.usherb.ca

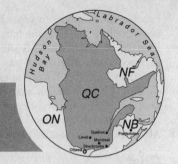

The Faculty of Medicine at the University of Sherbrooke was founded in 1961. It is a French-speaking institution that is involved in medical research and that strives to meet the medical needs of its community. The Faculty of Medicine is one component of the Health Sciences Center, which also includes a School of Nursing and a large number of affiliated hospitals and health centers.

Academics

Sherbrooke offers a four-year curriculum leading to the M.D. degree. Educational methodology is based on small group discussions, case studies, audiovisual and computer assisted learning, and hands-on clinical experiences. Combined degree programs, such as the M.D./M.Sc. program are open to highly qualified students who have an interest in research.

BASIC SCIENCES: The first academic period begins in late August and spans 39 weeks. In general, students are in class or other scheduled session for approximately 30 hours per week. Courses are: Introduction to M.D. Program, Biological Medicine I and II, Clinical Immersion, Growth Development and Aging, Nervous System, Locomoter System, Pscyhosocial Sciences, Preventive Medicine and Community Health, Integration, and Clinical Skills. The second year is organized into blocks based on anatomical/physiological systems. These are: Cardiovascular System, Respiratory System, Urinary System, Gastrointestinal System, Hemato-Immunologic System, Infectious Disease, Endocrine System, Reproductive System, and Human Sexuality. In addition, students take part in a Rotation in Community Hospitals and a course in Clinical Skills.

CLINICAL TRAINING: The third and fourth years are organized into several components. These are: Required Courses, Required Primary Clerkships, Rotations in Community, Elective Programs, Integration Period, and Final Exam. Required Courses are: Interdisciplinary Concepts, Clinical Skills, and Introduction to Clerkships. The required Primary Clerkships are: Medicine (10.5 weeks); Surgery (7 weeks); Pediatrics (7 weeks); Psychiatry (7 weeks); Ob/Gyn (7 weeks); and Multidisciplinary—Anesthesia, Ophthalmology, Dermatology, ORL—(3.5 weeks). Rotations in Community are comprised of Family Medicine and Emergency (7 weeks) and Community Health (4 weeks). The Elective Program lasts 12 weeks, followed by the Integration Period (6 weeks) and the Final Exam Period (one week). Teaching hospitals are Cuse Fleurimont, Cuse Bowen, Hopital Charles Le Moyne, and Hopital Sainte-Croix.

Students

Each entering class has approximately 105 students. About 80 percent of students are from the Province of Quebec. Women account for 60 percent of students.

STUDENT LIFE: The University of Sherbrooke is a large university with many social, recreational and other extra-curricular activities for medical students. Medical students have both on campus and off campus housing options.

GRADUATES: Many graduates enter one of the residency programs offered at hospitals affiliated with Sherbrooke.

Admissions

REQUIREMENTS: Fluency in French is required. The minimum requirement for admissions is two years of university or a B.A. degree. Prerequisites are: General Biology (one year); General Chemistry (one year); Organic Chemistry (one year); Physics (three semesters); and Mathematics through Calculus. The MCAT is not required.

SUGGESTIONS: In addition to prerequisite courses, students should complete course work in the Humanities and in the Social Sciences. Priority is given to residents of Quebec, and 86 positions in each entering class are reserved for this group of applicants. Fifteen additional places are reserved for applicants from New Brunswick, one place is reserved for an applicant from Prince Edward Island, one from Nova Scotia, and two places are available for qualified foreign applicants. Overall, about 5% of applicants are admitted each year.

PROCESS: Applications are available from the Admissions Office at the address above. Following review of applications, qualified candidates are invited to a learning skills test (THAMUS)

Cost

Yearly tuition and fees (in Canadian dollars) is $3,127 per year for Canadian residents and $15,127 per year for nonresidents.

FINANCIAL AID: Canadian residents may qualify for financial aid offered by the Province of Quebec. Institutional funds also exist for those with financial need and those who have outstanding academic credentials.

UNIVERSITY OF SHERBROOKE

STUDENT BODY

Type	Public
*Enrollment	NR
*% male/female	NR
*% underrepresented minorities	NR
# applied (total/out)	1,401/199
% interviewed (total/out)	NR/NR
% accepted (total/out)	NR/NR
% enrolled (total/out)	NR/NR

ADMISSIONS

Average GPA and MCAT Scores

Overall GPA	NR	Science GPA	NR
MCAT Bio	NR	MCAT Phys	NR
MCAT Verbal	NR	MCAT Essay	NR

Score Release Policy

The school has not responded to our inquiry regarding withheld MCAT scores. Therefore, we advise caution. Contact the Admissions Office before withholding any scores.

Application Information

Regular application	3/1
Regular notification	5/1–8/1
Transfers accepted?	NR
Admissions may be deferred?	No
Interview required?	No
Application fee	$30

COSTS AND AID

Tuition & Fees

Tuition and fees (in/out)	$3,127/$15,127
Cost of books	NR

Note: All fees and expenses are listed in Canadian dollars
*Figures based on total enrollment

UNIVERSITY OF TORONTO

FACULTY OF MEDICINE

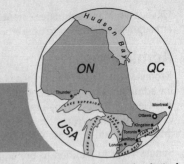

Toronto, Ontario M5S 1A8
Admissions: 416-978-2717 • Fax: 416-971-2163
Internet: ut//.library.utoronto.ca/www/medicine/ume.htm

The mission of the Faculty of Medicine of the University of Toronto is to achieve excellence in education, research, clinical care, and community health. The Faculty has been at the forefront of education and research for over 100 years, and has grown into one of the largest health sciences complexes in North America. In 1992, a revised curriculum was introduced, designed to prepare students for the lifelong learning required to be compassionate and informed physicians.

Academics

The curriculum is based on four guidelines: Patient-Centered Learning, Integrated and Multidisciplinary Content, Student-Motivated Learning, and Structured Problem-Based Learning. In addition to the four-year program leading to an M.D., a six-year M.D./Ph.D. program is offered jointly by the Faculty of Medicine and the School of Graduate Studies.

BASIC SCIENCES: The initial phase of the undergraduate medical program spans approximately 82 weeks. The curriculum consists of the following sequential blocks or units which focus on principles of medicine: Art and Science of Clinical Medicine; Brain and Behavior; Metabolism and Nutrition; Determination of Community Health; Structure and Function; Pathobiology of Disease; and Foundations of Medical Practice. Students meet actual as well as simulated patients, and are introduced to clinical medicine by faculty members in teaching hospitals. The emphasis is on student-centered, self-directed work and small group tutorials. Students are in scheduled sessions for approximately 35 hours per week. Most learning takes place in small group settings. Independent study is also important.

CLINICAL TRAINING: The third and fourth academic periods are comprised mainly of six-week clinical clerkships. These are: Medicine, Surgery, Ob/Gyn, Pediatrics, Family and Community Medicine, Psychiatry, Specialty Medicine, Specialty Surgery, Emergency Medicine and Anesthesia, Ambulatory and Community Experience, and three electives. Training takes place at a network of teaching hospitals and community-based health agencies. Affiliated hospitals include Baycrest Centre for Geriatric Care, Centre for Addiction and Mental Health (formerly Addition Research Foundation and the Clarke Institute of Psychiatry), The Hospital for Sick Children, Mount Sinai Hospital, St. Michael's Hospital, Toronto Rehabilitation Institute (formerly Hillcrest Hospital and Queen Elizabeth Hospital), Sunnybrook and Women's College Health Science Centre, The Toronto Hospital (formerly the Toronto Hospital and the Ontario Cancer Institute/Princess Margaret Hospital. Students are also able to learn in the community through participation in settings such as teaching health units and physicians' offices.

Students

About 15 percent of students are from outside of the province. Approximately 40 percent of students are women. Class size is 177.

STUDENT LIFE: One of the advantages of attending medical school at the University of Toronto is the City itself. The university campus is located within easy walking distance of the attractions and facilities of Toronto. Students enjoy clubs, concerts, museums, major league sporting events, and shopping. Just outside of the city, skiing and other outdoor sports are readily accessible. On- campus activities include pubs, concerts, special lectures, theaters, intramural sports, student government, special interest clubs, and the *Medical Journal*. Medical students benefit from the large campus of 55,000 students and its resources. Student support includes health services and a housing office that coordinates both on- and off-campus housing. Residence halls with meal plans are one of many housing options.

GRADUATES: A key aspect of the program is that it provides exposure to all medical career options. Graduates enter primary care fields, specialties, academic medicine, research, and leadership positions.

Admissions

REQUIREMENTS: Academic achievement is measured by grades and MCAT results. Prerequisite courses are at least two full course equivalents in Life Sciences and at least one full course equivalent in Humanities, Social Sciences, or Languages. These courses should provide applicants with an understanding of the basic principles and vocabulary of physics, chemistry, and biology, a working knowledge of statistics, and the ability to gather, interpret, and present information from complex texts both in writing and orally. Students must be in their third year or higher of university to be considered for admission.

SUGGESTIONS: Students from social sciences, humanities, and physical and life sciences are encouraged to apply. Demonstrated high-level proficiency in oral and written English is considered essential for success in the curriculum and in practice, and applicants are encouraged to have completed at least two full equivalents in course that require expository writing. Generally, minimum requirements are an average grade point average of 3.6/4.0 and a minimum of 8 on each section of the MCAT. Desired personal characteristics include a perceptive nature, strong commitment, high personal standards, and a history of academic and personal achievement.

PROCESS: Applications for admission to the medical school must be submitted by October 15 to:

> OMSAS, Ontario Universities Application Center
> PO Box 1328
> Guelph, Ontario N1H 7P4

The Faculty will invite selected applicants for an interview. Notices of acceptance are sent to students in the spring or summer prior to the proposed date of enrollment.

Cost

Cost of attendance (in Canadian dollars) is $14,000 for domestic students and $23,750 for international students. The average cost of residence with a full meal plan is approximately $7,000 for the eight-month session.

FINANCIAL AID: The Faculty of Medicine is committed to the University of Toronto policy which states that each student will have access to the resources necessary to meet his or her needs. Financial aid is available in the form of loans, grants, summer scholarships, and paid research opportunities. While most assistance is granted on the basis of need, a limited number of scholarships based on academic achievement and merit are also awarded each year to incoming students.

UNIVERSITY OF TORONTO

STUDENT BODY

Type	Public
*Enrollment	NR
*% male/female	NR
*% underrepresented minorities	NR
# applied (total/out)	1,731/NR
% interviewed (total/out)	22/NR
% accepted (total/out)	NR/NR
% enrolled (total/out)	NR/NR

ADMISSIONS

Average GPA and MCAT Scores

Overall GPA	NR	Science GPA	NR
MCAT Bio	NR	MCAT Phys	NR
MCAT Verbal	NR	MCAT Essay	NR

Score Release Policy

The school has not responded to our inquiry regarding withheld MCAT scores. Therefore, we advise caution. Contact the Admissions Office before withholding any scores.

Application Information

Regular application	10/15
Regular notification	5/31
Transfers accepted?	No
Admissions may be deferred?	Yes
AMCAS application accepted?	NR
Interview required?	Yes
Application fee	$75

COSTS AND AID

Tuition & Fees

Tuition (in/out)	$14,000/$23,750
Cost of books	NR
Fees (in/out)	$919/$1,498

Note: All fees and expenses are listed in Canadian dollars
*Figures based on total enrollment

UNIVERSITY OF WESTERN ONTARIO
FACULTY OF MEDICINE AND DENTISTRY

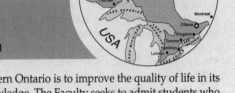

Medical Sciences Bldg., London, Ontario N6A 5C1

Admissions: 519-661-3744

Internet: www.med.uwo.ca • Email: admissions@med.uwo.ca

The mission of the Faculty of Medicine and Dentistry at the University of Western Ontario is to improve the quality of life in its community and beyond through the pursuit, discovery, and integration of knowledge. The Faculty seeks to admit students who demonstrate integrity, initiative, and productivity. One of the strengths of the curriculum is that it promotes early patient contact.

Academics

The Faculty of Medicine and Dentistry, along with the Faculty of Graduate Studies, has established a combined M.D.-Ph.D. program in which the research curriculum of the graduate program is integrated into the M.D. program. Applicants must be accepted to the medical school as M.D. candidates before entering the combined program.

BASIC SCIENCES: Introductory clinical training is an important part of the basic science curriculum, which spans the first two years. First-year courses are comprised of Anatomy; Biochemistry; Patient Centered Clinical Methods; Life Cycle; Health, Illness, Society; Microbiology and Immunology; General Pathology; and Physiology. The second year consists of Patient Centered Clinical Methods; Medicine; Diagnostic and Systemic Pathology; Pharmacology; and Health, Illness, and Society.

CLINICAL TRAINING: Year three is comprised of required clinical clerkships. These are: General Medicine (9 weeks), Physical Medicine and Rehabilitation and Geriatrics (2 weeks), Ophthalmology (4 weeks), General Surgery (6 weeks), Family Medicine (6 weeks), Ob/Gyn (6 weeks), Psychiatry (6 weeks), and Pediatrics (6 weeks). Year four consists of clinical electives and a Transition Period, which includes courses in Health Care Management, Ecosystem Health, Oncology, Advanced Communication Skills, and Medicine Review. Training takes place at a number of affiliated teaching hospitals, including London Health Sciences Center, St. Joseph's Health Center, Victoria Campus, University Campus, Children's Hospital of Western Ontario and affiliated health units and medical centers, Madame Vanier Children's Services, Parkwood Hospital, Thames Valley Children's Center, St. Thomas Psychiatric Hospital, and Byron Family Medical Center.

Students

Class size is 96.

STUDENT LIFE: The University of Western Ontario offers students a rich lifestyle. School-sponsored events and countless clubs and organizations are offered on campus. London is a small city of about 300,000 with a range of cultural and recreational activities. Both on- and off-campus housing is available.

GRADUATES: The curriculum is designed to allow graduates to enter any clinical or medical research field. A significant portion of graduates enter residency programs at hospitals affiliated with the University of Western Ontario.

Admissions

REQUIREMENTS: Enrollment is limited to Canadian citizens and permanent residents of Canada. Those who are in the third year or have successfully completed three full years of study in any degree program at a recognized university are eligible to apply. A minimum of five full or equivalent courses must be included in the final undergraduate year (September to April year only). Science prerequisites are one full course in Biology, one full course in Organic Chemistry, and one additional full science course. Nonscience prerequisites are two full nonscience courses from different disciplines and one senior-level course in one of these two subjects. Interested applicants should contact the Faculty for more detailed course requirements. The MCAT is required. The latest date that applicants should take the exam is August in the year of application. Only applicants who have achieved a certain grade point average and MCAT scores will be considered for admission. Typically, the minimum GPA is 3.50 and minimum MCAT scores are a 9 on Biological Sciences, an 8 on Physical Sciences, a 9 on Verbal Reasoning, and a Q on the Writing Sample. English proficiency is a requirement.

Suggestions: For entrance in the fall of 1999, there were 1725 applicants for 96 positions. Thus, admission is competitive. Apart from science prerequisites, there is no prescribed "pre-med program." Students at Western Ontario come from a variety of undergraduate programs and a wide range of disciplines. For those who have taken the MCAT more than once, only the most recent score is used.

Process: The deadline for application is October 15 for the following September. Applications are available by contacting:

> OMSAS
> Box 1328
> 650 Woodlawn Rd. West
> Guelph, Ontario N1H 7P4
> Phone: 519-823-1940

Those applicants who satisfy the course load, GPA, and MCAT requirements will be contacted for an interview. Letters indicating admissions decisions are sent to applicants beginning in the end of May and continuing until the class is full.

Cost

Tuition and student fees amount to about $11,000 (Canadian dollars) per year for Canadian residents.

Financial Aid: Grants, loans and paid research assistantships are offered to students who qualify. Eligibility is based on financial need and/or scholastic achievement.

University of Western Ontario

Student Body

Type	Public
*Enrollment	NR
*% male/female	NR
*% underrepresented minorities	NR
# applied (total/out)	1,847/587
% interviewed (total/out)	23/NR
% accepted (total/out)	NR/NR
% enrolled (total/out)	NR/NR

Admissions

Average GPA and MCAT Scores

Overall GPA	NR	Science GPA	NR
MCAT Bio	NR	MCAT Phys	NR
MCAT Verbal	NR	MCAT Essay	NR

Score Release Policy

The school has not responded to our inquiry regarding withheld MCAT scores. Therefore, we advise caution. Contact the Admissions Office before withholding any scores.

Application Information

Regular application	10/15
Regular notification	5/31 unitl filled
Transfers accepted?	NR
Admissions may be deferred?	No
AMCAS application accepted?	No
Interview required?	Yes
Application fee	$175 OMSAS, plus $75 for each school (subject to change)

Costs and Aid

Tuition & Fees

Tuition	$10,000
	($ amount subject to change)
Cost of books	NR
Fees	$722
	($ amount subject to change)

Note: All fees and expenses are listed in Canadian dollars

*Figures based on total enrollment

Puerto Rican Medical School Profiles

UNIVERSIDAD CENTRAL DEL CARIBE

SCHOOL OF MEDICINE

PO Box 60-327, Bayamon, PR 00960-6023

Admissions: 787-798-6732

Internet: www.uccaribe.edu

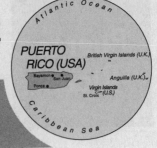

The School of Medicine at the Universidad Central del Caribe is a fully accredited medical school and a member of the AAMC. An important part of its mandate is the formation of committed health professionals who are sensitive to diverse patient and societal needs. The emphasis is on promoting critical thinking, integrated learning, and primary care. The school is entirely Spanish/English bilingual and serves an important role in training physicians to meet the medical needs of under-served populations.

Academics

The curriculum emphasizes techniques and values related to the provision of primary medical care. The first two years primarily teach basic medical sciences and an introduction to the clinical sciences through courses in community health, human behavior, clinical medicine, and clinical skills. The second two years are devoted to clinical rotations and to continuing interdisciplinary instruction.

BASIC SCIENCES: Basic sciences are taught primarily through lectures. Labs and small group sessions are also utilized. First year courses consist of Human Gross Anatomy, Histology, Community Health I, Physiology, Nutrition, Behavioral Sciences, Bioethics and Humanities in Medicine, Problem Base Learning I, Introduction to Clinical Skills, and Student Well-being Program. Second year courses are: Microbiology and Immunology, Psychopathology, Pharmacology, Pathology, Pathophysiology, Clinical Medicine, Clinical Skills, Community Health II, and Problem Based Learning II. Most instruction during the first two years takes place in the new Biomedical Sciences building, which also houses laboratories and research facilities.

CLINICAL TRAINING: Clinical clerkships begin in the third year. These are comprised of Radiology (1 week), Internal Medicine (11 weeks), Family Medicine and Geriatrics (7 weeks), General Surgery (6 weeks), Pediatrics (9 weeks), and Ob/Gyn (9 weeks). Fourth year clerkships are: Surgical Specialties (6 weeks), Community Health II (3 weeks), Psychiatry (6 weeks), Emergency Medicine (2 weeks), and 16 weeks of electives. Major teaching hospitals are the Dr. Ramon Ruiz Arnau University Hospital, San Pablo Hospital, and the Medical Psychiatric Center. Other affiliated institutions are San Juan Veterans Administration Hospital, I. Gonzalez Martinez Oncologic Hospital, and Alejandro Otero Lopez Hospital.

Students

About 40 percent of students are women. Virtually all students are from underrepresented minority groups.

STUDENT LIFE: To help students acclimate to medical school, an orientation is given to the entering first-year class. This also serves as an opportunity for students to interact with each other and with faculty members and administrators. Students are encouraged to develop an interest in culture and the arts. With this in mind, the Dean of Student Affairs sponsors social and cultural activities for medical students. Counseling services are aimed at helping students take advantage of the extensive educational opportunities at the Medical School. A comprehensive health plan is offered to all medical students. Housing facilities are available through individual arrangements in areas adjacent to the Medical School and the University Hospital.

GRADUATES: The Medical School has graduated about 1,500 physicians who serve the Commonwealth of Puerto Rico and Hispanic communities in the United States.

Admissions

REQUIREMENTS: Applicants must demonstrate proficiency in both Spanish and English. This is essential, as lectures are conducted in the language preferred by the respective professor, most often Spanish. In addition, Spanish is necessary for most clinical work. Applicants must complete a minimum of 90 credits at an institution of higher education. A baccalaureate degree is highly recommended. Required premedical course are: General Biology (8 semester hours), General Chemistry (8 hours), Organic Chemistry (8 hours), Physics (8 hours), college-level Math (6 hours), English (6 hours), Spanish (6 hours), and Behavioral Sciences and/or Humanities (6 hours). The MCAT is required. Officials exam results from within the past two years must be submitted to the School of Medicine.

PROCESS: The Universidad Central del Caribe School of Medicine participates in the American Medical College Application Service (AMCAS). All applicants must file an AMCAS application. In addition, applicants should contact the School of Medicine for an Institutional Application form. This form is returned with a processing fee, photographs, an essay, and a certificate of Good Conduct. After applications, MCAT scores, and transcripts are given an initial review, applicants who are under consideration will be invited for personal interviews with members of the Faculty.

Cost

Tuition for Puerto Rico residents is $8,500 per semester. For nonresidents, tuition is $12,000 per semester.

FINANCIAL AID: Several types of financial aid are available. For students of exceptional financial need (EFN) who are willing to commit to entering a primary health care field, EFN scholarships cover the cost of tuition, fees, and books. Financial Assistance for Disadvantaged Health Profession Students offers a similar package to eligible students. Residents of Puerto Rico with financial need may qualify for Legislative Scholarships, which are renewed on a yearly basis. In addition to scholarships, qualified medical students may apply for subsidized and unsubsidized loans.

UNIVERSIDAD CENTRAL DEL CARIBE

STUDENT BODY

Type	Private
*Enrollment	NR
*% male/female	NR
*% underrepresented minorities	NR
# applied (total/out)	1,009/618
% interviewed (total/out)	13/4
% accepted (total/out)	NR/NR
% enrolled (total/out)	NR/NR

ADMISSIONS

Average GPA and MCAT Scores

Overall GPA	NR	Science GPA	NR
MCAT Bio	NR	MCAT Phys	NR
MCAT Verbal	NR	MCAT Essay	NR

Score Release Policy

The school has not responded to our inquiry regarding withheld MCAT scores. Therefore, we advise caution. Contact the Admissions Office before witholding any scores.

Application Information

Regular application	6/1–12/15
Regular notification	10/15–varies
Admissions may be deferred?	No
AMCAS application accepted?	Yes
Interview required?	Yes
Application fee	$50

COSTS AND AID

Tuition & Fees

Tuition (in/out)	$17,000/$24,000
Cost of books	NR
Fees	$2,504

Financial Aid

% students receiving aid	NR
Average grant	NR
Average loan	NR
Average debt	NR

*Figures based on total enrollment

PONCE SCHOOL OF MEDICINE

PO Box 7004, Ponce, PR 00732

Admissions: 787-840-2575

Ponce School of Medicine is located in the southern part of the island of Puerto Rico, and benefits from the resources of the city of Ponce. The School strives to prepare primary care physicians to serve in Puerto Rico and among Hispanic communities in the continental United States. Along with fulfilling standard premedical school requirements, applicants should be bilingual in Spanish and English. Ponce promotes and sponsors scientific research.

Academics

The primary goal of the School of Medicine is to provide quality medical education to bilingual students, with an emphasis on primary care and family medicine. The curriculum includes a strong emphasis on basic sciences, enabling students to get the most out of their clinical training. Longitudinal programs in preventive medicine and medical ethics are integrated into the four-year curriculum.

BASIC SCIENCES: Basic sciences are taught during the first two years. Year one courses include: Gross Anatomy Imaging and Embryology, Cellular Biology and Histology, Neuroscience, Biochemistry, Microbiology and Immunology, Behavioral Science, Physiology, General Pathology, Bioethics, Human Genetics, and a year-long session devoted to clinical correlation. Second year courses are: Pathophysiology, Pathology, Pharmacology, Psychiatry, Introduction to Clinical Medicine, Infectious Diseases, Family and Community Medicine, and Bioethics. Instructional methods include computer-assisted learning, lectures, labs, and problem-based learning. Standardized patients are used for teaching and evaluation of basic clinical skills. During the first two years, students are in class or other scheduled sessions for about 30 hours per week. Students must pass Step I of the USMLE for promotion to year three.

CLINICAL TRAINING: The third year begins in July with two weeks of a course called Introduction to Hospital Life. Following this orientation, students begin required clerkships. These are: Internal Medicine (10 weeks), Surgery (10 weeks), Pediatrics (10 weeks), Ob/Gyn (5 weeks), Psychiatry (5 weeks), and Family Medicine (5 weeks). The third year also includes a Dean's Hour, which emphasizes Medical Humanities, Health Economics, Law, Bioethics, and Literature. In the fourth year, students participate in a required clerkship in Medicine (4 weeks), a Sub-internship (Medicine, Ob/Gyn, Pediatrics, or Family Medicine), a clerkship in Emergency Medicine (4 weeks), and a Primary Care Selective (4 weeks). Students are also required to complete 16 weeks of elective rotations, of which five weeks may be completed at sites other than Ponce. USMLE Step II must be passed prior to graduation.

STUDENT LIFE: The relatively small class size of 60 students encourages communication among students and faculty. The School's location is an asset, offering a pleasant environment for living and studying.

Admissions

REQUIREMENTS: Required undergraduate course work includes eight semester credits in Biology, General Chemistry, Organized Chemistry, and Physics in addition to six credits in Advanced Math and Spanish. Twelve credits in both Behavioral Sciences and English are also required. Behavioral science includes Psychology, Sociology, Anthropology, Political Sciences, Economics, and Anthropology. Applicants must have a minimum overall grade point average of 2.7 and an average of 2.5 in science courses. The MCAT is required, and scores should be from within one year of application. Applicants should have at least the mean on all sections of the MCAT.

SUGGESTIONS: In evaluating applicants, the Admissions Committee considers academic achievements, MCAT scores, interview reports, letters of recommendation, and other supplementary information. Preference is given to residents of Puerto Rico.

PROCESS: Ponce takes part in the AMCAS application process. The deadline for submission to AMCAS is December 15. Secondary applications are sent to all qualified applicants, and interviews are conducted throughout the spring.

Cost

Tuition for Puerto Rico residents is $16,973. For nonresidents, the cost is $25,304. Nonresident students can acquire resident status at the School after successful completion of the first two years of the medical program.

FINANCIAL AID: Assistance is primarily need-based. Most financial aid is in the form of loans.

PONCE SCHOOL OF MEDICINE

STUDENT BODY

Type	Private
*Enrollment	NR
*% male/female	NR
*% underrepresented minorities	NR
# applied (total/out)	989/638
% interviewed (total/out)	20/6
% accepted (total/out)	NR/NR
% enrolled (total/out)	NR/NR

ADMISSIONS

Average GPA and MCAT Scores

Overall GPA	3.37	Science GPA	NR
MCAT Bio	NR	MCAT Phys	NR
MCAT Verbal	NR	MCAT Essay	NR

Score Release Policy

The school has not responded to our inquiry regarding withheld MCAT scores. Therefore, we advise caution. Contact the Admissions Office before witholding any scores.

Application Information

Regular application	12/1
Regular notification	10/15 until filled
†Early application	6/1–8/1 (residents only)
†Early notification	10/1
Admissions may be deferred?	No
AMCAS application accepted?	Yes
Interview required?	Yes
Application fee	$50

COSTS AND AID

Tuition & Fees

Tuition (in/out)	$16,973/$25,304
Cost of books	NR
Fees	$1,761

Financial Aid

% students receiving aid	NR
Average grant	NR
Average loan	NR
Average debt	NR

†For Puerto Rico residents only

*Figures based on total enrollment

UNIVERSITY OF PUERTO RICO

SCHOOL OF MEDICINE

G.P.O. Box 365067, San Juan, PR 00936-5067

Admissions: 787-766-4992

Internet: www.upr.clu.edu

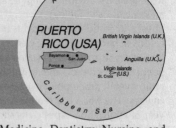

The Medical Sciences Campus at the University of Puerto Rico includes schools of Medicine, Dentistry, Nursing, and Pharmacy as well as the College of Health Related Professions, the Faculty of Biosocial Sciences, and the Graduate School of Public Health. The University of Puerto Rico strives to maintain a preeminent scientific and academic position by promoting medical education and research at local, national, and international levels.

Academics

Medical training is accomplished through a variety of educational experiences, both in the classroom and at multiple service settings in the public and private sectors of Puerto Rico. Medical students benefit from the resources of other health professional schools and from interaction with students at other schools. Through the Center for International Health, medical students gain exposure to the research and policy issues surrounding global health. Grading for all courses is on an A–F scale.

BASIC SCIENCES: Basic sciences are taught using a combination of lectures, small group discussions, labs, and exposure to clinical correlates. Required first year course are: Medical Gross Anatomy, Medical Histology, Medical Embryology, Medical Neuroscience, Introduction to Biochemistry, Human Physiology, Human Development I, Public Health and Preventive Medicine I, Integration Seminar I, Behavioral Sciences, and Introduction to Clinical Diagnosis. Second year courses consist of Pathobiology-Introduction to Laboratory Medicine, Infectious Diseases, Medical Pharmacology, Fundamentals of Clinical Diagnosis, Human Development II, Public Health and Preventive Medicine II, Basic Clinical Clerkship, Mechanisms of Disease, Psychopathology, and Integration Seminar II. Outside of the classroom, students learn in the Learning Resources Center, the Standardized Patient Laboratory, and the Clinical Learning Laboratory,

CLINICAL TRAINING: The third year is comprised of clinical rotations. These are: Radiology (2 weeks), Psychiatry (4 weeks), Medicine (12 weeks), Family Medicine (4 weeks), Pediatrics (10 weeks), Surgery (10 weeks), and Ob/Gyn (6 weeks). During year four, clerkships are: Dermatology (1 week); Physical Medicine and Rehabilitation (1 week); Public Health (3 weeks); Legal, Ethical, and Administrative Aspects in Medicine (1 week); and Selective Clerkships (8 weeks). In addition, 18 weeks are open for clinical and research electives. Clinical education uses a variety of settings including University Hospital, University Pediatric Hospital, San Juan City Hospital, Veterans Administration Hospital, and the Oncology Hospital. In addition, the school uses certain private hospitals, clinics, and public health facilities. Some electives may be taken at institutions other than those affiliated with the University of Puerto Rico, such as hospitals in other regions of Puerto Rico and in other countries.

Students

Each entering class has about 100 students. Students come from foreign countries and the mainland United States as well as Puerto Rico. Fifty percent of students are women.

STUDENT LIFE: Recreational facilities on campus include the Sports and Gym Center. The medical school promotes student health through its exercise/wellness program and by sponsoring a range of student activities and events. When they have free time, medical students enjoy the city of San Juan and its surroundings.

GRADUATES: The University of Puerto Rico and its affiliated hospitals offer residency programs in most major medical fields.

Admissions

REQUIREMENTS: With few exceptions, entering students must have completed their Bachelors degree. Prerequisite courses are one year each of Biology, General Chemistry, Physics, and Organic Chemistry. The MCAT is required, and August in the year prior to admission is the latest acceptable test date.

SUGGESTIONS: Both residents of Puerto Rico and nonresidents are considered for admission. Grade point average and MCAT scores are important in admissions decisions. In addition to academic credentials, the University of Puerto Rico looks for integrity and motivation in its students.

PROCESS: All applicants are encouraged to visit the campus. Candidates for the M.D. program must submit an application by December 1. Those who qualify are invited to interview after their applications are reviewed. Final decisions and notifications are made throughout the year and are completed in the spring.

Cost

Tuition for the School of Medicine is $5,000 per year for residents and $10,500 per year for nonresident students. However, nonresident students from the United States pay fees equal to the amount they would pay in their home state.

FINANCIAL AID: Honor students who are in the upper 5 percent of their class and who have a GPA of at least 3.5 are exempt from tuition after the first year. University employees and the children of permanent university employees do not pay tuition. Currently, about 60 percent of medical students receive financial aid, which is given in the form of grants or loans.

UNIVERSITY OF PUERTO RICO

STUDENT BODY

Type	Public
*Enrollment	NR
*% male/female	NR
*% underrepresented minorities	NR
# applied (total/out)	970/624
% interviewed (total/out)	15/1
% accepted (total/out)	NR/NR
% enrolled (total/out)	NR/NR

ADMISSIONS

Average GPA and MCAT Scores

Overall GPA	NR	Science GPA	NR
MCAT Bio	NR	MCAT Phys	NR
MCAT Verbal	NR	MCAT Essay	NR

Score Release Policy

The school has not responded to our inquiry regarding withheld MCAT scores. Therefore, we advise caution. Contact the Admissions Office before witholding any scores.

Application Information

Regular application	12/1
Regular notification	3/31
Admissions may be deferred?	Yes
AMCAS application accepted?	Yes
Interview required?	Yes
Application fee	$15

COSTS AND AID

Tuition & Fees

Tuition (in/out)	$5,000/$10,500
Cost of books	NR
Fees	$844

Financial Aid

% students receiving aid	NR
Average grant	NR
Average loan	NR
Average debt	NR

*Figures based on total enrollment

7 Osteopathic Profiles

ARIZONA COLLEGE OF OSTEOPATHIC MEDICINE

Office of Admissions, 19555 North 59th Avenue, Glendale, AZ 85308
Admission: 623-572-3215 • Fax: 623-572-3229

The Arizona College of Osteopathic Medicine (AZCOM) was founded in 1995. The College, along with its sister college, the Chicago College of Osteopathic Medicine (CCOM), is part of Midwestern University. In addition to the Colleges of Osteopathic Medicine, Midwestern University also includes a college of pharmacy and a college of health sciences. The school is located on a 124-acre site in scenic Glendale, Arizona, a suburb of Phoenix. Facilities include three main academic centers housing lecture halls, conference rooms, a student services facility, numerous lecture and laboratory classrooms boasting the finest in educational equipment, cadavers for anatomy laboratories rather than plastic models, on-campus housing which features one- and two-bedroom student apartments and a heated pool, a comprehensive library with computer resources and study rooms, a research facility, a clinic, and a student clubhouse. The mission of the Arizona College of Osteopathic Medicine of Midwestern University responds to the contemporary societal need for physicians by emphasizing primary care and education experiences needed to serve in rural and underserved urban communities.

Admissions

REQUIREMENTS: As a private institution, the college attracts a national applicant pool, and out-of-state residents account for over 80 percent of the group. Only 125 positions are available in each class, and in recent years there have been over 3,000 applicants. The average GPA of successful applicants is about 3.4 in both Sciences and overall. Minimum course work includes six semester hours in English and eight semester hours in each of the following: biology, inorganic chemistry, organic chemistry, and physics. The MCAT is required and must be no more than three years old. In addition to the AACOMAS application, applicants must submit a supplemental application (provided by the College after the AACOMAS application has been received).

STUDENT BODY	
Type	Private
*Enrollment	125
*% male/female	60/40
*% underrepresented minorities	3
# applied (total/out)	2,700/NR
% interviewed (total/out)	13/NR
% accepted (total/out)	10/NR
% enrolled (total/out)	46/NR
Average age	27

*Figures based on total enrollment

ADMISSIONS		
Average GPA and MCAT Scores		
Overall GPA 3.44	Science GPA 3.39	
MCAT Bio 9.10	MCAT Phys 8.33	
MCAT Verbal 8.28	MCAT Essay Q	
Application Information		
Regular application		2/1
Regular notification		NR
*AMCAS application accepted?		No
Application fee		$50

*AACOMAS application is required.

COSTS AND AID	
Tuition & Fees	
Tuition	$25,000
Cost of books	$2,060
Fees	$1,619
Financial Aid	
% students receiving aid	90
Average grant	$9,270
Average loan	$33,000
Average debt	$130,000

CHICAGO COLLEGE OF OSTEOPATHIC MEDICINE
MIDWESTERN UNIVERSITY

Office of Admissions, 555 31st Street, Downers Grove, IL 60515
Admission: 800-458-6253 or 630-515-6171 • Internet: admiss@midwestern.edu

Midwestern University administers the Chicago College of Osteopathic Medicine (CCOM), the Chicago College of Pharmacy, and the Chicago College of Allied Health Professions, in addition to related programs in Glendale, Arizona. The MWU campus is located in a western suburb of Chicago, Illinois. Clinical training takes place at various sites around the city and throughout the Midwest region. Students enjoy early clinical exposure through volunteering, preceptor programs, and formal patient contact in the second semester of year one. Research is also important at CCOM, which offers a combined D.O./Ph.D. program and has summer research awards for medical students. The Downers Grove campus offers modern academic and recreational facilities, in addition to on-campus housing. The male/female ratio is 60/40, and the average age of incoming students is about 25.

Admissions

REQUIREMENTS: The college receives between 4,000 and 5,000 applications each year to fill a class of 160 students. All AACOMAS applicants who meet minimum qualifications receive a secondary application, but only about 10 percent of applicants are interviewed. Interviews begin in September, and use a panel format. Notification occurs on a rolling basis, with about 60 percent of interviewees accepted. Science preparation must include two semesters or three quarters of Biology, Chemistry, Organic Chemistry, and Physics. To be competitive in the admissions process, candidates should have a minimum 3.0 GPA. The MCAT is required and should be no more than three years old. For applicants who have retaken the exam, the best set of scores is used. Though the school is private, some preference is given to Illinois residents.

STUDENT BODY	
Type	Private
*Enrollment	630
*% male/female	60/40
*% underrepresented minorities	8
# applied	3,935
% interviewed	10
% accepted	65
% enrolled	61
Average age	25

*Figures based on total enrollment

ADMISSIONS			
Average GPA and MCAT Scores			
Overall GPA	3.5	Science GPA	3.4
MCAT Bio	10	MCAT Phys	9
MCAT Verbal	9	MCAT Essay	NR
Application Information			
*Regular application			2/1
Regular notification			NR
AMCAS application accepted?			No
Application fee			$50

*Applicants are encouraged to apply early

COSTS AND AID	
Tuition & Fees	
Tuition (in/out)	$21,938/$26,645
Cost of books	$2,060
Fees	$280
Financial Aid	
% students receiving aid	91
Average grant	NR
Average loan	$38,500
Average debt	$109,222

DES MOINES UNIVERSITY
COLLEGE OF OSTEOPATHIC MEDICINE AND SURGERY

3200 Grand Avenue, Des Moines, IA 50312

Admission: 515-271-1400 • Fax: 515-271-1578

Email: doadmit@dsmu-edu • Internet: www.dsmu.edu

The College of Osteopathic has a flexible program, which allows students to meet a range of professional goals. Medical students study alongside other health-professions students, giving them a more complete picture of health care provision. The first-year curriculum is primarily basic-science instruction, with a clinically based course focusing on the physical diagnosis beginning in the second semester. The second-year curriculum uses a systems-based approach that integrates clinical and basic sciences. Third- and fourth-year rotations may be selected from sites across the country. Des Moines is a city of 450,000 and is an affordable, convenient place to live. The average age of incoming students is about 24, and the male/female ratio is 60/40.

Admissions

REQUIREMENTS: Eight semester hours (with lab) each in biology, chemistry, organic chemistry, and physics are required. In addition, applicants must have taken six semester hours of English. We accept students without regard to legal state of residence. Usually 75 percent of students are from states other than Iowa. You can apply while working on your undergraduate degree but you should have plans to receive it by the time you register with the College. The MCAT (taken within the last two years) is required. Those AACOMAS applicants who meet the minimum requirements for GPA and MCAT are sent secondary applications and about half of those who return secondary applications are invited for an interview. Notification occurs on a rolling basis.

STUDENT BODY

Type	Private
*Enrollment	796
*% male/female	60/40
*% underrepresented minorities	19
# applied (total/out)	1,379/952
% interviewed (total/out)	27/70
% accepted (total/out)	27/70
% enrolled (total/out)	15/69
Average age	24

*Figures based on total enrollment

ADMISSIONS

Average GPA and MCAT Scores

Overall GPA	3.45	Science GPA	3.37
MCAT Bio	8.95	MCAT Phys	7.64
MCAT Verbal	7.93	MCAT Essay	O

Application Information

Regular application	2/1
Regular notification	Rolling
Transfers accepted?	Yes
Admissions may be deferred?	Yes
AMCAS application accepted?	No
Interview required?	Yes
Application fee	$50

COSTS AND AID

Tuition & Fees

Tuition	$23,900
Cost of books	$2,600
Fees	$75

Financial Aid

% students receiving aid	95
Average grant	$26,723
Average loan	$40,202
Average debt	$124,012

UNIVERSITY OF HEALTH SCIENCES
COLLEGE OF OSTEOPATHIC MEDICINE

2105 Independence Avenue, Kansas City, MO 64106-1453
Admission: 816-283-2000 or 800-234-4847
Internet: www.aacom.org/uhscom.htm

UHS-COM is both the largest medical school in the state of Missouri and the oldest in Kansas City, Missouri. Affordable and friendly, Kansas City's metropolitan area encompasses counties in the states of Kansas and Missouri. The College as stated in the mission statement ". . . prepare(s) men and women to be exceptionally competent osteopathic physicians. . . ." For 1999, 42 percent female of the entering class was female, and the average age was 26. The age range was 21–42, and class size is 220. For its exemplary curriculum devoted to understanding the relationship between healing and a patient's spiritual beliefs, the University received the coveted Spirituality and Medicine Award from the John Templeton Foundation.

Admissions

REQUIREMENTS: As a private school, no preference is given to Missouri residents. Course requirements are 15 semester hours of biology, 3 of which must be in genetics; 16 semester hours of chemistry, 3 of which must be in biochemistry; 8 semester hours of physics; and 6 semester hours of English and/or literature. It is expected that required science courses have labs. The MCAT is required and must be no more than three years old. For those who have retaken the exam, the best set of scores is considered. AACOMAS applicants who meet minimum requirements are sent secondary applications. About 15 percent of applicants are interviewed, with interviews occurring between September and April. The interview consists of one session with a group of faculty members including osteopathic physicians on staff. Applicants are advised to know the history and tenets of osteopathic medicine and to be able to articulate their personal motivation for osteopathic medicine. About 85 percent of interviewees are accepted, with notification occurring on a rolling basis. The average GPA of successful applicants is about 3.5, and the average MCAT is 8.5.

STUDENT BODY	
Type	Private
*Enrollment	864
*% male/female	65/35
*% underrepresented minorities	10
# applied (total/out)	3,060/2,899
% interviewed (total/out)	14/NR
% accepted (total/out)	13/NR
% enrolled (total/out)	7/NR
Average age	26

*Figures based on total enrollment

ADMISSIONS	
Average GPA and MCAT Scores	
Overall GPA 3.48	Science GPA 3.46
MCAT Bio 8.82	MCAT Phys 8.11
MCAT Verbal 8.39	MCAT Essay O
Application Information	
Regular application	2/1
Regular notification	Rolling
Transfers accepted?	Yes
Admissions may be deferred?	No
AMCAS application accepted?	No
Interview required?	Yes
Application fee	$35

COSTS AND AID	
Tuition & Fees	
Tuition	$27,775
Cost of books	$1,075 (4-yr. avg.)
Fees	$50
Financial Aid	
% students receiving aid	94
Average grant	$1,500
Average loan (UHS Loan)	$4,000
Average debt	$140,000

KIRKSVILLE COLLEGE OF OSTEOPATHIC MEDICINE

Office of Admissions, 800 West Jefferson, Kirksville, MO 63501
Admission: 660-626-2237 • Fax: 660-626-2969 • Internet: www.kcom.edu

The Kirksville College of Osteopathic Medicine is the founding school of osteopathic medicine, and is distinguished by offering an education firmly based on holistic care, wellness, and academic excellence. Kirksville has a reputation for training physicians in primary care areas, as well as providing a strong clinical and basic science education for specialization. Though the first two years are reserved for basic science instruction, a clerkship with a primary care physician is included in the first-year curriculum. Traditional tenets of osteopathic medicine are coupled with the use of all modern technology, thus providing a well-rounded, comprehensive education. Problem solving and critical thinking are emphasized in both the basic science courses and clinical training. Clinical rotations take place in one of the following areas: Arizona, Michigan, Missouri, Ohio, and Utah. Additional fourth-year rotations take place in Georgia, New York, and Texas. Kirksville is a community of approximately 20,000 residents. With a 1999 class size of 170, the average age is 26 with a composite MCAT of 27 and an overall GPA of 3.41.

Admissions

REQUIREMENTS: As a private institution, no preference is given to Missouri residents, and almost all states are represented in the student body. Course requirements are Biology (8 semester hours); Chemistry (8 hours); Organic Chemistry (8 hours); Physics (8 hours); and English (6 hours). To be considered for admission, applicants should have a minimum GPA of 2.5 in both the sciences and overall. The MCAT is required and scores must be no more than three years old. About 10 percent of AACOMAS applicants are interviewed, with interviews consisting of two sessions with faculty or administrators. Financial aid, both merit- and need-based, is available in the form of grants and loans.

STUDENT BODY	
Type	Private
*Enrollment	608
*% male/female	72/28
*% underrepresented minorities	1.5
# applied (total/out)	3,054/2,900
% interviewed (total/out)	15/91
% accepted (total/out)	NR/NR
% enrolled (total/out)	50/90
Average Age	26

*Figures based on total enrollment

ADMISSIONS			
Average GPA and MCAT Scores			
Overall GPA 3.41		Science GPA 3.32	
MCAT Bio 9.46		MCAT Phys 8.99	
MCAT Verbal 8.98		MCAT Essay Q	
Application Information			
Regular application			2/1
Regular notification			NR
EDP application deadline			8/1
EDP notification decision			10/15
Deferred admissions			Yes
Transfers accepted?			Yes
AMCAS application accepted?			No
Application fee			$50

COSTS AND AID	
Tuition & Fees	
Tuition	$24,400
Cost of books	NR
Fees	NR
Financial Aid	
% students receiving aid	93
Average grant	$4,900
Average loan	$36,500
Average debt	$112,618

LAKE ERIE COLLEGE OF OSTEOPATHIC MEDICINE

Office of Admissions, 1858 West Grandview Boulevard, Erie, PA 16509

Admission: 814-866-8111 • Fax: 814-866-8123 • Internet: www.lecom.edu

Lake Erie College of Osteopathic Medicine is located in Erie, Pennsylvania. Its mission is to train primary care physicians to serve the needs of Northwestern Pennsylvania as well as underserved and rural areas. The curriculum is divided into three phases: Introduction to the Basic Sciences, Correlated Systems, and Clinical Experience. Clinical exposure is offered in the second semester of the first year.

Admissions

REQUIREMENTS: LECOM is a private college; no preference is given to state resident applicants. Science course requirements are: 8 semester hours of Biology, Chemistry, Organic Chemistry, and Physics. In addition, 6 semester hours of English and Behavioral Science are required. The MCAT is required and must be no more than three years old. Students are required to apply through AACOMAS, the central processor for osteopathic colleges. Secondary applications are sent to students after their AACOMAS applications are received. Applicant interviews are scheduled between October and March. Acceptance notification occurs on a rolling basis.

STUDENT BODY	
Type	Private
*Enrollment	498
*% male/female	65/35
*% underrepresented minorities	12.5
# applied (total/out)	3,350/2,861
% interviewed	17
% accepted (total/out)	6/44
% enrolled (total/out)	64/43
Average age	25

*Figures based on total enrollment

ADMISSIONS

Average GPA and MCAT Scores

Overall GPA	3.3	Science GPA	3.2
MCAT Bio	8.09	MCAT Phys	7.58
MCAT Verbal	7.87	MCAT Essay	O

Application Information

Priority application	2/1
Regular application	3/15
Regular notification	Rolling
AMCAS application accepted?	No
Application fee	$50

COSTS AND AID

Tuition & Fees

Tuition (in/out)	$21,760/$22,760
Cost of books	$1,000
Fees	$1,000

Financial Aid

% students receiving aid	90
Average grant	NR
Average loan	$36,000
Average debt	$126,000

UNIVERSITY OF MEDICINE AND DENTISTRY OF NEW JERSEY
SCHOOL OF OSTEOPATHIC MEDICINE

Admissions Office, Academic Center
One Medical Center Drive, Suite 162A, Stratford, NJ 08084
Admission: 609-566-7050 • Fax: 609-566-6222 • Internet: www.aacom.org/umdnjsom.htm

The UMDNJ School of Osteopathic medicine is a state-affiliated institution, focused on training primary care physicians to help meet the health care needs of the New Jersey population. Although most students follow a four-year curriculum leading to the D.O., a newly implemented D.O./Ph.D. program is suitable for students with interest and experience in research. Contiguous to the School of Medicine are the clinical facilities of the University Medical Center at Stratford. First- and second-year medical students benefit from this proximity, with clinical exposure integrated into basic science studies. Third- and fourth-year students rotate to teaching sites around the state. Affiliated teaching facilities are: University Medical Center divisions at Cherry Hill and Washington Township; Atlantic City Medical Center (615 beds); Christ Hospital (400 beds); and Our Lady of Lourdes Hospital (200 beds). Among all students, the male/female ratio is about 55/45. Underrepresented minorities make up approximately 10 percent of each class. Class size is 75.

Admissions

REQUIREMENTS: Residents of New Jersey account for 90 percent of the student body and are given priority in admissions. The minimum course requirements are eight semester hours of Biology, Physics, Chemistry, and Organic Chemistry, all with associated labs, and six semester hours each of English, Math, and Social Sciences. Applicants should have at least a 3.0 GPA in both sciences and overall, as the average GPA of successful applicants is about 3.4. The MCAT is required, and must be no more than three years old. The average MCAT of successful applicants is in the 8–9 range. Just under 10 percent of approximately 3,200 applicants are interviewed, with interviews taking place between August and April. About one-third of interviewees are accepted. Wait-listed candidates may send supplementary information to update their files.

STUDENT BODY	
Type	Public
*Enrollment	NR
*% male/female	55/45
*% underrepresented minorities	10
# applied (total/out)	NR/NR
% interviewed (total/out)	NR/NR
% accepted (total/out)	NR/NR
% enrolled (total/out)	NR/NR

*Figures based on total enrollment

ADMISSIONS			
Average GPA and MCAT Scores			
Overall GPA	NR	Science GPA	NR
MCAT Bio	NR	MCAT Phys	NR
MCAT Verbal	NR	MCAT Essay	NR
Application Information			
Regular application			2/1
Regular notification			NR
AMCAS application accepted?			NR
Application fee			$125

COSTS AND AID	
Tuition & Fees	
Tuition (in/out)	$14,492/$22,679
Cost of books	NR
Fees	NR
Financial Aid	
% students receiving aid	NR
Average grant	NR
Average loan	NR
Average debt	NR

MICHIGAN STATE UNIVERSITY
COLLEGE OF OSTEOPATHIC MEDICINE

Director of Admissions, C110 East Fee Hall, MSUCOM, East Lansing, MI 48824
Admission: 517-353-7740 • Fax: 517-355-3296
Email: comadm.@com.msu.edu • Internet: www.com.msu.edu

The College of Osteopathic Medicine at Michigan State University is focused on meeting the health care needs of the state's population. Training primary care physicians both at the undergraduate and residency level and contributing to interdisciplinary research are key elements of the College's mission. The curriculum emphasizes early patient care, behavioral aspects of medicine, and lifelong learning. An unusual feature is the opportunity for students to jointly pursue Ph.D./D.O. degrees. The College shares some facilities with other MSU academic programs, such as nursing, veterinary medicine, and allopathic medicine. In total, MSU enrolls 40,000 students. Clinical training takes place throughout Michigan, in community hospitals, clinics, and other health care provider environments. In a recent class, the male/female ratio was 53/47, and the average age was about 26. Underrepresented minorities account for 15 percent of the students, most of whom are African American.

Admissions

REQUIREMENTS: Requirements are eight semester hours of Biology, Chemistry, Organic Chemistry, and Physics, in addition to six hours of English and Behavioral Science. Grades in these courses must be a 2.0 or better, and the combined science and overall GPAs must be a 2.5 or better. The MCAT is required, and scores can be no more than three years old. For those who have taken the exam more than once, all results are considered. All in-state residents, and about a quarter of out-of-state residents who submit preliminary applications through AACOMAS, receive secondary applications. About 10 percent of those returning secondaries are interviewed, and about 25 percent of those interviewed are accepted. Interviews take place from October through March and consist of two sessions with faculty members or administrators. About 80 percent of the 125 positions are reserved for Michigan residents.

STUDENT BODY	
Type	Public
*Enrollment	NR
*% male/female	53/47
*% underrepresented minorities	15
# applied (total/out)	3,164/NR
% interviewed (total/out)	NR/NR
% accepted (total/out)	NR/NR
% enrolled (total/out)	NR/NR
Average age	26

*Figures based on total enrollment

ADMISSIONS	
Average GPA and MCAT Scores	
Overall GPA 3.40	Science GPA 3.40
MCAT Bio 8.40	MCAT Phys 8.40
MCAT Verbal 8.40	MCAT Essay NR
Application Information	
Regular application	12/1
Regular notification	NR
Early application	9/15
Early notification	10/15
AMCAS application accepted?	No
Interview required?	Yes
Application fee	$60

COSTS AND AID	
Tuition & Fees	
Tuition (in/out)	$15,432/$32,829
Cost of books	NR
Fees	NR
Financial Aid	
% students receiving aid	NR
Average grant	NR
Average loan	NR
Average debt	NR

UNIVERSITY OF NEW ENGLAND
COLLEGE OF OSTEOPATHIC MEDICINE

11 Hills Beach Road, Biddeford, ME 04005
Admission: 207-283-0171, ext. 2212 or 800-477-4863 • Fax: 207-286-3678
Email: llacroix@mailbox.une.edu • Internet: www.une.edu

The UNE College of Osteopathic medicine is a private, nonprofit institution, focused largely on training physicians for Family Practice and other primary health care fields. Also emphasized is rural medicine, with the goal of graduating health practitioners who will help meet the health care needs of underserved populations in the New England region. A portion of the basic science curriculum at UNE uses a body systems approach and incorporates osteopathic principles and topics like human behavior, community health, health maintenance, and ethics. Clinical rotations begin midway through the third year, and take place in over 20 community hospitals and medical centers throughout the Northeast. The UNE campus offers a health science library, computer resources, a fitness center, and university-owned apartments. Biddeford is a small city situated on the water, with a population just under 20,000. The male/female ratio is about 55/45 and the average age of entering students in a recent class was 28. Underrepresented minorities account for about 4 percent of the student body. Class size is 115.

Admissions

REQUIREMENTS: Residents of New England are given some preference in admissions, though qualified applicants from other regions are considered. The minimum course requirements are one year each of Biology, Physics, Chemistry, and Organic Chemistry, all with associated labs. Applicants should have at least a 2.7 GPA in both sciences and overall, as the average overall GPA of successful applicants is about 3.3. The MCAT is required, and must be no more than two years old. The average MCAT of successful applicants is in the 8–9 range. Most of the 2,700 ACOMAS applicants receive secondary applications. Of those returning secondaries, approximately 10 percent are interviewed, with interviews taking place between August and April. The interview consists of one session, usually with a team of interviewers. About 80 percent of interviewed candidates are accepted on a rolling basis. Wait-listed candidates may send supplemental information to update their files.

STUDENT BODY

Type	Private
*Enrollment	438
*% male/female	58/42
*% underrepresented minorities	9
# applied	1,000
% interviewed (total/out)	4/2.7
% accepted	15
% enrolled	85
Average age	27

*Figures based on total enrollment

ADMISSIONS

Average GPA and MCAT Scores

Overall GPA	3.38	Science GPA	3.23
MCAT Bio	8.67	MCAT Phys	7.83
MCAT Verbal	8.50	MCAT Essay	P

Application Information

Regular application	1/2
Regular notification	Rolling
Transfers accepted?	Yes
Admissions may be deferred?	No
AMCAS application accepted?	No
Interview required?	Yes
Application fee	$55

COSTS AND AID

Tuition & Fees

Tuition	$26,220
Cost of books	NR
Fees	$260

Financial Aid

% students receiving aid	91
Average grant	$1,000
Average loan	NR
Average debt	NR

NEW YORK COLLEGE OF OSTEOPATHIC MEDICINE
NEW YORK INSTITUTE OF TECHNOLOGY

Box 170, Old Westbury, NY 11568
Admission: 516-626-6947 • Fax: 516-686-3831 • Internet: www.nyit.edu/nycom

The New York College of Osteopathic Medicine is part of the New York Institute of Technology, an independent institution that encompasses numerous academic and professional programs at the undergraduate and graduate level. In conjunction with some of these programs, medical students may pursue joint degrees, such as a D.O./M.B.A. or D.O./M.S. The College of Medicine is located 22 miles east of New York City and uses more than 20 clinical facilities in and around Manhattan, on Long Island, in upstate New York, and in northern New Jersey. With such a diverse patient population, students learn to be excellent clinicians in both primary and specialty fields. The medical student population itself is diverse, largely as a result of special efforts at recruiting women, minorities, and immigrants who were trained as physicians in other countries. Women account for 48 percent of the student body, and underrepresented minorities account for about 13 percent.

Admissions

REQUIREMENTS: Course requirements are 8 semester hours of Biology, Chemistry, Organic Chemistry, and Physics in addition to 6 semester hours of English. A minimum grade of 2.75/4.0 is expected in all of the required courses, and applicants' combined Science and overall GPAs must be higher than 2.75 for serious consideration. The MCAT is required as well as a baccalaureate degree. About 20 percent of AACOMAS applicants are interviewed, with interviews taking place between November and May. The supplementary application is given to candidates at the time of interview. Interviews are conducted with basic science faculty and/or osteopathic physicians from the community. About two-third of those interviewed are accepted. Preference is given to New York residents and to residents of states in the northeastern United States.

STUDENT BODY

Type	Private
*Enrollment	1,007
*% male/female	52/48
*% underrepresented minorities	13
# applied (total/out)	32/4
% interviewed (total/out)	17/NR
% accepted (total/out)	14/NR
% enrolled (total/out)	56/NR

*Figures based on total enrollment

ADMISSIONS

Average GPA and MCAT Scores

Overall GPA	3.45	Science GPA	3.30
MCAT Bio	8.7	MCAT Phys	8.4
MCAT Verbal	7.4	MCAT Essay	NR

Application Information

Regular application	2/1
Regular notification	Rolling
AACOMAS application accepted?	Yes
Supplemental application fee	$60

COSTS AND AID

Tuition & Fees

Tuition	$24,000
Cost of books and supplies	$1,520
Fees	$726

Financial Aid

% students receiving aid	90
Average grant	NR
Average loan	NR
Average debt	NR

UNIVERSITY OF NORTH TEXAS HEALTH SCIENCE CENTER AT FORT WORTH

TEXAS COLLEGE OF OSTEOPATHIC MEDICINE

3500 Camp Bowie Boulevard, Fort Worth, TX 76107-2699
Admission: 800-535-TCOM (8266) or 817-735-2204 • Fax: 817-735-2225
Internet: www.hsc.unt.edu/education/tcom/admis.html

The Texas College of Osteopathic Medicine and the Graduate School of Biomedical Sciences comprise the University of North Texas Health Science Center, a state-supported institution known for education, research, and patient care. The College utilizes a modified systems approach in its curriculum, which examines the human body through nine distinct systems. Students enrolled during their first two years of study are taught anatomy, physiology, pharmacology and other basic sciences as related to each body system. At the same time, students develop an understanding of clinical applications on how to diagnose and treat patient illnesses. During the third and fourth year of study, students are able to pursue a number of clinical training programs throughout the state at university sites, clinics, and affiliated teaching hospitals. A rural medicine track that provides extensive preparation for those who wish to practice in small communities is also available. Approximately 75 percent of graduates enter a primary care field. Dual degree program options, including a D.O./Ph.D., D.O./M.S., D.O./M.P.H., and D.O./Dr.P.H. are also offered in conjunction with the Graduate School and School of Public Health.

Admissions

REQUIREMENTS: At least 90 percent of the positions in each class of 115 are reserved for Texas residents. One year of traditional pre-medical sciences is required, in addition to one year of English Composition. The MCAT is required, and scores must be from within the past three years. The average MCAT score of accepted applicants is 9 on each part. Applications are accepted through the Texas Medical and Dental Schools Application Service (TMDSAS). Selected applicants are invited to interview between August and December. Initial offers of acceptance are sent on January 15 and continue until the incoming class is full.

STUDENT BODY

Type	Public
*Enrollment	453
*% male/female	55/45
*% underrepresented minorities	11
# applied (total/out)	1,261/730
% interviewed (total/out)	23/5
% accepted (total/out)	14/2
% enrolled (total/out)	69/43
Average age	25

*Figures based on total enrollment

ADMISSIONS

Average GPA and MCAT Scores

Overall GPA	3.58	Science GPA	3.55
MCAT Bio	9.32	MCAT Phys	8.67
MCAT Verbal	7.4	MCAT Essay	NR

Application Information

Regular application	10/15
Regular notification	1/15
Early application	8/1
Early notification	10/1
Transfers accepted?	Yes
Admissions may be deferred?	Yes
AMCAS application accepted?	No
Interview required?	Yes
Application fee	$0

COSTS AND AID

Tuition & Fees

Tuition (in/out)	$6,550/$19,650
Cost of books	$2,110
Fees	$780

Financial Aid

% students receiving aid	5
Average grant	NR
Average loan	NR
Average debt	$72,554

NOVA SOUTHEASTERN UNIVERSITY
HEALTH PROFESSIONS DIVISION
COLLEGE OF OSTEOPATHIC MEDICINE

3200 S. University Drive, Fort Lauderdale, FL 33328
Admissions: 954-262-1101
Fax: 954-262-2282 • Internet: www.com.msu.edu

The Colleges of Osteopathic Medicine, Optometry, Allied Health, Pharmacy, and Biomedical Science are among the many schools featured at Nova Southeastern University, which is situated on a 232-acre campus in Fort Lauderdale. The curriculum includes two years of basic science instruction, followed by two years of clinical training. One of the required clinical rotations is a three-month clerkship in a rural, underserved area. Some students are admitted to a special seven-year primary medicine track that ensures residency placement, and others jointly pursue an M.P.H. along with the D.O. Seventy percent of graduates enter primary care fields. The male/female ratio is about 70/30, and the average age of incoming students is approximately 26.

Admissions

REQUIREMENTS: Typically, the College receives over 3,700 applications each year to fill a class of 150 students. All AACOMAS applicants receive a secondary application, but only a small percentage of applicants are interviewed. Interviews begin in September and consist of a session with a panel of health professionals. Notification occurs on a rolling basis. The minimum undergraduate GPA is 2.0. Science preparation must include eight semester hours each in Biology, Chemistry, Organic Chemistry, and Physics. In addition, three semester hours of English Literature and three of English Composition are required. The MCAT is required and should be no more than three years old. For applicants who have retaken the exam, the best set of scores is used. Though the school is private, preference is given to Florida residents, who comprise about 80 percent of the student body.

STUDENT BODY	
Type	Private
*Enrollment	585
*% male/female	67/33
*% underrepresented minorities	28
# applied (total/out)	NR/NR
% interviewed (total/out)	NR/NR
% accepted (total/out)	NR/NR
% enrolled (total/out)	NR/NR
Average age	26

*Figures based on total enrollment

ADMISSIONS		
Average GPA and MCAT Scores		
Overall GPA 3.45	Science GPA	3.30
MCAT Bio 8	MCAT Phys	8
MCAT Verbal 8	MCAT Essay	NR
Application Information		
Regular application		1/15
Regular notification		NR
AMCAS application accepted?		NR
Application fee		$50

COSTS AND AID	
Tuition & Fees	
Tuition (in/out)	$19,340/$22,720
Cost of books	NR
Fees	100
Financial Aid	
% students receiving aid	87
Average grant	$19,050
Average loan	$27,285
Average debt	$118,498

OHIO UNIVERSITY
COLLEGE OF OSTEOPATHIC MEDICINE

102 Grosvenor Hall, Athens, OH 45701
Admission: 740-593-4313 or 800-345-1560 • Fax: 740-593-2256
Internet: www.oucom.ohiou.edu

Though all students at the Ohio College of Osteopathic Medicine are encouraged to consider careers in primary care, a special track is offered to those who show particular enthusiasm for primary care. During the first two years, most students follow a clinical presentation curriculum. About 20 percent of the students follow an alternative, primary care-oriented curriculum that emphasizes problem-solving and lifelong-learning skills. All students begin to acquire patient skills during the first year in a Patient Simulation Program and through direct contact with patients at local ambulatory care sites. During the third and fourth years, those in the primary care track participate in longer-term, integrated clinical training sessions in addition to discrete rotations. Clinical education takes place at Centers for Osteopathic Regional Education (CORE), which are health care facilities grouped into five regions within the state. Students have the opportunity to enhance research skills in college-sponsored summer research programs. Women account for about 46 percent of students, and underrepresented minorities account for about 18 percent. The average age of incoming students is 25.

Admissions

REQUIREMENTS: Eight semester hours each in Biology, Chemistry, Organic Chemistry, and Physics are required. In addition, applicants must have taken six semester hours of English and Social Science. As a state-affiliated institution, the college gives preference to Ohio residents, who make up about 80 percent of the student body. About 50 percent of AACOMAS applicants are sent supplemental applications. About 10 percent of those who submit supplemental applications are invited to interview. Interviews take place from October through April, and consist of three 30-minute sessions with members of the faculty or administration. Approximately one-third of interviewees are accepted, with notification occurring on a rolling basis. In the past, successful candidates have had a mean GPA of 3.4 and an average of at least 8 on each section of the MCAT.

STUDENT BODY

Type	Public
*Enrollment	404
*% male/female	54/46
*% underrepresented minorities	23
# applied (total/out)	2,404/1,925
% interviewed (total/out)	NR/NR
% accepted (total/out)	6/1
% enrolled (total/out)	57/61
Average age	25

*Figures based on total enrollment

ADMISSIONS

Average GPA and MCAT Scores

Overall GPA	3.50	Science GPA	3.39
MCAT Bio	8.72	MCAT Phys	8.11
MCAT Verbal	8.24	MCAT Essay	O

Application Information

Regular application	1/2
Regular notification	Rolling
Transfers accepted?	Yes
Admissions may be deferred?	Yes
AMCAS application accepted?	No
Interview required?	Yes
Application fee	$25

COSTS AND AID

Tuition & Fees

Tuition (in/out)	$10,929/$10,929
Cost of books	$2,738
Fees (in/out)	$1,065/5001

Financial Aid

% students receiving aid	89
Average grant	$2,500
Average loan	$20,358
Average debt	$95,000

OKLAHOMA STATE UNIVERSITY
COLLEGE OF OSTEOPATHIC MEDICINE

1111 West 17th Street, Tulsa, OK 74107
Admission: 918-561-8421 or 800-677-1972 • Fax: 918-561-8250
Email: Labgood@osu-com.okstate.edu • Internet: http://osu.com.okstate.edu/osucom.html

The curriculum at the College of Osteopathic Medicine includes hands-on clinical experiences, student-centered, and problem-based methods of instruction, as well as frequent consultation with faculty and community-based physicians. The first year focuses on biomedical sciences, and the second year emphasizes case-based learning and problem solving as it relates to conditions seen in primary care environments. The third and fourth years are composed of clinical rotations, most of which take place at Tulsa Regional Medical Center, the country's largest osteopathic hospital (521 beds). Students also rotate to adjacent rural areas, and they may fulfill requirements at various medical institutions across the country. Although 64 percent of graduates enter primary care, they are prepared to enter residencies in all medical specialty fields. The medical school, a college of Oklahoma State University, is located in Tulsa, a very livable city of about 500,000.

Admissions

REQUIREMENTS: Of the 88 positions in a class, 73 are reserved for Oklahoma residents. Prerequisites for application are 8–10 semester hours of Biology, Physics, Chemistry, and Organic Chemistry with labs, in addition to 6–8 hours of English, and 1 upperlevel science course. The minimum undergraduate GPA is 3.0, and an average of 7.0 on the MCAT is required. All AACOMAS applicants meeting these requirements receive a secondary application, but only about 10 percent of applicants are interviewed. Interviews begin in October, and continue until early March. Interviews are one on one, and typically each applicant will have two interviews. Notification occurs on a rolling basis, and about 35 to 40 percent of interviewees are accepted.

STUDENT BODY

Type	Public
*Enrollment	350
*% male/female	64/36
*% underrepresented minorities	19
# applied (total/out)	1,161/914
% interviewed (total/out)	NR/NR
% accepted (total/out)	88/14
% enrolled (total/out)	NR/NR
Average age	26

*Figures based on total enrollment

ADMISSIONS

Average GPA and MCAT Scores

Overall GPA	3.53	Science GPA	3.35
MCAT Bio	8.30	MCAT Phys	8.08
MCAT Verbal	8.85	MCAT Essay	Q

Application Information

Regular application	1/15
Regular notification	Rolling
Transfers accepted?	Yes
Admissions may be deferred?	Yes
AMCAS application accepted?	No
Interview required?	Yes
Application fee	$25

COSTS AND AID

Tuition & Fees

Tuition (in/out)	$9,552/$24,244
Cost of books	$1,400
Fees	$836

Financial Aid

% students receiving aid	90
Average grant	$5,800
Average loan	$24,482
Average debt	$97,500

PHILADELPHIA COLLEGE OF OSTEOPATHIC MEDICINE

Office of Admissions/Registrar, 4170 City Avenue, Philadelphia, PA 19131
Admission: 800-999-6998 or 215-871-6700 • Fax: 215-871-6719
Email: admissions@pcom.edu • Internet: www.pcom.edu

Philadelphia College of Osteopathic Medicine (PCOM) is among the five-largest medical schools in the country, with 250 students per class. Early clinical exposure through community service activities and formal course work complement basic science instruction. The curriculum is interdisciplinary, includes topics such as medical ethics and medical law, and emphasizes primary care and prevention. Clinical training takes place at 33 affiliated institutions in and around Philadelphia. In addition, students may arrange to fulfill elective requirements in other states or in other countries. Joint-degree programs lead to the D.O./M.B.A. or D.O./M.P.H. The entering class of 1999 included students from 20 states. The male/female ratio was 55/45, and the average age was 25.

Admissions

REQUIREMENTS: As a private institution, PCOM accepts applicants from all over the country and does show preference for Pennsylvania residents. Science preparation must include 8 semester hours each in Biology, Inorganic Chemistry, Organic Chemistry, and Physics. In addition, 6 hours of English Literature/Composition are required. The MCAT is required, and for applicants who have retaken the exam, the best set of scores is used. All AACOMAS applicants receive secondary applications. Of the approximately 4,000 applicants returning secondaries, about 18 percent are invited to interview on campus, with interviews beginning in September. The interview consists of one session with a panel that could include faculty, students, and administrators. Notification of committee decision occurs on a rolling basis. In a recently accepted class, the average GPA was 3.33 overall, and the average combined MCAT score was 26.

STUDENT BODY	
Type	Private
*Enrollment	996
*% male/female	55/45
*% underrepresented minorities	14
# applied (total/out)	3,855/2,676
% interviewed (total/out)	300/273
% accepted (total/out)	6/3
% enrolled (total/out)	77/71
Average age	26

*Figures based on total enrollment

ADMISSIONS			
Average GPA and MCAT Scores			
Overall GPA	3.33	Science GPA	3.25
MCAT Bio	8.50	MCAT Phys	8.00
MCAT Verbal	8.10	MCAT Essay	O
Application Information			
Regular application			2/1
Regular notification			Rolling
Early application			9/1
Early notification			11/1
Transfers accepted?			No
Admissions may be deferred?			No
AMCAS application accepted?			No
Interview required?			Yes
Application fee			50

COSTS AND AID	
Tuition & Fees	
Tuition	$23,500
Cost of books	$1,465
Fees	$225
Financial Aid	
% students receiving aid	89
Average grant	$8,951
Average loan	$37,000
Average debt	$147,600

PIKEVILLE COLLEGE
SCHOOL OF OSTEOPATHIC MEDICINE

147 Sycamore Street, Pikeville, KY 41501
Admissions: 606-432-9617 • Internet: www.pc.edu

Pikeville is the newest school of osteopathic medicine in the country, and is devoted primarily to meeting the demand for primary care practitioners in the Appalachian region. Teaching lifelong-learning skills is an important aspect of the School's program, as is integrating behavioral and social aspects of medicine into basic science and clinical training. Patient contact begins during the first two years, when students learn to take medical histories by working with community physicians and their patients one afternoon each week. About 20 percent of contact hours are focused on community and behavior medicine. In support of a commitment to primary care, about 30 percent of required clinical rotations take place in ambulatory primary care settings such as physician's offices and rural clinics. At least 90 percent of this training occurs at sites in the Appalachian region.

Admissions

Pikeville does participate in the AACOMAS application process. Requirements for admission include twelve hours of Biology, four hours of Chemistry, eight hours of Physics, and eight hours of Organic Chemistry. The MCAT is required.

STUDENT BODY

Type	Private
Enrollment	240
*% male/female	53/47
*% underrepresented minorities	2
# applied (total/out)	1,598/115
% interviewed (total/out)	7/NR
% accepted (total/out)	81/NR
% enrolled (total/out)	60/NR
Average age	28

*Figures based on total enrollment

ADMISSIONS

Average GPA and MCAT Scores

Overall GPA	3.33	Science GPA	3.25
MCAT Bio	7.70	MCAT Phys	7.10
MCAT Verbal	7.50	MCAT Essay	O

Application Information

Regular application	2/1
Regular notification	Rolling
Transfers accepted?	Yes
Admissions may be deferred?	No
AMCAS application accepted?	No
AACOMAS accepted	Yes
Interview required?	Yes
Application fee	$75

COSTS AND AID

Tuition & Fees

Tuition	$23,100
Cost of books	$0
Fees	$0

Financial Aid

% students receiving aid	96
Average grant	$12,457
Average loan	$25,900
Average debt	NR

TOURO UNIVERSITY COLLEGE OF OSTEOPATHIC MEDICINE
SAN FRANCISCO

Dr. Donald Haight, Dir. of Admissions
Mare Island, CA 94592
Admisssions (CA): 888-880-7336 (outside CA): 888-887-7336
Internet: www.tucom.edu

The Touro University College of Osteopathic Medicine, San Francisco, is located in the northeast part of San Francisco Bay, on Mare Island. Touro University is an international institution based in New York, with branches in Israel and the Russian Federation. The mission of the TUCOM is to train osteopathic, family practice physicians to help meet the need for primary care practitioners in California and throughout the country. Though preventative medicine and primary care are emphasized, graduates are also prepared to enter residency programs that train osteopathic specialists. Patient contact begins in the first year, and clinical training takes place at sites throughout the greater Bay Area including hospitals, clinics and physicians' offices. Students have the opportunity to experience both urban and rural patient populations.

Admissions

Requirements are eight semester hours of Biology, Physics, Chemistry, and Organic Chemistry. Six semester hours each of English, Humanities, and Behavioral Sciences are also required. Computers are considered an important educational and informational tool, making computer literacy advisable. Touro participates in AACOMAS. The MCAT is required, and scores must be no more than three years old. In the past, successful applicants have had a 3.0 GPA in both the Sciences and overall, and an average score of 8 on the MCAT.

STUDENT BODY

Type	Private
*% male/female	57/43
*% underrepresented minorities	3
# applied	NR
% interviewed	NR
% accepted	NR
% enrolled	NR
Average age	26.2

*Figures based on total enrollment

ADMISSIONS

Average GPA and MCAT Scores

Overall GPA	3.5	Science GPA	3.4
MCAT Bio	10	MCAT Phys	9
MCAT Verbal	8	MCAT Essay	NR

Application Information

Regular application	Yes
Regular notification	NR
Transfers accepted?	No
Admissions may be deferred?	No
AMCAS application accepted?	No
Interview required?	Yes
Application fee	$100

COSTS AND AID

Tuition & Fees

Tuition	$25,000
Cost of books	$1,500
Fees	$1,965

Financial Aid

% students receiving aid	92
Average grant	$0
Average loan	$44,000
Average debt	NR

WEST VIRGINIA SCHOOL OF OSTEOPATHIC MEDICINE

Director of Admissions/Registrar, 400 North Lee Street, Lewisburg, WV 24901
Admission: 304-647-6251 • Fax: 304-645-4849 • Internet: www.wvsom.edu

The West Virginia School of Osteopathic Medicine is part of the West Virginia State System of Higher Education. As a state school located in rural Appalachia, it is geared towards meeting the needs of West Virginia's significantly rural population. Nine other states have loose affiliations with the School and are also served by its programs. The curriculum includes an organ-based approach to learning basic sciences, and clinical training at community sites. Among all students, the average age is 28, and the male/female ratio is 59/41.

Admissions

REQUIREMENTS: Residents of West Virginia account for 70 percent of the student body and are given priority in admissions. Residents of Alabama, Georgia, Mississippi, Maryland, Virginia, North and South Carolina, Tennessee, and Kentucky are then considered. The minimum course requirements are eight semester hours of Biology, Physics, General Chemistry, and Organic Chemistry, all with associated labs, and six semester hours of English. The average GPA of successful applicants is about 3.3 in both Sciences and overall. The MCAT is required and must have been taken between spring 1991 to the present. The average MCAT of successful applicants is in the 7–8 range. About 14 percent of approximately 1,700 applicants are interviewed, with interviews taking place between August and March. About one-third of interviewees are accepted. Wait-listed candidates may send supplementary information to update or strengthen their files.

STUDENT BODY

Type	Public
*Enrollment	261
*% male/female	59/41
*% underrepresented minorities	7
# applied (total/out)	1,630/1,437
% interviewed (total/out)	NR/NR
% accepted (total/out)	NR/2.4
% enrolled (total/out)	65/50
Average age	28

*Figures based on total enrollment

ADMISSIONS

Average GPA and MCAT Scores

Overall GPA	3.40	Science GPA	NR
MCAT Bio	7.30	MCAT Phys	6.90
MCAT Verbal	7.90	MCAT Essay	NR

Application Information

Regular application	1/2
Transfers accepted?	Yes
Admissions may be deferred?	No
Interview required?	Yes
Regular notification	NR
AMCAS application accepted?	NR
Application fee	$50

COSTS AND AID

Tuition & Fees

Tuition (in/out)	$11,490/$28,990
Cost of books	NR
Fees	NR

Financial Aid

% students receiving aid	95
Average grant	NR
Average loan	NR
Average debt	NR

WESTERN UNIVERSITY OF HEALTH SCIENCES
COLLEGE OF OSTEOPATHIC MEDICINE OF THE PACIFIC

Office of Admissions, 309 East College Plaza, Pomona, CA 91766-1889
Admission: 909-623-6116 • Fax: 909-469-5570
Internet: www.westernu.edu

The Western University of Health Sciences (Western U.) is comprised of five Colleges—College of Osteopathic Medicine of the Pacific (COMP), Allied Health Professions, Graduate Nursing, and Pharmacy. A college of Veterinary Medicine will welcome its first students in fall 2001. Western U. is a leader in training primary care practitioners, including nurses, osteopathic physicians, physician assistants, physical therapists, pharmacists, and family nurse practitioners. Clinical training facilities include Arrowhead Regional Medical Center and many affiliated ambulatory sites. The university is located 35 miles east of Los Angeles.

Admissions

REQUIREMENTS: Course minimum requirements are one year each of Biology, Chemistry, Organic Chemistry, Physics, English, and Behavioral Science. The MCAT is required and must be no more than 3 years old. In a recent class, accepted students had an average GPA of 3.3 both in the Sciences and overall, and an average MCAT score of 8.33. Applicants are advised that they must have a minimum GPA of 2.50 in the Sciences and overall to be considered for admission. Secondary applications may be sent to candidates meeting minimum requirements as determined by the AACOMAS application. The AACOMAS deadline is January 15.

STUDENT BODY

Type	Private
*Enrollment	695
*% male/female	55/45
*% underrepresented minorities	16
# applied (total/out)	2,912/NR
% interviewed (total/out)	15/NR
% accepted (total/out)	67/NR
% enrolled (total/out)	59/NR

*Figures based on total enrollment

ADMISSIONS

Average GPA and MCAT Scores

Overall GPA	3.4	Science GPA	3.3
MCAT Bio	9	MCAT Phys	9
MCAT Verbal	8	MCAT Essay	P

Application Information

Regular application	1/15
Regular notification	NR
AMCAS application accepted?	No
Application fee	$60

COSTS AND AID

Tuition & Fees

Tuition	$24,720
Cost of books	$2,076
Fees	$665

Financial Aid

% students receiving aid	95
Average grant	NR
Average loan	NR
Average debt	$124,039

8 Post-baccalaureate Pre-medical Programs

Colleges and universities offer organized post-baccalaureate pre-medical programs. Although this list is quite comprehensive, it is likely to be incomplete because many schools have just recently adopted post-bacc programs. In addition, many undergraduate institutions that do not offer formal programs have flexible enrollment policies that facilitate post-bacc studies.

For further listings of post-bacc programs, Syracuse University Health Professions Advisory Program (315-443-2321) has an online compilation at: www-hl.syr.edu/hpap.

The AAMC also has an up-to-date listing. See: **www.aamc.org/stuapps/appinfo/postbac.htm.**

AKRON UNIVERSITY

Richard Mostardi, Ph.D.
Department of Biology
Akron, OH 44325
216-972-7152

UNIVERSITY OF ALABAMA AT BIRMINGHAM

Minority Medical Education Program
1400 University Boulevard, 241 HUC
Birmingham, AL 35294-1150
800-707-3579

ALBRIGHT COLLEGE

Dr. Richard Heller
Chief Health Professions Advisor
Department of Biology
P.O. Box 19612
Reading, PA 19612-5234

AMERICAN INTERNATIONAL COLLEGE

Dr. Alan Dickinson
Chief Health Professions Advisor
1000 State Street
Springfield, MA 01109
413-737-7000, Ext. 379

ARIZONA STATE UNIVERSITY

Brice W. Corder, Assistant Dean
College of Liberal Arts and Sciences
Tempe, AZ 85287-1701
609-965-2365

ARMSTRONG STATE COLLEGE

Dr. Henry E. Harris
Department of Chemistry/Physics
Savannah, GA 31419-1997
912- 927-5304

Open to students who lack prerequisites basic to medicine.

AUGUSTA COLLEGE

John B. Black, Ph.D.
Professor of Biology
Department of Biology
2500 Walton Way
Augusta, GA 30910
404-737-1539

Open to students who lack prerequisites basic to medicine.

ALLEGHENY UNIVERSITY OF THE HEALTH SCIENCES

MCP Hahnemann School of Medicine
Medical Science Preparatory Program
  (attn. Gerald Soslau, Ph.D.)
Broad and Vine, Mail Stop 344
Philadelphia, PA 19102-1192
215-762-7864

Two programs are offered to help students enhance their credentials for entrance to medical school. The Medical Science Preparatory Program is a year-long, nondegree program for students who have completed the pre-medical science requirements but need to enhance their preparation. The Interdepartmental Medical Science program involves actual medical school course work.

ASSUMPTION COLLEGE

Dr. Allan Barnitt, Jr.
Division of Natural Sciences
Worcester, MA 01615-0005
508-752-5616, Ext. 293

AVILA COLLEGE

Dr. C. Larry Sullivan, Pre-medical Advisor
11901 Wornall Road
Kansas City, MO 64145
816-942-8400, Ext. 225

Program for underrepresented minorities and disadvantaged students who have been previously unsuccessful in gaining admission to medical school.

BARNARD COLLEGE

Associate Dean of Students and Chief Pre-medical Advisor
3009 Broadway
New York, NY 10027-6598
212-854-2024

Program offered to Barnard alumnae or female graduates of Bryn Mawr, Mount Holyoke, Radcliffe-Harvard, Smith, Vassar, or Wellesley.

BARRY UNIVERSITY

Dr. Elizabeth Hays
Biology Department
Miami Shores, FL 33161
305-899-3204

BEAVER COLLEGE

Dr. C. Mikulski
Chief Medical Professions Advisor
Glenside, PA 19038
215-572-2129

BENNINGTON COLLEGE

Post-baccalaureate Admissions
Bennington, VT 05201
802-442-5401

Bennington's full-time program is designed for students who have completed a bachelor's degree and have subsequently decided to pursue a career in medicine or allied health sciences. Generally, post-bacc studies require two years. Those who complete the program receive a comprehensive letter of evaluation. Qualified students may apply for direct acceptance to Allegheny University of the Health Sciences (MCP Hahnemann School of Medicine).

BOSTON UNIVERSITY

Dr. Glen B. Zamansky
Health Science Program Office
College of Liberal Arts
725 Commonwealth Avenue, Room B-2
Boston, MA 02215
617-353-4866

THE BOWMAN GRAY SCHOOL OF MEDICINE

Office of Minority Affairs
Post-baccalaureate Development Program
Medical Center Blvd.
Winston-Salem, NC 27157-1037
910-716-4201

The program is open to minority and disadvantaged students with a bachelor's degree from an accredited U.S. school; undergraduate GPA of 2.5 or better; total MCAT score of 21 or above and at least an N on the writing sample; and 8 semester hours each of Biology, Chemistry, Organic Chemistry, and Physics.

BRANDEIS UNIVERSITY

Post-baccalaureate Pre-medical Studies
Joy Paradissis Playter
Assistant Dean
Academic Fairs
Kutz 108
Waltham, MA 02254
617-736-3460

Open to students who lack prerequisites basic to medicine.

BRESCIA COLLEGE

Pre-professional Advisor
Biology/Medical Technology
717 Frederica Street
Owensboro, KY 42301
502-686-4276

BROWN UNIVERSITY

Pre-medical Special Student Program
Dean Mark Curran
Box 1959
Providence, RI 02906
401-863-3452

Program for Rhode Island residents and Brown alumnae. Possible direct admissions to Brown University School of Medicine.

BRYN MAWR POST-BACCALAUREATE PREMEDICAL PROGRAM

Canwyll House
Bryn Mawr College
101 North Merion Ave.
Bryn Mawr, PA 19010-2899
610-526-7350

Since 1972, Bryn Mawr has helped adults achieve their goal of becoming physicians. The Post-bacc program is selective, and most participants have little or no prior science background. Generally, courses are completed in one year, plus one or two summers. Bryn Mawr offers pre-medical advising, a composite letter of recommendation, and the possibility of direct entrance to several medical schools. These are MCP Hahnemann; Temple; Jefferson; University or Rochester; Brown; Dartmouth; and SUNY Stony Brook.

SAN JOSE STATE UNIVERSITY (CALIFORNIA STATE)

Post-baccalaureate Pre-medical studies
College of Science, Dept. of Biological Science
One Washington Square
San Jose, CA 95192-0100
408-924-4840

The Post-bacc program at San Jose State University is flexible, enrolling students with and without prior science course work. Post-bacc students study alongside undergraduates and benefit from pre-medical advisors.

SAN FRANCISCO STATE UNIVERSITY (CALIFORNIA STATE)

Dr. Barry S. Rothman
Health Professions Advising Committee
School of Science and Engineering, TH 323
1600 Holloway Avenue
San Francisco, CA 94132
415-338-2410

Open to students who lack prerequisites basic to medicine and/or who have been previously unsuccessful in gaining admission to medical school.

CALIFORNIA STATE UNIVERSITY—DOMINGUEZ HILLS

James Lyle, Pre-medical Advisor
Department of Chemistry
Carson, CA 90747
310-516-3376

CALIFORNIA STATE UNIVERSITY—FULLERTON

Albert Flores, Health Professions Coordinator
800 North State College Boulevard
Mail Stop KH203
Fullerton, CA 92634
714-773-3980

Offers pre-medical courses to college graduates interested in careers in medicine.

CALIFORNIA STATE UNIVERSITY—HAYWARD

Dr. Edward B. Lyke
Director Pre-professional Health Advisory Program
Hayward, CA 94542
510-885-2366

CALIFORNIA STATE UNIVERSITY—LONG BEACH

John J. Baird, Professor Emeritus
Department of Biology
1250 Bellflower Boulevard
Long Beach, CA 90840
213-985-4693

UNIVERSITY OF CALIFORNIA—DAVIS

School of Medicine
Post-baccalaureate Re-applicant Program
Office of Minority Affairs
Davis, CA 95616
530-752-1852

Eligibility for the program requires: prior rejection from a AAMC-affiliated medical school; a socio- and/or economically disadvantaged background; completion of an undergraduate degree from an accredited American college or university; California residency; minimum GPA of 2.7; and minimum MCAT average of 6.0.

UNIVERSITY OF CALIFORNIA—IRVINE

Eileen Munoz, Program Coordinator
E108A, Medical Science I
UC—Irvine College of Medicine
Irvine, CA 92717
714-856-4603

Aimed at underrepresented minorities and/or economically disadvantaged students who have been previously unsuccessful in gaining admission to medical school.

UNIVERSITY OF CALIFORNIA—SAN DIEGO SCHOOL OF MEDICINE

Health Careers Opportunity Program
9500 Gilman Drive #0655
La Jolla, CA 92093-0655
619-534-4170

The Post-baccalaureate Program for qualified re-applicants to medical school is a one-year course of academic study, clinical and/or research experience, medical school reapplication strategies, counseling, test-taking, and study skills workshops. The program is aimed at culturally diverse and/or disadvantaged students.

CARSON-NEWMAN COLLEGE

Director of Health Pre-Professions
Carson-Newman College
Box 71992
Jefferson City, TN 37760
423-471-3257

CHADRON STATE COLLEGE

Jay Dee Druecker, Ph.D.
Health Professions Advisor
10th and Main
Chadron, NE 69337
308-432-6278

CHAPMAN UNIVERSITY

Dr. Virginia Carson, Pre-medical Advisor
Post-baccalaureate Pre-professional Health Science
  Program
Orange, CA 92666
714-997-6696

Open to students who lack prerequisites basic to medicine.

CHRISTIAN BROTHERS UNIVERSITY

Dr. Stan Eisen, Head
Biology Department
650 East Parkway South
Memphis, TN 38104
901-722-0447

CUNY—CITY COLLEGE

Dr. Robert Goode, Director
Program in Premedical Studies
J-529
Convent at 138th Street
New York, NY 10031
212-650-6622

CUNY—HERBERT LEHMAN COLLEGE

Frederick Downs, Ph.D.
Pre-medical Advisor
Bedford Park Boulevard West
Bronx, NY 10468
212-960-8757

CUNY—Hunter

Professor C. Howard Krukofsky
Pre-professional Office
695 Park Ave.
New York, NY 10021
212-772-5244

CUNY—Queens College

Daniel Marien, Chair
Health Professions Advisory Committee
Department of Biology
Flushing, NY 11367
718-997-3470

CUNY—York College

Dr. Jack Schlein
9420 Guy Brewer Boulevard
Jamaica, NY 11451
718-262-2716

Columbia University

Post-baccalaureate Pre-medical Program
School of General Studies
408 Lewisohn Hall
2970 Broadway, Mail Code 4101
New York, NY 10027
212-854-3777

Columbia's program is flexible, offering courses during the day and at night. In addition to medical school prerequisites, students may enroll in other relevant more advanced science courses. Columbia has linkages with Brown University School of Medicine; Jefferson Medical College; MCP Hahnemann School of Medicine; SUNY at Stony Brook School of Medicine, SUNY at Brooklyn; and Temple University School of Medicine.

Cleveland State University

Madeline Hall, Ph.D.
Associate Professor
Department of Biology
24th and Euclid
Cleveland, OH 44115

Program for students who lack prerequisites basic to medicine and/or who have been previously unsuccessful in gaining admission to medical school.

University of Connecticut Postbaccalaureate Program

UCT Health Center
School of Medicine
Farmington Ave.
Farmington CT 06030-1905

The College of Arts and Sciences of the University of Connecticut at Storrs, in cooperation with the school of Medicine, in Farmington offers two nondegree study programs for capable college graduates wishing to prepare for application to schools of medicine. Program A serves students who have little or no science preparation, while Program B serves students who have completed science prerequisites and wish to demonstrate academic excellence in upper division science coursework.

Dowling College

Dr. Stephen J. Shafer
Chief Health Professions Advisor
Department of Biology
Oakdale, NY 11769
516-244-3185

Open to students who lack prerequisites basic to medicine.

Drake University

Dr. Rodney A. Rogers
Department of Biology
Drake University
2507 University Avenue
Des Moines, IA 50311
515-271-3925

Duquesne University

B101 Bayer Learning Center
Pittsburgh, PA 15282
412-396-6335

Open to students who lack prerequisites basic to medicine and/or who have been previously unsuccessful in gaining admission to medical school. Qualified students may apply for a linkage program with Allegheny University of the Health Sciences (MCP Hahnemann), Temple University School of Medicine, or Lake Erie College of Osteopathic Medicine.

EL CAMINO COLLEGE

Madeline Carteron, Counselor
16007 Crenshaw Boulevard
Torrance, CA 90506
310-715-3551

Open to students who lack prerequisites basic to medicine.

FAYETTEVILLE STATE UNIVERSITY

Dr. Pinapaka Murthy
Chair and Pre-medical Advisor
Department of Natural Sciences
1200 Murchinson Road
Fayetteville, NC 28301-4298

FISK UNIVERSITY

Mary McKelvey, Ph.D.
Director, UNCF Premedical Summer Institute
Nashville, TN 37208-3051
615-329-8796

FLORIDA STATE UNIVERSITY

Kathleen S. Smith
Program in Medical Sciences
R-115, 34 Montgomery
Tallahassee, FL 32306
904-644-1855

Open to Florida residents who lack prerequisites basic to medicine and/or who have been previously unsuccessful in gaining admission to medical school. Pre-medical advising is offered.

GEORGETOWN UNIVERSITY

Richard H. Sullivan, Associate Dean
College Dean's Office
Attention: Special Student Applications
White-Gravenor
Washington, DC 20057

Georgetown offers a flexible program, allowing students to fulfill pre-medical requirements. Pre-medical advising is available.

GLENVILLE STATE COLLEGE

Dr. Mary Jo Pribble
Glenville, WV 26351
304-462-7361

GOUCHER COLLEGE

Liza Thompson, Director
Post-baccalaureate Pre-medical Program
1201 Dulaney Valley Road
Baltimore, MD 21204
800-697-4646
pbpm@goucher.edu

Goucher offers an intensive, comprehensive post-baccalaureate pre-medical program for college graduates who have not fulfilled pre-medical requirements. Students complete all medical school prerequisites in one year. Advising and MCAT preparatory courses are important components of the program. Goucher offers links with MCP Hahnemann, Temple University School of Medicine, SUNY Stony Brook, and Tulane. In some cases, students have arranged direct admissions with other medical schools as well. Among post-bacc programs, Goucher's medical school acceptance rate is unsurpassed.

HARVARD EXTENSION SCHOOL

Health Careers Program
51 Brattle St.
Cambridge, MA 02138-3722
617-495-2926

The Health Careers Program is designed to helps students who already have earned a bachelor's degree to return to school and complete the necessary requirements for admission to medical school. Students may take courses on an as-needed basis, or may apply to be sponsored which involves a more structured program. Most post-baccalaureate students require about two years to complete requirements, although a few students are able to do so in a year and a summer.

ILLINOIS INSTITUTE OF TECHNOLOGY

Dr. Robert Roth, Chair and Chief Health Professions Advisor
Department of Biology
Chicago, IL 60616
312-567-3480

Open to students who lack prerequisites basic to medicine and/or who have been previously unsuccessful in gaining admission to medical school.

IMMACULATA COLLEGE

Dr. Barbara Piatka
Biology Department
Immaculata, PA 19345
215-647-4400

INDIANA UNIVERSITY—PURDUE UNIVERSITY AT INDIANAPOLIS

Post-baccalaureate Pre-medical Program
Dr. Ralph Ockerse, Pre-medical Advisor
Biology Department
723 West Michigan Street
Indianapolis, IN 46202-5132
317-274-0586

Open to students who lack prerequisites basic to medicine and/or who have been previously unsuccessful in gaining admission to medical school.

IOWA STATE UNIVERSITY

Dr. Heidi H. Saikaly, Coordinator
Pre-medical and Pre-professional Health Programs
102 Carrie Chapman Catt Hall
Ames, IA 50011
515-294-4841

Open to students who lack prerequisites basic to medicine.

JOHNSON COUNTY COMMUNITY COLLEGE

Darwin Lawyer, Counselor
GED 155
12345 College at Quivira
Overland Park, KS 66210-1299
913-469-3809

LAMAR UNIVERSITY

Hugh Akers, Chair
Pre-professional Advisory Committe
Department of Chemistry
Beaumont, TX 77710
409-880-8275

LA SALLE UNIVERSITY

Geri Seitchik, Ph.D., Chair
Pre-Health Professions Advisory Committee
Department of Biology
1900 West Onley
Philadelphia, PA 19141-1199
215-951-1245

LONG ISLAND UNIVERSITY—BROOKLYN CAMPUS

Dr. A. A. Zavitsas, Pre-professional Advisor
Science Division
University Plaza
Brooklyn, NY 11201

LOYOLA MARYMOUNT UNIVERSITY

Dr. Anthony P. Smulders
Loyola Boulevard at West 80th Street
Los Angeles, CA 90045-2699
310-338-5954

Open to students who lack prerequisites basic to medicine, but who have completed a bachelor's degree. Admission is selective.

LOYOLA UNIVERSITY OF CHICAGO

Margaret J. O'Brien, Ph.D., Director
Post-baccalaureate Pre-professional Health Sciences Program
6525 North Sheridan Road
Chicago, IL 60626
773-508-6054

Open to students who lack prerequisites basic to medicine. Loyola offers a flexible, comprehensive program including advising.

LUTHER COLLEGE

Dr. Russell Rulon
Biology Department
700 College Drive
Decorah, IA 52101
319-387-1552

Open to students who lack prerequisites basic to medicine.

MADONNA COLLEGE

Florence Scholdenbrand
36600 Schoolcroft Road
Livonia, MI 48150-1173
313-591-5100

MANHATTANVILLE COLLEGE

Dr. Sheila Morehouse
Chairman, Pre-med Committee
Department of Chemistry Box 76
Purchase, NY 10577
914-694-2200 Ext. 401/320

MANKATO STATE UNIVERSITY

Ronald Hybertson
Pre-medical Advisor
Box 34, Department of Biological Sciences
Mankato, MN 56002-8400
507-389-5732

UNIVERSITY OF MASSACHUSETTS—AMHERST

W. Brian O' Conner, Chair
c/o Department of Biology
Amherst, MA 01003
413-545-3674

Open to students who lack prerequisites basic to medicine.

UNIVERSITY OF MASSACHUSETTS—BOSTON

Grace McSorley
Pre-medical Advisor
Career Services
Harbor Campus
Boston, MA 02125
617-287-5514
mcsorley@umbsky.cc.umb.edu

UNIVERSITY OF MIAMI

Deborah Paris-Herbert, Director
Committee on Premedical Studies
P.O. Box 248004
Coral Gables, FL 33124
305-284-5176

Open to residents who lack prerequisites basic to medicine and/or who have been previously unsuccessful in gaining admission to medical school. Admissions to the program is selective

MICHIGAN STATE UNIVERSITY

College of Human Medicine
A-239 Life Sciences
East Lansing, MI 48824
517-389-5732

MSU's program is for underrepresented minority and disadvantaged students who apply for admission to MSU's College of Human Medicine

MILLS COLLEGE

Office of Graduate Studies
Post-baccalaureate Pre-medical Program
5000 MacArthur Blvd.
Oakland, CA 94613
510-430-3309

The Mills College Post-bacc Pre-med program is designed for highly motivated men and women who did not intend to pursue a career in health care as undergraduates and who have not yet completed the courses in science and mathematics required for entrance to medical school.

UNIVERSITY OF MONTANA

Dr. Galen Mell, Director
Pre-medical Sciences
Division of Biological Sciences
Missoula, MT 59812
406-243-6333

MOUNT HOLYOKE

Frances Perkins Fellows Program
Kay Althoff, Director
South Hadley, MA 01075
413-538-2077
frances-perkins@mtholyoke.edu

New York University

Pre-health Advisement Office
College of Arts and Science
Main Building
100 Washington Square East
Room 904
New York, NY 10003-6688
212-998-8160

The Pre-medical Program at NYU offers college graduates with nonscience backgrounds the opportunity to pursue a career in medicine. The program is tailored to meet the needs of participants. Post-bacc students attend classes alongside undergraduates. Most post-baccs study part-time for approximately two years.

University of North Dakota

School of Medicine and Health Sciences
Indians Into Medicine (INMED) Program
Box 9037
Grand Forks, ND 58202-9037
701-777-3037

INMED assists Native American college students and graduates in medical school preparation. These students can enroll in University of North Dakota undergraduate or graduate courses to strengthen their medical science backgrounds and to complete medical school admissions requirements.

University of North Carolina—Greensboro

Robert E. Cannon, Chair
Pre-medical Advisory Committee
Department of Biology
Greensboro, NC 27412
919-334-5391

Ohio State University

Bruce A. Biagi, Ph.D.
MEDPATH Office
College of Medicine
1178 Graves Hall
333 West 10th Avenue
Columbus, OH 43210-1239
614-292-3161
biagi.1@osu.edu

MEDPATH offers three post-bacc programs, including a Career Change Option, which is designed for individuals who are changing careers or who have not taken or completed pre-medical requirements. The program includes all medical school prerequisites and MCAT preparation. Other programs offered through MEDPATH are aimed at medical school applicants who have completed basic prerequisites and wish to improve their credentials and preparation.

Old Dominion University

Dr. Paul Kirk, Jr.
Pre-health Advisor
Department of Biological Sciences
Mills Goodwin Room 110
Norfolk, VA 23529-0266
804-683-3595

Olivet Nazarene University

Larry G. Ferren
Chemistry Box 6047
Kankakee, IL 60901

Open to students who lack prerequisites basic to medicine

University of Oregon

Marliss G. Strange, Associate Director
Academic Advising and Student Services
164 Oregon Hall
Eugene, OR 97407

Pennsylvania State University

Dr. Robert B. Mitchell
Health Professions Office
224 Pond Lab
University Park, PA 16802
814-865-7620

Philadelphia College of Pharmacy and Science

Dr. Margaret Kasschau, Director
Post-baccalaureate Program
600 South 43rd Street
Philadelphia, PA 19104
215-596-8508

University of Pennsylvania

Post-baccalaureate Pre-health Program
School of Arts and Sciences
College of General Studies
3440 Market St. Suite 100
Philadelphia, PA 19104-3335
215-573-2053

Penn offers several programs. The Post-Baccalaureate Pre-Health Program serves adults interested in pursing careers in medicine who have not taken the basic sciences required for admission to medical school. The Special Science Program is designed for those who wish to enhance or complete an already existing science record. The Post-bacc program participates in an early decision arrangement with Jefferson Medical College, MCP/Hahnemann School of Medicine, and Temple University School of Medicine.

University of Pittsburgh

Richard S. Wood, Program Advisor
Non-degree Studies
College of Arts and Sciences
252 Thackeray Hall
Pittsburgh, PA 15260
412-624-6787/Fax 412-624-8265
dickwood+@pitt.edu

Rensselaer Polytechnic Institute

Dr. Michael Hanna
Department of Biology
Rensselaer Polytechnic Institute
Troy, NY 12180-3590
518-276-6000

Ramapo College

T. Sall
Professor of Life Science
Mahwah, NJ 07430-1680
201-529-7731

University of Rhode Island

C. Christian Goertemiller, Ph.D.
Chair, Pre-medical Advising Committee
Biological Science Center, B-106
Kingston, RI 02881
401-792-2670

Roosevelt University

Dr. Johnathan Green, Chair
Biology Department
430 South Michigan
Chicago, IL 60605
312-341-3676/3683

Rosary College

Sister Mary Woods
7900 West Division Street
River Forest, IL 60305
708-366-2490

Rutgers University

Health Professions Advising Center
Nelson Biological Laboratories, Room A-119
P.O. Box 1059
Piscataway, NJ 08855-1059
908-445-5667

Rutgers University—Newark

Dr. John M. Maiello, Chair
Pre-health Advisory Committee
Department of Biological Sciences
306 Hill Hall
360 Martin Luther King Blvd.
Newark, NJ 07102
973-353-5705

Saint Xavier University

Sister Marion Johnson, Chair
Pre-medical Committee/Science Department
3700 West 103rd Street
Chicago, IL 60655
312-298-3521

Seattle University

Dr. Margaret Hudson, Ph.D.
Chief Pre-medical/Pre-dental Advisor
Biology Department
Seattle University
Seattle, WA 98122
206-296-5486

Scripps College

Post-baccalaureate Pre-medical Program
W.M. Keck Science Center
925 North Mills Ave.
Claremont, CA
91711-5916
909-621-8764

Scripps offers both one- and two-year programs for candidates who have earned their B.A. or B.S. degree, but have not taken required pre-medical science courses. It has linkages with Temple University School of Medicine in Philadelphia, Pennsylvania and with the Western University of Health Sciences, College of Osteopathic Medicine in Pomona, California.

Simmons College

Carol Pooler, Director
Continuing Education
300 The Fenway
Boston, MA 02125
617-738-2141

Open to students who lack basic prerequisites.

Southern Illinois University at Carbondale School of Medicine

Medical/Dental Education Preparatory Program
  MEDPREP
Wheeler Hall
Carbondale, IL 62901-4323
618-536-6671

MEDPREP is a program for minority and disadvantaged (economic or rural) students who wish to strengthen their credentials for a health professional program.

Spalding University

Math/Science Department
851 South 4th Street
Louisville, KY 40203
502-585-9911

SUNY—Stony Brook

Sandra Bruner
Faculty Committee on Health Professions
Office of Undergraduate Academic Affairs
Melville Library E3320
Stony Brook, NY 11794-3351
516-632-7080

Temple University School of Medicine

Health Professions Advisor
Sullivan Hall
Academic Advising Center
Philadelphia, PA 19122
215-204-8669

Texas Christian University

Dr. Phil Hartman
Department of Biology
Fort Worth, TX 76129
817-921-7196

Open to students who lack prerequisites basic to medicine.

University of Houston

Diane Dorris
Health Professions Advisor
University Studies Division
Houston, TX 77204-3243
713-743-8586

Open to minority students (African American and Mexican American) who have previously applied to the College of Medicine at the University of Texas Medical Branch at Galveston.

University of Texas—Arlington

Assistant Dean of Science for Student Affairs
College of Science
P.O. Box 19047
Arlington, TX 76019
817-273-2310

University of Texas—Permian Basin

Professor and Chair, Life Sciences
Box 8397
Odessa, TX 79762-8301
915-367-2242

Towson State University

Dr. Caryl Peterson
Department of Biology
Towson, MD 21204
410-830-3131
peterson-c@toa.towson.edu

The program is designed for students whose career goals shifted to medicine or dentistry following completion of the bachelor's degree. Most post-bacc students enroll full-time at Towson State, for a 12- or 14-month period. However, a less-intensive two-year program is also offered.

Trinity College

Post-baccalaureate Pre-medical Certificate Program
Division of Natural Sciences and Mathematics
125 Michigan Avenue, NE
Washington, DC 20017
202-884-9484

A flexible program open to women who lack prerequisites basic to medicine.

Trinity College

Dr. Virginia Lyons
Health Professions Advisor
208 Colchester Avenue
Burlington, VT 05401
802-658-0337

Tufts Premedical Program

Professional and Continuing Studies
Tufts University
112 Packard Ave.
Medford, MA 02155
617-627-3562

Tufts Pre-medical Program is designed for students who did not intend to pursue a career in health care as undergraduates, or who have not completed pre-medical requirements. The program is flexible, but requires a minimum number of credits. Applicants to the Pre-medical Program may simultaneously apply to Tufts School of Medicine for matriculation the following fall.

University of Vermont

Polly Allen or Beth Taylor-Nolan
UVM Student Services Advisors
802-656-2085/Fax: 800-639-3210

Wayne State University

Julia M. Simmons
Director of Minority Recruitment and Pre-Matriculation Programs
540 East Canfield Ave.
Detroit, MI 48201
313-577-1598

To be eligible, applicants must complete an undergraduate degree from an accredited institution by June of the year for which admission is requested; have only two basic science deficiencies; have taken the MCAT and have an overall GPA of 2.20–3.30; and be a Michigan resident.

Wellesley College

Judith Rich, Coordinator
Office of the Dean of Continuing Education
Wellesley, MA 02181
617-235-0320, Ext. 2660

Advising services available. Students who complete minimum course work requirements are eligible for a composite letter.

University of West Florida

Dr. William Halpern, Associate Professor
Department of Chemistry
1100 University Parkway
Pensacola, FL 32514
904-474-2741
whalpern@uwf.edu

Open to students who lack prerequisites basic to medicine.

West Chester University

Dr. Philip Rudnick, Director
Pre-medical Program
West Chester, PA 19383
610-436-2978

WESTERN ILLINOIS UNIVERSITY

P. James Nielsen
Pre-medical Advisor
Department of Biology
Macomb, IL 61455
309-298-1483

Open to Illinois residents who lack prerequisites basic
to medicine and/or who have been previously unsuccessful gaining admission to medical school.

WILLIAM PATERSON COLLEGE

Dr. Donald Levine, Chairman
Pre-professional Committee
300 Pompton Road
Wayne, NJ 07470
201-595-3453/2245

WORCESTER STATE COLLEGE

Dr. Allan Cooper
Pre-medical Advisor
486 Chandler Street
Worcester, MA 01602
508-793-8000, Ext. 8600

WRIGHT STATE UNIVERSITY

Robert A. Wood, Director
Office of Pre-professional Advising
College of Liberal Arts
445 Millett Hall
Dayton, OH 45435
513-873-3181

ALPHABETICAL INDEX

REGIONAL INDEX

ABOUT THE AUTHOR

Malaika Stoll is a first-year student at Stanford Medical School. She grew up in Berkeley, California, and graduated from Dartmouth College. After college she worked for two years as a Health Educator with the Peace Corps in Zaire. She earned a master's degree in public affairs from Princeton University, and went on to work in international health and development for the World Bank and the United States Agency for International Development. She completed her science requirements at Goucher College's Post-bacc Pre-medical Program. While applying to medical school, she taught for The Princeton Review in Berkeley, worked at UC Berkeley School of Public Health, and wrote this book.

Notes

Notes

Notes

Notes

Notes

Notes

Notes

Notes

Notes

Notes

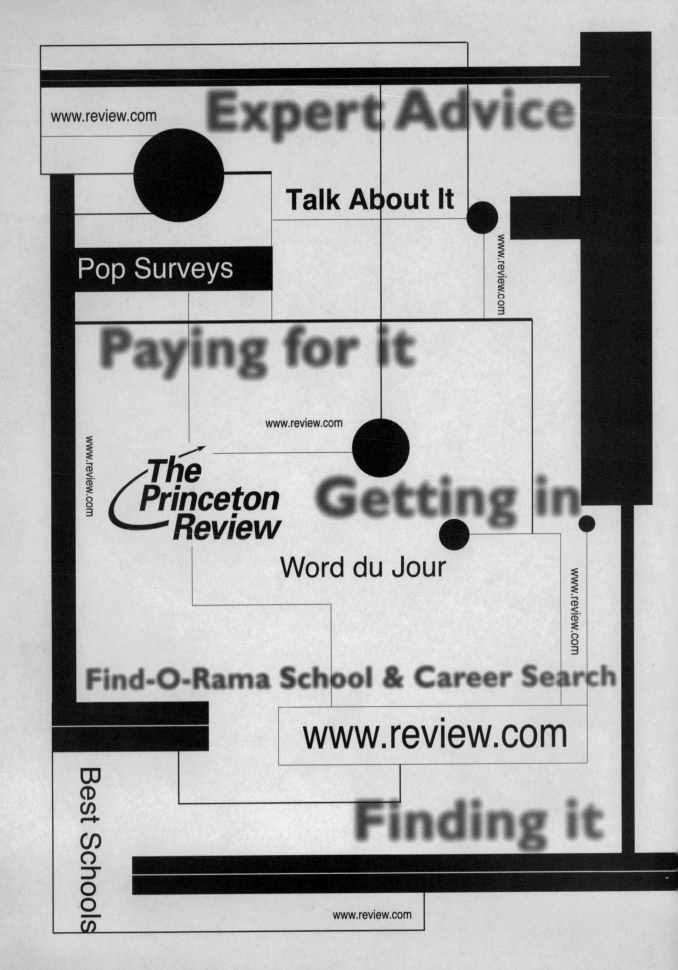

FIND US...

International

Hong Kong
4/F Sun Hung Kai Centre
30 Harbour Road, Wan Chai,
Hong Kong
Tel: (011)85-2-517-3016

Japan
Fuji Building 40, 15-14
Sakuragaokacho, Shibuya Ku,
Tokyo 150, Japan
Tel: (011)81-3-3463-1343

Korea
Tae Young Bldg, 944-24,
Daechi- Dong, Kangnam-Ku
The Princeton Review- ANC
Seoul, Korea 135-280,
South Korea
Tel: (011)82-2-554-7763

Mexico City
PR Mex S De RL De Cv
Guanajuato 228 Col. Roma
06700 Mexico D.F., Mexico
Tel: 525-564-9468

Montreal
666 Sherbrooke St.
West, Suite 202
Montreal, QC H3A 1E7 Canada
Tel: (514) 499-0870

Pakistan
1 Bawa Park - 90 Upper Mall
Lahore, Pakistan
Tel: (011)92-42-571-2315

Spain
Pza. Castilla, 3 - 5° A, 28046
Madrid, Spain
Tel: (011)341-323-4212

Taiwan
155 Chung Hsiao East Road
Section 4 - 4th Floor,
Taipei R.O.C., Taiwan
Tel: (011)886-2-751-1243

Thailand
Building One, 99 Wireless Road
Bangkok, Thailand 10330
Tel: (662) 256-7080

Toronto
1240 Bay Street, Suite 300
Toronto M5R 2A7 Canada
Tel: (800) 495-7737
Tel: (716) 839-4391

Vancouver
4212 University Way NE,
Suite 204
Seattle, WA 98105
Tel: (206) 548-1100

locations

National (U.S.)
We have over 60 offices around the U.S. and
run courses in over 400 sites. For courses and locations
within the U.S. call 1 (800) 2/Review and you will be
routed to the nearest office.

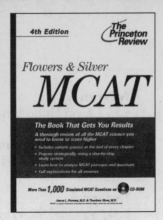
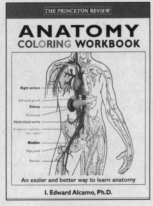
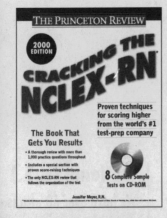